Tourette's Syndrome—Tics, Obsessions, Compulsions

Developmental Psychopathology and Clinical Care

James F. Leckman and Donald J. Cohen

with colleagues from the Yale Child Study Center

JOHN WILEY & SONS, INC.

New York • Chichester • Weinheim • Brisbane • Singapore • Toronto

Library of Congress Cataloging-in-Publication Data:

Leckman, James F.
    Tourette's syndrome—tics, obsessions, compulsions : developmental psychopathology and clinical care / James F. Leckman and Donald J. Cohen.
        p. cm.
    Includes bibliographical references and index.
    ISBN 0-471-16037-7 (cloth : alk. paper)
    1. Tourette syndrome. 2. Tic disorders. 3. Obsessive-compulsive disorder. 4. Symptomatology. I. Cohen, Donald J. II. Title.
    [DNLM: 1. Tourette Syndrome. 2. Tic Disorders. 3. Obsessive –Compulsive Disorder. 4. Attention Deficit Disorder with Hyperactivity. WM 197 L461t 1998]
    RC375.L43 1998
    616.8'3—dc21
    DNLM/DLC
    for Library of Congress   98-9988

In memoriam
Arthur K. Shapiro, M.D., and Bill Pearl
Two pioneers

Editors

James F. Leckman, M.D.
Neison Harris Professor of Child
   Psychiatry and Pediatrics
Yale Child Study Center
New Haven, Connecticut

Donald J. Cohen, M.D.
Irving B. Harris Professor of Child
   Psychiatry, Pediatrics, and
   Psychology
Yale Child Study Center
New Haven, Connecticut

Contributors

John P. Alsobrook II, Ph.D.
Associate Research Scientist
Yale Child Study Center
New Haven, Connecticut

George M. Anderson, Ph.D.
Senior Research Scientist
Yale Child Study Center
New Haven, Connecticut

Alan Apter, M.D.
Professor of Psychiatry
Sackler School of Medicine
Tel-Aviv University, Israel

Amy Arnsten, Ph.D.
Associate Professor of Neurobiology
Yale University
New Haven, Connecticut

Richard A. Bronen, M.D.
Associate Professor of Neurosurgery
   and Diagnostic Radiology
Yale University
New Haven, Connecticut

Linda L. Carpenter, M.D.
Assistant Professor of Psychiatry
Brown University School of Medicine
Providence, Rhode Island

Alice S. Carter, Ph.D.
Associate Professor of Psychology
Yale Child Study Center
New Haven, Connecticut

Elisabeth M. Dykens, Ph.D.
Professor
Neuropsychiatric Institute
University of California at Los Angeles
Los Angeles, California

Diane Findley, Ph.D.
Associate Research Scientist
Yale Child Study Center
New Haven, Connecticut

Nancy J. Fredine, M.A.
Research Associate
Yale Child Study Center
New Haven, Connecticut

Joel Gelernter, M.D.
Associate Professor of Psychiatry
Yale University
New Haven, Connecticut

John C. Gore, Ph.D.
Professor of Diagnostic Radiology and
   Applied Physics
Yale University
New Haven, Connecticut

Shahzad Khan, M.D.
Weems Community Mental Health
   Center
Meridian, Mississippi

Robert A. King, M.D.
Professor of Child Psychiatry
Yale Child Study Center
New Haven, Connecticut

Paul J. Lombroso, M.D.
Associate Professor
Yale Child Study Center
New Haven, Connecticut

Kimberly Lynch, M.S.N.
Clinical Nurse Specialist
Yale Child Study Center
New Haven, Connecticut

Robert Malison, M.D.
Assistant Professor of Psychiatry
Yale University
New Haven, Connecticut

Christopher J. McDougle, M.D.
Raymond E. Houk Professor of
    Psychiatry, Pediatrics and
    Neurobiology
Riley Hospital for Children
University of Indiana
Indianapolis, Indiana

Sharon I. Ort, M.P.H.
Assistant Clinical Professor
Yale Child Study Center
New Haven, Connecticut

Young-Suk Paik, M.D.
Assistant Professor of Child Psychiatry
Department of Neuropsychiatry
Wonkwang University School of
    Medicine, Republic of Korea

David L. Pauls, Ph.D.
Professor
Yale Child Study Center
New Haven, Connecticut

Bradley S. Peterson, M.D.
House Jameson Assistant Professor of
    Child Psychiatry
Yale Child Study Center
New Haven, Connecticut

**Lawrence Scahill, M.S.N., M.P.H.,
    Ph.D.**
Assistant Professor
Yale School of Nursing and the Yale
    Child Study Center
New Haven, Connecticut

Linda Schuerholz, Ed.D.
Developmental Cognitive Neurologist
Kennedy Kreiger Institute
Baltimore, Maryland

Robert T. Schultz, Ph.D.
Assistant Professor
Yale Child Study Center
New Haven, Connecticut

Sara S. Sparrow, Ph.D.
Professor
Yale Child Study Center
New Haven, Connecticut

Lawrence H. Staib, Ph.D.
Assistant Professor of Diagnostic
    Radiology
Yale University
New Haven, Connecticut

Kathryn A. Taubert
Retired Management Education
    Executive, The Travelers Insurance
    Companies and former Training
    Director for the March of Dimes
    Birth Defects Foundation
Newtown, Connecticut

Kenneth E. Towbin, M.D.
Professor of Psychiatry and
    Behavioral Sciences and Pediatrics
The George Washington University
    School of Medicine
Washington, DC

John T. Walkup, M.D.
Associate Professor of Psychiatry
Division of Child Psychiatry
Johns Hopkins Medical Institutions
Baltimore, Maryland

Heping Zhang, Ph.D.
Assistant Professor of Biostatistics
Department of Public Health
Yale Child Study Center
New Haven, Connecticut

Lynne Zimmerman, Ph.D.
Assistant Clinical Professor
Yale Child Study Center
New Haven, Connecticut

Ada H. Zohar, Ph.D.
Research Affiliate
Yale Child Study Center
Lecturer of Psychology
The Scheinfeld Center for Human
    Genetics in the Social Sciences
Hebrew University, Israel

Preface

Tourette's syndrome is a developmental, neuropsychiatric disorder defined by persistent, motor and vocal tics, frequently associated with obsessions, compulsions, and attentional difficulties. Often based upon a multigenerational, genetic predisposition, the multifaceted symptoms of Tourette's syndrome unfold during the first years of life as an interaction between biological vulnerability and adverse environmental events. The range and combinations of symptoms are unique, and no two individuals are identical. During the past decades, clinical and basic researchers from throughout the world have been studying Tourette's syndrome as an important and potentially disabling disorder, in its own right, and as a model disorder for the investigation of multigenerational, developmental psychopathology. Investigations of Tourette's syndrome have generated a rich array of neurobiological, genetic, and therapeutic findings, and new hypotheses are guiding more focused investigations of pathogenesis and treatment. In ongoing international collaborations, clinical and basic researchers are pooling data in the search for the genetic basis of the disorder. Recent progress provides good reason to be hopeful that further scientific advances will illuminate the genetic vulnerability, the neurobiological and psychological processes underlying the natural history, and approaches to prevention and more effective treatments.

For almost 25 years, the research group in the Yale Child Study Center has had the privilege of being part of the new epoch of research on Tourette's syndrome and associated disorders. The research program began with the efforts of a small group of clinical investigators who drew together in 1972 to study childhood neuropsychiatric disorders. Soon, other child psychiatrists and a range of other scientists joined the research group. Within a decade, the group included child and adolescent psychiatry, clinical psychology, neuropsychology, neurochemistry, genetics, nursing, neuropharmacology, neuro-imaging, epidemiology, education, psychoanalysis, molecular developmental biology, biostatistics, and communication disorders. Each clinician, clinical investigator, and basic scientist brought special talents and interests, and new energy to the research program. A steady stream of undergraduates, medical students, post-doctoral fellows and visiting faculty from the United States and abroad have enriched our efforts.

Over the years, members of the group moved on from Yale to join other academic departments or industry, as did many of the residents and post-doctoral fellows. They brought with them the ideas, methods, and clinical interests to other academic centers in the United States and internationally, and helped to shape a vibrant community without walls. A host of collaborations emerged from the research group, both within the Yale Child Study Center and with colleagues in many other universities and other nations including the United Kingdom, the Netherlands, Turkey, Israel,

Japan, Korea, Brazil, and Canada. This book reflects the more than 25 years of our research program—which the two of us have had the privilege of heading—and the many colleagues who have joined in the process. In a real sense, the research program has become a central part of the life's work of many of us and a source of intellectual and personal challenge and enrichment.

This book was written by members of our extended collegial group—individuals who have joined together over many years for clinical work and scholarship. We have many different backgrounds and our interests differ in emphasis. However, we believe that there are major commonalties that can accurately be called the Yale Child Study Center approach. This approach has developed, over the years, on the basis of shared respect for the basic principles and phenomena of developmental psychopathology—the ongoing interaction between biological and experiential factors over the course of development. Also, the approach has been firmly based on a shared commitment to understanding and caring for children and families as whole people. While we have pursued a range of quite basic, biological and psychological studies, the Yale Child Study Center approach has always maintained a feeling for the clinical context, the attempt to understand and help individuals, who are suffering from Tourette's syndrome, obsessive-compulsive disorder, and associated disorders. All of us—clinicians and basic scientists, alike—know the patients whom we care for and study as full people, and we have matured and learned in partnership with them. Finally, we share a belief in the value of multiple perspectives and the multidisciplinary study of phenomena. We have learned to appreciate and share each discipline's languages, literatures, and special concerns and contributions.

During these decades, the clinicians within the Yale Child Study Center and the researchers who have studied children and adults have cared for and evaluated literally thousands of patients and families. The precise number is hard to define since children and families have been seen in several different contexts: within the Tourette's Syndrome and Obsessive Compulsive Clinic and other clinical settings in the Child Study Center, including our specially designed Child Psychiatry Inpatient Service in Yale-New Haven Children's Hospital; in the adult Obsessive-Compulsive Disorder Clinic at the Connecticut Mental Health Center; in research programs on genetics, pharmacology, neuropsychology, neuro-imaging, and other areas; and in consultation with other colleagues throughout the world. We have heard about and discussed patients in many parts of the United States and internationally. The advent of the Internet and the worldwide web have increased these opportunities, and we invite our readers to visit our web site at *info.med.yale.edu/chldstdy/tsocd.htm* to learn more about ongoing research and to share their own observations.

The goal of this book is to review what we have learned and to suggest the many important questions that remain open. This is a work in progress. We are far from unraveling the pathogenesis of Tourette's syndrome and the associated disorders, and also from having truly effective, rational therapies or preventive interventions. Yet, it has seemed to us timely to bring together our thoughts and findings. In doing so, we have described and reviewed work from within the Child Study Center as well as the major currents and data from investigators throughout the world. When there are open questions, there are also going to be differences of opinion. We hope that we have handled issues that remain controversial in a fair fashion, while indicating our own views clearly.

Our discussions of therapy also convey a particular emphasis. Basically, we have been less interested in suppressing tics—although we want to accomplish this, when possible—than in supporting children and family as they navigate through life. While we have been very much involved in basic and applied neuropsychopharmacology research, and have written our share of prescriptions, we see medications as only one part of treatment, and not the mainstay. Today, there are rather sharp differences among clinicians and investigators in relation to the balance between psychosocial and developmental considerations and pharmacological interventions. These issues are the focus of much discussion, not only in relation to Tourette's syndrome but also to other childhood neuropsychiatric disorders. Hopefully, the discussions will lead to well-defined hypotheses that can formally be investigated in the treatment of Tourette's syndrome and other conditions. The systematic study of the formation of clinician-family relationships and the process of clinical care can add a great deal to our understanding of development as well as a theory of therapeutic change.

The content of this book reflects our major concern with understanding and caring for individuals with Tourette's syndrome as whole people whose inner worlds are vulnerable to a bewildering array of unwanted urges, images, and thoughts that consistently call for action. With the onset of tics, obsessions, and compulsions, the child experiences a threat to his sense of autonomy and personal integrity—a siege against the self. The loss of control and mastery over his inner world and behavior and his oversensitivity to the outside world are traumatic. They are a threat to feeling whole. Yet, this threat also may reflect a vulnerability or "weakness" in the integrative structure of the self. The clinician must appreciate both sides of the threat—the intrusions from the inner world of thoughts and feelings that usually are censored and remain unconscious and preconscious, as well as the vulnerability of the structure of self. In the image of warfare, the siege is aimed at the weakest points of an already vulnerable fortress. The metaphors of aggression and warfare are drawn from the accounts of patients, who often feel that there is a battle inside their heads between opposing wills, the desire to tic and the wish to remain still. They attempt to beat down or overpower their compulsions. They feel that they lose many small battles a day, but those who are able to move ahead in their lives feel like victors. The late Joseph Bliss was a pioneer in describing these experiences and his seminal report (1980) continues to be a source of insight and revelation.

In using the term *self* we do not have in mind a metaphysical claim or theory. We mostly wish to point out the importance of caring for a person who is caught in a struggle with forces inside himself. The clinician joins the struggle as a collaborator. In a way, though, *self* is too static a concept, since the children and adults we care for, just as all people, have evolving selves and different selves in different contexts. One goal of our approach to therapy is to help patients maintain this openness and flexibility and not to crystallize their selves around the role of being victims of a disorder or its treatment.

This book is organized in several sections. An initial introductory chapter provides a broad perspective on the history of the research program and the framework of our current understanding of the disorders and therapeutic interventions. The theoretical and empirical themes discussed in this chapter are elaborated throughout the book. Section One describes individuals, clinical symptoms, and the major categories of disorders (Tourette's syndrome, obsessive-compulsive disorder, attention deficit hyperactivity disorder, learning disabilities). At the end of this part, we discuss strengths and adaptation of individuals with Tourette's syndrome and consider the possibility that a vulnerability to develop Tourette's syndrome may also be associated with certain adaptive advantages. Section Two presents a broad and detailed discussion of pathogenesis, including studies in epidemiology, genetics, epigenetic factors, neuroanatomy, and neurochemistry. Section Three focuses on assessment and treatment. We titled this section "Partnerships for making the best of Tourette's syndrome" to highlight the necessary partnerships between children, families, and clinicians in the struggle to achieve wished for outcomes.

To link the individual chapters into a coherent whole, we provide a brief summary at the end of each chapter. The summary highlights the themes that have been covered. Immediately after this, we provide a preview of the next chapter. In a book such as this, where the same phenomena are taken up from differing perspectives, there must be some duplication of material. We have tried to keep this to a minimum while still making it possible to read each chapter as a freestanding entity.

There are many individuals, foundations, and government agencies that have been essential to the research program. The names of many individuals who have worked within the research program over the years will be found in the list of authors in the References. To mention any is to run the risk of slighting many more. Yet, we would like to acknowledge with gratitude the very first members of the research program: Bennett Shaywitz (pediatric neurology), Malcolm Bowers (psychiatry), J. Gerald Young (child and adolescent psychiatry), and Kenneth K. Kidd (genetics). We also wish to note the individuals who have been most central to the continuing success of the research program. Two have been leaders within the program for almost 20 years: David Pauls (genetics) and George Anderson (neurochemistry), both of whom joined soon after earning their doctorates and have risen to the top of their fields. Others have been working with the group for about a decade, give or take a few years: Robert King (child and adolescent psychiatry and medical director of the Tic Disorders and Obsessive-Compulsive Disorder Specialty Clinics), Lawrence Scahill (nursing and clinical trials), and Bradley Peterson (child and adolescent psychiatry and neuro-imaging). Some individuals have held us together over the course of the years, including Sharon Ort, Maureen McSwiggin-Hardin, and Jill Detlor (nursing); Charles Hurst (genetics); and Shana Wildstein, Ramona Bachmann, and Monique Staggers (administration). We would also like to acknowledge the efforts of our colleagues Kenneth E. Towbin, Mark A. Riddle, Wayne K. Goodman, Phillip B. Chappell, and Christopher J. McDougle—each of whom had a major and lasting impact on the research program during their years at Yale. We are also grateful to the contributions of our many colleagues who have served in supporting roles as research studies were conceived, fought for, implemented, written-up for publication and translated into clinical care.

In the preparation of this book we are appreciative of the support and intellectual challenge provided to one of us (JFL) during a sabbatical leave at The Neurosciences Institute in San Diego. Within that extraordinary scientific community particular thanks go to Gerald M. Edelman (director), George Gabor Miklos (a senior fellow and evolutionary biologist), and Esther Thelen (a visiting fellow). On the practical side, we are both grateful for the devoted efforts of Tammy Babitz who helped to coordinate and organize this multifaceted endeavor.

All researchers in the field of Tourette's syndrome and all families are indebted to the Tourette Syndrome Association (TSA). Mr. Bill Pearl, the founder, was a cherished friend, and through the Gateposts Foundation he helped us to provide care to all children and families who needed it. The unique director of scientific and medical affairs of the TSA, Ms. Sue Levi-Pearl, has been a constant supporter and guide. Dr. Arthur Shapiro, whose research initiated the modern history of the field, was an early supporter and critic. We are very grateful for the long-term support of the National Institutes of Health—National Institute of Mental Health, National Institute of Child Health and Human Development, and National Institute of Neurological and Communicative Disorders and Stroke. We also acknowledge the timely support for new ideas and new investigators provided by the TSA, the W. T. Grant Foundation, National Alliance for Research on Schizophrenia and Depression, the March of Dimes, the Stanley Foundation, and many private individuals and family foundations.

Within the Child Study Center and the Yale School of Medicine, colleagues have been generous with their ideas, encouragement, and research collaboration. Our most senior child psychiatric colleagues—Drs. Albert J. Solnit, Samuel Ritvo, and John E. Schowalter—have been our teachers and steady companions.

We feel blessed to have been and to remain surrounded by such extraordinary colleagues; to have had the chance of learning and working with young and older friends we admire; to have had the confidence and trust of patients we have cared about; and to still have the energy and enthusiasm to look forward to tomorrow's patients and the findings from next week's experiments. We are confident that the next two decades will be even more interesting than the past, and that we will all be surprised by what is finally learned about the causes and cure of Tourette's syndrome and associated disorders.

Clinical research is demanding and not always productive. Yet, it is also a privilege to be able to try to add to knowledge that may help a child grow to a more healthy outcome. We have experienced the hard work as well as the joys, and we hope that, in addition to the facts and findings about Tourette's, this volume will convey the excitement and importance of clinical research. We also hope that this volume will convey the respect we have felt for those who have shared in this enterprise with us—our students, colleagues and the families that we serve.

JAMES F. LECKMAN AND DONALD J. COHEN

Contents

SECTION THREE
PARTNERSHIPS FOR MAKING THE BEST OF TOURETTE'S

CHAPTER 1

Introduction: The Self under Siege

DONALD J. COHEN and JAMES F. LECKMAN

The human body is the best picture of the human soul.

—*Ludwig Wittgenstein, 1958*

When Georges Gilles de la Tourette and Sigmund Freud were young, clinical scholars in Charcot's clinic in the Salpetriere at the end of the nineteenth century, they were introduced to patients with complex tic syndromes. Gilles de la Tourette became acquainted with the case of a fascinating Princess with many years of motor and very colorful vocal tics. Although she was never treated directly by him, this individual and a small handful of other patients became the basis for his clinical description in 1885 of the syndrome that carries his name. This work launched a line of neurological investigations on the organization and nature of tics, obsessions, and compulsions that continues until today.

In Paris, Freud was also introduced to Charcot's methods, his findings on hysteria, and the studies on tics. Back in Vienna, he continued to investigate the origin and symptoms of patients with the vast array of symptoms that constituted turn-of-the-century "hysteria." These clinical disorders illuminated the permeable boundaries between voluntary and involuntary, conscious and unconscious, and meaningful and meaningless mental disorders. In 1893, Freud included a detailed report of his treatment of Frau Emmy von N whose complex emotional disorder included dramatic tic symptoms (1953a). As with Gilles de la Tourette, Freud's work also launched a new field and a continuing line of psychoanalytic investigation of the psychology of the inner world.

In Freud's theory, there was an intrinsic relationship between neurological and constitutional factors, on one hand, and the dynamic processes of the unconscious mental life. Both normal development and neurosis expressed both types of forces and, he believed, eventually science would be

1

able to create more accurate maps of the brain and behavior that would be complementary perspectives on human mental life and behavior (Mayes & Cohen, 1995).

Throughout this century, these two traditions—the neurological view of Gilles de la Tourette and the psychological one of Freud—occasionally came into contact, in the work of particular clinicians and theorists. Yet, they were mainly divergent and hard to integrate. Tourette's syndrome hovered between the two domains of study, sometimes located more in the territory of the brain and sometimes that of the mind.

TOURETTE'S SYNDROME AND THE INTEGRATION OF BIOLOGY AND PSYCHOLOGY

In the 1970s, biological and psychological perspectives began to converge and form a vigorous new hybrid—the investigation of brain-behavior relations in neuropsychiatric disorders. Freud's vision of complementarity had appeared to become a more likely prospect. In this rapprochement, the strange clinical syndromes of mind and body that fascinated Freud and Gilles de la Tourette have served as a valuable nodal point.

Throughout most of the century, Tourette's syndrome was considered a rare and exotic condition, seen by a clinician only a few times in a career. However, the availability of a new medication, haloperidol, and the pioneering work of Drs. Arthur and Elaine Shapiro suddenly focused attention on Tourette's syndrome as an easily diagnosed and not so rare condition (A. Shapiro & Shapiro, 1968; A. Shapiro, Shapiro, Bruun, & Sweet, 1978). Soon, the Tourette Syndrome Association (TSA) succeeded in generating a far greater awareness of the diagnosis among physicians and the public, and patients recognized themselves in the clinical accounts and came for treatment. The century-long tradition of two points of view continued, as they do today: Tourette's syndrome was conceptualized as a neurological disorder with psychological consequences when seen by neurologists, or a psychiatric disorder with a biological basis when seen by psychiatrists.

In the early 1970s, a good deal of biologically oriented, psychiatric research focused on brain neurochemistry because of the increasing understanding of the synthesis, release, and metabolism of neurotransmitters and the affects of medication on these systems. Clinical researchers searched for biological correlates of rigorously defined conditions. The research program on Tourette's syndrome and associated disorders described in this volume originated in this intellectual milieu. The studies from this program are leading exemplars of a new paradigm: the field of research and care that integrates the neurology of Gilles de la Tourette, the phenomenology of Freud, and the advances in the developmental biological and behavioral sciences.

Through listening to, caring for, and studying patients, a new perspective on Tourette's syndrome began to arise. This view of Tourette's syndrome was within the clinical framework of developmental psychopathology and was based on the cross-fertilization of developmental neuroscience, developmental psychology, and child psychiatry (Cicchetti & Cohen, 1995a). Tourette's syndrome became the model neuropsychiatric disorder for studying the interacting contributions of genetic vulnerability and varied experiences, from gestation through the course of the first years of life, in the shaping of the lines of personal development of the individual and the nature and severity of a psychiatric disorder (Mayes & Cohen, 1996b). In a sense, Tourette's syndrome became our hysteria—the model disorder for exploring mind-brain relationships in health and disease. As we have been exploring these themes in empirical and theoretical work, we have been working on the current volume for more than 20 years (Cohen, Bruun, & Leckman, 1988).

In the middle 1970s, the patients with the most severe forms of Tourette's syndrome were just beginning to be seen and treated by a very few physicians, particularly those who worked initially with Dr. Arthur Shapiro. Initially, huge doses of haloperidol (up to 200 mg/day) were used along with other compounds, but clinicians soon settled down on a general standard of evaluation and care. Along with the expansion of clinical engagement with families with Tourette's syndrome, investigators in the United States and abroad soon started to systematically study the symptoms, treatment, and, to a limited extent, biological correlates of the disorders. In addition to Arthur Shapiro, some of the early leaders in this field were Ruth D. Bruun, Gerald S. Golden, C. D. Marsden, Gerald Erenberg, Arnold J. Friedhoff, Masaya Segawa, Harold H. Klawans, Yishiko Nomura, Roger Freeman, and Harvey S. Singer among others. Over a few years, Tourette's syndrome emerged as an often undiagnosed, or wrongly diagnosed, but rather common condition.

The research program within the Yale Child Study Center on childhood neuropsychiatric disorders started in 1972, with a focus on children and adolescents with autism, pervasive developmental disorders, developmental language disorders, attentional disorders, and other complex conditions (Cohen, 1974). Our founding, small research group included child and adolescent psychiatrists, a pediatric neurologist, and an adult psychiatrist. Soon, specialists in developmental neurochemistry and then a range of other fields joined in, including human genetics, nursing, psychology, neuro-radiology, pharmacology, and education. We were especially interested in disorders that seemed to reflect disturbance in the unfolding of biological endowment and that, like Tourette's syndrome, hovered between developmental neurology and child psychiatry, between body and mind. Tourette's syndrome became the model system for testing new methods in the investigation of biological endowment and for charting the unfolding of developmental competence and dysfunctions in maturational processes.

The program in the Yale Child Study Center was especially influenced by the Center's commitment to doing research within the context of providing clinical care. In an important way, this tradition opened special opportunities for intensive observation and engagement with families over long periods of time.

In medical research, clinicians have a particular, privileged epistemological position. Because of their primary responsibility for providing care, they are allowed access to patients in privacy, to hear about all aspects of their lives, and to be with and observe patients at their most vulnerable and intimate moments. Clinicians may intervene with guidance and specific treatments, even when knowledge is limited; and the systematic observation of the impact of interventions offers further data about the underlying processes. A clinician's data are as rich as the lived experience of the patients and the physician's own ability to sustain the relationship, be curious and remain observant. In this process, the clinician-investigator can and should include all aspects of human biology and psychology as potentially relevant to understanding the patient and providing suitable treatment.

This breadth of the clinical epistemology contrasts with the needs of a laboratory scientist to concentrate on a small domain to test specific hypotheses with a sharply defined methodology. The clinical perspective that has provided the tone for our research program on Tourette's syndrome has encouraged multiple disciplines and perspectives to pool knowledge and methods while, at the same time, keeping the patient and family at the center of attention. Just as the clinician has the task of integrating history, current findings, and laboratory tests into a coherent, narrative, clinical formulation, in our research program the varied and always changing methodologies of clinical and basic research have been integrated by the clinician's concern for the whole patient, living in a family and society.

The first patients with Tourette's syndrome that we saw, in the middle 1970s, were referred most often as clinical enigmas. They were among the most seriously impaired patients we have ever seen. They suffered from painful, extreme forms of the disorder that we now recognize in far milder variants. Arthur Shapiro referred to some of these patients as "polymorphous" because of their range of symptoms; active clinicians shared a small number of such patients who made the rounds among the "experts" and taught many of us a good deal—including humility. We were keenly aware of how much there was to be learned. In the Child Center, we learned a great deal from these patients about the onset and progression of symptoms, the range and fluctuation of tics, the emergence of obsessions and compulsions, their inner experiences and the traumas they experienced with parents, teachers, and society, and from within themselves.

Much of the early work within the Center was descriptive of these remarkable phenomena. Even today, after having cared for thousands of patients and families, we remain intrigued by the clinical phenomenology—the clinical surface of signs and symptoms, as well as the patient's experiences and the underlying processes. In teaching medical students, residents, and fellows, we have an opportunity to return to the lived phenomena again and to see them vividly through fresh eyes. Are the tics voluntary or involuntary, physical or mental? Why do they come and go? If patients don't have them when they are in the office, why do tics appear as soon as they walk down the hall to the elevator? What accounts for the specific symptoms, the virtuosity with which they are chosen and executed? What makes the patient feel better when the tic is finally emitted? Are tics, then, like sneezes or masturbation? Like an itch or a scratch? Why do patients curse? How do they learn the curse words? Why are mothers so often the target of aggressive attacks—attacking words, pinching, yelling, and controlling? When a child is doing something his parents and he hate, can he control it? How do you know what is intentional and what is beyond control? Is Tourette's syndrome organic or functional?

THE PSYCHOBIOLOGY OF TOURETTE'S SYNDROME: CLINICAL FEATURES, NEUROBIOLOGY, AND GENETICS

The organizing biological hypothesis in the 1970s was the concept of dopaminergic over-reactivity or hypersensitivity of dopamine receptors. The remarkable therapeutic benefits of haloperidol and other neuroleptics—and our recognition of the exacerbation of tics by stimulants—seemed to clearly support the role of dopamine excess at some point in the pathophysiology, if not as the cause. At Yale, the methods were being developed for studying central catecholamine and serotoninergic functioning through sampling of cerebrospinal fluid (CSF) for the major metabolites, homovannillic acid (HVA) and 5-hydroxyindoleacetic acid (5-HIAA), respectively (Cohen, Shaywitz, Young, & Bowers, 1980). At that time, loading with probenecid was used to prevent their egress from the CSF and increase their concentration; 5 ml of CSF fluid or more was needed for the assays that can now be performed on a drop.

The findings of these studies on cerebrospinal fluid metabolites, at Yale and elsewhere, supported the dopaminergic hypothesis and propelled the field forward (Cohen, Shaywitz, et al., 1979; Cohen, Shaywitz, Caparulo, Young, & Bowers, 1978). We were thrilled with these first studies—not only with the results but also with the ability to study something in the CSF that appeared to be related to profound psychological processes. Whether the findings have stood the test of time (Leckman, Goodman, et al., 1995) is less important than the impetus they provided for using current methods of biological psychiatry in the study of developmental, child psychiatric disorders.

We did not just study neurochemical systems, such as CSF metabolites in bodily fluids. The clinical needs of the children and families, and the breadth of their difficulties as well as their capacity for personal engagement captivated us. These sensitive, intelligent, and tormented children and their distressed families were remarkably evocative of our clinical empathy and intellectual interest. In Tourette's syndrome, we found a disorder that had an immediate demand on our clinical conceptualization of the mysterious leap between mind and body. Patients described the origin of their tics from within, from an urge that could not be resisted to which they eventually capitulated; they thought that in some way the tic was voluntary; and yet it was not at all wished for, and was the result, in some inscrutable way, of forces in the brain-mind that were below the surface of consciousness, just as the forces described one century earlier by Freud in his research on hysteria (Bliss, 1980).

During the next several years, we felt like explorers in a new world in which neurobiology and depth psychology were being joined. Very intensive, clinical discussions with parents and patients suggested that tics, obsessions, and compulsions were not isolated to the patient but seemed to occur among other family members. The classic literature reported that there were rare situations in which a father and son both had Tourette's syndrome, but the common wisdom was that Tourette's syndrome had no specific genetics. Yet, in case after case, we would sit with parents and hear a different family saga. Sometimes, a father would deny having had any tic symptoms only to have them recalled, often quite gently, by his wife, or to "remember" a period in childhood when he, too, had eyeblinking and sniffing, or more. As we became more adept, the histories became richer and the multigenerational nature of tic symptoms became clear. Also, another theme emerged. In clinical cases, it was already recognized that some patients had not only motor and vocal tics, but also more complex behaviors, complex tics, and mental symptoms that could be considered mental tics or obsessions. Deeper study of individual patients made clear that they had all the symptoms and signs of obsessive-compulsive disorder and, more interesting, that their family histories were filled with obsessive-compulsive disorder as well as tic symptoms. For generations, there had been debate about whether Tourette's syndrome could be seen as a motor form of obsessive-compulsive disorder, or whether obsessive-compulsive disorder was a mental form of Tourette's syndrome. Our careful clinical studies of individual patients and their families revealed that the epistemological issues could be addressed differently by appreciating that these were two perspectives on the same set of phenomena.

The clinical observations became scientific hypotheses that were amenable to rigorous testing (Kidd, Prusoff, & Cohen, 1980; Pauls, Cohen, Heimbuch, Detlor, & Kidd, 1981). This translation of clinical observations to formal scientific scrutiny is precisely the reason for having research clinics that bring physician/clinicians into close contact with basic researchers from various disciplines.

Advances in the field of Tourette's syndrome exemplify this back-and-forth movement from clinic to laboratory to clinic. Soon, with the great boost of the TSA, rigorous genetic research using formal methods of assessment and analysis confirmed the clinical impressions of the familiality of Tourette's syndrome and its association with obsessive-compulsive disorder. The first, quick-and-dirty genetic studies were strongly supportive of a familial and genetic nature of Tourette's syndrome and very quickly led to great interest in genetic factors in Tourette's syndrome among other research groups and in relation to other disorders. The first pedigrees so much resembled classic depictions of dominant genetic transmission that we were surprised the genetics of Tourette's syndrome had for so long gone unappreciated. Now, almost 18 years later, the genetic story continues to unfold its complexities.

Another example of clinical and basic research converging came from the studies of the neuropharmacology of neuronal activity. In the late 1970s and early 1980s, basic neurobiological researchers at Yale were engrossed in studies of the locus ceruleus (LC), a small neuronal center deep in the brain that serves as a switching station for many neurotransmitter systems and regulates the noradrenergic system outflow. Basic investigators studied the regulation of the firing rate of the LC in exquisite recordings. Clonidine, an anti-hypertension medication that stimulates the inhibitory, presynaptic, adrenergic receptors, sharply reduced the rate of LC firing and the functioning of the noradrenergic system, the neuronal pathways intimately involved in arousal and anxiety.

Within a very short time, the basic laboratory studies of noradrenergic regulation were translated into clinical practice. The earliest clinical translations were in the treatment of individuals who were suffering from the terrible withdrawal symptoms from narcotics. Dramatically, clonidine blunted their autonomic over-responsivity and the pains of withdrawal. Shortly after that, we wondered if some aspect of Tourette's syndrome might also reflect the over-activity of the noradrenergic system. For the first trial, we selected one of the most profoundly impaired youngsters, a boy who engaged in nonstop yelling, a myriad of tic movements and aggressive outbursts. We estimated the dose and then gathered around his bedside. Forty minutes after the first dose, he fell asleep. When he awoke in one hour, he was already calmer. Over the next days, his symptoms abated, and he became more easily engaged socially and in treatment. The clinical benefits of clonidine in the treatment of the disorder seemed apparent in other patients, as well. (D. Cohen, Detlor, Young, & Shaywitz, 1980; D. Cohen, Young, Nathanson, & Shaywitz, 1979). Later, more rigorous, systematic trials continued to demonstrate a clinical effectiveness for clonidine, although, as in much else in life, further knowledge complicated the story (Leckman et al., 1991).

Almost 20 years later, it still appears that clonidine has a clinical role, perhaps through its inhibition of the LC and reduction of stress responsivity and hyperarousal, or by acting on other brain regions. Yet, the specific value of clonidine was perhaps less critical than the fact that it opened up a new approach to studying a well-defined brain system related to anxiety and arousal in a child psychiatric disorder. We used clonidine as a provocative agent to study the degree of reduction of the major metabolite of norepinpehrine, 3-methoxy, 4-hydroxyphenylene glycol (MHPG); degree of lowering of blood pressure; and extent of increase in a hormonal system (growth hormone) regulated in part by norepinephrine (NE) (Leckman, Cohen, Gertner, Ort, & Harcherik, 1984; Selinger, Cohen, Ort, Anderson,

& Leckman, 1984; J. Young et al., 1981). In these early studies of Tourette's syndrome, biological systems could be monitored along with clinical changes in tic frequency and severity, and improvements in a child's attention and overall functioning (Harcherik, Leckman, Detlor, & Cohen, 1984; Leckman et al., 1989). The new field of biological child psychiatry envisioned the possibility of integrating biological systems and behavioral change (Leckman, Cohen, et al., 1986). These studies suggested that this promissory note could be fulfilled, suggested new studies, and shaped strategies of rigorous psychobiological research. The significance of this impact can be estimated by comparing the research that was now possible with the state of investigation in child psychiatry one decade earlier. Even in the 1970s, broad-based, psychobiologically oriented research on child psychiatric disorders was limited to only a few sites that were, like us, helping to shape a field of research and the methodologies for studying and understanding child psychiatric disorders in general. Each new methodology—from studying cerebrospinal fluid and metabolites in urine and plasma, to investigation of hormonal response, enzymes, developmental changes in measures of behavior and biology—had to be approved for use with children, studied in normal and contrast groups, and refined as an instrument while, at the same time, being used to explore the disorders.

During the 1980s, research on Tourette's syndrome became increasingly robust and popular throughout the world. A new cadre of investigators from around the world began to make their voices heard, including Christopher G. Goetz, David E. Comings, Joseph Jankovic, Thomas N. Chase, Anthony E. Lang, Mary M. Robertson, Roger Kurlan, Ben J. M. van de Wetering, Paul R. Sanberg, Ari Rothenberger, Alan Apter, and Amos D. Korczyn. By 1982, there was sufficient research underway for the TSA to organize the first international scientific congress (Friedhoff & Chase, 1982). Many of the papers were quite preliminary. Our paper conveyed the flavor of the research program, "Interaction of biological and psychological factors in the natural history of Tourette's syndrome: a paradigm for childhood neuropsychiatric disorders" (D. Cohen, Detlor, Shaywitz, & Leckman, 1982). At this time, we began to describe Tourette's syndrome as a model neuropsychiatric disorder. This status also justified the degree of research and clinical attention that this remarkable condition was receiving. We felt that the methods and findings of research on Tourette's syndrome would have implications for many other conditions. One decade after the first international congress, a second international symposium brought together the burgeoning field of systematic research on Tourette's syndrome (Chase, Friedhoff, & Cohen, 1992).

The Tourette's syndrome research portfolio in the Child Study Center was richly expanded during the 1980s. The advent of brain imaging—computerized tomography—offered the chance to study brain structure and search for possible major alterations that could underlie the diathesis to Tourette's syndrome and other neuropsychiatric disorders. The first computerized axial tomograms (CAT) scans were done in a state of great awe;

a group of clinicians and neuroradiologists gathered around the machine and waited expectantly for the images to be developed (Caparulo et al., 1981; Harcherik et al., 1985). Each new technological advance in imaging—including the most recent functional magnetic resonance imaging (MRI) methodologies—has generated the same breath-holding expectation as we wait to see if *the* lesion will finally be revealed (B. Peterson, Riddle, Cohen, Katz, Smith, & Leckman, 1993; Peterson et al., 1998).

Twin studies at this time supported the role of genetic factors, and also gave some room to think about non-genetic, environmental sources of variance (Price, Kidd, Cohen, Pauls, & Leckman, 1985). The importance of nongenetic, environmental factors (Leckman et al., 1990) was consistent with the general models of developmental psychopathology, which guided our understanding not only of Tourette's syndrome but the broad range of childhood disorders (Cicchetti & Cohen, 1995a, 1995b; Leckman, Peterson, et al., 1997; Peterson, Leckman, & Cohen, 1995).

The Child Study Center research program on the genetics of Tourette's syndrome discovered that the clinical impressions about the close relation between tics and obsessive-compulsive disorder actually could be documented in rigorous clinical studies (Pauls, Towbin, Leckman, Zahner, & Cohen, 1986). The family genetic methodology and genetic modeling quickly moved to the center of research interest worldwide (Pauls & Leckman, 1986). During the last few years, an international genetics collaboration has worked energetically to obtain DNA from well characterized patients and families, and many laboratories in the United States and Europe are collaborating in the search for the genetic locus or loci. So far, no genetic linkage or strong genetic candidate gene has emerged, but both are only a matter of time. Perhaps it is naive to predict—especially since we made the same prediction five years ago—that within a few years, there will be important discoveries of a gene or small set of genes that convey vulnerability to Tourette's syndrome. Yet, we will make the prediction and feel quite certain that we are not being mislead by false optimism.

As more children were being seen clinically and in research projects, the severity of patients' symptoms, as a group, seemed to decrease; patients were receiving the diagnosis of Tourette's syndrome who were not markedly impaired. This trend has continued until today, and we are no longer quite sure where to draw the line between the quite frequent, rather innocent appearing tics of young schoolchildren—exhibited at some point by perhaps 10% of all children in the first grades of elementary school—and a "true" case of a tic syndrome or even Tourette's syndrome. If every child with a few tics is diagnosed as having Tourette's syndrome, then it is among the most common of conditions and might drift into expected normalcy (just like a few freckles are part of the normal variations in biology). Yet, there are children who clearly do not seem to be just on the normal distribution but for whom the frequency and vigor of the tics leads to real disruption of functioning. However valuable for the purposes of defining a case and need for treatment, any demarcation may seem arbitrary (e.g., that the tics must persist for more than a year or that there is some degree of real clinical impairment, or both). Diagnostic issues are not just scholastic exercises, as they enter importantly into rigorous research studies of genetics, neurochemistry, and treatment, as well as practical decisions about reimbursement for care. Diagnostic issues also are central to epidemiology, which requires clear specification of what will constitute a case (Apter et al., 1992).

In the middle 1980s, clinicians caring for children with Tourette's syndrome were delighted with the availability of a new agent that could be used in the treatment of obsessive-compulsive disorder. Alongside haloperidol and pimozide for tics, clinicians could try a medication that operated on a problem that was often even more disabling. When clomipramine became available in the United States, we could see for ourselves that it actually could liberate some children who were frozen with obsessions and compulsions. The rapid introduction of the serotonin re-uptake inhibitors (SRIs) a few years later greatly expanded the possibilities for pediatric psychopharmacology of Tourette's syndrome and obsessive-compulsive disorder. The availability of new medications was coupled with the commitment within the Center and in other academic departments of child psychiatry to systematic, rigorous psychopharmacological research on short- and long-term efficacy, effectiveness, and side effects of medication. Today, with available medications, most patients who require pharmacological intervention for tics, obsessions, compulsions, attentional problems, and aggressiveness can be offered some degree of relief. Yet, no medication is ideal, nor are the clinical improvements often complete. There is thus continuing hope that genetic and developmental neuroscience research will reveal new targets for molecular intervention, just as the basic work on the LC was a critical step on the road to trying clonidine in patients.

CLINICAL UNDERSTANDING AND CARE

Every year there are patients who come for care who open up new ideas for research and treatment. One decade ago, we reviewed our understanding of clinical care (D. Cohen et al., 1988). Since then, our understanding has continued to be deepened by clinical immersion, especially with those patients with Tourette's syndrome whom we have followed closely for many years and who stand as our own, internal representational images of the mechanisms and processes expressed in the clinical disorder.

Each clinician in the Tourette's syndrome program in the Child Study Center has had a small group of patients with whom we have shared our lives; we have learned more than usual from these patients because of our closeness and concern, and the frequency of our meetings, especially during crises. They have served as the basis for our theorizing about the integration of biology and psychology over the course of development (D. Cohen, 1991a). Abe has been one such patient:

Case Example. At age 17, Abe's parents brought him for evaluation tied to a chair to prevent his horrible, self-injurious behavior. He lurched forward, banged his head, threw whatever came to reach, yelled, and cursed. At his worst, he was tied to a bed or allowed to simply thrash about for hours. His mind and body were trapped by rituals of touching one part of the body and then another, repeating, jerking, calling out. His eyes would be magnetically attracted to particular patterns, especially intersecting lines and squares, from which he could not dis-engage. For an hour or two, he would sit in frozen concentration, moving his eyes from one corner to another of the pattern, unable to detach. He would become drenched with sweat and finally would be able to pull himself back by a force of great will when he felt, for some reason, that he had done the pattern " just right" and "correctly." He had "crazy" ideas that he had to hold himself back from. Between paroxysms of tics and compulsions, he begged for help.

*   *   *   *   *

For more than 18 years, Abe has been in our office two to four times a week for discussion and treatment. During these almost two decades, we have jointly gone through very long and difficult periods. When things were at their worst, Abe was in nonstop movement. He had tics of every part of the body, gyrations of the trunk, head and body banging, and dystonic tensing of his upper torso. He would get stuck in postures, and yell so loudly at the top of his lungs that his face would puff up and be beet red and he would seem about to burst. He was frightening and frightened, and when he really banged at his face, to the point of breaking his nose, he looked like a prizefighter who had just lost a major match.

Abe was a good describer of his inner world. Inside his mind, there were two bulls that attacked each other—pulling and pushing in opposite directions—and he was caught in between. He could not clear his mind of crazy ideas, and the only way to soothe the crescendos of tension was to do something strong, powerful, and abrupt like yelling or banging. His mind became glued to a particular thought, and he had to think the thought or do the actions that were incessantly on his mind. For years, he had to search his body for each and every pubic hair that had then to be pulled; during many months, he felt compelled to stick his finger up his nose until blood gushed; he could not shower without spending hours in washing rituals. He became obsessed with the number three. He had to count: 1, 2, 3, and then be sure that he did not stop on 3, and so return to: "1,2,3853,4,5, 6. No: not 3, back to 1." In any internal conflict, the victory of one force left the other force defeated, and Abe was on both sides of the battle and thus always a looser.

From Abe, we learned about the nonstop, every-minute burden of feeling overwhelmed from within by attacking forces that were within one's self and, at the same time, outside of it.

Over months and then years, Abe became increasingly the winner against the internal demons that possessed his mind. His courage was stunning in this many-year war. He had tremendous pride in his achievements and maintained the sense that he would, eventually, move ahead in his life to fulfill his ambitions in sports and business. His warm heartedness, humor, and concern for others—including a genuine and deeply touching concern for his clinicians and their families—brought him a circle of friends and enduring relations. Although as a young adult, he has not achieved the goals he set for himself, he does not stop trying or hoping. Dressed in a handsome suit, he is a good looking, strong young man whose physical and emotional scars are badges of his heroic combat.

One of us (DJC) read the above account to Abe (not his real name) to obtain consent for publication. Abe appreciated hearing the description: "I want others to know what I have gone through and what I have achieved. Especially younger children." He discussed his feeling that although he is now about to be engaged to a very caring woman, he would not want to have children after they were married. "I wouldn't want my son to have to go through what I have." And then daydreamed about what it would be like to have a son to teach football, to take places, to make into a strong man, as he himself is. He then retold the story of the bulls that were locked in combat inside of his mind: "One of the bulls is the mind and the other bull is the body. They are charging each other with their horns, inside my mind. I can see them banging against each other, and I am both of them. They keep attacking until they get caught in each other, their horns are locked. And then I can stop." With this, Abe, a bull of a man whose avocation is weight lifting, embraced his scholastic clinician and lifted him from the floor. "You are just like my father." The embrace represented a respite—the mind-body coming together, for both of them.

We have seen literally hundreds of schoolage boys and girls who offer poignant accounts of their internal experiences of tics and obsessions. They draw their tics for us (sometimes, with spidery legs just like forest tics) and provide their own accounts of the "abnormal pathways in their brains" that have been explained to them by their doctors and the pamphlets they have read. They blame that " dopamine stuff " that poisons them inside and that can be stopped by medications. One sweet child offered a theory that his tic started as mucous in his throat and then went into his brain, where the tics really came from. We have heard teenagers describe that they know that they are thinking too much about something—a girl who is perfect in every way, a fearful thought that they will hurt someone, a dread that they might have come into contact with AIDS by sitting near someone on the bus—but who, in spite of knowing their thoughts are not rational, are not able to use their reason to subjugate the worries. They know and do not know.

Often, the children with Tourette's syndrome become expert observers of their own experiences. Indeed, we have often felt that they become too good at this and spend too much time engaged in focusing attention on the self and inner experiences. They think about their minds in the same way that a child with a chronic physical condition, such as diabetes, may become too good a biologist and too preoccupied with how his body works. Children should take their bodies and minds more for granted. While increasing meta-representation is a developmental achievement that allows for self-reflection, too much reflection on the self is a heavy burden and can lead to a narcissistic over-investment in the self. This introspection and reflection may also be an aspect of the diathesis, itself, as if inner attunement and outward sensitivity to details are both a gift and a curse. When other schoolage children use their energy and channel their aggression into learning, sports, and figuring out the outer world, these children are caught up prematurely in focusing on how their minds work and what to do about their impulses. This preoccupation with their own feelings and responses may lead them to premature thoughtfulness and a remarkable ability and openness to portray the flow of their thoughts, feelings, and fantasies. This skill in free association and description is acquired by more constricted adults only after years of psychoanalytic therapy, if then.

We have also learned the many ways that Tourette's is a family affair. When we say that tics, obsessions, and compulsions run in families, this may seem blandly true. But the full implications of familiality are profound. Imagine the pain of a father who himself has tics when he sees that his beloved son is beginning to clear his throat one morning at breakfast, and then cannot stop the noise. Another father described that he saw his daughter get up from bed, go to the closet and straighten her shoes. At that moment, he knew that she, too, had Tourette's syndrome, and that her life, and the life of the family, would never be quite the same.

The parents of children with Tourette's syndrome, who themselves have had similar symptoms or saw them in their own families, are often doubly burdened. Like all parents, a child's illness or troubles are a great distress for the parent, especially when the difficulties are persistent, impairing, and socially painful. But when there is a hereditary factor, the parent's unhappiness may be compounded by personal guilt as well as the anger that may come from the partner—and the partner's family—who may feel free of the pathogenic taint. Converting the parental knowledge of his or her own experiences with tics and parental guilt into helpful concern is part of the therapeutic process. Indeed, most children who are afflicted with tics and associated problems are reassured that even with such difficulties, one may grow up to be like a beloved parent. And parents, too, can use their own coping and overcoming as reassurance for their child and themselves.

One of the pleasures of a long involvement with children with Tourette's syndrome has been to see that this optimistic attitude is quite often empirically valid. Indeed, most children with Tourette's syndrome, even those with the most severe difficulties in the schoolage years, develop into functioning and competent adults. Often, they are free of tics, or virtually free of them, unless under stress. Their tics become less noticeable as they are no longer under the microscopic scrutiny of parents and other adults who often see a child's imperfections under a high degree of magnification. Even those with persistent obsessions, compulsions, and tics, generally are able to cope and move ahead in their lives—to finish school, go on to college or a job, to marry, and then to have their own families. It is when they are about to marry or are just married, that many of these children now return, with fiancé or spouse, to discuss the implications of their disorder for the next generation. Then a special opportunity is provided to help the patient reflect on and integrate childhood experiences and to share them with his or her chosen life partner. Current genetic information can be conveyed that can be supportive of the young family in their considerations about their own children's fate. While there is no genetic marker that allows for prenatal diagnosis, most families can be told that available knowledge suggests that only a small percentage of the children of individuals with Tourette's syndrome are likely to have any clinically significant symptoms or any symptoms at all. Hopefully, when tics do emerge in a family that we have been caring for, and this has happened often enough, the young parents can work with us to reduce the likelihood of a devastating outcome by keeping the focus on the child, not the tics.

This can serve as the mantra for our approach to clinical care. For any illness that cannot be cured—and even for those that can but where the treatment is painful or prolonged—a major responsibility of the clinician is to help maintain the child's development on course. This means keeping the clinical eye on the child, *not* the symptoms. Children with many tics may do quite well at home, with friends, and in school, and feel good and effective. In such a situation, allowing nature to run its course is probably a reasonable option. In any case, all treatment needs to be assessed by its impact on social, emotional, and cognitive development, and the adequacy of a child in meeting the various tasks of development. Over the long-haul, we have seen very good therapeutic results, even for those children who still have troubling symptoms, with education of the family, support, guidance, psychotherapy, cognitive behavioral therapy, and judicious use of medication, in various combinations.

Yet, all too often, we have seen development become derailed not only because of the severity of symptoms and the repercussions in family and community of tics and obsessive-compulsive disorder, but because of the pursuit of "cure" through many treatments, including zealous use of medication. In the 1970s, we saw children and adolescents who had not received timely, sufficient, or appropriately targeted therapy; their Tourette's syndrome was not diagnosed or managed. Today, we see children who have had many medications started, raised, and lowered in rapid succession, without careful monitoring, and who are receiving four, five, or six medications concurrently. They become confused about their bodily states, what and why they feel the way they do, and what is under their control. Their sense of autonomy becomes eroded. Helping a child remain a person through the process of being a patient is an important part of clinical care.

Clinicians can learn a great deal about neurobiology and about the broad principles of clinical care by being part of the lives of children and families dealing with Tourette's syndrome and its treatment. With the involvement of many professionals in the care of a patient—teachers, therapists, pediatrician, psychiatrist—the clinician also can hold the parts together for the child and help the child in his attempts to integrate all of the experiences into an understanding of what is being done to and for him.

THE DEVELOPMENT AND MAINTENANCE OF THE SELF

Our theoretical understanding of the experience of Tourette's syndrome, and thus our guide to treatment, derives from developmental, behavioral, and neurosciences, as well as psychoanalysis. In our theories, we attempt to understand the patient's inner experiences in a manner that will also help the patient and family understand what they are living through. A major part of mental life is devoted to understanding life as it is being lived and has been experienced. This task of understanding is a central developmental process for all children. In normal development, children from the first months of life start to build up a sense of coherence. They feel the security that comes from being cared for by loving parents, who have continuity in space and time, and are there for them when they are expected. They relate this moment to what just happened, and they learn to anticipate the next steps in a sequence. They experience that their various sensations—touch, taste, sight, sound—are related to each other, and are different aspects of their perceptions of a person or thing in the outside world. They trust in the veridicality of their senses and mental constructions, and feel that they can count on their perceptions and ideas to guide them safely.

Even in the first year of life, children learn about their own intentionality. They anticipate the future and act as agents to achieve immediate and then increasingly distant goals. They have internal representations and plans. They know they need others to achieve their goals, at times, but also that they can get things on their own: They can wish for something, act on the wish, and reach a target. They know their desire may differ from their parents' desires for them, and they can assert their right to pursue their goal, even when this means recognizing and dealing with conflict. They develop a sense of independence and of autonomy, of being a separate person. They progressively develop a folk psychology, a "natural" psychological theory that explains behavior on the basis of desires and intentions. They thus evolve a theory of how their own mind and the minds of others work. As they do, they grow to recognize that they may be of two minds; when they have to choose between one option and another, they learn to deal with internal as well as external conflicts.

In all these ways, children develop a conscious sense of who they are as individuals and an unconscious, not fully represented sense of self—of an internal locus of integration of desires, abilities, values, and intentions that is suffused with feelings of pride and competence. At times of great stress or illness, or when falling asleep, children will fall apart, and the coherent sense of self as stable over time and within itself may break down. When children do not develop a sense of the psychological functioning of others or an understanding of their own minds, when they break down acutely or persistently, they lose their grasp on the coherence of the outer and inner worlds, which become unpredictable and frightening (Baron-Cohen, Tager-Flusberg, & Cohen, 1993; Mayes & Cohen, 1996a).

These natural, developmental processes occur so effortlessly and smoothly for most children that the complexities of building a stable sense of self are not visible on the surface. Children just seem to become more and more like little people—they know and act like themselves. How this comes about, biologically and psychologically, is a fascinating story that is only beginning to be approached empirically. In this epic, prominent roles are played by neurobiological mechanisms for the operation of each of the perceptual and cognitive modules and the integration into wholes of the various subsystems of perception, attention, emotion, and cognition and their shaping into patterns of intention and memory. Some of these activities are performed by specific cortical areas and by the parallel neuronal systems that connect the cortex and midbrain structures, the cortico-striatal-thalamo-cortical pathways (CSTC).

The overlapping CSTC pathways subserve subsystems such as the regulation of attention, perception, motor control, and the coordination of emotion with the internal and external situation. The systems are brought together into a harmoniously orchestrated whole by brain centers, which serve integrative roles, including cortical, thalamic, amygdala, and other regions. (Leckman, Peterson, et al., 1997). The functioning of these integrated neuronal systems, in normal children and adults and in those with various types of disorders, can now be studied using neuro-imaging techniques (such as functional MRI) (Peterson et al., 1998).

The unfolding of a coherent sense of self—based on an integrated functioning CNS—occurs when a child has the normal, developmental preconditions: the normal genetic endowment that shapes brain maturation during gestation and postnatally; an appropriate or good-enough environment, particularly the necessary continuity of loving care; protection from adversity; good health; and luck. (Cicchetti & Cohen, 1995a).

THE SELF UNDER SIEGE

The normal processes that lead to integrated, coherent, historical experience and stable self-representation provide a theoretical and emotional foundation for understanding the self (D. Cohen, 1980, 1991b). Developmental psychopathology utilizes these concepts as a framework for understanding and treating disorders (Peterson & Cohen, 1998). For children with Tourette's syndrome, disturbances in the regulation of attention and behavior may appear during the first years of life, before tics, as a harbinger of early dysfunctions in CNS maturation and integration. In these children, the tics may emerge gradually, as if restless overactivity and fidgeting were prodromal to the full disorder. For other children, the onset of tics at ages 6, 7, or 8 years may occur as if a genetic switch were thrown. A parent described looking out the window one morning and to her horror, she thought her perfectly well child was starting to have a seizure. His paroxysmal movements were the first signs of a tic disorder, which persisted for many years.

The unfolding of tics, obsessions, and compulsions can heuristically be related to the elaboration and recruitment of various CSTC connections. Metaphorically, the symptoms appear to reflect patterns of breakdown in the normal grammar or intrinsic rules that govern the relations of experience and behavior. When the normal grammar of integrated CNS and self-functioning break down, the individual experiences and emits fragments of normal behavioral patterns, disjoined from their normal syntax and thus out of context and apparently meaningless. Or recursive cycles of behavior become activated (Peterson & Leckman, in press), as if a feedback system starts to function and cannot be terminated at reaching its normal end, a satisfactorily completed action; the child never feels fully satisfied, the behavior does not fully match the internal template that initiated the behavior (Leckman, Walker, & Cohen, 1993; Leckman, Walker, Goodman, Pauls, & Cohen, 1994). The child thus stops only with exhaustion or the activation of a competitive response. The "electrical shorts" between CSTC mechanisms (B. Peterson et al., 1998), the recruitment of inappropriate pathways, as in cardiac arrhythmias, lead the child to feel bewildered by what he is feeling, thinking, and needing to do.

Models such as these suggest the nature of the psychological challenge to a child and adolescent who must try to make sense of an experiential world that is not governed by the usual rules, a world in which his thoughts and actions are both his and also alien to him. His self is under siege from forces within and yet out of his own sphere of autonomy. There are eruptions into consciousness and behavior of feelings, thoughts, and acts that are deeply encoded and yet normally not within consciousness, including sexual and aggressive fantasies; there is overuse of mechanisms that in other contexts may serve an adaptive role, such as cleaning, checking, repeating, and undoing, but which now over-carry their purpose and are impairing rather than adaptive; and there are tiny, repetitive sensations that normally are below the perceptual threshold or that might signal a need for action but that now lead to funny feelings in different parts of the body, relieved only by the sudden movement that is a tic (Leckman, Walker, & Cohen, 1993).

THE THERAPEUTIC PROCESS AND THE COHERENCE OF THE SELF

The therapeutic process for children with these breakdowns in internal integration, who feel they are possessed and going crazy, is aimed at reconstitution of coherence and meaningfulness. Thus, at the very start, explanations, education, and guidance are meant to reduce anxiety and the feeling of isolation. In the relationship with a family, the clinician creates an external, prosthetic integration—a holding of the patient and parents and a containment of their anxiety. As the child and family come to identify with the therapist's goals and attitudes, including his lack of anxiety or need to immediately do something, they can regain their own composure. The process of listening to the child and family's stories, in depth and over time, is an important aspect not only of obtaining their histories, but also helping to shape their current adaptation. Often, these stories are already quite distorted by the period of uncertainty before diagnosis, which now is becoming shorter; ill-advised interventions, including overuse or misuse of medications; and the familial tensions and peer difficulties that often accompany the disorders.

More specific therapeutic interventions then can occur in the clinical context of the relationship, with fully shared concern and knowledge. These include a range of options—cognitive and behavioral approaches, psychotherapy, school interventions, and, of course, medication. Taken together, available interventions are effective for the majority of individuals. Even those patients whose tics, obsessions, and compulsions persist can be offered support and optimism to cope with their troubles, including the consolation that childhood is usually harder than adulthood. We know that adult adaptation—vocation, intimacy, marriage, and life satisfactions—is far more a function of personal coping and development than of the severity of tics, as such (Towbin, Riddle, Cohen, & Leckman, 1988).

The self, once formed, needs a great deal to maintain its vigorous functioning as the locus of integration of desires, abilities, and values and as an experiential core of coherence in time and space. While the self of a child grows out of his biological endowment and intimate experiences, it is reinforced by the achievements at each phase of development, including mastering the basic tasks of development (learning, peer relations, and pleasure in activities).

In subtle ways, a touch of the Tourette's syndrome/obsessive-compulsive diathesis may help provide a particular flavor to self-development, one marked by increased awareness of one's own feelings and of the feelings of others. This diathesis may also have some adaptive functioning in relation to conscientiousness, attentiveness to vital details and changes, orderliness, regularity, cleanliness, and other useful traits (Leckman & Mayes, in press-a, in press-b). CSTC pathways and specific brain centers that subserve neurobiological integration may also help to structure the self in these domains of functioning. However, when the Tourette's syndrome diathesis becomes a full-blown disorder, the underpinnings of the self are attacked. Therapeutic goals must then be aimed at helping the individual to regain a sense of his or her autonomous and coherent self and to resume development.

ng the past 20 years, we have accompanied hundreds of children, ents, and adults through this therapeutic process. As is true generally of children with Tourette's syndrome, the majority have done nicely as whole people (Leckman et al., 1998). Advances in genetics, neuroimaging, neuropharmacology, and behavioral research will, no doubt, enhance the therapeutic possibilities. And, who knows, developmental neuroscience and prenatal diagnosis may actually reduce the incidence of Tourette's syndrome and associated disorders or virtually eliminate the disorders all together. If so, there will be a reduction in the burden of illness experienced by many children and families. In a strange way, there may also be a loss to humanity, since the biological vulnerability may also have adaptive value. There are some redeeming features—energy, talents, humor, zest for life, as well as conscientiousness and orderliness—that seem to accompany and grow out of the vulnerability to Tourette's syndrome and in the ways that individuals with Tourette's syndrome learn to successfully cope with their adversity. It is the task of clinicians to help preserve these gifts in children and adults with Tourette's syndrome who come for their care.

SUMMARY OF CHAPTER 1

The self under siege—a model of Tourette's syndrome gained from the care of hundreds of patients and decades of programmatic research is offered in this introductory chapter that blends psychoanalytic perspectives with recent advances in genetics and the developmental neurosciences. The meanings of this metaphor are explored in Section One, elaborated in Section Two, and put to the test in Section Three where guidelines for treatment are presented. However, as with any model or metaphor, it does not tell the whole story of individuals with Tourette's syndrome as they struggle to find pathways to healthy outcomes despite the burden of this disease.

PREVIEW OF CHAPTER 2

Tic symptoms—the hallmark of the Tourette's syndrome phenotype—are considered in this chapter. Emphasis is given to the sensory urges that precede many of the motor and phonic tics as well as the heightened sensitivity to external stimuli seen in many Tourette's syndrome patients. Competing diagnostic schemata are presented and discussed. Next, natural history of Tourette's syndrome is reviewed. Curiously, in order to understand the waxing and waning course of Tourette's syndrome and the natural history of tic disorders, it may be important to appreciate the fractal nature of tics. A consideration of what regularly makes tics better or worse may provide clues concerning the underlying neurobiology of this condition.

Individuals, Symptoms, and Diagnoses

Tourette's syndrome appears to be due to a disturbance in inhibition which affects the modulation of impulses, motor activity, thought, attention, and complex actions.

—Donald J.Cohen, J. Gerald Young, J. A. Nathanson, and Bennett A. Shaywitz, 1979

The idea of a disease-entity is not an objective to be reached, but our most fruitful point of orientation.

—Karl Jaspers, 1923

CHAPTER 2

Tics and Tic Disorders

JAMES F. LECKMAN, ROBERT A. KING, and DONALD J. COHEN

> Tics are rapid, coordinated caricatures of normal motor acts.
>
> —*A. J. Lees, 1985*

> There is really no adequate description of the sensations that signal the onset of the actions. The first one seems irresistible, calling for an almost inevitable response. . . . The end of the Tourette's syndrome action is the "feel" that is frequently accompanied by a fleeting and incomplete sense of relief.
>
> —*Joseph Bliss, 1980*

> Nature is inhabited by patterns in time.
>
> —*Esther Thelen and Linda B. Smith, 1994*

WHAT ARE TICS?

To the naïve observer, tics are a bewildering assemblage of abrupt movements and sounds. James Boswell characterized Samuel Johnson's tics as "convulsive starts and odd gesticulations, which tended to excite at once surprise and ridicule" (quoted in Murray, 1982). The same is true today. Working in close collaboration with patients and their families, we and other clinical investigators have endeavored to characterize both the overt features of tics and the associated mental states. Insights gained in these areas have deepened our understanding of tics and may illuminate some of the mysteries of their usual waxing and waning course as well as features of their natural history and neurobiology.

Definition

Tics are often more easily recognized than precisely defined. They are isolated disinhibited fragments of normal motor or vocal behaviors. Said

23

another way, tics are sudden, repetitive, stereotyped motor movements or phonic productions that involve discrete muscle groups. They can be easily mimicked and are often confused with normal coordinated movements or vocalizations.

From an Aristotelian perspective, tics can be characterized by their anatomical location, number, frequency, and duration. Another useful descriptor is the intensity or forcefulness of the tic, as some tics call attention to themselves simply by virtue of their exaggerated, forceful character. Finally, tics are also frequently described in terms of their complexity. Complexity, as it is commonly used, refers to how simple or involved a movement or sound is, ranging from brief, meaningless, abrupt fragments (simple tics) to ones that are longer, more involved, and seemingly more purposive in character (complex tics). As described in Chapter 15, each of these elements has been incorporated into ordinal rating scales that have proven to be useful in estimating and monitoring tic severity (Leckman et al., 1989; also see rating instruments in Appendix 1).

Clinical descriptions from the nineteenth century onward, including those of J. M. G. Itard (1825) and Georges Gilles de la Tourette (1885/1982), have focused on cataloguing and classifying tics as viewed from the outside. Partially in homage to our scholarly forebears, we discuss the overt phenomena of tics before considering the sensory and mental states that surround them.

Motor Tics

Motor tics usually begin with brief bouts of transient tics involving the face or head. A typical report involves bouts of eye blinking of variable intensity

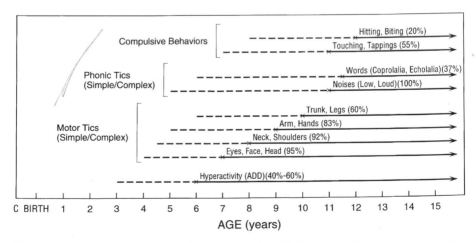

Figure 2.1   Natural history of tics and associated behaviors. The occurrence of tics progressing at different ages from transient episodes (broken lines) to sustained periods (solid lines). Adapted from Jagger et al., 1982.

beginning in kindergarten or the early school years. These symptoms often disappear after a few weeks, only to reappear later (Figure 2.1). Some authors report a rostral-caudal progression of motor tics, with tics of the face, head, and shoulders appearing earlier and in a higher proportion of patients than motor tics involving the extremities or the torso (Jagger et al., 1982). The observed range of motor tics is extraordinary, so that virtually any voluntary motor movement can emerge as a motor tic. Table 2.1 presents a brief compendium of some of the more common motor tics.

Motor tics may be described as simple or complex. *Simple motor tics* are sudden, brief (usually less than 1 second in duration), meaningless movements. Common examples include eye blinking, facial grimacing, mouth movements, head jerks, shoulder shrugs, and arm and leg jerks. Younger patients often are totally unaware of their simple motor tics.

Over time, many patients develop *complex motor tics,* which are sudden, more purposive-appearing, stereotyped movements of longer duration. Examples are myriad. Facial gestures and grooming-like movements such as brushing hair back are commonplace. Gyrating, bending, and more dystonic-appearing movements of the head or torso are also seen. These complex motor tics rarely are seen in the absence of simple motor tics. Paroxysms of several tics occurring at the same time or in rapid succession afflict more severe cases. Lewd and obscene gestures with hands or tongue (copropraxia) and self-abusive acts (hitting the face, biting a hand or wrist) are observed in a small number of patients. At times, it may be

TABLE 2.1   Examples of Simple and Complex Motor and Vocal Tics

Tic Symptom Dimensions	Examples
Simple Motor Tics: Sudden, brief, meaningless movements	Eye blinking, eye movements, grimacing, nose twitching, mouth movements, lip pouting, head jerks, shoulder shrugs, arm jerks, abdominal tensing, kicks, finger movements, jaw snaps, tooth clicking, rapid jerking of any part of the body.
Complex Motor Tics: Slower, longer, more purposeful movements	Sustained looks, facial gestures, biting, touching objects or self, throwing, banging, thrusting arms, gestures with hands, gyrating and bending, dystonic postures, copropraxia (obscene gestures).
Simple Phonic Tics: Sudden, meaningless sounds or noises	Throat clearing, coughing, sniffling, spitting, screeching, barking, grunting, gurgling, clacking, hissing, sucking, and innumerable other sounds.
Complex Phonic Tics: Sudden, more meaningful utterances	Syllables, words, phrases, statements such as "shut up," "stop that," "oh, okay," "I've got to," "okay honey," "what makes me do this," "how about it," or "now you've seen it," speech atypicalities (usually rhythms, tone, accents, intensity of speech); echo phenomenon (immediate repetition of one's own or another's words or phrases); and coprolalia (obscene, inappropriate, and aggressive words and statements).

difficult to distinguish complex tics from motor dyskinesias and other choreas and hyperkinetic movement disorders (Fahn & Erenberg, 1988; Jankovic, 1997).

The degree of impairment and disruption associated with particular motor tics is variable and a salient clinical feature. Partly dependent on frequency, forcefulness, complexity, and duration of specific tics, estimates of impairment also need to include the impact on the individual's self-esteem, family life, social acceptance, school or job functioning, and physical wellbeing. For example, a very frequent simple motor wrist tic may be less impairing than an infrequently occurring, forceful copropraxic gesture. Patients are often painfully aware of their complex motor tics and their unsettling impact on other people. The self-recriminations associated with these behaviors may also have a detrimental effect on self-esteem and limit socialization. Finally, physical injuries, including blindness from retinal detachment, occur in a small minority of adolescent and adult cases secondary to severe self-abusive tics.

Phonic Tics

Phonic or vocal tics usually appear after the onset of motor tics. In most cases, onset is between 8 and 15 years of age. Fewer than 5% of patients have isolated phonic tics in the absence of motor symptoms. Phonic tics often show a similar progression from transient episodes to more sustained periods of phonic symptoms (Figure 2.1). Again, the range of possible phonic symptoms is extraordinary, with any noise or sound having the potential to be enlisted as a tic (Table 2.1). Phonic symptoms are characterized by their number, frequency, duration, volume, and complexity (noises versus syllables or words).

Simple phonic tics are fast, meaningless sounds or noises that can be characterized by their frequency, duration, volume intensity, and potential for disrupting speech. Sniffing, throat clearing, grunting, barks, and high-pitched squeaks are common simple phonic symptoms. *Complex phonic tics* are quite diverse and can include syllables, words, or phrases, as well as odd patterns of speech in which there are sudden changes in rate, volume, and/or rhythm. Immediate echo phenomena such as repeating words and phrases are common in some patients (echolalia and palilalia). A minority of patients exhibit coprolalia, in which obscene or socially inappropriate syllables, words, or phrases are expressed, at times in a loud explosive manner. Complex phonic tics are rarely if ever present in the absence of simple phonic tics and motor tics of one sort or another. Provocative and insulting phonic symptoms have a high potential for stigmatizing the patient and his or her family and can lead to social isolation.

In summary, tics present as fragments of innate behavioral routines that are expressed in a disinhibited fashion. This viewpoint leads naturally to questions about the neurobiological substrates of Tourette's syndrome and related conditions, as discussed in Chapters 13 and 14.

Faint Signals, Sensory Urges, and Momentary Relief

Many patients with tic disorders report being besieged by a variety of sensory and mental states associated with their tics. Eloquent descriptions of these phenomena have appeared in first-person and biographical accounts of celebrated ticquers (Lees, 1985). These phenomena are more frequently reported by adults and include premonitory sensory urges that are reported to prompt the tics, complex states of inner conflict over if and when to yield to these urges, and a sensation of relief that frequently accompanies the performance of a tic.

Joseph Bliss, a lifelong sufferer of Tourette's syndrome, drew the attention of the medical community to what he called "faint signals" in an article published in 1980. In that seminal paper, he set down the knowledge he had gained from his lifelong effort to understand the sequence of events that leads to tics. To quote Bliss:

> There is really no adequate description of the sensations that signal the onset of the actions. The first one seems irresistible, calling for an almost inevitable response. . . . Intense concentration on the site can, in itself, precipitate the action. . . . Tourette's syndrome movements are intentional body movements. . . . The end of a Tourette's syndrome action is the "feel" at the terminal site of the movement, a feel that is frequently accompanied by a fleeting and incomplete sense of relief. (p. 1334)

This description is wholly congruent with those of others (Leckman, Walker, & Cohen, 1993, p. 102): "A need to tic is an intense feeling that unless I tic or twitch I feel as if I am going to burst. Unless I can physically tic, all of my mental thoughts center on ticking until I am able to let it out. It's a terrible urge that needs to be satisfied"; "A feeling of pressure—a need that's very hard to describe, like something itches deep inside you—but no place you can describe; and the only way you can relieve this need is by tics. It's like your brain itches, or your insides are being tickled"; "I guess it's sort of an aching feeling, in a limb or a body area, or else in my throat if it precedes a vocalization. If I don't relieve it, it either drives me crazy or begins to hurt (or both)—in that way it's both mental and physical." Much of what we have learned since 1980 are footnotes to Bliss's lucid exposition. All of what we have learned has come from Tourette's syndrome sufferers who have been willing to share their experience.

Young children under the age of 10 years with simple tics—a forceful eye blink or a quick head jerk—usually do not have or are totally unaware of these sensory urges. For them, Tourette's syndrome is truly an involuntary movement disorder. The awareness of these urges typically shows up later, on average more than 3 years after the onset of the tics. On the other hand, precocious children as young as 7 years old have spontaneously offered compelling descriptions of this phenomenon. We vividly recall one boy of 7 describing his "Tourette's" and his "cocky" going to his lips and making him grimace.

A second point is that having premonitory urges does not mean that every tic is preceded by such a conscious urge. More than 90% of the 134 Tourette's syndrome patients that participated in a study of these premonitory urges reported having experienced such urges during the past week, but often tics involving more automatic behaviors, like eye blinking, do not have urges that precede them (Leckman, Walker, & Cohen, 1993).

Third, the shoulder girdle, throat, hands, midline of the stomach, and front of the thighs and feet are "hot spots" for such urges (Leckman, Walker, et al., 1993; Figure 2.2). The urges are often located in a small discrete area that can be readily identified. For others, these urges are more generalized and are best captured by a building sense of inner tension. Many individuals will report having both types of sensations.

Fourth, these urges are sometimes more troublesome than the tics. This is true particularly for some adults who are able partially to resist the tics but are left with these distracting urges. We have wondered whether these urges could contribute to the attentional problems that so frequently accompany Tourette's syndrome. A corollary to this point is that usually

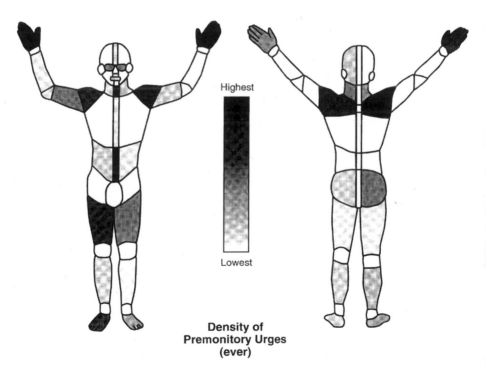

**Density of
Premonitory Urges
(ever)**

Figure 2.2   Density of premonitory urges. The densities of premonitory urges for each of 89 anatomical regions are depicted. The highest density on the scale represents 0.40 total premonitory urges per region per person, the lowest 0 urges per region per person, and the midpoint 0.20 urges per region per person. These data are based on premonitory urges ever experienced as assessed in a self-report questionnaire (N = 132). See Leckman, Walker, and Cohen (1993) for details.

when the tics get better, so do the urges. During the waxing and waning course of Tourette's syndrome or with medications or other treatments, as the tics improve, so do the urges.

A full consideration of these premonitory urges brings us face-to-face with another troublesome aspect of Tourette's syndrome: that the tics themselves are at least partially voluntary acts, or as Bliss said, "intentional" capitulations to these virtually irresistible sensory invitations. Indeed, in our study of premonitory urges (Leckman, Walker, et al., 1993) we found that 92% of the subjects reported that they experienced their tics to be partly or wholly voluntary in character. Taken out of context, this forced intentionality can be misunderstood and a source of anguish and guilt: Why can't I resist? What's wrong with me?

As we wonder about the origins of these urges, it seems clear that these pestering signals are likely to arise within the inner space of our bodies. We may all be able to experience them, but those without Tourette's syndrome may need to sit in a quiet room without distractions. They are signals emanating from the body that are ordinarily screened out of conscious awareness. Viewed from this perspective, Tourette's syndrome is a sensori-motor disorder characterized by a heightened sensitivity to a changeable set of somatic stimuli.

Advances in the neurosciences have also helped us realize how plastic the brain is, how a distributed set of neurons originally engaged in one function can, over the course of days, be reprogrammed to attend to another related function. How this plasticity arises remains in doubt. But the selective modification of premonitory sensory urges over time suggests that a deeper understanding of the mechanisms involved may lead to novel therapeutic interventions. For example, one severely affected patient went from a dreadful, stigmatizing laugh to a less noticeable throat clearing over the course of a week; this change coincided with an upper respiratory tract infection. Similar accounts are commonplace and suggest that experiential events associated with correlated firing in sensorimotor systems can reorganize an individual's tic repertoire.

Too Easily Captured by External Perceptions

In a comparable fashion, many patients with Tourette's syndrome are remarkably sensitive to perceptions arising in the external world (A. Cohen & Leckman, 1992). As first noted by Gilles de la Tourette, patients may unconsciously mirror the behavior (echopraxia) and speech (echolalia) of others as well as of themselves (palilalia): they do and say what they have just seen or heard.

Other instances include site sensitization: being unusually aware of, distracted and distressed by particular somatic stimuli. The classic example is tags in new clothing that in some remarkable way serve as a distracting focus of attention; unless they are removed, the child has difficulty attending to other things. A related phenomenon is triggering perceptions; one example of this was reported by a man who goes into a bout of severe vocal tics if he hears the cough of a particular woman who rides the same bus with him in the morning. Other disinhibited behaviors seen in a minority of Tourette's syndrome patients also appear to be perceptually mediated. Some patients report the emergence of urges to perform more complex acts that are dangerous, forbidden, or simply senseless and bizarre in response to proscriptive injunctions. An extreme example was told by a retired physicist, who during World War II, had to give up a job in high energy physics because whenever he saw the sign "Danger: High Voltage," he had the urge to touch the apparatus. Related phenomena may include the urge to touch a hot iron, to put the car in reverse gear while driving down a highway, to touch the breast of an unknown woman in an adjacent seat, and to shout out in a quiet church service. Finally, some of the just right phenomena that we associate with obsessive-compulsive behavior may also belong in this category (see Chapter 3). For example, the need for things to be arranged over and over until they look just right is dependent on visual perceptions.

This stimulus-dependent property of tics and related obsessive-compulsive phenomena provides intriguing parallels with animal studies, in which investigators have documented plasticity of neural firing in monkey striatum during a sensorimotor conditioning task as well as other reward-conditioned stimuli (Aosaki, Kimura, & Graybiel, 1995; Rolls, Thorpe, & Maddison, 1983). They are also at the essence of what we mean when we characterize Tourette's syndrome as the self under siege.

DIAGNOSIS AND CLASSIFICATION OF TIC DISORDERS

There is no sensitive and specific diagnostic test for Tourette's syndrome or other tic disorders at present. The diagnosis is based solely on the individual's history and clinical presentation. Consequently, the current diagnostic classifications of tic disorders are based on the conventional wisdom of experts in the field. Readers interested in the art and limitations of diagnostic estimates are also referred to Chapter 7, where the fine points of differential diagnosis are discussed.

Diagnostic categories can be useful to families, educators, and other professionals. They provide a common basis for discussion and are an essential tool in epidemiological and clinical research. They are what Richard Dawkins (1976) has termed *memes,* complex ideas that form themselves into distinct memorable units. According to Dawkins, such ideas have a certain self-replicating character based on their utility. They evolve and are subject to the same laws of natural selection that genes are subject to. The variation and competition among current classification systems provide a clear example of this evolutionary process.

Several widely used diagnostic classifications currently include tic disorders, including the classification system offered by the American Psychiatric Association (1994; Table 2.2) in the *Diagnostic and Statistical*

TABLE 2.2   *DSM-IV* Tic Disorder Classification

I. Diagnostic Criteria for Tourette's Syndrome (307.23)
   A. Both multiple motor and one or more vocal tics have been present at some time during the illness, although not necessarily concurrently.
   B. The tics occur many times a day (usually in bouts), nearly every day or intermittently throughout a period of more than a year; and during this period, there was never a tic-free period of more than three consecutive months.
   C. The disturbance causes marked distress or significant impairment in social, occupational, or other areas of functioning.
   D. Onset before age 18 years.
   E. The disturbance is not due to the direct physiological effects of a substance (e.g., stimulants) or a general medical condition (e.g., Huntington's chorea or post-viral encephalitis).

II. Diagnostic Criteria for Chronic Motor or Vocal Tic Disorder (307.22)
   A. Single or multiple motor or vocal tics, but not both, have been present at some time during the illness.
   B. The tics occur many times a day, nearly every day, or intermittently throughout a period of more than a year. During this period there was never a tic-free interval of more than three months.
   C. The disturbance causes marked distress or significant impairment in social, occupational, or other areas of functioning.
   D. Onset before age 18 years.
   E. The disturbance is not due to the direct physiological effects of a substance (e.g., stimulants) or a general medical condition (e.g., Huntington's chorea or post-viral encephalitis).
   F. Criteria have never been met for Tourette's Disorder.

III. Diagnostic Criteria for Transient Tic Disorder (307.21)
   A. Single or multiple motor and/or vocal tics.
   B. The tics may occur many times a day, nearly every day for at least four weeks, but for no longer than 12 consecutive months.
   C. The disturbance causes marked distress or significant impairment in social, occupational, or other areas of functioning.
   D. Onset before age 18 years.
   E. Disturbance is not due to the direct physiological effects of a substance (e.g., stimulants) or a general medical condition (e.g., Huntington's chorea or post-viral encephalitis).
   F. Criteria have never been met for Tourette's Disorder or Chronic Motor or Vocal Disorder.

IV. Diagnostic Criteria for Tic Disorder Not Otherwise Specified (307.20)
   This category is for a tic disorder that does not meet the criteria for a specific tic disorder. Examples include tics lasting less than four weeks or tics with an onset after age 18 years.

Source: Diagnostic and Statistical Manual of Mental Disorders, 4th ed. Copyright 1994 American Psychiatric Association.

Manual of Mental Disorders, 4th edition (*DSM-IV*); criteria by the World Health Organization (1992) in the *International Classification of Disease and Related Health Problems,* 10th revision (*ICD-10*); and the Classification of Tic Disorders (CTD) by the Tourette's Syndrome Classification Group (1992; Table 2.3). Although clear differences exist among these classification schemes, they are broadly congruent, with each containing three major, well-specified categories: Tourette's syndrome or its equivalent; chronic motor or vocal tic disorder or its equivalent; and transient tic disorder or its equivalent.

Transient Tic Disorder

Almost invariably a disorder of childhood, transient tic disorder is usually characterized by one or more simple motor tics that wax and wane in severity over weeks to months. The anatomical distribution of these tics is usually confined to the head, neck, and upper extremities. Transient phonic tics, in the absence of motor tics, can also occur, though more rarely. Although sound epidemiological studies have not focused on this category, this is a common condition affecting a sizable percentage of all children (for more detail, see Chapter 10). The age of onset is typically 3 to 10 years; boys are at greater risk; and the initial presentation may be unnoticed. If medical consultation is sought, family practitioners, pediatricians, allergists, and ophthalmologists are typically the first to see the child. Missed diagnoses are common, particularly as the symptoms may have completely disappeared by the time of the consultation. As set forth in the prevailing diagnostic criteria, the subsequent natural history of this condition is limited to fewer than 12 consecutive months of active symptomatology. As such, this is often a retrospective diagnosis, as the clinician is unable to know ahead of time which children will show progression of their symptoms and which children will display a self-limiting course. This uncertainty points to the value of deferring the diagnosis, as codified in the Tourette Syndrome Classification Study Group criterion F (Table 2.3, VI).

Chronic Motor or Vocal Tic Disorder

This chronic condition can be observed among children and adults. The prevalence of this disorder among school-age children may be as high as 3% or 4% (Costello, Angold, Burns, Stangl, Tweed, & Erkanli, 1996; see Chapter 10). As with other tic disorders, it is characterized by a waxing and waning course and a broad range of severity. Chronic simple and complex motor tics are the most common manifestations. A majority of tics involve the head, neck, and upper extremities. Although some children may display other developmental difficulties, such as attention-deficit/hyperactivity disorder, the disorder is not incompatible with an otherwise normal course

TABLE 2.3   Classification of Tic Syndromes (The Tourette Syndrome Classification Study Group)

I. Diagnostic Criteria for Tourette Syndrome (A-1 & A-2)

   A. Both multiple motor and one or more vocal tics have been present at some time during the illness, although not necessarily concurrently.

   B. The tics occur many times a day, nearly every day, or intermittently throughout a period of more than a year.

   C. The anatomic location, number, frequency, complexity, type, severity of tics changes over time.

   D. Onset before age 21.

   E. Involuntary movements and noises cannot be explained by other medical conditions.

   F. Motor and/or vocal tics must be witnessed by a reliable examiner directly at some point in the illness or be recorded by videotape or cinematography (for Definite Tourette's Syndrome, A-1) or tics were not witnessed by a reliable examiner, but tics were witnessed by a reliable family member or close friend; and description of tics as demonstrated is accepted by reliable examiner (for Tourette's Syndrome by History, A-2).

II. Diagnostic Criteria for Chronic Multiple Motor Tic or Phonic Tic Disorder (B-1 & B-2)

   A. Either multiple motor or vocal tics, but not both, have been present at some time during the illness.

   B. The tics occur many times a day, nearly every day, or intermittently throughout a period of more than a year.

   C. The anatomic location, number, frequency, complexity, or severity of tics changes over time.

   D. Onset before age 21.

   E. Involuntary movements and noises cannot be explained by other medical conditions.

   F. Motor and/or vocal tics must be witnessed by a reliable examiner directly at some point in the illness or by videotape or cinematography (Definite Chronic Multiple Motor Tic or Phonic Tic Disorder, B-1) or tics were not witnessed by a reliable examiner, but tics were witnessed by a reliable family member or close friend; and description of tics as demonstrated is accepted by a reliable examiner (Chronic Multiple Motor Tic or Phonic Tic Disorder by History, B-2).

III. Diagnostic Criteria for Chronic Single Tic Disorder (C-1 & C-2)

   A. Same as in II (B-1 & B-2), but with single motor or vocal tic.

IV. Diagnostic Criteria for Transient Tic Disorder (D-1 & D-2)

   A. Single or multiple motor and/or vocal tics.

   B. The tics occur many times a day nearly every day for at least 2 weeks, but for no longer than 12 consecutive months, although the disorder began over a year ago.

   C. The anatomic location, number, frequency, complexity, or severity of tics changes over time.

   D. No history of Tourette's Syndrome or chronic motor or vocal tic disorders.

   E. Onset before age 21.

   F. Motor and/or vocal tics must be witnessed by a reliable examiner directly at some point in the illness or by videotape or cinematography (Definite

Continued

TABLE 2.3   *(Continued)*

Transient Tic Disorder, D-1) or tics were not witnessed by a reliable examiner, but tics were witnessed by a reliable family member or close friend; and description of tics as demonstrated is accepted by a reliable examiner (Transient Tic Disorder by History, D-2).

V. Diagnostic Criteria for Nonspecific Tic Disorder (E-1 & E-2)
    A. Tics that do not meet the criteria for a specific tic disorder; an example would be a tic disorder with the tics lasting less than 1 year, and without any change over that period of time.
    B. Motor and/or vocal tics must be witnessed by a reliable examiner directly at some point in the illness or by videotape or cinematography (Definite Nonspecific Tic Disorder, E-1) or tics were not witnessed by a reliable examiner, but tics were witnessed by a reliable family member or close friend; and description of tics as demonstrated is accepted by a reliable examiner (Nonspecific Tic Disorder by History, E-1).

VI. Diagnostic Criteria for Definite Tic Disorder, Diagnosis Deferred (F)
    A. Meets all criteria of definite Tourette's Syndrome (first definition), but duration of illness has not yet extended to 1 year.

VII. Diagnostic Criteria for Probable Tourette Syndrome (G)
    A. Type 1: Fulfills all criteria for definite Tourette's Syndrome (first definition) completely, but excludes the third and fourth criteria; or
    B. Type 2: fulfills all criteria for definite Tourette's Syndrome (first syndrome) except for the first criterion; this type can be either a single motor tic with vocal tics or multiple motor tics with possible vocal tic(s).

VIII. Diagnostic Criteria for Probable Multiple Tic Disorder—Motor and/or Vocal (H)
    A. Fulfills all criteria for definite multiple tic disorder (second definition) completely, except for the third and/or fourth criteria.

Adapted from The Tourette Syndrome Classification Study Group (1993). Definitions and classification of tic disorders. *Archives of Neurology, 50,* 1013–1016. Criteria A, B, & D are based on *Diagnostic and Statistical Manual of Mental Disorders, 3rd ed., rev.* Copyright 1987 American Psychiatric Association.

of development. This condition can also appear as a residual state, particularly in adulthood. In such instances, a predictable repertoire of tic symptoms may only be seen during periods of heightened stress or fatigue. Chronic vocal tic disorder by all accounts is a rare condition. Some authors exclude chronic cough of adolescence from this category (A. Shapiro et al., 1988).

Tourette's Syndrome (Chronic Motor and Phonic Tic Disorder)

The most severe tic disorder is best known by the eponym Gilles de la Tourette's syndrome. Typically, the disorder begins in early childhood with transient bouts of simple motor tics such as eye blinking or head jerks. These tics may initially come and go, but eventually they become persistent and begin to have adverse effects on the child and his or her family. As noted above, the repertoire of motor tics can be vast, incorporating virtually any voluntary movement by any portion of the body. Although some authors have drawn attention to a rostral-caudal progression of motor tics (head, neck, shoulders, arms, torso), this course is not predictable. As the syndrome develops, complex motor tics may appear. Often they have a camouflaged appearance (e.g., brushing hair away from the face with an arm) and can only be distinguished as tics by their repetitive character. Rarely, complex motor tics can be self-injurious and further complicate management (e.g., punching one side of the face or biting a wrist).

On average, phonic tics begin one to two years after the onset of motor symptoms and are usually simple in character (e.g., throat clearing, grunting, squeaks). More complex vocal symptoms such as echolalia, palilalia, and coprolalia occur in a minority of cases. Other complex phonic symptoms include dramatic and abrupt changes in rhythm, rate, and volume.

The forcefulness of motor tics and the volume of phonic tics can also vary tremendously, from behaviors that are barely noticeable (a slight shrug or a hushed guttural noise) to strenuous displays (arm thrusts or loud barking) that are frightening and exhausting.

In addition to the tic behaviors, associated behavioral and emotional problems frequently complicate Tourette's syndrome or other chronic tic disorders. These difficulties range from impulsive, disinhibited, and immature behavior to compulsive touching or sniffing. There is no clear dividing line between these abrupt and disruptive behaviors and complex tics on the one hand and comorbid conditions of attention-deficit/hyperactivity disorder and obsessive-compulsive disorder on the other.

Other Tic Disorder Diagnoses

These classification systems also include one or more additional diagnostic categories. The CTD includes five additional categories: definite single tic disorder, nonspecific tic disorder, definite tic disorder–diagnosis deferred, probable Tourette's syndrome, and probable multiple tic disorder (Table 2.3). The major virtue of these additional categories is that they provide the clinician or the researcher with a more precise system for classifying cases that do not fit neatly into one of the principal categories. The *DSM-IV* and *ICD-10* classifications employ fewer diagnostic options and tend to lump the remaining cases into "not otherwise specified," "other," or "unspecified" categories.

Nosological Controversies

With the publication of *DSM-IV* in 1994, a notable difference between the CTD and *DSM* classification schemes emerged, namely, the *DSM-IV* requirement that the tic symptoms "cause marked distress of significant impairment in social, occupational or other important areas of functioning" (p. 103). This criterion is based on a conceptualization of mental disorder articulated by the framers of the *DSM-IV* and was intended to distinguish between normality and pathology. Unfortunately in the case of tic disorders, this criterion is vague and open to widely varying interpretation. For example, it is not clear who needs to be distressed or for how long. The frequent presence of comorbid diagnoses that in combination with the tic symptoms may cause distress or impairment may result in additional difficulties in applying the *distress* criterion of *DSM-IV*. Finally, problems arise in research settings in which all of the *DSM-IV* criteria are satisfied save the distress criterion, leaving open how such cases should be classified.

Another minor but substantive difference between the *DSM-IV* and the Tourette Syndrome Classification Study Group criteria is the age of onset criterion (tic onset prior to age 18 years in *DSM-IV* and prior to 21 years in the Tourette Syndrome Classification Group). Until a more objective diagnostic test is developed, this difference is likely to remain unresolved. However, as the vast majority of individuals report the onset of their tic symptoms in the first decade of life, this 3-year difference is unlikely to have much practical impact.

Caveats on the Topic of Diagnostic Categories

Before leaving the discussion of diagnostic categories, a few caveats are in order. First, it is important to recognize that diagnostic categories, despite their value, can be misapplied and misused. Thus, it is crucial to consider the alternative diagnostic possibilities, as reviewed in Chapter 7.

Second, even if Tourette's syndrome is the correct diagnosis, it will be important for families, educators, and clinicians to focus on the whole person with Tourette's rather than the relevant diagnostic category. Preoccupations with the disorder potentially have a number of adverse consequences, not the least of which is the implicit message to the patient concerning his or her identity. As discussed in the previous chapter, to place Tourette's syndrome at the center of one's identity is to invite distortion and a negative expectancy rather than a more adaptive outcome. For example, it is common for families to arrive at an initial consultation with the firmly held belief that their child, who today has a few troublesome tics, is destined to become someone on a daytime television talk show whose life has been devastated by Tourette's syndrome. Active clinical intervention is required to adjust and correct these potentially harmful expectancies.

Third, the potential explanatory power of diagnostic categories, at times, can lure families and professionals into attributing more to the disorder than is reasonable. In our experience, this is particularly true when a child's development has been encumbered with other difficulties such as pervasive developmental disorders, dyslexia, or disruptive behavior problems.

THE OCCURRENCE OF TICS IN BOUTS: A CLUE TO THE WAXING AND WANING COURSE OF TICS AND TIC DISORDERS

The onslaught of tics and urges is not steady. Individual tics tend to occur in bouts with brief intertic intervals that can be measured in seconds. These bouts themselves occur in bouts and may account for transient periods of tic exacerbation that occur during the course of a typical day. Empirical studies of this phenomenon are just getting underway (B. Peterson & Leckman, in press). Speculation has focused on the fractal occurrence of tics. This fractal quality means that regardless of the time increments studied—seconds, minutes, hours, days, weeks, or years—the nonlinear temporal patterning of tics or bouts of tics or bouts-of-bouts of tics or bouts-of-bouts-of-bouts of tics or bouts-of-bouts-of-bouts-of-bouts of tics remains basically the same (Figure 2.3). This quality, if confirmed, may elucidate a fundamental property of tics and tic disorders. For example, the well-known waxing and waning course of tics may simply be another way to refer to bouts-of-bouts-of-bouts-of-bouts of tics and the time interval between them. At the other end of the time scale, it is possible that an examination of the neural mechanisms underlying this fractal phenomenon may identify related events that can be measured in milliseconds or even shorter intervals that are associated with the generation of tic phenomena.

Tics then might be best understood as being the product of nested processes that unfold over many time scales, from milliseconds to years or even decades. As such, they may be exemplars of a dynamical system at work in the development of the CNS (Thelen & Smith, 1994).

The Natural History of Tics and Tic Disorders

Tics usually have their onset in the first decade of life. Most investigators report a median onset of simple motor tics at 5 or 6 years of age (Erenberg, Cruse, & Rothner, 1987; Goetz, Tanner, Stebbins, Leipzig, & Carr, 1992; Sandor, Musisi, Moldofsky, & Lang, 1990; A. Shapiro et al., 1988). Figure 2.4 presents age of onset data for 221 patients with Tourette's syndrome evaluated at Yale.

Subsequently, the classic history includes a waxing and waning course and a changing repertoire of tics. Typically in cases of Tourette's syndrome, the symptoms multiply and worsen, so that even during the waning phases the tics are troublesome. In our experience for a majority of patients, the period of worst tic severity usually falls between the ages 7 and 15 years, following which there is a steady decline in tic severity (Leckman, Zhang, et al., 1998; Figure 2.5). This fall-off in tic symptoms is consistent with available epidemiological data that indicate a lower prevalence of Tourette's syndrome among adults compared to children (see Chapter 9). It is also typical of the findings reported in follow-up studies of clinically referred Tourette's syndrome patients (Erenberg et al., 1987;

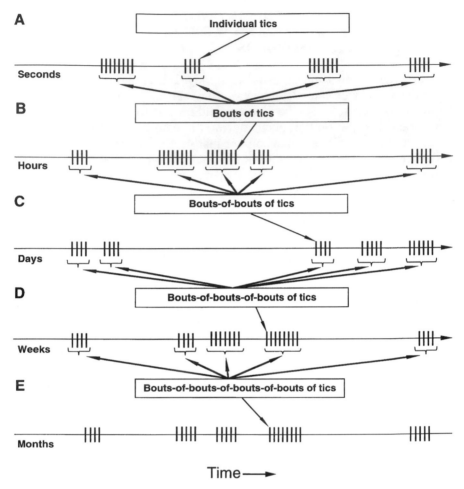

Figure 2.3   Fractal character of the temporal occurrence of tics. Progressively longer time dimensions (seconds to months) are heuristically depicted in this figure (A–E). Tics occur in bouts (A) and bouts of tics occur in bouts (B). We predict that regardless of the temporal dimension, the boutlike appearance of tics (or higher-order combinations of bouts and bouts-of-bouts of tics) will be observed. This fractal quality may well underlie the waxing and waning of tics observed over weeks to months (E) as well as other features of the natural history of Tourette's syndrome. For additional information, see B. Peterson & Leckman, in press.

Goetz et al., 1992; Sandor et al., 1990; Table 2.4). In many instances, the phonic symptoms become increasingly rare or may disappear altogether, and the motor tics may be reduced in number and frequency.

In adulthood, a patient's repertoire of tics usually diminishes in size and becomes predictable during periods of fatigue and heightened emotionality. Complete remission of both motor and phonic symptoms has also been reported, but estimates vary considerably, with some studies reporting rates

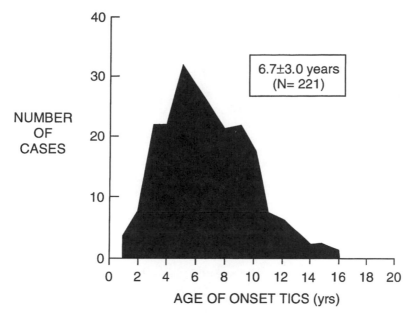

Figure 2.4 Age of onset distribution. This figure presents the age of onset of tics in a series of 221 individuals with Tourette's syndrome evaluated at the Yale Child Study Clinic (unpublished data). These data were influential in resetting the age of onset criterion in the *DSM-IV* for Tourette's disorder to 18 years of age rather than 21 years of age.

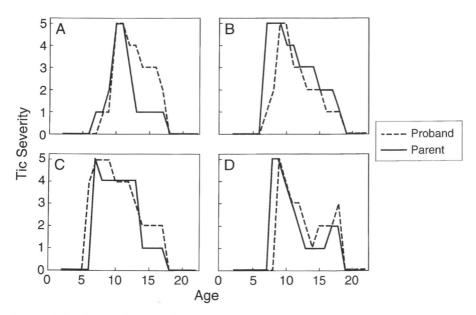

Figure 2.5 Onset of tic severity over the first two decades. Data on the relative severity of tics are presented for four patients (A–D). The relative tic severity scale goes from 0 (no tics) to 5 (severe tics). Estimates from the patient and a respective parent were obtained independently. For details, see Leckman, Zhang, et al., 1998.

TABLE 2.4   Summary of Follow-Up Studies of Tourette's Syndrome

Studies	N (RR) (Sex Ratio, M:F)	Mean (Range): Current Age & FUI (Yrs.)	Tic Severity (%)	Psychosocial Outcomes (%)	Prognostic Factors
Mahler & Luke (1946)	10 (All males)	18 (12–23) FUI: NA (1.5–12)	Remission: 30; improved: 40; NC/worse: 30	*Occupational:* Student: 30; employed: 50; unemployed: 20 *Social:* Excellent/good: 60; fair/poor: 40 *Personality:* Good: 40; fair: 30; poor: 30	Tics better with outdoor physical activity; no relationship to type or duration of therapy.
Zausmer (1954)	41 (2:1)	NA (11–12.2) FUI: 2.6 (NA)	Remission: 13; improved: 66; NC/worse: 21	NA	Better in females.
Torup (1962)	220 (3:1)	18 (6–16) FUI: 9 (2–16)	Remission: 50; improved: 46; NC/worse: 4	NA	Worse if parents had tics that have persisted into adulthood; worse if conflicts at home.
Lucas et al. (1967)	15 (65) (3:1)	19 (11–29) FUI: 6 (2–15)	Remission: 7; improved: 73; NC/worse: 20	*Social:* Excellent/good: 53; fair/poor: 47	NA
Corbett et al. (1969)	73 (82) (4:1)	15 (6–29) FUI: 5.4 (1–18)	Remission: 40; improved: 54; NC: 6	NA	Better prognosis the longer the FUI; worse if body tics and/or coprolalia; worse if comorbid depression or OCD.
Bruun et al. (1976)[Q]	78 (98) (3:1)	NA (6–67) FUI: 2.7 (0.5–8.5)	Remission: 5; improved: 86; NC: 8; worse: 1	NA	NA
A. Shapiro et al. (1978)	50 (NA)	NA (20–85) FUI: NA (13–20)	Remission: 8; periods of remission: 54; improved: 34; NC/worse: 4	NA	Better prognosis among high SES families; less waxing and waning associated with worse outcomes and vigorous tics.
Asam (1982)	16 (7:1)	27 (15–44) FUI: 17 (5–38)	Remission: 13; improved: 56; NC/worse: 31	*Educational:* Jr HS: 19; voc: 6 *Marital Status:* Married: 25; divorced: 6; unmarried: 69 *Social:* Good: 34; fair/poor: 66	NA
Mak et al. (1982)	15 (NA)	18 (11–35) FUI: 5.8 (3–12)	Remission: 7; improved: 47; NC/fluctuations: 46	*Social:* Good: 47; fair: 20; poor: 33 *Marital Status:* Married: 13; divorced/unmarried: 87	Poorer social prognosis associated with lower IQs, abnormal EEGs, and poor school adjustment.
Nee et al. (1982)	30 (3:1)	NA (21–71) FUI: NA (NA)	Remission: NA; improved: 67; NC/worse: 33	NA	NA
Erenberg et al. (1987)[Q]	58 (59) (NA)	18 (10–21) FUI: NA (NA)	Almost no tics: 26; improved: 47; NC: 14; worse: 14	*Coping with Tics:* Well: 59; some difficulty: 36; severe difficulty: 5	Worst ever tic severity and drug response unrelated to outcome.
Bruun (1988a)	251 (NA)	NA (NA) FUI: NA (5–15)	Remission: 3; improved: 44; NC: 45; worse: 8	*Marital Status:* Married: 54; divorced: 9; widowed: 2; unmarried: 35 *Occupational:* Employed: 61; unemployed: 30; social security: 9	NA

TABLE 2.4   *(Continued)*

Studies	N (RR) (Sex Ratio, M:F)	Mean (Range): Current Age & FUI (Yrs.)	Tic Severity (%)	Psychosocial Outcomes (%)	Prognostic Factors
Sandor et al. (1990)	33 (44) (5.6:1)	25 (13–59) FUI: 7 (1–15)	Remission: 0; improved: 45; NC/worse: 55	*Marital Status:* Married: 18; divorced: 3; unmarried: 79 *Social Status:* Downward shift in social adaptation: 39; require ongoing social supports: 30	Medication did not alter psychosocial achievement.
Goetz et al. (1992)	58 (62) (2.4:1)	27 (21–62) FUI: 27 (21–62)	Remission: 0; mild: 76; mod/severe: 24	*Educational:* HS graduate: 98 *Occupational:* Full-time worker or student: 90	Tic severity during late youth predictive of adult severity; no predictive value associated with childhood tic severity.
Park et al. (1993)	101 (100) (9:1)	12 (8–21) FUI: 1.6 (0.5–7)	Remission: 2; improved: 81; NC/worse: 17	NA	NA

N, number of cases; RR, response rate (N/number of possible cases); M, male; F, female; FUI, follow-up interval; NA, data not reported in the article; NC, no change in clinical status; ^{Q} questionnaire study; OCD, obsessive-compulsive disorder. Dr. Young-shin Kim assisted in the preparation of this table.

of remission as high as 50% (Torup, 1962; Table 2.4). In such cases, the legacy of Tourette's syndrome in adult life is most closely associated with what it *meant* to have severe tics as a child. For example, individuals who were misunderstood and punished at home and at school for their tics or who were teased mercilessly by peers and stigmatized by their communities will fare worse than a child whose interpersonal environment was more understanding and supportive.

In contrast, adulthood is also the period when the most severe and debilitating forms of tic disorder can be seen. In this small minority of adult patients, severe tics can persist or reemerge with frightening intensity. At their worst, these tics can be self-injurious and disabling, placing in serious jeopardy an individual's accomplishments and aspirations.

A number of potential risk factors have been identified that may influence the patient's trajectory of tic severity, including a number of pre- and perinatal events, exposure to bacterial antigens provoking an autoimmune response, withdrawal from neuroleptic drugs, exposure to psychostimulants or androgenic steroids, physical fatigue and emotional stress, heat exposure, and the presence of a range of comorbid psychiatric disorders. A full consideration of these factors is beyond the scope of this chapter, but it is worth noting that what regularly makes tics better or worse may provide clues concerning the underlying neurobiology of this condition and may point the way to preventive interventions. Various risk and protective factors are discussed in detail in Chapters 6, 8, 9, and 11.

SUMMARY OF CHAPTER 2

Tic symptoms, the hallmark of the Tourette's syndrome phenotype, are best understood as fragments of innate behavioral programs that are normally assembled by the basal ganglia acting in concert with cortical and thalamic sites. The sensory urges that precede many of the motor and phonic tics may further illuminate the normal internal cues that typically aid in the assembly of these behavioral programs. Diagnostic schemata for tic disorders are presented and discussed as clinically useful, but evolving, conventions. The occurrence of tics in time appears to have fractal characteristics that may help to predict the waxing and waning course of chronic tic disorders and, surprisingly, may point the way to the identification of neurons with the same burst-pause pattern of reactivity that play a crucial role as tic generators. The natural history of tics usually shows a marked decline during the course of adolescence. Finally, a consideration of what regularly makes tics better or worse may provide clues concerning the underlying neurobiology of this condition.

PREVIEW OF CHAPTER 3

Like tics, obsessions and compulsions besiege the patient's inner world. It is an unsettling onslaught that can leave in doubt a person's sense of wholeness and control. Chapter 3 provides a detailed description of these phenomena before turning to consider symptoms of depression and anxiety that frequently occur as complications in the course of Tourette's syndrome.

CHAPTER 3

Obsessive-Compulsive Disorder, Anxiety, and Depression

ROBERT Λ. KING, JAMES F. LECKMAN, LAWRENCE SCAHILL,
and DONALD J. COHEN

> While talking or even musing as he sat in his chair, he commonly held his head to one side towards his right shoulder, shook it in a tremulous manner, moving his body backwards and forwards, and rubbing his left knee in the same direction, with the palm of his hand. . . . He had another peculiarity, of which none of his friends even ventured to ask an explanation. It appeared to me some superstitious habit, which he had contracted early, and from which he had never called upon his reason to disentangle him. This was his anxious care to go out or in at a door or passage, by a certain number of steps from a certain point, or at least so as that either his right or his left foot . . . should constantly make the first actual movement when he came close to the door or passage.
>
> —*James Boswell,* Life of Johnson, *quoted by Murray, 1982*

Although motor and vocal tics are the pathognomonic symptoms of Tourette's syndrome, other associated difficulties such as obsessions, compulsions, anxiety, depression, emotional lability, attentional deficits, and learning problems may be an equal or greater source of distress and impairment to individuals with Tourette's syndrome than tics per se. The present chapter focuses on obsessive-compulsive symptoms and related anxiety and affective problems that may accompany Tourette's syndrome. Attention-deficit/hyperactivity disorder, learning difficulties, and related problems are considered in Chapter 4.

OBSESSIONS AND COMPULSIONS

In his original description of the disorder, Gilles de la Tourette (1885/ 1982) noted obsessive-compulsive symptoms in several of the patients he

43

studied. Subsequent studies have shown rates of obsessive-compulsive features ranging from 11% to 80% of individuals with Tourette's syndrome (Table 3.1), with more recent studies reporting higher rates (Robertson & Yakeley, 1993). As reviewed in Chapter 10, this wide range in prevalence appears to reflect differences not only in sample composition, but also in the assessment instrument and criteria used. Although obsessive and compulsive features are common in individuals with Tourette's syndrome, the proportion whose symptoms are sufficiently severe to warrant a diagnosis of obsessive-compulsive disorder is considerably smaller, with only about 30% of adults with Tourette's syndrome meeting the full criteria for obsessive-compulsive disorder.

This elevated prevalence of obsessive-compulsive symptoms is found not only in clinical samples of patients with Tourette's syndrome, but also in nonreferred individuals with tics identified in community samples (Apter et al., 1993), as well as in the first-degree relatives of individuals with tics (see Chapters 10 and 11). Although the nature of the association between obsessive-compulsive symptoms and Tourette's syndrome remains a matter of some controversy (Pauls, Leckman, & Cohen, 1994), there is a growing consensus in the scientific community that in many instances obsessions and compulsions are integral features of the experience of patients with Tourette's syndrome. With increasing clarity we are beginning to trace this relationship from the level of vulnerability genes to the neural circuitry and the distressing complexities of the clinical presentation.

TABLE 3.1   Occurrence of Obsessive-Compulsive Symptoms (OCS) or Obsessive-Compulsive Disorder (OCD) in Patients with Tourette's Syndrome

Study	N	OCS/OCD[†]
D. Cohen, 1980; D. Cohen et al., 1978	25	56%
Nee et al., 1980, 1982	5	68
Montgomery et al., 1982	12	67
Lees et al., 1984	53	61
Grad et al., 1984	25	28
Comings & Comings, 1985	250	35
Frankel et al., 1986	63	52
A. Shapiro et al., 1988	666	3–63
Brunn, 1988b	350	16–42
Robertson et al., 1988b	90	37
Bornstein et al., 1990	763	8–85
Pauls, Raymond, et al., 1991	86	36
Coffey et al., 1992	84	13
Apter et al., 1993*	12	42
Leckman, Walker, et al., 1994	134	23–69
Spencer et al., 1995	32	23

[†] Variable definitions used to define OCS or OCD (see text).
* Community-based survey of 28,037 adolescents ages 16 to 17.

Definitions

Obsessions are persistently recurring thoughts, impulses, or images that are experienced as intrusive, inappropriate, and distressing and which are not simply excessive worries about realistic problems (APA, 1994). *DSM-IV* defines compulsions as repetitive behaviors or mental acts that the person feels driven to perform according to a rigidly applied rule in order to reduce distress or to prevent some dreaded outcome, albeit one not realistically related to the action. As we discuss below, this definition of compulsions may not adequately describe the driven repetitive acts and compulsive urges associated with Tourette's syndrome. The current *DSM-IV* diagnostic criteria for obsessive-compulsive disorder are shown in Table 3.2.

To meet the full criteria for a diagnosis of obsessive-compulsive disorder, *DSM-IV* severity criteria require that the obsessions or compulsions

TABLE 3.2   *DSM-IV* Diagnostic Criteria for Obsessive-Compulsive Disorder

A. Either Obsessions or Compulsions

Obsessions are defined by:
1. Recurrent and persistent thoughts, impulses, or images that are experienced, at some time during the disturbance, as intrusive and inappropriate and that cause marked anxiety or distress.
2. The thoughts, impulses, or images are not simply excessive worries about real-life problems.
3. The person attempts to ignore or suppress such thoughts, impulses, or images, or to neutralize them with some other thought or action.
4. The person recognizes that the obsessional thoughts, impulses, or images are a product of his or her own mind (not imposed from without as in thought insertion).

Compulsions as defined by:
1. Repetitive behaviors (e.g., handwashing, ordering, checking) or mental acts (e.g., praying, counting, repeating words silently) that the person feels driven to perform in response to an obsession, or according to rules that must be applied rigidly.
2. The behaviors or mental acts are aimed at preventing or reducing distress or preventing some dreaded event or situations; however, these behaviors or mental acts either are not connected in a realistic way with what they are designed to neutralize or prevent or are clearly excessive.

B. At some point during the course of the disorder, the person has recognized that the obsessions or compulsions are excessive or unreasonable. *Note:* This does not apply to children.

C. The obsessions or compulsions cause marked distress, are time consuming (take more than 1 hour a day), or significantly interfere with the person's normal routine, occupational (or academic) functioning, or usual social activities or relationships.

D. If another Axis I disorder is present, the content of the obsessions or compulsions is not restricted to it.

The disturbance is not due to the direct physiological effect of a substance (e.g., a drug of abuse, a medication) or a general medical condition.

Source: American Psychiatric Association, 1994.

cause marked distress, consume more than an hour daily, or significantly interfere with routine functioning or relationships. The severity threshold of at least one hour appears to be somewhat arbitrary (Apter et al., 1996). Many individuals with Tourette's syndrome have clinically significant obsessions or compulsions that do not cause enough impairment or distress to meet these criteria. This subsyndromic level of symptoms is sometimes termed *subclinical obsessive-compulsive disorder*. Because obsessions and compulsions appear to occur on a spectrum of severity and are relatively common in the general population (Apter et al., 1996; Rachman & deSilva, 1978), it is often not clear when to regard the mildest forms of obsessions and compulsions as psychopathological.

The descriptive range of common obsessions and compulsions is shown in Table 3.3, adapted from the Yale-Brown Obsessive Compulsive Scale (W. Goodman, Price, Rasmussen, Mazure, et al., 1989; W. Goodman, Price, Rasmussen, Mazure, Delgado, et al., 1989). This scale also has items for quantifying the time spent, degree of control and resistance, associated impairment and distress, and overall severity of reported obsessions and compulsions. Although patients with Tourette's syndrome can present with any of these obsessive-compulsive symptoms, certain constellations are more common than others. In our experience, obsessions with violent and aggressive themes, obsessional worries about symmetry and exactness, and compulsions involving ordering, arranging, counting, touching, and doing and redoing are commonplace in Tourette's syndrome. In contrast to other patients with obsessive-compulsive disorder, patients with Tourette's syndrome only occasionally present with isolated contamination worries and cleaning compulsions.

Distinguishing between Tics and Compulsions

Many individuals with Tourette's syndrome report repetitive behaviors that are preceded by a perceptual awareness that something in the immediate environment is not just right. These phenomena bear some similarity to the premonitory urges that frequently accompany tics (Leckman, Walker, Goodman, Pauls, & Cohen, 1994; Miguel et al., 1995; Scahill, Leckman, & Marek, 1995; Scahill et al., 1997). Indeed, taken in isolation, it may be impossible to distinguish meaningfully whether a given symptom, such as repetitive or symmetrical touching or tapping, should be considered a complex tic or a simple compulsion. The patient with such repetitive touching or arranging is usually unable to adduce any motive for the action other than an urge to do it or to get it right. Attempts to suppress the behavior voluntarily or to prevent its performance generally produce what patients describe as a profoundly unpleasant, mounting tension or sense of frustration. Performance of the stereotypic behavior produces a momentary feeling of relief, completion, or satisfaction that is often only transient and followed sooner or later by a mounting need to repeat the action.

TABLE 3.3   Examples of Obsessions and Compulsions

Obsessions

Aggressive Obsessions[†]
  Fear might harm self.
  Fear might harm others.
  Violent or horrific images.
  Fear of blurting out obscenities or insults.
  Fear will act on unwanted impulses (e.g., hit/run motor vehicle accident).
  Fear will steal things.
  Fear will harm others because not careful enough (e.g., hit/run motor vehicle accident).
  Fear will be responsible for something else terrible happening (e.g., fire, burglary).

Separation Obsessions[*]
  Loss or injury to significant attachment figures.

Sexual Obsessions[†]
  Forbidden or aggressive sexual thoughts, images, or impulses.
  Content involves children or incest.

Religious Obsessions (Scrupulosity)[†]
  Concerned with sacrilege and blasphemy.

Obsessions with Need for Symmetry or Exactness[†]
  Accompanied by magical thinking (e.g., concerned that mother will have accident unless things are in the right place).
  Not accompanied by magical thinking.

Contamination Obsessions[‡]
  Concerns or disgust with bodily waste or secretions (e.g., urine, feces, saliva).
  Concern with dirt or germs.
  Excessive concern with environmental contaminants (e.g., asbestos, radiation, toxic waste).
  Excessive concern with household items (e.g., cleansers, solvents).
  Excessive concern with animals (e.g., insects).
  Bothered by sticky substances or residues.
  Concerned will get ill because of contaminant.
  Concerned will get others ill by spreading contaminant.

Hoarding/Saving Obsessions
  Concerned with the need to collect or hoard items.

Somatic Obsessions
  Concern with illness or disease.[*]
  Excessive concern with body part or aspect of appearance (e.g., dysmorphophobia).[*]

Other Obsessions
  Need to know or remember.
  Fear of saying certain things.
  Fear of not saying just the right thing.
  Fear of losing things.
  Intrusive (nonviolent) images.
  Intrusive nonsense sounds, words, or music.
  Lucky/unlucky numbers.
  Colors with special significance.

Continued

TABLE 3.3   (*Continued*)

Compulsions

Checking Compulsions
Checking locks, stove, appliances, etc.
Checking that did not/will not harm others.
Checking that did not/will not harm self.
Checking that nothing terrible did/will happen.
Checking that did not make mistake.
Checking tied to somatic obsessions.

Repeating Rituals[†]
Re-reading or re-writing.
Need to repeat routine activities (e.g., in/out door, up/down from chair).

Counting Compulsions[†]
Repeating actions or counting items in odd or even sets or by special numbers (e.g., 4s, 7s).

Ordering/Arranging Compulsions[†]
Arranging closets, room, cabinets, or other items in excessive or idiosyncratic manner.

Cleaning/Washing Compulsions[‡]
Excessive or ritualized handwashing.
Excessive or ritualized showering, bathing, toothbrushing, grooming, or toilet routine.
Cleaning of household items or other inanimate objects.
Other measures to prevent or remove contact with contaminants.

Hoarding/Collecting Compulsions
Distinguish from hobbies and concern with objects of monetary or sentimental value (e.g., carefully reads junkmail, piles up old newspapers, sorts through garbage, collects useless objects).

Other Compulsions
Mental rituals (other than checking/counting).
Excessive list making.
Need to tell, ask, or confess.
Need to touch, tap, or rub.*[†]
Symmetrical or counted touching or tapping.[†]
Rituals involving blinking or staring.*[†]
Measures to prevent: harm to self, harm to others, terrible consequences.
Ritualized eating behaviors.*
Superstitious behaviors.*
Trichotillomania,* skin or scab picking.

* May or may not be OCD phenomena.
[†] Commonly associated with TS and chronic tic disorders.
[‡] Uncommonly associated with TS and chronic tic disorders.
Adapted from Y-BOCS, Goodman, Price, Rasmussen, Mazure, et al., 1989; Goodman, Price, Rasmussen, Mazure, Delgado, et al., 1989.

For example, many of Samuel Johnson's eccentricities noted by contemporaries appear to have been compulsions and complex tics related to Tourette's syndrome. In addition to the compulsions noted in the epigraph of this chapter, Johnson was careful never to walk on the cracks of paving stones and touched every post as he walked down the street, returning to go back and touch any that he had missed. Asked by a young child why he made such strange gestures, he replied, "From bad habit. Do you, my dear, take care to guard against bad habits" (Murray, 1982, p. 30).

The elusive sense of completion or closure that the patient seeks in the performance of compulsive habits often requires some specific tactile, somatosensory, or visual symmetry or order. As one man put it, "If they don't sound or feel or look right, then I perform these actions until they are" (Leckman, Walker, et al., 1994, p. 677). Table 3.4 shows the distribution across the different perceptual modes of the just right phenomena experienced by one group of patients with Tourette's syndrome and obsessive-compulsive disorder or recurrent obsessive-compulsive symptoms.

Symmetry, order, or alignment in the visual mode is perhaps the commonest mode of perceptual completion sought. For example, one boy spent over three hours each morning trying to get the part of his hair exactly straight (Scahill, Walker, Lechner, & Tynan, 1993); another spent hours trying to get his tapes and books precisely arranged on his desk. Just right phenomena in the tactile mode may involve symmetry, as with the patient who has to repeat with the left hand actions done with the right, or even up shoelace length and tension to be precisely the same on both feet. In other patients, the desired somatosensory experience may be harder to specify, as with the teenage girl who had to bang her glass on the table top until it

TABLE 3.4   Perceptual Modes in "Just Right" Perceptions

Mode	OCD without Tics (%)*	OCD with Tics (%)[†]
Looks only	33 (30)	11 (21)
Feels only	15 (14)	5 (10)
Sounds only	2 (2)	0
Looks and feels	21 (19)	12 (23)
Looks and sounds	2 (2)	4 (8)
Feels and sounds	0	0
Looks, feels, and sounds	14 (13)	11 (21)
Any looks	70 (63)	38 (73)
Any feels	50 (45)	28 (54)
Any sounds	18 (16)	15 (29)
Any mode	91 (82)	47 (89)

*Obsessive-compulsive disorder without tics ($n = 121$), of which 111 reported "just right" perceptions at some point in their illness.
[†]Tic-related obsessive-compulsive disorder ($n = 56$) of which 52 reported "just right" perceptions at some point in their illness. The numbers in parentheses are the percentage of patients in each diagnostic group who reported ever having "just right" perceptions. No significant differences were observed based on tic status.
Adapted from Leckman, Walker, et al., 1994.

felt just right, frequently resulting in spills and breakage; asked how she knew when she got it right, she replied, "I can't put it into words, but I know it when I do it." More worrisome, the desired sensation may be nociceptive, as with patients who must jam their finger up their nose or hit themselves until it feels just right. Like the patients described by Bruun (1988b) who compulsively filed their teeth until they felt and looked even, the motive is not deliberate self-injury, but a driven pursuit of an all too often evanescent sense of getting it right.

The just right desiderata may also be auditory, as with the child who insists on his parents repeating a phrase over and over until they get it precisely right in some idiosyncratically specified way. Although the content and context of these phrases may seem emotionally neutral, the child's insistence is often reminiscent of many preschoolers' need to have a parent repeat some stock phrase in just the right way at bedtime.

Many compulsive behaviors involve a blend of somatosensory and visual modes, such as going back and forth through a doorway until passing exactly through the middle of the portal, or, like Samuel Johnson as described at the beginning of this chapter, on a specific foot.

The desired goal or subjective perfection sought may be more mental than sensory, requiring just the right concentration or act of volition. One patient noted that he stopped only "when I have reached a level of concentration on the action that assures me the action was completed satisfactorily" (Leckman, Walker, et al., 1994, p. 677). If interrupted or distracted, for example, by the impingement of intrusive "bad thoughts," such as injury to a loved one, the patient may need to repeat the routine until free of the bad thought, or even perhaps while thinking a countervailing good thought (Leckman, Grice, et al., 1995; Leckman, Walker, et al., 1994).

Despite the frequent similarities between the tics and the compulsions of individuals with Tourette's syndrome in terms of these perceptually tinged urges and just right phenomena, some patients do distinguish clearly between their complex tics and their compulsions. Although premonitory urges are most often described as straddling the physical and mental (Scahill, Leckman, et al., 1995), many subjects experience (or define) tics as movements prompted by or accompanied by a bodily sensation, whereas compulsions are preceded by more of a mental phenomenon (Miguel et al., 1995). As one 11-year-old boy with Tourette's syndrome and obsessive-compulsive symptoms put it, "The tic is more of an itch, and a compulsion is a want. A tic is physical and the compulsion is a mental feeling." A 35-year-old man observed similarly, "The urge to tic is a release of a buildup of physical energy; the compulsive urge is a buildup of emotional energy" (Leckman, Walker, et al., 1994, p. 678).

Careful inquiry by a clinician who conveys familiarity with the inner world of Tourette's syndrome and an interest in learning about the patient's experience often is rewarded by detailed descriptions of these complex phenomena that straddle the boundary between tics and compulsions:

Case Example. Father Brown, a Jesuit high school teacher with Tourette's syndrome, led an orderly and devout life. In addition to a panoply of simple motor and phonic tics, he had a shifting repertoire of complex tics, obsessions, and compulsions. Among his current repetitive behaviors (that illustrated the difficulty of distinguishing complex tics from simple compulsions) was the need to stretch his right hand out, cock his head, and look through his right eye, so that his extended middle and forefinger were lined up against some intersecting set of lines in the background; this had to be repeated until a certain visual alignment and feeling of muscular tension in his arm were achieved. Father Brown also had a shifting repertoire of phrases, such as "Oh, you dirty dog," which, under the guise of humor, he would compulsively have to repeat or get others to repeat. He could distinguish between his ordinary but strenuous religious devotions and a form of prayer that he considered a compulsion, consisting of having to recite the Ave Maria in a special way while fastening his eyes to the right on a statue of the Virgin Mary. If not done "just right," he would have to repeat his prayers all over again. Unlike the scrupulosity of Ignatius Loyola, his order's founder, who feared blasphemy were he to step accidentally on straw lying on the floor in a cross, there was no theology to Father Brown's compulsion; he just had to do it. Although his colleagues regarded his lesson plans as exemplary, he would have to spend hours filling them out in compulsive detail, retyping his lists until the margins were perfect, and arranging his desk and room precisely.

Some articulate youngsters may imaginatively elaborate these urges and obsessions in an attempt to give them meaning:

Case Example. In a playroom interview, Richard, a bright, nonpsychotic 10-year-old boy with Tourette's syndrome and obsessive-compulsive disorder, repetitively enacted a scenario with plastic figures in which, after great struggle, the lone hero would finally corral the bad guys into jail, only to have them break out and attack him, necessitating his beginning his struggles all over again. Sympathizing with the hero's Sisyphean struggles, the clinician asked whether Richard ever had similar problems. Richard immediately described his own struggles over his compulsive need to "even up" his actions, including his motor tics. To represent these struggles, he had elaborated, over the years, an imaginary world of warring good and bad figures. Perry, the King of the Evens, was the leader of the good guys, because he urged Richard to repeat actions an even number of times, which produced a sense of completeness and relief. Arrayed against Richard and Perry was the evil King of the Odds, who tormented Richard with feelings of incompleteness and subversively urged him to repeat a movement, such as a head-turning tic, "just one more time." Richard confided, however, that he was considering defecting to the Odds side, because 1 was an odd number and he would desperately like to be able to do something only once and be done with it.

Although many young children are fussy about the texture and feel of clothing, some children with Tourette's syndrome and/or obsessive-compulsive disorder have exquisite tactile hypersensitivity concerning their clothing. These children may become increasingly restrictive in the items they will wear. Periodic crises may ensue as they are unable to go to school after hours of being unable to find clothes, socks, or shoes whose touch, texture, or fit seem tolerable or feel right.

Dysmorphophobia may be another form of just right phenomenon, whose relationship to Tourette's syndrome and obsessive-compulsive disorder remains unclear. Dysmorphophobia is characterized by the anxious preoccupation with some minor or imagined physical imperfection. For example, a 15-year-old boy with a strong family history of Tourette's syndrome brooded for hours in the mirror over his imagined receding hairline, anxiously requiring weekly close-to-the-scalp haircuts so that he could feel and see that he was not going bald. A 15-year-old girl with Tourette's syndrome and obsessive-compulsive disorder was preoccupied with a small, cosmetically inconspicuous scar, whose raised surface, uneven texture, and altered tactile sensitivity led her to pick at it repetitively and to ruminate about the need for surgery. These tactile and visual phenomena are not unlike the descriptions of young female patients with trichotillomania in terms of the way they feel a given hair calls to them (R. King et al., 1995).

TIC-RELATED VS. NON-TIC-RELATED OBSESSIVE-COMPULSIVE DISORDER

The obsessions and compulsions found in individuals with Tourette's syndrome cover a broad range in terms of content, intensity, persistence, impairment, degree of perceived ego-syntonicity, and relationship to the individual's tic symptoms. A growing number of studies examining symptom type, natural history, sex ratio, family genetic data, neurobiological correlates, and treatment response lend increasing support to the hypothesis that tic-related obsessive-compulsive disorder constitutes a distinctive obsessive-compulsive disorder phenotype. Compared to obsessive-compulsive disorder in individuals without a history of tics, this subtype appears to be characterized by an earlier age of onset, a greater proportion of males, a more frequent family history of chronic tics, higher afternoon plasma prolactin levels and more normal CSF oxytocin levels (Leckman, Goodman, North, et al., 1994a, 1994b), and a poorer therapeutic response to monotherapy with serotonin-reuptake inhibitors, albeit with marked improvement with the addition of a neuroleptic (McDougal et al., 1994; McDougle, Goodman, Leckman, Barr, et al., 1993).

Clinical Features

Although there is considerable overlap in the obsessive-compulsive symptoms of individuals with and without Tourette's syndrome, recent studies, summarized in Table 3.5, have examined whether there are systematic phenomenological differences between the two groups. Most of these

TABLE 3.5 Tic-Related vs. Non-Tic Related Obsessive-Compulsive Disorder (OCD)

Study	N	Sex (% Female)	Onset (Years)	Distinctive Symptoms
George et al., 1993				
Tic-related OCD	15	26	NA	Touching, symmetry, sexual, and violent obsessions, blinking/staring rituals.
Non-tic related OCD	10	60	NA	Contamination fears and cleaning compulsions.
Holzer et al., 1994				
Tic-related OCD	35	23	13.2	Touching, tapping, repeating, blinking/staring rituals.
Non-tic related OCD	35	23	16.1	Cleaning compulsions.
Leckman, Pauls, et al., 1995				
Tic-related OCD	56	41	13.4	Violent and religious obsessions, checking, counting, hoarding, intrusive images, or sounds.
Non-tic related OCD	121	61	15.9	Cleaning compulsions (trend).
de Groot, Bornstein, et al., 1995				
Tic-related OCD	21	24	NA	Somatic obsessions, intrusive images or sounds.
Non-tic related OCD	37	65	21.3	Contamination fears and cleaning compulsions, checking.
Zohar et al., 1997				
Tic-related OCD	15	7	NA	Aggressive and sexual images and obsessions.
Non-tic related OCD	25	64	NA	
Eapen et al., 1997				
Tic-related OCD	16	44	NA	Symmetry, evening up, "just right" actions, touching.
Non-tic related OCD	16	50	NA	Washing, cleaning.
Leckman, et al., 1997				
Tic-related OCD	93	—	—	Sexual, aggressive, religious obsessions, checking, symmetry, and ordering.
Non-tic related OCD	198	—	—	

studies, conducted largely in adults, have found that current severity of obsessive-compulsive symptoms does not discriminate between tic- and non-tic-related types of obsessive-compulsive disorder. Touching compulsions, however, appear to be characteristic of the tic-related subtype of obsessive-compulsive disorder. Thus, the need to tap, touch, or rub is found in 70–80% of patients with comorbid tics, but only 5–25% of subjects in the non-tic-related obsessive-compulsive disorder subgroup. Compared to other obsessive-compulsive disorder patients, patients with tic-related obsessive-compulsive disorder more frequently report intrusive violent and/or aggressive thoughts and images, sexual and religious preoccupations, and concerns about symmetry and exactness. In contrast, patients with non-tic-related obsessive-compulsive disorder more frequently report contamination worries and cleaning compulsions. The two types of obsessive-compulsive disorder, however, do not appear to differ with regard to the presence of "just right" phenomena.

A factor-analytic study of two large samples of patients with obsessive-compulsive disorder, with and without Tourette's syndrome, examined lifetime scores on the symptom checklist categories of the Yale-Brown Obsessive Compulsive Scale (Leckman, Grice, et al., 1997). Largely paralleling earlier studies (Baer, 1994), four factors emerged, accounting collectively for more than 60% of the variance: (a) aggressive, sexual, religious, and somatic obsessions and checking; (b) symmetry and ordering; (c) cleanliness and washing; and (d) hoarding (Figure 3.1). Individuals with Tourette's syndrome or chronic tic disorder scored significantly higher on the obsessions and checking factor, the symmetry and ordering factor, and the hoarding factor than did subjects without a chronic tic disorder.

In addition to delineating distinct subtypes of obsessive-compulsive disorder with potentially important etiologic and therapeutic implications, these studies also suggest important refinements in the instruments used to assess obsessive-compulsive disorder. For example, scales that rely solely on current symptoms; omit hoarding, concerns about symmetry, exactness, and ordering; or use global severity ratings, may obscure the rich diversity of obsessive-compulsive disorder symptomatology over time (Leckman, Grice, et al., 1997).

Intrusive aggressive obsessions or compulsions are often extremely disturbing to patients with Tourette's syndrome and may bear little apparent descriptive relationship to their tics:

Case Example. Steve, a 19-year-old, had experienced since age 7 severe motor and vocal tics, which caused him much social embarrassment. Despite a harsh working-class upbringing, he had finished high school and found work as a manual laborer. His precarious adjustment, however, was shaken by the acute appearance of frightening ego-alien obsessive-compulsive symptoms. These consisted of horrific intrusive images of his violently attacking loved ones (against whom he had no other conscious hostile feelings), accompanied by a powerful compulsive urge, against which he had to struggle intensely. For example, he felt overwhelmed by a compulsion to punch his frail, cherished, elderly aunt in the face, to hit his

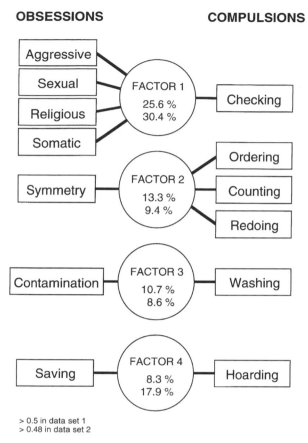

OBSESSIONS   **COMPULSIONS**

> 0.5 in data set 1
> 0.48 in data set 2

Figure 3.1   Varimax rotated factor structure for Yale-Brown Obsessive Compulsive Scale symptom checklist category scores. The same four factors (depicted as circles) were identified in two independent sets of data. Symptom categories (boxes) associated with each factor are presented. The percentages refer to the proportion of the variance that is associated with each factor by data set. For additional details, see text and Leckman, Grice, et al. (1997).

kindly female boss, and to kick his pregnant sister in the stomach. These urges were so frightening that he contemplated moving across the country or committing suicide to protect his loved ones. In contrast to the pleasure and excitement with which Steven related the damage he had inflicted in fist fights with peers, he experienced these new violent images and impulses as intrusive, senseless, and upsetting.

Still other children may suffer from sticky perseverative behaviors or preoccupations that may be more distressing to others than to the child, who may deny seeing them as problematic. These behaviors may occur against a background of temperamental difficulties, including inflexibility, intolerance of frustration, and difficulty shifting activities or tolerating changes in schedule (Garland & Weiss, 1996):

Case Example. David, a bright 15-year-old student with Tourette's syndrome, had always had a difficult time shifting activities and coping with frustration or changes in routine, often responding with tantrums. As an adolescent, his escalating oppositional behavior, including physical confrontations with parents, teachers, and even police, finally culminated in hospitalization. His frequent, stubbornly defiant behavior led to much difficulty at school, despite his superior intelligence. Although his avowedly deliberate oppositional behaviors were disruptive and maladaptive, David denied any distress over them. In contrast, however, he described some of his most extreme episodes as due to "traps," the term he used for compulsive behaviors that he recognized as senseless or extreme, but which he felt compelled to pursue regardless of consequences. For example, he had insisted on going next door to pet a neighbor's dog in the middle of the night, leading to a physical struggle with his father, who attempted to restrain him. During such episodes, which could last up to an hour, David reported, "I think, 'I've just *got* to do it, no matter what.'" Afterward, in contrast to many of his other deliberately oppositional behaviors that were quite ego-syntonic, David would be apologetic and remorseful. David also had a variety of rituals that involved his parents, for example, insisting his mother stand in a particular spot while he reported the day's events in order without error. If he could not get the order right or if she refused to cooperate, or failed to make the precisely prescribed reply he demanded, David would become angry and agitated. David's parents, teachers, and clinicians were confused as to how to understand or respond to these episodes.

Developmental and Evolutionary Perspectives

Some just right phenomena associated with Tourette's syndrome are reminiscent of the preschool child's insistent preference for things to look, feel, or sound just right. Bedtime rituals, involving toys or room having to be arranged just so, or a particular sequence of songs and goodnights precisely repeated, may serve to bind anxiety at times of transition or separation. Obsessive concerns about sameness or symmetry, order in certain situations, and upset if thwarted are found in as many as two-thirds of preschoolers as an apparently normal developmental phenomenon, appearing with greatest intensity between age 2 and 4 years (Evans et al., 1997). For example, the same outfit may have to be worn or the same sandwich, cut precisely in two, prepared daily. This developmental observation brings us again to an evolutionary perspective, first discussed in Chapter 1 and later in Chapter 8. From this viewpoint, obsessions and compulsions—of any sort—might be usefully considered to be disinhibited fragments of a highly conserved core bio-psycho-behavioral process involved in the maintenance of secure environments.

Natural History

Retrospective surveys of clinical samples of Tourette's syndrome patients suggest that compulsive behaviors usually make their onset later than simple motor and vocal tics. Thus, in one sample of 75 subjects, the mean age of onset of motor tics was 8.7 years; in contrast, the mean age of compulsive actions (head banging; kissing; touching objects, self, or sexual organs; mimicking others) was 10.8 years (Jagger et al., 1982). In prospectively followed subjects, however, obsessive-compulsive symptoms may predate the onset of tics. In a prospective longitudinal study of 21 children at high risk for Tourette's syndrome (younger siblings of Tourette's syndrome probands) who were without tics at entry into the study, obsessive-compulsive symptoms, obsessive-compulsive personality, or obsessive-compulsive disorder were apparent at follow-up in 4 (19%) of the children (age 6.5–9.1 years); 2 of these 4 children did not have tics (Carter, Pauls, Leckman, & Cohen, 1994). Leonard et al. (1994) observed that some children with early-onset obsessive-compulsive disorder later developed tics.

In contrast to non-tic-related obsessive-compulsive disorder, tic-related obsessive-compulsive disorder appears to be characterized by an early age of onset and more males than females affected. Although in most individuals with Tourette's syndrome, the severity of motor and phonic tics appears to wane by later adolescence (Goetz et al., 1992; Leckman, Zhang, et al., 1998; Chapter 2), the developmental time course of obsessions and compulsions has not been well studied. Clinically, we have the impression that the course of obsessions and compulsions is at least partially independent of that of tics and that these symptoms may remain distressing in adulthood even as motor and phonic tics have largely remitted.

COMORBID ANXIETY, DEPRESSION, AND OTHER INTERNALIZING DISORDERS

In our clinical experience, children and adults with Tourette's syndrome appear to be at risk for increased depression and non-obsessive-compulsive disorder anxiety symptoms in addition to the comorbid attentional and learning difficulties discussed in Chapter 4. Occasionally, the florid disinhibition seen in a few individuals with very severe tics and family histories of bipolar disorder also raises the question of a bipolar spectrum disorder and issues regarding the possible benefits of mood stabilizers.

Systematic studies employing diverse assessment techniques confirm these clinical impressions of elevated levels of psychopathology in individuals with Tourette's syndrome (see reviews by Carter et al., 1994; Coffey & Park, 1997).

Uncontrolled Studies

In an uncontrolled survey (Stefl, 1984), responded to by 431 of 555 members of the Ohio chapter of the Tourette Syndrome Association (74% of the respondents being under 19 years of age), the following symptoms were endorsed as occurring "often": extreme anxiety (31.6% of respondents), extreme mood swings (32.7%), trouble getting to sleep (22.4%) or staying asleep (10.6%), and bed-wetting (8.4%). Sleepwalking and bad dreams/ night terrors were reported as "sometimes" occurring by 14.7% and 40%

of respondents, respectively. Coffey (1993) and colleagues studied 103 adult and child patients with Tourette's syndrome and found 37% had obsessive-compulsive disorder or obsessive-compulsive symptoms and 30% met criteria for a non-obsessive-compulsive anxiety disorder, including 8% each for generalized anxiety disorder and overanxious disorder, 5% for panic disorder or attacks, 5% for separation anxiety disorder, 3% for simple phobia, and 1% for posttraumatic stress disorder. An additional 8% had significant anxiety symptoms that were not sufficiently impairing to warrant a categorical diagnosis. Some studies suggest that bipolar disorder may be overrepresented in community (Kerbeshian, Burd, & Klug, 1995) and clinic (Berthier, Kulisevsky, & Campos, 1998) samples of subjects with Tourette's syndrome.

Other studies, although uncontrolled, have employed instruments with well-established norms. For example, using parental Child Behavior Checklist (CBCL, Achenbach & Edelbrock, 1983) reports on 186 children with Tourette's syndrome, L. Rosenberg, Brown, and Singer (1995) found elevated scores (T score ≥ 70) in the following percentage of children, age 6–11 years: schizoid anxious, 39%; uncommunicative, 38%; somatic complaints, 28%; depressed, 30%; social withdrawal, 26%; and total internalizing problems, 45%. Among the adolescents, age 12–16 years, the percentage with elevated scores in each area were schizoid anxious, 34%; uncommunicative, 34%; somatic complaints, 42%; and immature, 37%; total internalizing problems, 37%. Using the parent report alone (Frank, Sieg, & Gaffney, 1991) or in conjunction with the Teacher's Report Form version of the instrument (Nolan, Sverd, Gadow, Sprafkin, & Ezor, 1996), other studies have found comparable levels of psychopathology.

Reflecting the difficulties in peer relations and relative social skill deficits observed in many school-age children with Tourette's syndrome (Dykens et al., 1990; Chapter 6), classmates rate children with Tourette's syndrome as less popular and more withdrawn than their peers (Stokes et al., 1991). The language ability scores of these children with Tourette's syndrome correlated positively with ratings of likability and negatively with ratings of aggressivity, suggesting that language skills play a role in regulating aggressive drives and mediating social interactions.

In contrast to parents', teachers', and peers' ratings, children's own self-reports may reveal less psychopathology. Comparing self-reports on the Youth Self-Report version of the scale to parental ratings on the CBCL for 25 children with Tourette's syndrome (mean age 12 years), L. Rosenberg, Brown, and Singer (1994) found that the children rated themselves as significantly less symptomatic on the Internalizing, Externalizing, and Total Problems scales than did their parents. Edell and Motta (1989) found no significant differences between children with Tourette's syndrome and controls on self-rated measures of trait anxiety and self-concept.

Studies of adults with Tourette's syndrome also show elevated levels of emotional difficulty. Using the Minnesota Multiphasic Personality Inventory, Grossman, Mostofsky, and Harrison (1986) found increased ideational disturbances, social alienation, angry and guilty preoccupations, depressive affect, and somatic concerns, as well as fear of impulses being expressed at embarrassing moments. In a study of 90 adults with Tourette's syndrome using the Mood Adjective Checklist, Robertson, Trimble, and Lees (1988b) found elevated levels of anxiety, depression, and hostility; 25% of the subjects had severe anxiety and 17% were clinically depressed, with depression correlated with earlier onset and longer duration of the tic disorder.

Controlled Studies

Controlled studies also concur that individuals with Tourette's syndrome appear to have increased rates of anxiety disorder and mood disorders (Pauls et al., 1994; Robertson, Channon, Baker, & Flynn, 1993). Pitman, Green, Jenike, and Mesulam (1987) found lifetime prevalences of 44% for both generalized anxiety and unipolar depression in patients with Tourette's syndrome, which was significantly higher than normal controls but lower than a contrast group of subjects with obsessive-compulsive disorder alone. Comings and Comings (1987c, 1987e) studied 246 patients with Tourette's syndrome and 47 normal controls using a questionnaire; they found that the patients with Tourette's syndrome had significantly elevated frequency of panic disorder (16% with three or more panic attacks a week), impairing phobia (19%), and multiple phobias (26%). Depression was not correlated with tic severity.

Pauls and coworkers (1994) compared a group of 85 probands with Tourette's syndrome, 27 control probands, and their respective first-degree relatives. Compared to the control subjects, the probands with Tourette's syndrome showed elevated frequency of major depressive disorder (40.7%), obsessive-compulsive disorder (36%), panic disorder (12.8%), and simple phobia (18.6%), but not social phobia or generalized anxiety disorder. Compared to the first-degree relatives of the control probands, the first-degree relatives of the probands with Tourette's syndrome had significantly elevated prevalences of major depressive disorder, panic disorder, simple phobia, social phobia, and generalized anxiety disorder. However, these higher-than-expected prevalences were significantly elevated only in those relatives who themselves had a tic disorder or obsessive-compulsive disorder, suggesting that although these affective and anxiety disorders are often associated with tics and obsessive-compulsive disorder, they are not variant phenotypic expressions of the putative Tourette's syndrome gene(s).

Etiology of Comorbid Anxiety and Mood Problems

The reasons for the higher-than-expected frequencies of anxiety, depression, and other emotional difficulties in individuals with Tourette's syndrome remain unclear. One common possible explanation is the chronic debilitating burden of disruptive, potentially stigmatizing tic and obsessive-compulsive symptoms. At least from preadolescence onward, many individuals with Tourette's syndrome are uncomfortably aware of premonitory urges that are often experienced as feelings of mounting tension or anxiety and may be more distressing than the tics per se (Leckman, Walker, et al., 1993; Chapter 2). Furthermore, the constant vigilance and energy deployed in an attempt to suppress tic symptoms in potentially embarrassing social situations may contribute to chronic anxiety, social withdrawal, self-preoccupation, and fatigue. As tics can rarely be completely suppressed, self-reproach over tic breakthroughs and the perceived criticism of family or peers may result in low self-esteem and hopelessness. Finally, learning and attentional difficulties, when present, may expose the child to more adverse academic and social experiences, while leaving him or her poorly equipped to develop adequate coping mechanisms.

By late adolescence, youngsters with tics may show impairment in several adaptive realms. In an epidemiologic study of Israeli adolescents screened for compulsory military service, subjects with tics scored significantly lower than controls on a variety of measures of cognitive, academic, language, and overall adaptive competence and physical fitness for military service (Apter et al., 1992).

Limitations to a purely experiential explanation of the origin of the emotional difficulties accompanying Tourette's syndrome, however, are suggested by the observation that it is not unusual, in clinical practice, to see resilient children and adults with few behavioral problems despite severe tics, as well as more vulnerable patients with multiple emotional problems despite relatively mild tics. Systematic quantitative studies have yielded conflicting data regarding the correlation between psychopathology and tic severity. Using complex statistical modeling, de Groot, Janus, and Bornstein (1995) found a relationship between tic severity and anxiety and psychosomatic symptoms in older children. Nolan and colleagues' (1996) study of children with Tourette's syndrome and ADHD found that the children with more severe tics had significantly higher scores on the depressed, uncommunicative, obsessive-compulsive, aggressive, and internalizing scales of the CBCL. In contrast, other studies have failed to find a clear relationship between tic severity and children's social-emotional functioning (Edell & Motta, 1989; Frank et al., 1991; L. Rosenberg et al., 1995; Stokes et al., 1991).

The exacerbating effect on tics of stress, anxiety, pleasurable excitement, and, in some cases, thermal stress, is well documented (Bornstein, Stefl, & Hammond, 1990; Leckman, Cohen, et al., 1986; Lombroso, Mack, Scahill, King, & Leckman, 1991; Silva, Munoz, Barickman, & Friedhoff, 1995; Surwillo, Shafii, & Barrett, 1978). These findings, taken together with the evidence cited above that many individuals with Tourette's syndrome experience difficulty in modulating anxiety, arousal, and mood, have led to the suggestion that Tourette's syndrome may be associated with increased stress-induced reactivity of the hypothalamic-pituitary-adrenal axis and increased central and peripheral noradrenergic sympathetic activity. For example, comparing subjects with Tourette's syndrome and normal controls during the day preceding an anticipated research lumbar puncture, the subjects with Tourette's syndrome excreted significantly more ACTH and norepinephrine and reported higher levels of anticipatory anxiety (Chappell, Riddle, et al., 1994; Leckman, Goodman, et al., 1995).

Neurobiological deficits in the basal ganglia, limbic system, and cerebral cortex, the sites most often implicated in the pathogenesis of Tourette's syndrome, may also underlie the vulnerability to comorbid depression, anxiety, and stress reactivity seen in Tourette's syndrome (Leckman, Walker, et al., 1994; Lombroso, Scahill, Chappell, et al., 1995). Other basal ganglia-related movement disorders, such as Huntington's disease and Meige's syndrome (idiopathic orofacial dystonia), are associated with high rates of prodromal depression, anxiety, and other emotional disturbance which often predate the motor symptoms or other manifestations of these disorders (Cummings, 1995; Tolosa, 1981). The premorbid personality of individuals who later develop Parkinson's disease tends to be quiet, introverted, and low in novelty seeking; although depression occurs in 20–90% of individuals with the disorder, it often predates the motor symptoms and bears no simple relationship to their severity (R. Brown & Jahanshahi, 1995; Mayberg & Solomon, 1995).

A variety of other basal ganglia disorders are associated with cognitive and affective difficulties, leading to speculation concerning the far-reaching effects of basal ganglia pathology on neurotransmitter regulation and projections to the frontal cortex, limbic system, and related structures (Saint-Cyr, Taylor, & Nicholson, 1995). Of particular interest in relationship to Tourette's syndrome is the finding that major depression, ADHD, and vocal tics are significantly more common in children with Sydenham's chorea compared to children with rheumatic fever without Sydenham's chorea (Mercadante, Campos, Marques-Dias, Leckman, & Miguel, 1997). Medication-related side effects may be yet another source of depression or anxiety in patients with Tourette's syndrome. In addition to cognitive blunting and sedation (Bruun 1988b), neuroleptics can produce a picture of weepy dysphoria and intensified or de novo separation anxiety in children (Mikkelsen, Deltor, & Cohen, 1981); akathisia may also manifest itself as acute, anxious restlessness. Clonidine also can produce sedation and a subdued mood. Although some children with Tourette's syndrome on stimulants may become activated and experience an increase in tics, stimulants can also produce dysphoria, crying jags, and overfocused or compulsive behavior following acute administration, as well as depressive "let down" as the dose wears off (Borcherding, Keysor, Rapoport, Elia, & Amass, 1990; J. Rapoport et al., 1980). Although most often at higher doses, serotonin-reuptake inhibitors can produce akathisia, restlessness, disinhibition, agitation, and even disorganized, hypomanic, or psychotic behavior (R. King, Leckman, & Cohen, 1991; R. King, Segman, & Anderson, 1994; Riddle et al., 1991).

SUMMARY OF CHAPTER 3

There is a remarkable variety of obsessive-compulsive symptoms that can accompany Tourette's syndrome or that can appear in close family members even in the absence of tics. Some of these obsessive-compulsive symptoms blend with complex motor and vocal tics, making the boundary between these symptom domains indistinct and arbitrary. Some portion of the cognitive and perceptual symptoms of obsessive-compulsive disorder are likely to reflect the forceful and untimely appearance in consciousness of innate fears that under normal circumstances provide cues for the assemblage of harm-avoidant behaviors. Other symptoms may be understood as inappropriate release or failure to terminate various basic mammalian behavioral fixed-action routines related to grooming, nesting, attachment, pair-bonding, and so on. Still other compulsions associated with symmetry or other just right phenomena may be related to dysfunction of basic sensorimotor processing circuits that compare expectations of how things should look, feel, or sound with what is actually experienced with the completion of an act. Although such feedback mechanisms usually serve an adaptive function by providing an ongoing assessment of disparity between acts and their intended goal, their dysfunction may lead to pathologically prolonged, repetitive behavioral routines in an attempt to obtain an elusive just right sense of closure. Other forms of psychopathology commonly associated with Tourette's syndrome—notably depression and anxiety—appear to represent the combined effects of constitutional and experiential factors. Some of these symptoms may represent the cumulative effects of adverse social interactions secondary to the tic, obsessive-compulsive, attentional, and learning difficulties associated with Tourette's syndrome. On the other hand, vulnerability to anxiety, and perhaps mood difficulties as well, may also reflect underlying defects in neuroregulation.

PREVIEW OF CHAPTER 4

A number of individuals with Tourette's syndrome present with symptoms of distractability, impulsivity, and motoric hyperactivity. In clinically referred groups, this figure is often above 50%; in population-based samples, the figure is substantially lower. This chapter reviews these data as well as discussing the available information concerning the occurrence of various forms of learning disability.

CHAPTER 4

Phenomenology and Natural History of Tic-Related ADHD and Learning Disabilities

JOHN T. WALKUP, SHAHZAD KHAN, LINDA SCHUERHOLZ, YOUNG-SUK PAIK, JAMES F. LECKMAN, and ROBERT T. SCHULTZ

> Inattention, impulsiveness, and hyperactivity can be reduced to a delay in the development of inhibition of behavior.
>
> —*Russell Barkley, 1995*

Attention-deficit/hyperactivity disorder (ADHD) and learning disorders (LD) are common childhood problems that can continue to impact on functioning in adulthood. ADHD and LD often occur together and can occur in combination with other psychiatric disorders, including Tourette's syndrome. Rates of ADHD in clinically ascertained Tourette's syndrome subjects range from 50% to 90%. The nature of the relationship between Tourette's syndrome and ADHD and LD continues to be a subject of controversy. We concur with Russell Barkley (1995) that ADHD is best viewed as a delay in being able to inhibit environmentally cued behavioral responses. As such, it constitutes another example of the basic problem of not being able to inhibit adequately components of an evolutionarily conserved core process. In the case of ADHD, this leads to difficulties in being able to separate facts from feelings, to consider past actions or anticipate future reactions, and to make full use of one's working memory.

Regardless of the nature of the relationship, problems with inattention, impulsivity, motor overactivity, and learning in the classroom and later the workplace can be the most disabling symptoms persons with Tourette's syndrome experience, often more disabling than the tic symptoms themselves. In this chapter, we review the symptoms of ADHD and LD as observed in children and adults with Tourette's syndrome.

HISTORICAL PERSPECTIVES

Georges Gilles de la Tourette (1885/1982) stated in his initial article that his subject's "mental state was perfectly normal." Tourette's case series focused on adults with severe tic symptoms and noted that children with Tourette's syndrome often had less disability (due to tics) than adults. Tourette noted that over time, disability increased as tic symptoms' severity increased and complications in living developed. Tourette did not describe his adult patients as having problems with attention, concentration, or activity level, but he did refer to problems some children had with coping and functioning in school.

In contrast to Gilles de la Tourette's clinical experience, many of the Tourette's syndrome patients who present today are children with mild to moderate tic symptoms and an array of problems in the school setting. In the classroom, problems with inattention, impulsivity, overactivity, learning, and behavior can be particularly acute and, at times, disabling for children with Tourette's syndrome (Table 4.1). As the medical community and the public have become more aware of ADHD and LD in children, an increasing number of adults with Tourette's syndrome are assessing the possible impact ADHD and LD may have had on their early life, education, and current functioning and are seeking evaluation and treatment.

ATTENTION-DEFICIT/HYPERACTIVITY DISORDER

Diagnosis

The diagnosis of ADHD subsumes the broad problem areas of inattention, impulsivity, and hyperactivity. The symptom complex now known as ADHD was first described in the 1920s after a number of children developed hyperactivity, impulsivity, and inattention as a consequence of an encephalitis epidemic (Ebaugh, 1923). A variety of terms have been used to define this clinical entity: *organic drivenness* (Kahn & Cohn, 1934); *minimal brain dysfunction* (Clements, 1966); *hyperkinetic syndrome of childhood* (*DSM-II*, American Psychiatric Association, 1968); *hyperactivity; attention deficit disorder with and without hyperactivity* (*DSM-III*, American Psychological Association, 1980); *attention-deficit hyperactivity disorder* (*DSM-III-R*, American Psychiatric Association, 1987); and *attention-deficit/hyperactivity disorder, predominantly inattentive type, predominantly hyperactive-impulsive type, and combined type* (*DSM-IV*, American Psychiatric Association, 1994; Table 4.2). Although the diagnosis is readily accepted in the United States, there is still disagreement

TABLE 4.1   Frequency of ADHD in Tourette's Syndrome (TS)

Author	N	N with TS	N with TS/ADHD
Epidemiological studies that included some assessment of ADHD symptoms.			
Apter et al., 1992	28,037	12	1 (8.3%)
Caine et al., 1988	142,000	41	11 (27%)
Robertson et al., 1994	3.35 million	40	10 (25%)
School-based studies of TS that included an assessment of ADHD symptoms.			
Comings et al., 1990	3,034	15	10 (66%)
Kurlan et al., 1994	35	9	4 (44%)
Clinic-based surveys of TS patients that included an assessment of ADHD symptoms.			
Comings & Comings, 1985		250	135 (54%)
Park et al., 1993		101	55 (55%)
Kurlan et al., 1996		87	65 (75%)
Singer and Rosenberg, 1989			
6–11 yr olds			(24%)
12–16 yr olds			(43%)
Family studies using TS probands that included an assessment of ADHD symptoms.			
Pauls et al., 1993		85	46 (54%)
Comings et al., 1995		353	215 (60.9%)

internationally about the validity of the syndrome. Debate focuses on whether hyperactivity in the sense these diagnostic terms imply is truly valid and also whether the inattentiveness in ADHD is the underlying neuropsychological deficit in these patients (E. Taylor, 1994).

As discussed in Chapter 7, a number of issues complicate the differential diagnosis of ADHD. The symptoms of ADHD need to be differentiated from developmentally appropriate levels of inattention, impulsivity, and overactivity. This differential diagnosis is not as significant an issue for school-age children, as it is for children less than five years of age, where there is considerably more difficulty making a definitive diagnosis.

Among school-age children there can be considerable situationally based variability in ADHD symptoms. Some children do not appear inattentive in one-on-one learning experiences, but do have difficulties in larger classroom settings. Similarly, it is common for children to not appear hyperactive in the clinician's office when problems are clearly evident in the home and/or school. Further, if ADHD is based on a normally distributed vulnerability (which it may not be), then it is possible that the differential diagnosis is complicated by variability in the placement of the diagnostic threshold and the presence of a large number of children with subthreshold symptomatology.

Many other psychiatric disorders impact on attention and concentration in children. With careful assessment, it is possible to differentiate ADHD from other psychiatric disorders. Less than careful assessments, however, can lead to misdiagnosis and inappropriate treatments. This problem is

TABLE 4.2   *DSM-IV* Criteria for ADHD for Attention-Deficit/ Hyperactivity Disorder

A. Either (1) or (2):

(1) Six (or more) of the following symptoms of inattention have persisted for at least 6 months to a degree that is maladaptive and inconsistent with developmental level:

Inattention

(a) Often fails to give close attention to details or make careless mistakes in schoolwork, work, or other activities.

(b) Often has difficulty sustaining attention in tasks or play activities.

(c) Often does not seem to listen when spoken to directly.

(d) Often does not follow through on instructions and fails to finish schoolwork, chores, or duties in the workplace (not due to oppositional behavior or failure to understand instructions).

(e) Often has difficulty organizing tasks and activities.

(f) Often avoids, dislikes, or is reluctant to engage in tasks that require sustained mental effort (such as schoolwork or homework).

(g) Often loses things necessary for tasks or activities (e.g., toys, school assignments, pencils, books, or tools).

(h) Is often easily distracted by extraneous stimuli.

(i) Is often forgetful in daily activities.

(2) Six (or more) of the following symptoms of hyperactivity-impulsivity have persisted for at least 6 months to a degree that is maladaptive and inconsistent with developmental level:

Hyperactivity

(a) Often fidgets with hands or feet or squirms in seat.

(b) Often leaves seat in classroom or in other situations in which remaining seated is expected.

(c) Often runs about or climbs excessively in situations in which it is inappropriate (in adolescents or adults, may be limited to subjective feelings of restlessness).

(d) Often has difficulty playing or engaging in leisure activities quietly.

(e) Is often "on the go" or often acts as if "driven by a motor."

(f) Often talks excessively.

Impulsivity

(g) Often blurts out answers before questions have been completed.

(h) Often has difficulty awaiting turn.

(i) Often interrupts or intrudes on others (e.g., butts into conversations or games).

Some hyperactive-impulsive symptoms that caused impairment were present before age 7 years.

C. Some impairment from the symptoms is present in two or more settings (e.g., at school [or work] and at home).

D. There must be clear evidence of clinically significant impairment in social, academic, or occupational functioning.

E. The symptoms do not occur exclusively during the course of a Pervasive Developmental Disorder, Schizophrenia, or other Psychotic Disorder and are not better accounted

TABLE 4.2   (*Continued*)

for by another mental disorder (e.g., Mood Disorder, Anxiety Disorder, Dissociative Disorder, or a Personality Disorder).

Code based on type:

314.01 Attention-Deficit/Hyperactivity Disorder, Combined Type: If both Criteria A1 and A2 are met for the past 6 months.

314.00 Attention-Deficit/Hyperactivity Disorder, Predominantly Inattentive Type: If Criterion A1 is met but Criterion A2 is not met for past 6 months.

314.01 Attention-Deficit/Hyperactivity Disorder, Predominantly Hyperactive-Impulsive Type: If Criterion A2 is met but Criterion A1 is not met for the past 6 months.

Coding note: For individuals (especially adolescents and adults) who currently have symptoms that no longer meet full criteria, "In Partial Remission" should be specified.

more acute now that an increasing number of professionals from various backgrounds are offering ADHD assessment and treatment services. The presentation of many psychiatric disorders in children ages four to seven years is very similar and overlaps with ADHD. For example, the assessment of young children with anxiety is difficult, as often the most readily observable symptoms of anxiety are similar to ADHD: inattention, decreased concentration, agitation, and irritability. It is only with careful screening that the more internalizing symptoms of anxiety are elicited. Perhaps even more confusing is the fact that the earliest presentation of many more serious psychiatric disorders is similar to that of ADHD. For example, children with depression, before they have clearly depressed mood, may present with decreased attention and concentration and mild agitation, similar to symptoms in children with ADHD. Similarly, the tic symptoms of Tourette's syndrome can be of such frequency that maintaining attention and concentration is difficult. Premonitory sensations, which often precede tic symptoms, can also account for problems with attention and concentration in children with tic disorders (Leckman, Walker, et al., 1993). It is beyond the scope of this chapter to comment on the relationship of ADHD to bipolar disorder; however, it is not inconceivable that at its onset in childhood, bipolar disorder may present with symptoms only of impulsivity and motor overactivity—indistinguishable from ADHD.

The diagnosis can also be difficult to establish if the child has two (or more) disorders that have an impact on attention, concentration, and motor activity. Persons with Tourette's syndrome, ADHD, and obsessive-compulsive disorder may have three different kinds of problems with inattention, impulsivity, and overactivity (M. Silverstein, Como, Palumbo, West, & Osborn, 1995). As discussed in Chapter 7, in this situation the differential diagnostic question is to identify the presence of all three conditions and their respective impact on attention and concentration and to develop a treatment program that is consistent with the hierarchy of impairment (Walkup & Riddle, 1997).

Phenomenology of ADHD in Tourette's Syndrome

By definition, the phenomenology of ADHD symptoms in persons with Tourette's syndrome is similar to ADHD symptoms in persons without Tourette's syndrome. Some experts, however, have speculated that Tourette's syndrome plus ADHD subjects may have more impulsivity and overactivity and fewer problems with inattention than subjects with ADHD alone, yet there are no studies that have rigorously compared subjects with Tourette's syndrome plus ADHD to those with ADHD alone to determine differences in ADHD symptoms. Factor or cluster analyses of obsessive-compulsive symptoms in persons with and without Tourette's syndrome have been conducted (Leckman, Grice, et al., 1997), but similar studies have not been done with ADHD symptoms. The goal of the few studies that have compared subjects with Tourette's syndrome plus ADHD to subjects with ADHD alone has been to identify neuropsychological and attentional factors that are unique to Tourette's syndrome (e.g., cognitive slowness; Schuerholz, Baumgardner, Singer, Reiss, & Denckla, 1996).

Research studies comparing subjects with Tourette's syndrome plus ADHD to subjects with Tourette's syndrome alone have attempted to identify the neuropsychological contribution of ADHD to Tourette's syndrome. (See Chapter 5 for a more complete review of the neuropsychology of Tourette's syndrome and ADHD.) These studies have identified subtle differences in some aspects of cognition and attention. Most of the differences can be attributed to the diagnosis of ADHD (Dykens et al., 1990) or ADHD and comorbid conditions such as obsessive-compulsive disorder (Yeates & Bornstein, 1994). It is logical that ADHD symptoms would have neuropsychological correlates, and the finding that obsessive-compulsive disorder accounted for problems with attention is intriguing and has been observed by others (Channon, Flynn, & Robertson, 1992). The presence of obsessive-compulsive disorder in Tourette's syndrome may impact on reaction time (M. Silverstein et al., 1995), but there are too few studies to clearly identify the relationship between obsessive-compulsive disorder and other psychopathology on measures of attention.

The presence of ADHD in Tourette's syndrome may also account for the pattern of comorbid psychiatric problems commonly seen in Tourette's syndrome. Compared to children with Tourette's syndrome only, children with Tourette's syndrome plus ADHD and those with only ADHD share a similar profile of comorbid conditions—depression, anxiety, and disruptive behavior—suggesting that the presence of multiple comorbidities in Tourette's syndrome is perhaps a function of the presence of ADHD and not specific to Tourette's syndrome. Obsessive-compulsive disorder, however, is clearly more frequent in subjects with Tourette's syndrome than in subjects with ADHD (Spencer et al., in press). Attempts to identify factors in children with Tourette's syndrome that impact negatively on peer relationships also identify a significant association between ADHD and peer problems (Stokes et al., 1991) and diffusely elevated scores on the Child Behavior Checklist (Yeates & Bornstein, 1996).

There has been considerable debate as to the relationship of Tourette's syndrome to ADHD. Some authors have suggested that Tourette's syndrome and ADHD are not related, but that the co-occurrence often described in clinical populations is the result of ascertainment bias (Pauls, Leckman, & Cohen, 1993). Others have suggested that Tourette's syndrome and ADHD are the overt manifestation of a genetically determined dysregulation of serotonin and dopamine metabolism (Comings et al., 1996). The very frequent co-occurrence of Tourette's syndrome and ADHD in clinical populations suggests, however, that there must be some relationship between Tourette's syndrome and ADHD. As discussed in Chapter 11, based on the results of a family genetic study, it has been hypothesized that there are two types of ADHD in persons with Tourette's syndrome (Pauls et al., 1993). When ADHD symptoms begin before Tourette's syndrome symptoms develop, the disorders do not appear to be related; when ADHD symptoms have an onset after the development of Tourette's syndrome, the disorders do appear to be related. This conclusion was based on the observation that ADHD and Tourette's syndrome did not cosegregate in relatives of children whose ADHD started before their tics. In contrast, ADHD and Tourette's syndrome did cosegregate in relatives of children whose ADHD started after their tics. Stated another way, when ADHD precedes the development of Tourette's syndrome, it appears that the child has inherited two different disorders that co-occur by chance, whereas when the ADHD follows the development of tics, ADHD and Tourette's syndrome appear to be related (Pauls et al., 1993). The authors of this study caution against overinterpretation of this finding given their small sample size. However, the study does raise questions about the etiology of attention deficits in Tourette's syndrome and suggests other possible etiologies.

Natural History of ADHD in Tourette's Syndrome

Few studies of the natural history of ADHD in Tourette's syndrome have been published. ADHD symptoms often precede the onset of tic symptoms by as much as 2.5 years. On the other end of the age spectrum, the neuropsychological studies referenced above noted that some adults with Tourette's syndrome had ADHD symptoms as children that persisted into adulthood with an observable impact on functioning. What is less clear, however, is how frequently children's ADHD symptoms resolve in adolescence and how many continue to experience symptoms into adulthood. Most epidemiological studies of adult psychiatric disorders have not been sufficiently sensitive to the diagnosis of ADHD and LD, so that published prevalence rates are likely to be underestimates of the true prevalence (see Chapter 10).

Follow-up studies of children with ADHD, but without Tourette's syndrome, suggest that symptoms in a significant minority of children resolve without long-term sequelae. Individuals whose symptoms continue past adolescence often remain symptomatic throughout adulthood. At long-term follow-up, subjects with ongoing symptoms of ADHD had lower academic achievement, fewer years of school completed, and increased rates of substance abuse and serious behavior problems in adulthood (G. Weiss, Hechtman, Perlman, Hopkins, & Werner, 1979). For those children who did not appear to be symptomatic at follow-up, the risk for serious adjustment problems in adulthood was comparable to normal controls (Gittelman-Klein, Mannuzza, Shenker, & Bonagura, 1985; Mannuzza, Gittelman-Klein, Bonagura, Konig, & Shenker, 1988). It is clear from these long-term studies that symptoms in adulthood are associated with increased morbidity. What is unclear from these studies is the phenotype of childhood ADHD that is associated with continued symptoms into adulthood and poorer prognosis. As these long-term outcome studies were done in the 1970s; it is not clear if long-term studies today would have the same outcome. Diagnostic practices have changed since these studies were completed. One might speculate that more children are being diagnosed and treated for ADHD now and that many of the children have milder symptom profiles. It is possible that those youngsters with milder symptoms and earlier intervention may comprise a group of children who will do better in adulthood.

Clinically, the presentation of ADHD in Tourette's syndrome varies over the lifetime. Although it is not common, some parents describe their ADHD child as having problems with impulsivity and activity level starting as early as infancy. Other children have a more typical onset around age 4 or 5 years. Parents often comment on their children's having boundless energy, intense persistence, low frustration tolerance, and "a certain look in their eyes." Some children show little fear, take inappropriate risks, and can be considered accident-prone. Children may be manageable at home, but in daycare or preschool these children may have more problems following directions and playing well with others. Often, the children can make friends but then have difficulty keeping friends due to problem behaviors. Some children can become destructive and aggressive, and on rare occasions, these children are asked to leave their daycare or preschool.

In the school setting, teachers describe how the children's behaviors impact on their ability to learn and on the classroom environment. Children with ADHD have trouble remaining seated, talk out of turn, and respond impulsively to stimulating academic activities. They are impatient and quick to lose their temper. Problems with parenting can also occur, as children with ADHD can provoke power struggles with parents and other adults, escalating to temper tantrums and aggression. Monitoring the behavior of these children can require almost constant attention; lapses in parental monitoring can be associated with accidents and problems secondary to risk-taking behaviors.

Some children with milder symptom presentations or the inattentive subtype of ADHD do not have significant problems prior to school and may have only mild restlessness and inattentiveness in the school setting. Because these children do not have hyperactivity symptoms, their academic deficits may not come to the attention of school personnel. They are often described as "spacey," "uncooperative, but not naughty," or "unfocused." If children with the inattentive subtype are intelligent and achieve academically, they may not be identified with ADHD until middle or high school, when academic challenges are significant enough that their intelligence and learning style are overwhelmed. Children with milder forms of ADHD may also evidence impairment if they become focused on more salient nonacademic interests such as peer relationships and athletics.

Adults can also have ADHD. Some adults pursue an evaluation for ADHD after their children have been diagnosed. Parents of children with ADHD may comment that they had similar problems as a child and have a sense that those problems have some impact on their current functioning. Adults who pursue an evaluation will not only describe present-day symptoms, but may also describe early life experiences consistent with a diagnosis of ADHD. Many of these adults struggled academically as children but received no help; others were diagnosed but not treated; and others were treated as children, but treatment was discontinued during their early teenage years, as they were thought to have "outgrown" their need for medication. There are few studies of adult ADHD, but it is an area of increasing research and clinical interest.

LEARNING DIFFICULTIES

Learning disorders are diagnosed when there is a substantial discrepancy between standardized scores of academic achievement and a child's ability to learn based on the child's age, intelligence, and educational experience. By far the most common type of LD is reading disability, most often caused by a fundamental difficulty with phonetic decoding and segmentation (Pennington, 1991). Although nonprofessionals may speak of disorders of attention as a LD, the term should be reserved for specific academic skill areas, including mathematics, reading, spelling, and written language, though from a neuropsychological perspective, this list is arbitrary and not prescribed in any way by the functional organization of the brain (Table 4.3).

The underlying assumption is that LDs are caused by a primary, presumably brain-based, deficit that impacts the ability to perform in certain academic areas. Methods used to define LD vary based on local school board or state statutes rather than specific neuropsychological criteria; however, efforts to develop procedures that assess the strengths of various cognitive processes are increasingly used to define the limits of an individual's ability. Most states define a LD in terms of a discrepancy score between

TABLE 4.3 *DSM-IV* Diagnostic Criteria for *DSM-IV* Learning Disorders

Diagnostic Criteria for 315.00 Reading Disorder

A. Reading achievement, as measured by individually administered standardized tests of reading accuracy or comprehension, is substantially below that expected given the person's chronological age, measured intelligence, and age-appropriate education.
B. The disturbance in criterion A significantly interferes with academic achievement or activities of daily living that require reading skills.
C. If a sensory deficit is present, the reading difficulties are in excess of those usually associated with it.

Diagnostic Criteria for 315.1 Mathematics Disorder

A. Mathematical ability, as measured by individually administered standardized tests, is substantially below that expected given the person's chronological age, measured intelligence, and age-appropriate education.
B. The disturbance in Criterion A significantly interferes with academic achievement or activities of daily living that require mathematical ability.
C. If a sensory deficit is present, the difficulties in mathematical ability are in excess of those usually associated with it.

Coding note: If a general medical (e.g., neurological) condition or sensory deficit is present, code the condition on Axis III.

Diagnostic Criteria for 315.2 Disorder of Written Expression

A. Writing skills, as measured by individually administered standardized tests (or functional assessments of writing skills) are substantially below those expected given the person's chronological age, measured intelligence, and age-appropriate education.
B. The disturbance in Criterion A significantly interferes with academic achievement or activities of daily living that require the composition of written texts (e.g., writing grammatically correct sentences and organized paragraphs).
C. If a sensory deficit is present, the difficulties in writing skills are in excess of those usually associated with it.

Coding note: If a general medical (e.g., neurological) condition or sensory deficit is present, code the condition on Axis III.

315.9 Learning Disorder Not Otherwise Specified

This category is for disorders that do not meet criteria for any specific Learning Disorder. This category might include problems in all three areas (reading, mathematics, written expression) that together significantly interfere with academic achievement even though performance on tests measuring each individual skill is not substantially below that expected given the person's chronological age, measured intelligence, and age-appropriate education.

achievement test results and IQ test results, provided that the child has had access to formal education and the opportunity to learn the academic skills being assessed. Often a discrepancy of 1.5 *SD*s or 22 points is used as a cutoff for classification. Although this definition has the virtue of being easy to calculate, it fails to consider the correlation between achievement tests and IQ tests, which will vary somewhat by test instrument and age of the child. Thus, increasingly, states are moving toward regression-based discrepancy definitions. However, many professionals argue that low achievement scores, regardless of IQ, should constitute a LD, because by definition these children are not learning as well as the average child. It remains to be seen whether there are profile or etiologic differences between garden-variety learning disabled individuals and those with IQ-achievement discrepancies.

Prevalence of Learning Disabilities in Tourette's Syndrome

A variety of LDs have been described in clinical samples of Tourette's syndrome patients, but the lack of control for other psychiatric disorders and differing approaches to assessment make it difficult to identify the learning problems specifically associated with Tourette's syndrome. In more recent studies that have controlled for the presence of other disorders, there is increasing evidence that the prominent learning differences in subjects with Tourette's syndrome are often highly correlated with the presence of ADHD and not necessarily related to Tourette's syndrome itself. Comings, Himes, and Comings (1990) conducted an epidemiological study of Tourette's in a single school district in California comprising about 3,000 students. A total of 12% of children in special education classes were identified as having Tourette's syndrome. Similarly, Kurlan, Whitmore, Irvine, McDermott, and Como (1994) estimated the prevalence of definite or probable tics in students enrolled in full-time special education in a single school district in New York State to be 26%. Although these studies document the higher than expected rate of special education needs among children with Tourette's or tics, the reasons for the special education placement remain unclear. Poor school performance may be related to a true LD, or it could be a manifestation of emotional difficulties, ADHD, or some other neuropsychological difficulty for which children with Tourette's are at increased risk (e.g., R. Schultz et al., 1998; Singer & Rosenberg, 1989; Walkup, Rosenberg, Brown, & Singer, 1992; Walkup, Scahill, & Riddle, 1995).

Erenberg, Cruse, and Rothner (1986) were perhaps the first to estimate the frequency of true LDs in Tourette's syndrome. They surveyed 200 children and adolescents with Tourette's syndrome and found that 22% of their sample identified themselves as having a LD. Although this methodology allows collection of a large sample of data, it risks inaccuracy due to inherent problems in self-labeling. However, a recent retrospective chart review of 138 children with Tourette's also estimated the prevalence of LDs to be 22% (Abwender et al., 1996). Neither of these studies specified the nature of the LDs, for example, reading or math disorder. Abwender and colleagues also reported that among children without a specific LD, 38% experienced school difficulties and/or special educational placement. As the authors acknowledge, it is likely that these figures are an overestimation of the true rate of school problems in the general population of Tourette's syndrome, as all participants were drawn from a specialty clinic. ADHD (but not obsessive-compulsive disorder) symptomatology was a significant predictor of school problems. Children with ADHD symptoms had an almost fourfold increased risk for academic difficulty, compared to those children with Tourette's alone.

Smaller studies that directly measured the achievement and IQ of children with Tourette's syndrome provide a range of prevalence estimates. In an early study, Hagin, Beecher, Pagano, and Kreeger (1982) described a sample of 10 children with Tourette's between the ages of 7 and 13. Achievement test results using the Woodcock-Johnson Psychoeducational Battery suggested stronger reading skill than math or written language, but "few cases of scores below expectancy" (p. 325). In contrast to this report, Burd, Kauffman, and Kerbeshian (1992) reviewed the records of 104 consecutive clinical cases with Tourette's. The sample was highly impaired, with 10% being blind and about 25% with mental retardation. After excluding these and others with serious neurological or psychiatric impairment, they assessed the frequency of LD in a final sample of 42 children (35 males), between the ages of 7 and 18, using a 1.5 *SD* discrepancy score between IQ and achievement. They reported that 51% of this sample met criteria for a specific LD. Math LDs were most common (35%) and reading comprehension least common (13%). The authors caution that their clinic services children with severe Tourette's syndrome and high rates of comorbidity, including LD, and hence the findings may overestimate the population base rate. Brookshire, Butler, Ewing-Cobbs, and Fletcher (1994) studied reading, spelling, and arithmetic abilities using the Wide Range Achievement Test (WRAT) with a sample of 32 children with Tourette's. Mean spelling and reading scores were nominally higher than full-scale IQ (FSIQ) for the sample, suggesting the absence of LDs in these areas. The mean arithmetic score, on the other hand, was about 10 standard score points lower than FSIQ, and the pattern of academic performance was consistent with a math LD comparison group. Several other studies with the WRAT have found relative weakness in arithmetic in Tourette's syndrome samples (Bornstein, King, & Carroll, 1983; Golden, 1984; Incagnoli & Kane, 1981). Using the Woodcock-Johnson Psychoeducational Battery, Dykens and colleagues (1990) reported significant weaknesses in arithmetic and a strength in reading (single-word decoding) in a group of 30 children with Tourette's syndrome. This group of studies is consistent in demonstrating arithmetic weakness relative to other academic skills and/or FSIQ, and a relative strength in decoding skills. However, these studies did not define LDs by discrepancy criterion. Lower mean math scores for a group do not necessarily equate to a high prevalence of math LDs.

Schuerholz et al. (1996) recruited 65 children (age 6 to 14) with Tourette's syndrome for a series of related studies on the pathobiology of LD through the Kennedy Krieger Learning Disabilities Research Center. Although the authors did not recruit subjects for the study on the basis of learning difficulties, given the nature of the Research Center and its priorities, there would appear to be the opportunity for self-selection by families with concerns about learning problems, which would inflate the frequency of LD. Using the Woodcock-Johnson Psychoeducational Battery–Revised and a regression-based discrepancy formula of 1.5 *SD*s, they reported an overall frequency of any learning disability to be 23%, which is consistent with the data of Abwender et al. (1996) and Erenberg et al. (1986). Nevertheless, these estimates are generally commensurate with the population base rate of LDs, estimated at between 15% and 20% (Berger, Yule, & Rutter, 1975; Pennington, 1991). Fourteen of the 15 children identified with a LD were found to have written language disorder (21.5% of the sample), four children had a math LD (6%), and one had a reading LD. Consistent with the findings of Abwender et al., LDs were only present in children with comorbid ADHD.

In an ongoing study at Yale of 50 children with Tourette's. R. Schultz and colleagues (1998) assessed reading, mathematics, and spelling achievement with the Kaufman Test of Education Achievement–Brief Form (KTEA; A. Kaufman & Kaufman, 1985), and IQ with the Kaufman Brief Test of Intelligence (KBIT; A. Kaufman & Kaufman, 1990). The sample was recruited from an outpatient clinic not offering a specialized evaluation of learning problems, and thus recruitment biases in favor of comorbid learning disabilities may have been minimized. Moreover, the recruitment of controls, but not Tourette's syndrome cases, screened for the presence of learning disabilities, thus inflating the odds of finding significant group differences in achievement test scores. In this study, there were no differences in reading and spelling achievement scores between the overall Tourette's sample and the controls. However, controlling for verbal IQ, children with Tourette's plus ADHD scored significantly lower than those with Tourette's syndrome without ADHD on both reading and spelling. This is consistent with the results of Schuerholz et al. (1996) and Abwender et al. (1996) just described. Although the study found overall group differences on tests of mathematics achievement (controlling for IQ), these were due to unusually high scores among the control subjects, and not poor performance by the children with Tourette's syndrome. Children with Tourette's had a mean math score of 110, which was equal to their composite IQ and 10 points higher than the standardization sample mean.

This study at Yale also evaluated the likelihood of a reading, spelling, or math LD in a case-by-case manner, using both an absolute cutoff of a standard score below 85, and with a regression-based 1.5 standard error achievement–composite IQ discrepancy definition. The results differed subtly. Five children (10%) with Tourette's syndrome were identified as having a math learning disability with each definition, though the same five were not identified by both methods. For reading, four children (8%) met the regression-based criterion, and three (6%) met the cutoff criterion. Two children were identified as having a spelling learning disability (4%) with the regression-based definition, but eight (16%) met the absolute cutoff criterion. All of the children with standard scores below 85 on reading, math, or spelling had comorbid ADHD. However, only 50–75% of children satisfying the regression-based criteria were diagnosed with ADHD, a range of figures not substantially different from the composition of this

Tourette's syndrome sample with comorbid ADHD (70%). Overall, 4–16% of the Tourette's samples met at least one criterion for a specific learning disability, a rate not substantially different from that of the general population. Thus, this recent data from the Yale study suggest a somewhat lower frequency of LDs in Tourette's syndrome than others have found. This might be due to the nature of the clinic from which these subjects were recruited. Alternatively, these figures might have been somewhat higher had we also assessed written language skills, which in at least one study was the single most prevalent form of LD. Consistent with other reports, the Yale study confirmed that children with comorbid ADHD were at the greatest risk for a LD.

The literature on LDs in Tourette's syndrome suggests that there is an increased risk for school-related problems, but the nature of these problems is surely multifactorial. Formal LD, defined by discrepancy criteria, probably does not affect more than 25% of the Tourette's population who participate in research studies. The true rate in the general Tourette's population may be less. In contrast to the non-Tourette's population, where reading disabilities are several times more common than other LDs, in persons with Tourette's syndrome arithmetic and written language skills appear to be the most likely areas of weakness. However, reliable estimation of the prevalence of these types of LDs must await more rigorously controlled studies, preferably with epidemiologically ascertained samples.

Natural History of Learning Disorders in Tourette's Syndrome

Clinically, the recognition of a LD can occur at almost any age. Children with severe LD are identified early, whereas children with milder LD may present later. Some very bright children may escape detection until late childhood, adolescence, or even during college. It is also not uncommon for some young adults to pursue an evaluation as a result of a personal sense that they are not functioning at their potential or when work demands change, challenging their underlying LD. As with ADHD, parents of children with LD often identify a similar pattern of learning weakness in themselves and pursue an evaluation.

There are no long-term outcome studies of the learning patterns in persons with Tourette's syndrome. Most experts agree that individuals who do well long term have successfully made some accommodation to their disability by developing learning strategies that decrease the impact of the disability or by focusing on their learning strengths and avoiding situations that challenge their learning weaknesses. Sometimes individuals who are successful in adult life carry with them self-esteem problems from their early learning difficulties. More tragic is the individual with more severe LD who has not had remedial attention and enters adult life undertrained and poorly adapted to the demands of work and life-long learning.

Problems with ADHD and LD are significant contributors to the morbidity associated with Tourette's syndrome. To date, we are increasing our understanding and awareness of ADHD and LD and their impact on living. It is also increasingly clear that Tourette's syndrome without ADHD and LD is not associated with significant problems with cognition or learning. Interestingly, a few studies suggest that the presence of other comorbid conditions such as obsessive-compulsive disorder adds to problems with attention concentration and learning. Assessment procedures are now more standardized and can provide a more sophisticated map of cognitive functioning, and computerized testing can identify problems in various aspects of attention. Intervention strategies are also better defined, if not always available for every child in need. Subsequent chapters in Section Three describe these advances in more detail.

Other Causes of School Underachievement

In practical terms, LDs are diagnosed when there is evidence that a person is underachieving, that is, when academic functioning is less than what would be expected based on ability or when there is a substantial discrepancy in functioning in one academic domain compared to another. A wide disparity between subtests of intelligence tests is often used as evidence that problems with achievement are reflective of an underlying disability. To meet requirements for special services in educational or work settings, however, more stringent and often arbitrary criteria are used. In many municipalities, it is not uncommon for a disparity of two years between achievement and intellectual potential to be required for children to receive special education services, for example, children in the third grade who are achieving at the first-grade level. This standard is common and easily operationalized and implemented, but some children with a bona fide LD may not receive appropriate interventions. For example, by this criterion, children in first grade cannot have a LD, as they are not far enough along in school to be two years behind in academic achievement. Similarly, children with superior intellectual functioning, but who are achieving at grade level, would also not necessarily be considered to have a LD, because their academic achievement is consistent with their grade level, if not with their intellectual potential.

In contrast, children may underachieve for reasons other than a brain-based cognitive abnormality and be considered for special education services. Markedly inadequate educational environments, psychosocial problems, and the functional impact of psychiatric disorders can be considered non-brain-based causes of underachievement. Also, those children who underachieve but are working to their capacity should not necessarily be considered to have a LD and placed in environments that expect them to achieve above their potential; these children should be identified and offered educational assistance appropriate to their intellectual capacity. With increasing diagnostic sophistication, neuropsychological specialists are providing a detailed map of cognitive function. Such efforts will make it easier to identify individuals at risk and develop programs of remediation.

One specific issue concerns the likelihood that there are other psychiatric disorders that impact on learning without a corresponding prominent disturbance in cognitive function. For example, depression and anxiety can impact more generally on a child's ability to learn. Similarly, externalizing disorders can lead to problems in classroom behavior and result in academic underachievement to a level consistent with a diagnosis of a LD. When differences in learning ability are combined with other disorders, it can be quite difficult to assess the relative contribution of the various disorders to the inability to learn. This may be a special problem in the case of children and adults with Tourette's syndrome, especially when their clinical picture includes symptoms of anxiety and depression. Again, as with ADHD, it is important to develop a hierarchy of conditions that impact on learning. Identifying the disorder with the most impact on learning is critical to the development of an appropriate treatment plan.

Finally, some differences in learning potential are related to what might be considered normal differences in academic potential. Although most conceptual models of LD suggest a categorical difference in functioning between those with and without LD, some authors have suggested that differences in learning exist along a continuum (Shaywitz, Fletcher, & Shaywitz, 1995); only when differences in learning potential become pronounced is there a categorical difference in ability to learn. It is also possible for subclinical learning weaknesses to be exacerbated by environmental or motivational factors, resulting in a more pronounced inability to learn.

RESEARCH PERSPECTIVES

As can be seen from the studies on Tourette's syndrome, ADHD, and LD, the advances in our understanding have occurred when the full complexity of the phenotype has been defined and the contributions of the various comorbid conditions have been identified. It is probably no longer appropriate, in any research study, to simply compare Tourette's syndrome subjects to controls and not account for the presence of other comorbid conditions in the Tourette's syndrome group. For example, ongoing neuropsychological and neuroimaging studies are comparing Tourette's syndrome alone, Tourette's syndrome plus ADHD, Tourette's syndrome plus ADHD and obsessive-compulsive disorder, Tourette's syndrome plus ADHD without obsessive-compulsive disorder, Tourette's syndrome and obsessive-compulsive disorder without ADHD, ADHD alone, and obsessive-compulsive disorder alone in an effort to critically define the contribution of each comorbid condition to clinical impairment. Although this is a positive advance in Tourette's syndrome research methodology, it is not without cost. Complex studies are difficult: their recruitment of subjects and data analysis and interpretation make them more difficult. However, as our awareness of the complexity of Tourette's syndrome increases, we will likely be forced to develop such studies, not only to examine phenomenology but also to explore the pathophysiology and treatment of Tourette's syndrome.

SUMMARY OF CHAPTER 4

Attention-deficit/hyperactivity disorder (ADHD) and learning disorders (LD) are frequently the major source of distress and impairment in clinically referred cases of Tourette's syndrome. We view ADHD as further evidence of evolutionarily conserved core processes that are revealed in the consulting room by a failure of their age-dependent inhibition. The fact that Tourette's syndrome, obsessive-compulsive disorder, ADHD, and LD are at times observed independently, argues that each domain may represent different core processes that to a degree are modular in character. Although the nature of the etiological relationship among Tourette's, ADHD, and LD is in dispute, it is essential to identify how these difficulties impact individual children and adults, and how to treat them effectively.

PREVIEW OF CHAPTER 5

Neuropsychological methods have been used to explore the broader phenotype in Tourette's and related disorders. Chapter 5 provides a comprehensive review of this literature. Given the primacy of motor symptoms in Tourette's syndrome, it is not surprising that this system has been the focus of many neuropsychological investigations. Visually guided complex movements appear to be one area of specific deficit among individuals with Tourette's. This chapter describes a component process model of visuomotor integration and reviews the evidence for Tourette's syndrome deficits in each of the component skills. Although symptoms in obsessive-compulsive disorder are cognitive in nature, here too there seem to be clear deficits in visuomotor integration. Evidence for other types of cognitive impairment in obsessive-compulsive disorder has not been consistently presented in the research literature to date. One area of functioning that has been studied in some detail is executive functioning. This is a broad domain, covering many different specific skills that are believed to be related through a common neural substrate in the prefrontal cortices and its connections with subcortical nuclei. Although this area of functioning has captured the fancy of many researchers in recent years, evidence is not currently consistent enough to allow clear conclusions about shared executive disability in these disorders. Rather, the research literature to date is considerably more clear with regard to visuomotor integration deficits in Tourette's syndrome and related disorders. This chapter closes with a description of the neural systems that contribute to visuomotor integration, and efforts are made to link obsessive-compulsive disorder and Tourette's syndrome by a common pathobiological substrate. In particular, dysfunction of the caudate nuclei might account for part of the overlap in symptoms and neuropsychological functioning in these disorders.

CHAPTER 5

Neuropsychological Findings

ROBERT T. SCHULTZ, ALICE S. CARTER, LAWRENCE SCAHILL, and
JAMES F. LECKMAN

> The motor centres and motor faculties, besides furnishing the conditions
> and possibilities of multiple and varied voluntary movements . . . enor-
> mously widen the field of sensory experience and complicate its results.
>
> —*David Ferrier, 1886*

Although motor and phonic tics constitute the core elements of the diagnostic criteria for Tourette's syndrome, perceptual and cognitive difficulties
are also common. These neuropsychological symptoms are potentially informative about the pathobiology of the disorder. Moreover, these associated difficulties can be more problematic for school and social adjustment
than the primary motor symptoms (D. Cohen, Friedhoff, Leckman, &
Chase, 1992). This chapter reviews the evidence on cognitive strengths and
weaknesses in Tourette's syndrome, including the neuropsychological profile of impaired visuomotor integration skill and executive functioning, and
the influence on this profile of comorbid conditions such as attention-
deficit/hyperactivity disorder (ADHD) and obsessive-compulsive disorder.
These difficulties are discussed in light of our emerging understanding of
the pathobiology of Tourette's syndrome and comorbid disorders. Although
neurobiological studies have focused on the role of the basal ganglia in the
pathogenesis of the primary motor symptoms, it now seems clear that these
neural systems also have an influential role beyond the motor system and
can help explain the neurocognitive signs that often accompany Tourette's
syndrome.

Family studies have established an etiologic link between Tourette's
syndrome and some forms of obsessive-compulsive disorder, and suggest
that tic-related obsessive compulsive disorder is a variant expression of a
common underlying genotype (Leckman, McDougle, et al., in press; Pauls,
Raymond, Leckman, & Stevenson, 1991; Pauls, Towbin, Leckman, Zahner,

& Cohen, 1986). The etiologic relationship between Tourette's syndrome and ADHD is less clear. Half or more of all clinic-referred cases of Tourette's syndrome also have comorbid ADHD (Robertson et al., 1988b; Walkup et al., 1995), and children with Tourette's syndrome and ADHD may have a different profile of cognitive abilities and worse social adjustment than children with Tourette's syndrome alone (Dykens et al., 1990; Stokes et al., 1991). Although this impressive comorbidity rate could suggest coupling of Tourette's syndrome and ADHD at a genetic level (Comings & Comings, 1985), referral biases to clinics favor the more severely impaired individuals (Caine et al., 1988), thus making it difficult to draw conclusions about the general population (Berkson, 1946). Initial epidemiological studies support the conclusion that referral bias may be an important factor (Apter et al., 1993). In contrast, family genetic studies have provided mixed evidence about the nature of this relationship. An earlier study (Pauls, Hurst, et al., 1986) found that ADHD (occurring alone) and Tourette's syndrome segregate independently, suggesting the absence of a genetically mediated relationship, whereas more recent evidence suggests that a subtype of ADHD seen in combination with Tourette's syndrome may be a variable phenotypic expression of the Tourette's syndrome vulnerability gene(s) (Pauls et al., 1993). The high rates of obsessive-compulsive disorder and ADHD comorbidity with Tourette's syndrome pose a challenge to the development of a Tourette's syndrome-specific neuropsychology; until very recently, studies did not attempt to account for comorbidities in their design and analysis.

Since the first psychological investigations of Tourette's syndrome, numerous domains of function have been targeted for study. Early studies tended to have small sample sizes and to focus on traditional subdomains of the Wechsler IQ tests and on drawing tasks (e.g., the Bender Gestalt and similar tests of visuomotor integration). More recent studies have focused on executive functions (EF), including measures of sustained attention and impulse control; planning, organization, and cognitive flexibility; visuomotor integration and its component processes; and various manifestations of school difficulties and learning disorders. The literature is a mixture of retrospective reporting of clinical case series with conventional test instruments and larger, hypothesis-driven studies of select abilities using experimental measures. Unfortunately, this literature has been bedeviled by methodological problems, some of which are more easily rectified than others. Although more recent studies have employed larger samples, with improved diagnostic characterization, all studies continue to draw subjects from mental health clinics and the membership rolls of advocacy groups, as opposed to epidemiologically ascertained samples. Members of advocacy groups and clinic-referred cases represent the more severely afflicted end of the Tourette's syndrome spectrum and more frequently have comorbid conditions, such as ADHD and obsessive-compulsive disorder. It is unlikely that the neuropsychological profile of the more severely afflicted is representative of the disorder in the general population. Moreover, pure obsessive-compulsive disorder and pure ADHD have their own neuropsychological signatures, and although the pathobiology and profile of functioning may be overlapping in these three conditions, comorbidity in samples has surely clouded our understanding of the neuropsychology of Tourette's syndrome. ADHD without Tourette's syndrome involves a variety of EF deficits (Barkely, 1997), whereas the neuropsychological profile in obsessive-compulsive disorder is punctuated by deficits in visuoperceptual processes (Boone, Ananth, Philpott, Kaur, & Djenderedjian, 1991; Hollander et al., 1993; Hollander, DeCaria, et al., 1990; Kuskowski et al., 1993; Zielinski, Taylor, & Juzwin, 1991). How these interact with or contribute to the Tourette's syndrome neuropsychological profile of visuomotor and EF deficits is not clearly understood at this time. Few studies have employed large samples and comprehensive assessment strategies that permit differentiation of specific impairments in functioning, identification of subpopulations of subjects with Tourette's syndrome, and identification of factors mediating individual differences in functioning within each diagnostic group. Multidisciplinary and comprehensive studies of Tourette's syndrome and related conditions, however, are currently underway at several major research centers, and these studies promise to redress many of the shortcomings in our knowledge base. Particularly exciting are studies on the relationships among neuropsychological phenotypes, neurobiological substrata, and genetic factors. With cross-discipline characterization of cases, it may soon be possible to describe the causal pathway from genetic and environmental influences to brain and to behavior.

VISUOMOTOR INTEGRATION

Neuropsychological studies of Tourette's syndrome have focused on a broad array of functions. Review of the literature, however, suggests that the most consistently observed deficits occur on tasks requiring the accurate copy of geometric designs, that is, visuomotor integration or visual-graphic ability. The ability to copy simple designs accurately has been investigated in 12 studies, excluding case reports. These are summarized in Table 5.1. Lucas, Kauffman, and Morris (1967) reported on 15 adolescents given the Bender Gestalt; in a qualitative analysis, 8 of the subjects were reported to have abnormal drawings, including poor motor control and size distortions. Like most studies in the literature, this one failed to incorporate a normal control group. E. Shapiro, Shapiro, and Clarkin (1974) studied 30 individuals with Tourette's syndrome. Two senior psychologists independently rated Bender Gestalt protocols for signs of organicity, with almost complete interrater agreement; 24 of the 30 subjects were judged to have mild to marked ratings of organicity. A replication study (Shapiro, Shapiro, Bruun, & Sweet, 1978) compared 50 subjects with Tourette's syndrome to 50 non-Tourette's syndrome psychiatric outpatients matched on

TABLE 5.1   Visual-Motor Integration Skill

Study	Sample	Age ± SD (Range)	Tests	TS Deficit/ Group Difference
Lucas et al. (1967)	15 TS	NA (11–18)	Bender Gestalt	Yes
Shapiro et al. (1974)	30 TS	NA	Bender Gestalt	Yes
Shapiro et al. (1978)	50 TS 50 psychiatric outpatients	22 children, 28 adults	Bender Gestalt	Yes
Incagnoli & Kane (1981)	13 TS	11.8 ± 1.1	Bender Gestalt	Yes
Hagin et al. (1982)	10 TS	10	Bender Gestalt	Yes
Sutherland et al. (1982)	32 TS 31 NC	14.7 14.2	Rey Osterrieth Copy	Yes
Ferrari et al. (1984)	10 TS	10.8 (7–14)	Bender Gestalt	Yes
Randolph et al. (1993)	12 TS	10.5 (8–16)	Rey Osterrieth Copy	No
Brookshire et al. (1994)	31 TS 20 nonTS sibs	11.4 ± 2.8 11.4 ± 2.9	VMI	Yes
Harris et al. (1995)	10 TS – ADHD 32 TS + ADHD	11.6 (8–14) 11.2 (7–14)	Rey Osterrieth Copy	No Yes
Schuerholz et al. (1996)	21 TS only 25 TS +/– ADHD 19 TS +ADHD 27 Controls	9.5 ± 1.9 9.9 ±1.7 10.9 ± 2.1 10.4 ± 2.6	Rey Osterrieth Copy	No*
Schultz et al. (1998)	14 TS – ADHD 34 TS + ADHD 23 NC	10.4 ± 1.4 11.0 ± 1.6 10.8 ± 1.7	VMI Rey Osterrieth	Yes No

Notes: For studies not employing a control group, deficit was indicated if more than 20% of the sample scored at least 1.5 *SD* below the mean. Unless otherwise specified, comorbidity with ADHD was not explicitly evaluated.

*The TS only group scored significantly higher than the other 3 groups.

Adapted with permission from Schultz et al. (1998).

Key:

NA	Not available
VMI	Beery Test of Visual Motor Integration
TS	Tourette syndrome
NC	Normal control
ADHD	Attention-deficit/hyperactivity disorder
TS + ADHD	TS with comorbid ADHD
TS – ADHD	TS without ADHD

sex, age, and overall IQ; visual-graphic ability was assessed with the Bender Gestalt. Significantly more Tourette's syndrome subjects in both age groups (40%) scored in the organically impaired range in comparison to the psychiatric control group (14%). Hagin and colleagues (1982) evaluated Bender Gestalt performance of 10 children (age 7 to 13) with Tourette's using the Koppitz scoring system; all but two children scored below age expectancy. Incagnoli and Kane (1981) reported on Bender Gestalt performance in 13 boys; these children scored an average of 16.5 months below their chronological age. Ferrari and colleagues (Ferrari, Matthews, & Barabas, 1984) studied 9 boys and 1 girl, between the ages of 7 and 14, diagnosed with Tourette's syndrome; compared to normative data, the group was significantly impaired on the Bender Gestalt, scoring an average of 23 months below chronological age. Brookshire and colleagues (1994) studied 31 subjects with Tourette's syndrome (age 6 through 16) using the Beery test of Visual-Motor Integration (VMI), a copying task similar to the Bender Gestalt. Although Wechsler Intelligence Scale for Children–Revised (WISC-R) IQ scores averaged about 100, the children with Tourette's syndrome scored 0.75 *SD* below the normative mean on the VMI. In comparison to a motor-free visual-perceptual test (Benton Judgment of Line Orientation), their scores on the VMI were significantly lower, suggesting impairment in the integration of visuoperceptual and motor functions, rather than a primary difficulty with visuoperceptual abilities earlier in the information-processing stream. Most recently, we studied the VMI performance of 50 children with Tourette's syndrome (34 with ADHD, and 16 without ADHD) and 23 age-matched controls (Schultz et al., 1998). Consistent with prior studies, we obtained significant group differences; children with Tourette's syndrome scored approximately 1 *SD* below the controls on the VMI. We found no evidence to suggest that comorbid ADHD or depressive symptomatology could account for the observed group differences.

A more difficult drawing test, the Rey Osterrieth Complex Figure (Rey), has been investigated in five prior studies. Whereas copying of simple designs requires the integration of visuoperceptual and fine motor skills, performance on the Rey is influenced by EF organizational skills in addition to visuomotor integration ability. Sutherland, Kolb, Schoel, Whishaw, and Davies (1982) compared the performance of 32 subjects with Tourette's syndrome, the majority under the age of 15, to 31 normal controls matched on age, full-scale IQ (FSIQ), and handedness; subjects with Tourette's syndrome were significantly impaired compared to the controls. Randolph, Hyde, Gold, Goldberg, and Weinberger (1993) studied 12 monozygotic twin pairs where at least one member of the pair was affected with Tourette's syndrome; all twins were between the age of 8 and 16 (mean 10.5). Using the 36-point Taylor (1959) scoring system, there was no significant difference between the less impaired (30.2 ± 6.6) and more impaired (28.8 ± 4.8) cotwin. Comparing these published means to normative data for children age 10 and 11 indicates that these subjects performed at the mean of unaffected subjects or slightly higher (our analysis). Harris and colleagues (1995) studied performance on the Rey in a sample of 42 children with Tourette's syndrome (age 8 through 14), 32 of whom had comorbid ADHD. Employing the organizational score of the Waber and Holmes scoring system (1985), they found that children without comorbid ADHD scored significantly higher on the Rey than those with both Tourette's syndrome and ADHD. Although those with Tourette's and not ADHD scored slightly above the normative mean, those with comorbid ADHD scored nearly 0.75 SD below the mean. Their interpretation emphasized EF deficits in children with Tourette's and ADHD. Also using the Waber-Holmes organizational score, Schuerholz and colleagues (1996) reported significantly superior Rey performance among a group of children with Tourette's syndrome alone, compared to children with Tourette's syndrome and ADHD symptoms and a group of unaffected control children. We recently studied 50 children with Tourette's syndrome, 34 with ADHD and 16 without, and compared performance on the Rey to 23 age-matched unaffected controls (Schultz et al., 1998). Using the Taylor scoring system, we reported that the Tourette's syndrome group performed significantly lower on copying the Rey, though the effect size was smaller (about 0.5 SD) than on the VMI and was reduced to a statistical trend when covarying the influence of general intelligence. There were no differences between children with and without comorbid ADHD. This is in contradiction to the findings of Harris et al. and Schuerholz et al., who found worse performance among those with comorbid ADHD using the Waber-Holmes organizational score. To further examine the nature of this discrepancy, we have now rescored all the Reys with two additional scoring systems, the Waber-Holmes and the Boston Qualitative Scoring System (Stern et al., 1994). Neither of these approaches revealed significant differences between patients and controls, or subtypes of Tourette's syndrome (Schultz, 1998).

In summary, there is unequivocal evidence for a deficit of about 1 SD in simple visuomotor integration skill in Tourette's syndrome. In contrast, there is mixed evidence for drawing deficits when EF demands are high. Moreover, Schultz et al. (1998) employed an extensive battery of neuropsychological measures; discriminate function analysis found that scores on the VMI were the single best predictor of diagnostic group membership, and although the Rey did not contribute significantly, a different dimension of EF did (see EF discussion below). Visuomotor integration, therefore, may be a clearer reflection of the underlying pathobiology in Tourette's syndrome than other neuropsychological measures. This interpretation, however, is complicated by the fact that most children with Tourette's syndrome have, at a minimum, some ADHD symptomatology. Children with ADHD alone also show deficits in visuomotor integration compared to unaffected controls (Campbell & Werry, 1986; Frost, Moffitt, & McGee, 1989), indicating that it might be the ADHD component and not Tourette's syndrome per se that is responsible for observed deficits in visuomotor integration. Ours is the only study to have examined the impact of comorbid ADHD on visuomotor integration scores, and although we found equally deficient performance in both subtypes, these data need replication. In addition, three studies examined the impact of comorbid ADHD on the Rey, with two of the three finding a significantly detrimental influence of ADHD on Rey drawings. Thus, although the literature on simple visuomotor integration is consistent in suggesting sizable deficits among children with Tourette's syndrome regardless of ADHD status, drawing tasks that tap EF may be preferentially sensitive to comorbid ADHD.

VISUOMOTOR INTEGRATION COMPONENT PROCESSES

Tests of visuomotor integration are compound measures, calling on visual-perceptual ability and fine motor coordination, in addition to the integration of visual-perceptual analyses into motor programs for successful performance (Figure 5.1). Deficient visual-motor integration could be a function of suboptimal capacity in one or more of these component processes. An important issue, therefore, is whether individuals with Tourette's syndrome have difficulty in these more rudimentary component processes that could explain their visuomotor integration performance, or whether the deficit is specific to the integration of visual and motor processes. In addition to separate visual and fine motor processes, performance on tests of visuomotor integration also requires intact sustained attention and motor impulse control. Vigilance and motor inhibition are the two pillars of attentional ability (Barkley, 1990, 1997; Barkley, Grodzinsky, & DuPaul, 1992). Effortful maintenance of attention is a prerequisite for adequate performance on any test. Motor inhibition can be distinguished from fine motor coordination

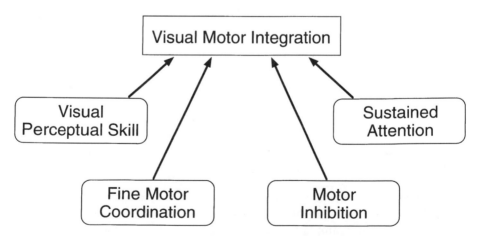

Figure 5.1   Component processes contributing to visual-motor integration skill. *Source:* From Schultz et al. (1998), with permission.

during a copying task in that the latter refers to the continuous coordination of the small muscle groups employed during a skilled pencil movement, and motor inhibition refers to both the cessation of activity when appropriate and the delayed onset of activity so as to allow for planning of the motor sequence. Thus, at least four separate subprocesses may contribute to visuomotor integration ability: visual-perceptual processes, fine motor coordination, sustained attention, and inhibitory motor processes.

Fine Motor Skill

The literature on fine motor coordination difficulties in Tourette's syndrome is nearly as compelling as that of visuomotor integration. However, only one report to date has studied the impact of fine motor coordination deficits on drawing ability (Schultz et al., 1998). Table 5.2 presents results from all studies that employed tests of motor speed (i.e., finger tapping) and motor coordination (i.e., the Grooved or Purdue Pegboard). Each of the eight studies produced evidence suggestive of motor skill difficulties, though some questions about laterality remain. As was true with the visuomotor studies, individuals with Tourette's syndrome were seldom directly compared to unaffected controls, but instead were frequently compared to normative data. Nevertheless, both types of studies yield consistent evidence for motor skill weakness.

On the Purdue Pegboard, Hagin et al. (1982) found that only one of the 10 children with Tourette's syndrome scored above the 50th percentile for their dominant hand, and only two did so for their nondominant hand. Randolph et al. (1993) studied performance on the Purdue in a sample of 12 identical twin pairs with Tourette's syndrome, and found significant impairment among the more severely affected sibling compared to the cotwin in the dominant hand condition. Our analysis of the reported means indicates that the average performance of all twins was about 0.75 SD below that of the normative mean for both the dominant and nondominant hand conditions. In the largest study to date, Bornstein (1990) found that about one-third of a sample of 100 children and adolescents with Tourette's syndrome scored more than 1.5 SDs below the mean on the Grooved Pegboard. In a follow-up study of a subset of these children (n = 82), Yeates and Bornstein (1994) examined the influence of comorbid ADHD on the neuropsychological functioning of children and adolescents affected with Tourette's syndrome. Both the Tourette's syndrome alone and the Tourette's syndrome plus ADHD subjects scored 0.5 to 2 SDs below the mean for the dominant and nondominant hand conditions of the Grooved Pegboard, but there was no significant difference between subtypes. In a follow-up study of 28 children with Tourette's syndrome, Bornstein and colleagues (Bornstein, Baker, Bazylewich, & Douglas, 1991) found average dominant and nondominant hand performance to be 0.5 and 1 SD below the normative mean. Comparing a sample of 36 adults with Tourette's syndrome to 15 unaffected controls, Bornstein (1991b) reported that only

TABLE 5.2   Fine Motor Skill

Study	Sample Size	Age ± SD	Test	Deficit/ Group Difference
Hagin et al. (1982)	10 TS	10	Purdue pegboard	Yes
Bornstein (1990)	100 TS	12.3 ± 3.3	Grooved pegboard	Yes
			Finger tapping	No
Bornstein et al. (1991)	28 TS	11.4 ± 3.9	Grooved pegboard	Yes— nondominant
			Finger tapping	Yes dominant
Bornstein (1991b)	36 TS	32.5 ± 11.4	Grooved pegboard	Yes— dominant
	15 NC	31.1 ± 9.9	Finger tapping	No
Randolph et al. (1993)	12 TS twin pairs (8 cases with comorbid ADHD)	10.5 (8–16)	Purdue pegboard	Yes[†]
			Finger tapping	No[†]
Brookshire et al. (1994)	31 TS 20 nonTS sibs	11.4 ± 2.8 11.4 ± 2.9	Grooved pegboard	Trend[‡]
Yeates & Bornstein (1994)*	82 TS (36 with comorbid ADHD)	11.7 ± 2.7	Grooved pegboard Finger tapping	No—TS + ADHD vs. TS-ADHD deficits
Schultz et al. (1998)	16 TS – ADHD 34 TS + ADHD 23 NC	10.4 ± 1.4 11.0 ± 1.6 10.8 ± 1.7	Purdue pegboard	Yes—TS ± ADHD vs. NC deficits No—TS + ADHD vs. TS-ADHD deficits

Notes: For studies not employing a control group, deficit was indicated if more than 20% of the sample scored at least 1.5 *SD* below the mean. Unless otherwise specified, comorbidity with ADHD was not explicitly evaluated.

* A subset of the 100 children studied by Bornstein (1990).

[†] Based on our comparison of reported scores to normative data. It is not clear whether a substantial minority (i.e., 20%) scored at least 1.5 *SD* below the mean on the finger tapping test.

[‡] The children with TS scored 0.50 to 0.67 *SDs* below the normative mean for the two conditions, but comparison to siblings without TS resulted in a statistical trend. The possibility of subsyndromal manifestations of the disorder in genetically related family members compromises the interpretability of this latter finding.

Adapted with permission from Schultz et al. (1998).

dominant hand performance was significantly lower, though the mean performance for the nondominant hand was in the impaired direction. Brookshire and colleagues (1994) also examined Grooved Pegboard performance in Tourette's syndrome. The 31 children with Tourette's syndrome in their sample scored 0.5 to 0.67 SD below the normative mean for each hand condition. Comparison to siblings without Tourette's syndrome resulted in a statistical trend, though the possibility of subsyndromal manifestations of the disorder in genetically related family members compromises the interpretability of this finding. Baron-Cohen, Cross, Crowson, and Robertson (1994) studied a different aspect of motor functioning. Using Luria's Hand Alteration Task, a measure of bimanual coordination, they found that children with Tourette's syndrome differed significantly from a younger control group. They interpreted the findings as representing a more general deficit in cognitive inhibition, introducing the term *intention editor*, though a fundamental deficit in motor function may represent a more parsimonious interpretation.

Pegboard tests involve visually guided movements and are dependent on adequate somatosensory ability. Nevertheless, these are primarily measures of relatively complex motor sequencing and dexterity, requiring fine manipulation by the fingers and quick, accurate, and coordinated arm and shoulder movements. Simple motor speed without visual-perceptual or somatosensory demands, as indexed by the Finger Tapping test, appears unimpaired in samples of subjects with Tourette's syndrome (Bornstein, 1990; Bornstein, 1991b; Bornstein et al., 1991; Randolph et al., 1993), suggesting that deficits in elementary motor skill cannot explain the deficits on the pegboard tests. Thus, the motor deficits in Tourette's syndrome appear to be at a level downstream from simple motor speed, involving more complex coordination of movements in space. We tested the hypothesis that motor coordination may account for a significant portion of visuomotor integration variance (Schultz et al., 1998). In agreement with previous studies, Tourette's syndrome children performed about 0.75 SD below that of controls on the Purdue Pegboard. There were no differences between children with ($n = 34$) and without ($n = 16$) comorbid ADHD, which is consistent with the Yeates and Bornstein study just described. Actual motor tics during the test did not occur, and thus cannot explain the impairment. Moreover, the number of times pins were dropped and the number of times set was lost (i.e., picking up two pins at once) was not different between the Tourette's syndrome and normal control groups, suggesting that the lower score represents a true impairment in coordinated purposeful movement. However, once the VMI was entered into the discriminate function analysis, the Purdue no longer contributed unique variance to distinguish the groups, suggesting that its predictive power was absorbed by its functional overlap with the VMI. Although we employed the Purdue Pegboard as a test of motor coordination, indisputably there is a visual component to the test. Indeed, it is difficult to conceive of meaningful tests of motor coordination that do not involve either direct visualization

TABLE 5.3   Visuoperceptual Ability

Study	Sample Size	Age ± SD	Test	Deficit/ Group Difference
Shapiro et al. (1978)	50 TS 50 psy outpt	22 children 28 adults	VIQ > PIQ	Yes
Incagnoli & Kane (1981)	13 TS	11.8 ± 1.1	VIQ > PIQ	No[a]
Sutherland et al. (1982)	32 TS 31 NC	14.7 14.2	PIQ Mooney closure R/L Differentiation Semmes	Yes[b] No No No
Golden (1984)	9 TS	13–20	VIQ > PIQ	No
Ferrari et al. (1984)	10 TS	10.8 (7–14)	Motor-free, Visual perception test VIQ > PIQ	Yes No[c]
Dykens et al. (1990)	19 TS + ADHD 11 TS – ADHD	10.5 (7–14)	PIQ	TS – ADHD impaired relative to TS + ADHD

Key:
NA	Not available
VMI	Beery Test of Visual Motor Integration
TS	Tourette syndrome
NC	Normal control
ADHD	Attention-deficit/hyperactivity disorder
TS + ADHD	TS with comorbid ADHD
TS – ADHD	TS without ADHD
VIQ	Verbal IQ
PIQ	Performance IQ
psy outpt	Psychiatric outpatients

or visual imagery (e.g., a motor test requiring blindfolding might still engage visual mapping and imagery of the physical environment). Comparisons of motor skill among the congenitally blind with and without Tourette's syndrome might adjudicate the issue, but such samples would be difficult to ascertain. Our findings are representative of the group of pegboard findings in the literature. Children and adults with Tourette's syndrome generally score about 0.5 to 1 SD below unaffected controls and are somewhat less impaired on these measures than on drawing tasks. Thus, even though both pegboard and drawing tasks share task demands, the greater sensitivity of drawing tasks suggests that visuomotor integrative processes, not purer motor processes, may be more fundamental to the disorder.

TABLE 5.3   (*Continued*)

Study	Sample Size	Age ± *SD*	Test	Deficit/ Group Difference
Bornstein et al. (1991)	28 TS	11.4 ± 3.9	VIQ > PIQ or PIQ >VIQ	Yes[d]
Bornstein (1991b)	36 TS 15 NC	32.5 ± 11.4 31.1 ± 9.9	PIQ	No[e]
Randolph et al. (1993)	12 TS twin pairs (8 cases with comorbid ADHD)	10.5 (8–16)	Facial recognition Block design	Yes[f] No
Lanser et al. (1993)	16 TS	10.4 (7–14)	VIQ > PIQ	No
Brookshire et al. (1994)	31 TS 20 nonTS sibs (including 5 "overactive" sibs)	11.4 ± 2.8 11.4 + 2.9	Judgment of line orientation	No (compared to sibling control)
Schultz et al. (1998)	16 TS – ADHD 34 TS + ADHD 23 NC	10.4 ± 1.4 11.0 ± 1.6 10.8 ± 1.7	BD (partialing voc), Matrices partialing voc)	Trend Yes

Notes: For studies not employing a control group, deficit was indicated if more than 20% of the sample scored at least 1.5 *SD* below the mean. Unless otherwise specified, comorbidity with ADHD was not explicitly evaluated.

[a] Four out of the 13 subjects had a VIQ-PIQ discrepancy of at least 15 points.

[b] For subjects 9 years or older.

[c] Five of the 10 subjects had a VIQ-PIQ discrepancy of at least 15 points.

[d] Five of 28 had VIQ at least 12 points greater than PIQ, and 5 had the opposite.

[e] VIQ-PIQ differences not reported, but PIQ not significantly lower than control group.

[f] Significantly impaired compared to less severely affected co-twin.

Adapted with permission from Schultz et al. (1998).

Visuospatial/Visuoperceptual Ability

The literature on potential visuoperceptual deficits in Tourette's syndrome is less extensive, less coherent, and less persuasive, largely because the measures employed have not been highly specific to this domain of functioning (Table 5.3). The early literature tended to focus on relative deficits in Wechsler Performance IQ (PIQ) compared to Verbal IQ (VIQ). Although Shapiro et al. (1978) and Sutherland et al. (1982) found significant PIQ deficits, Incagnoli and Kane (1981), Golden (1984), Ferrari et al. (1984), and Lanser and colleagues (Lanser, Van Santen, Jennekens-Schinkel, & Roos, 1993) did not. Dykens and colleagues (1990) found significantly lower PIQ among children with Tourette's syndrome without ADHD as compared to Tourette's syndrome with ADHD. Bornstein et al. (1991), on the other hand, reported greater VIQ-PIQ discrepancies in Tourette's syndrome, regardless of the direction. Schultz et al. (1998)

reported significantly lower Kaufman Brief Test of Intelligence (KBIT) Matrices scores (controlling for general intelligence) among children with Tourette's syndrome compared to age-matched controls, and a statistical trend in the same direction for the WISC-R Block Design subtest (also controlling for general intelligence). Other measures with a visuoperceptual or visuospatial component have also provided mixed results. With the exception of Brookshire et al. (1994), who used a motor-free test of visuospatial ability, no study has employed specific measures of visuoperceptual abilities unconfounded by intellectual reasoning or motor demands.

We recently tested a component process model of visuomotor integration (see Figure 5.1) in our sample of 50 Tourette's syndrome children and 23 age-matched controls (Schultz et al., 1998). As already described, visuomotor integration was assessed with the VMI. Visuoperceptual skill was assessed with the Block Design subtest of the WISC-R and the Matrices subtest of the KBIT. Because each of these subtests loads on general intelligence (g), covariance analyses with visuoperceptual measures and KBIT Vocabulary test scores created "purified" measures of visuo-perceptual skill. Vocabulary served as a proxy for g because it has the highest g loading of any individual intelligence subtest (Brody, 1992). Dominant, nondominant, and bimanual fine motor coordination were measured with the Purdue Pegboard (Tiffen, 1968). Motor inhibition and sustained attention were assessed with a computer-administered continuous performance test (CPT; Loong, 1991). Number of commissions (i.e., responses to nontarget letters) constituted the measure of motor inhibition; number of omissions (i.e., failures to detect the target) served as the measure of sustained attention. Scores on the VMI were significantly correlated with tests of visual-perceptual and fine motor coordination (controlling for g), providing partial support for our component process model of visuomotor integration. Moreover, three putative component processes—fine motor skill, visuoperceptual ability, and response inhibition—were also significant areas of weakness for children with Tourette's, irrespective of their ADHD status. However, none of the measures employed to assess these three component processes could fully account for the deficits in visuomotor integration. Even after controlling statistically for visuoperceptual skill, g, and fine motor control, children with Tourette's syndrome continued to perform worse than controls on the VMI, suggesting that the integration of visual inputs and organized motor output is a specific area of weakness in individuals with Tourette's syndrome. These conclusions are consistent with the data of Brookshire and colleagues (1994). In that study, low scores on the VMI by children with Tourette's syndrome could not be explained by their performance on a motor-free visual-perceptual test, suggesting a primary difficulty with the integration of visuoperceptual and motor functions, not visuoperceptual analyses.

VISUOMOTOR INTEGRATION DEFICITS IN OBSESSIVE-COMPULSIVE DISORDER

Deficits in visuomotor integration also have been reported in obsessive-compulsive disorder. We recently studied 24 children with obsessive-compulsive disorder but not Tourette's syndrome in comparison to 23 unaffected controls, matched on age and VIQ (Schultz, unpublished data). As was true for Tourette's syndrome, children with obsessive-compulsive disorder scored 1 *SD* below the controls on the VMI. The children with obsessive-compulsive disorder also performed more poorly on the Purdue Pegboard than controls, but the mean difference was less substantial than for Tourette's syndrome. Fine motor deficits have previously been reported by Hollander, Schiffman, et al. (1990). Comparing obsessive-compulsive disorder and Tourette's syndrome, there were no significant differences with regard to fine motor or visuomotor integration skills in our study, suggesting that the shared genetic diathesis results in functional commonalities. However, children with obsessive-compulsive disorder evidenced a specific impairment in visual-spatial skill (Block Design, controlling for *g*) in comparison to the controls and to the Tourette's syndrome children without obsessive-compulsive disorder. This finding is in agreement with the literature, as several studies have indicated that obsessive-compulsive disorder also involves deficits in visuomotor integration (Behar et al., 1984; Boone et al., 1991; Hollander et al., 1993; Hollander, Schiffman, et al., 1990), visuoperceptual ability (Aronowitz et al., 1994), and visuospatial reasoning (Head, Bolton, & Hymas, 1989; Savage et al., 1996). In fact, evidence for a deficit in visuoperceptual processes is more compelling for obsessive-compulsive disorder than for Tourette's syndrome. Although Tourette's syndrome and obsessive-compulsive disorder have deficits in the functionally related area of visuomotor integration and its component processes, obsessive-compulsive disorder appears to entail a relatively greater difficulty with visuoperceptual processing as opposed to the integration of visual percepts and motor output. A unique contributor to the impairment in obsessive-compulsive disorder, therefore, may be visuoperceptual processing difficulties, whereas for Tourette's syndrome visuomotor integration appears paramount.

NEURAL BASIS OF VISUOMOTOR INTEGRATION DEFICITS IN TOURETTE'S SYNDROME AND RELATED CONDITIONS

Considerable knowledge about neural systems subserving visuomotor integration and its component processes has been gleaned from lesions in adulthood. Both right- and left-hemisphere processes have been implicated in drawing ability, but the contributions of each to good performance is quite likely different. Right-hemisphere damage typically results in drawings with sufficiently accurate detail, but distorted spatial relations among the elements and a failure to capture the gestalt, whereas left-hemisphere lesions more often result in drawings that are slowly executed, oversimplified, lacking detail, but spatially intact (Gainotti & Tiacci, 1970; Marshall et al., 1994; McFie & Zangwill, 1960; Warrington, James, & Kinsbourne, 1966). The drawing dysfunction among right-hemisphere-damaged patients appears to be a result of a primary impairment in perception as it guides the movement of the hand in space (e.g., Kirk & Kertesz, 1989; Warrington & James, 1967). Interpretation of left-brain mechanisms in drawing disturbance is more difficult and in many cases is attributable to low-level errors of motor execution secondary to dominant hand hemiparesis (Carlesimo, Fadda, & Caltagirone, 1993; Gainotti, 1985; Kirk & Kertesz, 1989). However, ideomotor dyspraxia (deficits in selecting and sequencing movement elements) and ideational dyspraxia (deficits in the conceptual organization and planning of movement) can also cause the simplification of drawing seen in left-hemisphere constructional dyspraxics (Kirk & Kertesz, 1989; Piercy, Hécaen, & Ajuriaguerra, 1960; Warrington & James, 1967). Although both hemispheres may contribute to visuomotor integration, a more important role for the right is suggested by the greater frequency of drawing difficulties with right-hemisphere lesions (Damasio, 1985), especially when patients with global cognitive deficits are excluded (Villa, Gainotti, & De Bonis, 1986).

Lesions to the parietal cortex in humans produce impaired visual perception, particularly when the injury is in the right hemisphere (for a complete review, see Andersen, 1987). The integration of motor movements with visuoperception is conducted with body-centered representations of space (as opposed to retinotopic) within the posterior parietal cortex (Andersen & Zipser, 1988). Single-cell recording studies in nonhuman primates and functional neuroimaging studies in humans indicate that posterior parietal cortex codes for the position of body parts relative to one another and to the external world, and participates in planned movements in external space (Andersen, 1987; Bonda, Petrides, Frey, & Evans, 1995). These processes are essential for accurate drawing. Posterior parietal lobule lesions result in reaching errors and deficits in fine motor coordination with visual guidance (Andersen, 1987; Hyvärinen, 1982). Moreover, a small region within the posterior parietal cortex, the lateral intraparietal area, appears to be specialized for the visuomotor integration of saccadic eye movements, allowing location of targets in space and planning for subsequent movements (Andersen, Brotchie, & Mazzoni, 1992). Superior aspects of the right parietal lobe also subserve somatosensory processes (Mountcastle, Lynch, Georgopoulos, Sakata, & Acuña, 1975) that allow for feedback about the placement of the pencil on the fingertips and real-time adjustments for fine motor control during drawing.

Although considerable evidence documents the role of the nondominant parietal lobe in somatosensory and visuospatial processes contributing to visuomotor integration, it is also clear that drawing is a complex ability involving multiple brain regions. The integration of visuoperceptual, so-matosensory, and motor components in drawing is probably mediated by bidirectional exchange of information between parietal and motor areas of the frontal cortex (Quintana & Fuster, 1993), with a substantial integrative contribution from subcortical circuits (e.g., Alexander, DeLong, & Strick, 1986). Indeed, visuomotor integration deficits may arise from frontal and subcortical lesions, in addition to parietal lobe lesions. Marshall and colleagues (1994) studied drawing dysfunction in 37 patients with right-hemisphere stroke, with lesions distributed among subcortical, anterior cortical, and posterior cortical locations. When both drawing and visuoperceptual function were disturbed, lesions always involved the temproparietal-occipital junction. When visual-spatial functions were intact, but drawings were unrecognizable, lesion location more often was subcortical, with a point of lesion overlap across subjects in the anterior limb of the internal capsule and the lateral head of the right caudate nucleus. Thus, the basal ganglia may have a specific role in the synthesizing motor programming and perceptual inputs. This is consistent with other reports of constructional apraxia following subcortical lesions in the nondominant hemisphere (e.g., Agostini, Collette, Orlando, & Tredici, 1983; Lazar, Weiner, Wald, & Kula, 1995).

The role of the basal ganglia in drawing disturbance is particularly intriguing because neuroimaging, neuropathological, and phenomenological studies implicate the basal ganglia and functionally related cortical and thalamic structures in the pathobiology of Tourette's syndrome (Anderson et al., 1992a, 1992b; Balthazar, 1956; Hyde et al., 1995; Peterson, Riddle, Cohen, Katz, Smith, Hardin, et al., 1993; Singer, Hahn, & Moran, 1991; Singer et al., 1993; Wolf et al., 1996; also see Chapters 8, 12, and 13 for additional discussion). A specific role for the right caudate in the pathobiology of Tourette's is suggested by an MRI study of 10 pairs of monozygotic twins concordant for tics (Hyde et al., 1995). The size of the right caudate nucleus was significantly reduced in the more severely affected twin. Abnormalities of the right caudate, therefore, could have a primary role in both the tic behavior and the impaired visuomotor integration skills seen in Tourette's syndrome. In a recent follow-up study of these twins, Wolf et al. reported greater D_2 dopamine-receptor binding in the head of the caudate, bilaterally, using single photon emission computed tomography (SPECT) in the more severely affected cotwin. Intrapair binding differences accounted for nearly all of the variance in the corresponding within-pair differences in symptom severity. These bilateral findings are consistent with our findings of equivalent dominant and nondominant hand impairment on the Purdue Pegboard (Schultz et al., 1998).

Given the etiologic link between Tourette's syndrome and some forms of obsessive-compulsive disorder, and the possible genetic link between Tourette's syndrome and one form of ADHD seen in combination with Tourette's syndrome, it is informative to compare and contrast neuropsychological and neurobiological findings in these disorders. All three disorders share deficits in visuomotor integration. Moreover, neuroimaging findings also implicate the caudate nuclei in the pathobiology of obsessive-compulsive disorder (Baxter et al., 1992; Breiter et al., 1996; Luxenberg et al., 1988; Rauch et al., 1994; Robinson et al., 1995) and ADHD (Castellanos et al., 1994; Hynd et al., 1993), suggesting that the visuoperceptual and visuomotor integration deficit in Tourette's syndrome, ADHD, and obsessive-compulsive disorder could arise from a common abnormality in the basal ganglia, and more specifically in the caudate nuclei and their associated cortical-striatal networks. This is feasible because the caudate serves an integrative function, receiving input from motor areas of the frontal lobe (e.g., frontal eye fields, lateral orbital, supplementary motor and premotor areas) and visuoperceptual areas of the parietal lobe (Alexander et al., 1986; Gillman, Dauth, Frey, & Penny, 1987). In addition to having a role in motor planning (Caplan et al., 1990), the caudate is well situated to function as a control process for the integration of motor- and perceptual-processing streams important to visuomotor integration. It is also noteworthy that preliminary findings regarding lack of leftward asymmetry of the lenticular nuclei in Tourette's syndrome (Peterson, Riddle, Cohen, Katz, Smith, Hardin, et al., 1993; Singer et al., 1993) might be attributable to the comorbid ADHD condition and not to Tourette's syndrome per se (Aylward et al., 1996; Singer et al., 1993). This is consistent with other neuroimaging data suggesting a primary role for the basal ganglia in ADHD (e.g., Castellanos et al., 1994; Hynd et al., 1993; Lou, Henriksen, Bruhn, Borner, & Nielson, 1989). Thus, an overlapping set of subcortical circuits appears to be involved in the pathogenesis of Tourette's syndrome, obsessive-compulsive disorder, and ADHD, possibly accounting for the high rates of comorbidity and a shared neuropsychological phenotype.

EXECUTIVE FUNCTIONS

The neuropsychology of Tourette's syndrome has also focused on possible deficits in executive functioning (EF), a broad domain covering planning, goal-directed behavior, maintenance of cognitive set and cognitive flexibility, impulse control, sustained attention and effort, and self-regulation. EF does not refer to a single ability, but rather to a range of functions for which a suitable scientific taxonomy has yet to be developed. At the most general level, EF is synonymous with self-regulation of behavior and the ability to generate and execute goal-directed behavior (Pennington, 1991). EF is largely the purview of the frontal lobes (though with extensive interconnections to the basal ganglia), especially the nonmotor prefrontal cortex. Prefrontal cortex is important for the programming, initiation, regulation, and maintenance of behavior toward specific goals (Luria, 1980). Prefrontal cortex can be partitioned into different functional systems, including dorsolateral, orbital, and ventral-medial. The function of dorsolateral cortex is perhaps best understood. Extensive work by Goldman-Rakic and others (e.g., Fuster, 1995; Goldman-Rakic, 1987, 1988; Wilson, Scalaide, & Goldman-Rakic, 1993) has established that regions of the dorsolateral prefrontal cortex are deeply involved in working memory (WM), the maintenance of "online" representations (e.g., Brodman areas 46 and 9 appear specialized for visuospatial WM, whereas the lateral convexity is specialized for object feature WM). WM is critical for holding goal-related representations online so that problems can be solved without reliance on previously entrenched learned associations. Not only must goal-related memories be stored in an active buffer, but all the partial products of behavior and cognition during the process of solving goal-related problems must also be held for immediate accessibility. Although WM and the role of the dorsolateral prefrontal cortex currently dominate much of the discussion on EF, orbital and ventral-medial partitions are known to subserve important aspects of EF as well. Orbital frontal cortex, with its rich connections to limbic and paralimbic areas, cingulate gyrus, thalamus, and other prefrontal cortices, has an important role in judgment and planning, motivation, motor inhibition, response flexibility, and set shifting (Damasio, Tranel, & Damasio, 1990; Morecraft, Geula, & Mesulam, 1992; Passingham, 1972). The hallmark of posteromedial or "limbic" orbital frontal lesions is behavioral perseveration, implicating this region in motor control and inhibition (Butter, 1969; Mishkin, Vest, Waxler, & Rosvold, 1969). Ventral-medial prefrontal cortex may have a special role in mediating affective and social behavior (e.g., Damasio, 1994).

Compared to visuomotor integration, the literature on EF is less clear with regard to possible dysfunction in Tourette's syndrome subjects as a group. Although some studies find EF deficits on select measures, there is inconsistency across studies. Given that Tourette's syndrome is defined by an inability to inhibit the urge to move and vocalize, inhibitory processes and related EFs are logical targets of investigation. Moreover, involvement of corticostriatal pathways in the pathogenesis of Tourette's syndrome also suggests the likelihood of EF deficits in the disorder (see Chapter 12 for a more complete discussion of the neural circuitry implicated in Tourette's syndrome). The variable findings suggest substantial individual differences within the diagnostic group and the confounding effects of comorbid disorders, particularly ADHD. Inconsistency in the literature is probably also a function of conceptual ambiguity with regard to essential elements of this domain of neuropsychological functioning.

There have been at least 13 studies of Tourette's syndrome incorporating EF measures (Baron-Cohen et al., 1994; Bornstein, 1990, 1991b; Bornstein et al., 1991; Channon et al., 1992; Georgiou, Bradshaw, Phillips, & Chiu, 1996; Harris et al., 1995; Ozonoff, Strayer, McMahon, & Filloux, 1994; Randolph et al., 1993; Schultz et al., 1998; Shucard, Benedict, Tekokkilic, & Lichter, 1997; Silverstein et al., 1995; Sutherland et al., 1982; Yeates & Bornstein, 1994). The results vary by measure and by study. For example, tests of mental flexibility, such as the Wisconsin Card Sort (WCS), the Category test, and Trail Making have been employed in 8 of the 14 studies. For each of these most commonly employed measures of EF, no consistent finding has emerged. The one area of consistent findings across studies concerns response time (RT) during CPTs. Three studies reported that children with Tourette's syndrome respond significantly more slowly than expected during a CPT, suggesting difficulties with sustained attention (Como & Kurlan, 1991; Harris et al., 1995; Shucard et al., 1997). In addition, Harris and colleagues found that their subjects, regardless of comorbid ADHD status, exhibited significantly increased response time variability (RT SD) compared to test-normative data. Although RT measures appear sensitive to Tourette's syndrome, omission and commission error rate on the CPT have not shown a consistent relationship to diagnostic status (Como & Kurlan, 1991; Harris et al., 1995; Randolph et al., 1993; Schultz et al., 1998; Shucard et al., 1997).

Executive Functions and Attention-Deficit/ Hyperactivity Disorder

The importance of recognizing that the variability in EF findings may be influenced by the presence or absence of comorbid conditions such as ADHD cannot be overemphasized. Review of the neuropsychological profile of ADHD suggests that it is often associated with impaired EF (Barkley et al., 1992; Douglas, 1988). Interestingly, four studies compared Tourette's syndrome with ADHD to Tourette's syndrome without ADHD. Yeates and Bornstein (1994) found significantly greater impairment among those with comorbid ADHD on Trail Making A and B, but not the WCS or Category tests. In a comparison of 34 children with Tourette's syndrome alone and 16 children with Tourette's syndrome plus ADHD, we found no differences on Trail Making or the WCS (Schultz et al., unpublished). Harris et al. (1995) and Silverstein et al. (1995), on the other hand, found significantly greater impairment on the WCS among Tourette's syndrome with ADHD as opposed to Tourette's syndrome without ADHD. Commissions on a CPT have also been evaluated in Tourette's syndrome with and without ADHD. Harris et al. found significantly more impulsivity among those subjects with comorbid ADHD. Schultz et al. found that children with Tourette's syndrome were much more impulsive than the controls. Moreover, visuomotor integration skill and inhibitory control in combination were able to accurately classify 82% of the unaffected controls and 80% of the children with Tourette's syndrome. Commission error rate, however, was not predictive of comorbid ADHD among the children with Tourette's syndrome, as both subtypes of Tourette's syndrome had a significantly elevated number of commissions compared to normal controls. Como and Kurlan (1991) compared patients with Tourette's syndrome plus ADHD to children with ADHD alone to examine whether EF measures differed by ADHD subtype. The children with only ADHD performed significantly worse on a number of dimensions, including overall speed of response and number of CPT omission errors. Further studies comparing Tourette's syndrome and ADHD are needed to characterize the pattern of EF in these disorders. Moreover, careful examination of comorbid psychopathology, developmental history, clinical phenomenology, treatment response, brain structure and function, and family genetic history should help clarify how and when patients with Tourette's syndrome exhibit problems in the domain of EF.

Executive Functions and Obsessive-Compulsive Disorder

The literature on EF in obsessive-compulsive disorder is larger and more diverse in terms of measures. Although there is some good data pointing to EF deficits, findings are not consistent. Head and colleagues (1989) found deficits in set-shifting ability on the WCS in a sample of 15 adults with obsessive-compulsive disorder compared to matched controls. Hymas and colleagues (Hymas, Lees, Bolton, Epps, & Head, 1991), studied 59 patients with obsessive-compulsive disorder and found that a subset of 17 showed significant obsessional slowness and difficulties with cognitive set shifting. Martinot et al. (1990) studied 16 patients with obsessive-compulsive disorder and 8 controls using positron-emission tomography (PET) and neuropsychological assessments. They found some evidence for EF deficits, but more interestingly, found a significant correlation between poor Stroop Color Word Interference test performance and reduced lateral frontal lobe glucose metabolism. Hollander and Wong (1996) found set-shifting deficits on the Trail Making test in a group of 50 obsessive-compulsive disorder patients as compared to 31 controls. Moreover, set-shifting impairment was predicted by measures of serotonergic dysfunction. Most recently, Rosenberg, Dick, Ohearn, and Sweeney (1997) demonstrated deficits in occulomotor inhibition among 12 medication-free, nondepressed obsessive-compulsive disorder adults in comparison to 12 matched controls. These findings suggest that a variety of different EF deficits may exist in obsessive-compulsive disorder, and they implicate the orbital as well as the dorsal lateral prefrontal cortex in the pathobiology of the disease. In addition, these positive findings could also be attributed to basal ganglia dysfunction. In fact, Lopez-Villegas and colleagues (1996) demonstrated deficits in EF with a sample of 18 patients with basal ganglia calcification in comparison to 16 controls matched for age, IQ, and gender. Of the 18 patients with basal ganglia calcification, 6 met criteria for obsessive-compulsive disorder. These data are consistent with other reports that argue for a subcortical-prefrontal system of EF governance.

In contrast to these affirmative findings, Malloy (1987) found deficits on the WCS only among the less intelligent and more psychotic obsessive-compulsive disorder patients. Moreover, using another EF measure, the Controlled Oral Word Fluency Test, he failed to find EF deficits. Failure to identify EF deficits in obsessive-compulsive disorder using conventional neuropsychological measures such as the WCS has also been reported by Boone et al. (1991), Christensen, Kim, Dysken, and Hoover (1992), Martin et al. (1993), and Zielinski et al. (1991). A well-controlled study by Abbruzzese and colleagues (Abbruzzese, Ferri, & Scarone, 1995) contrasted WCS test performance among 33 patients with obsessive-compulsive disorder and 33 controls matched for age, sex, and education and also found no group differences. Cohen et al. (1996) compared EF among 65 obsessive-compulsive disorder patients, 32 controls, and 17 patients with another anxiety disorder, social phobia. Interestingly, only the patients with social phobia showed EF deficits.

A recent study has focused attention on mental speed during EF tests. Veal, Sahakian, Owen, and Marks (1996) studied 40 patients with obsessive-compulsive disorder in comparison to matched controls. Although there were no differences on the Tower of London test of planning with respect to accuracy, obsessive-compulsive disorder patients spent significantly more time generating alternative solutions and checking their own accuracy. Galderisi, Mucci, Catapano, D'Amato, and Maj (1995) specifically assessed the hypothesis that obsessional slowness would be most prominent on tests tapping frontal subcortical EF systems. They found no deficits with respect to EF accuracy among their group of obsessive-compulsive disorder patients but, consistent with their prediction, did find that obsessive-compulsive disorder patients were significantly slowed on EF tests and not on measures sensitive to temporal lobe functioning. Thus, measures that code performance in multiple ways may be best suited to revealing and characterizing the putative EF deficits in obsessive-compulsive disorder. Those that prove to be sensitive to the diagnosis of obsessive-compulsive disorder could be fruitfully used in comparison to groups of patients with Tourette's and/or ADHD to further specify the commonalities shared by these disorders.

IMPAIRED SUBPOPULATION

Several studies have noted that the majority of patients with Tourette's syndrome perform within normal limits on tests of neuropsychological functioning (±1.5 SDs from the mean), with only a subsample showing clinically meaningful impairments (Bornstein, 1990; Randolph et al., 1993; Schultz et al., 1998). For example, Bornstein showed that approximately 20% of his sample of 100 children with Tourette's syndrome showed impairment on a summary index of neuropsychological functioning, with impairments in sensory and motor functioning being the most common. Our data are in agreement with this assessment, as only a fraction of the subjects with Tourette's scored well below the normative mean on the visuomotor and fine motor measures (Schultz et al., 1998). For example, 32% of the children with Tourette's syndrome scored at least 1 SD below the mean on the VMI, and 78% scored below the mean. Thus, the entire distribution of scores appears to be shifted slightly downward toward more impaired performance on select neuropsychological measures.

The shift is small enough that the majority of children with Tourette's syndrome performed within normal limits, broadly defined. However, there are practical implications for these findings. Many children with Tourette's have great difficulty with penmanship, and this is likely a direct manifestation of visuomotor integration difficulties. The consistency with which drawing difficulties have been observed across all studies in the literature suggests that this domain of functioning be routinely assessed for all referrals with Tourette's syndrome, obsessive-compulsive disorder, or ADHD, as discussed in Chapters 15 and 17.

IMPACT OF PSYCHOTROPIC MEDICATIONS

A potential confound in all studies of academic and neuropsychological functioning is the active use of psychotropic medications among a portion of the sample under study. About half of clinic-ascertained samples of Tourette's syndrome subjects are treated with medications (Abwender et al., 1996; Schultz et al., 1998), and there is a risk that cognitive functioning could be altered. Although these concerns are justified, several reports provide evidence that medications are not creating the profile of neuropsychological functioning described in this review. Bornstein and Yang (1991) studied 96 children and adolescents with Tourette's syndrome, 51 of whom were taking a psychotropic medication, and found no difference in neuropsychological, intellectual, or educational functioning between the two groups. Schultz and colleagues (1998) studied the effects of medications on visuomotor integration, motor, visuoperceptual, motor inhibition, and sustained attention performance in a sample of 50 children with Tourette's; about half of the children were taking at least one medication to treat their tic symptoms. Only one variable, dominant hand performance on the Purdue Pegboard, differed significantly between the two groups. Moreover, when a Bonferroni correction was applied to adjust for the multiple comparisons, this failed to reach significance. Although psychomotor retardation with neuroleptics is typical after initiation of these agents or after a dosage increase (Cassens, Inglis, Appelbaum, & Gutheil, 1990; D. King, 1990), none of the children in this study had a recent medication change. Furthermore, dropping the nine children on neuroleptics from the data analyses did not change any of the results. Results from several other smaller studies support the conclusion that the neuropsychological deficits in Tourette's syndrome cannot be attributed to side effects of pharmacological treatments (Channon et al., 1992; Ferrari, Matthews, & Barabas, 1984; Golden, 1984; Shucard et al., 1997).

FUTURE DIRECTIONS

At present there is a great opportunity to explore neuropsychological functioning in Tourette's syndrome and related disorders with a combination of neurobehavioral and neuroimaging measures. As discussed in Chapter 12, the combination of approaches has clear and decided advantages over using either alone. Moreover, with the advent of functional MRI (fMRI), neuropsychological functioning can now be investigated *in vivo*. Although extremely powerful, fMRI technology remains in its infancy, especially regarding the statistical treatment of the data. However, by the turn of the century, fMRI capabilities should be firmly established in research medical centers as well as large metropolitan hospitals, making it the investigative tool of choice. Ultimately, patients will be tested with batteries of neurobehavioral probes during fMRI exams, and the profile of brain activations for each will be evaluated for significant deviance from normality. Once these techniques have been validated in large groups of patients with Tourette's syndrome and related conditions, there will be a time in the not too distant future when these methods will be the standard methodology for clinical neuropsychological assessment. The results will not only clarify the boundaries between these related disorders, they will also inform treatment and provide a mechanism to monitor progress across time.

Other promising research directions include efforts to take into account specific epigenetic factors that are likely to influence the course and severity of Tourette's, obsessive-compulsive disorder, and ADHD. As discussed in Chapter 12, a variety of adverse perinatal events have been implicated in the pathogenesis of Tourette's syndrome. These events and others that result in injury to the basal ganglia and their connection to thalamic and cortical sites are also likely to have a lasting impact on the individual's performance on the various neuropsychological measures. Indeed, some of the inconsistency and individual variation across studies may well be accounted for by including such factors in the analysis.

We anticipate that specific genotypes will be identified that confer an increased risk. As reviewed in Chapter 11, it seems likely that there will be multiple genes of both major and minor effect. Characterization of Tourette's syndrome patients with regard to these genotypes may well resolve some of the inconsistencies posed by the currently available neuropsychological studies. However, truly multidisciplinary studies that systematically collect relevant neuropsychological, neurobiological, genetic, and epigenetic data on well-characterized patient populations hold the greatest promise.

Clinically, the available neuropsychological data offer further challenges. Given the consistency of the visual-motor deficits in Tourette's syndrome, how can we be of assistance in informing educators and working with them to find ways to limit the impact of these weaknesses in academic settings? We return to this issue in Chapter 19, but much work remains to be done.

SUMMARY OF CHAPTER 5

Individuals with Tourette's syndrome frequently are observed to have difficulty in a variety of neuropsychological domains of functioning, including visuomotor integration and executive functioning. Visuomotor integration appears to be the domain of functioning most impaired. This difficulty usually takes the form of being unable to accurately copy simple and complex designs and figures. These deficits implicate neural circuits that link cortical and subcortical basal ganglia structures in the brain. It is informative that these same neuropsychological deficits are found in ADHD and OCD, suggesting commonality in brain mechanisms and neuropsychological expression in these related conditions.

PREVIEW OF CHAPTER 6

Given the overt nature of tic symptoms, it is not uncommon for individuals with Tourette's syndrome to become a public spectacle. Teasing by peers is also commonplace. Chapter 6 explores the areas of peer acceptance and adaptive functioning and returns to the theme of resilience.

CHAPTER 6

Peer Acceptance and
Adaptive Functioning

ELISABETH M. DYKENS, SARA S. SPARROW, DONALD J. COHEN,
LAWRENCE SCAHILL, and JAMES F. LECKMAN

> Social-emotional functioning refers to intra- and interpersonal regulation of
> emotion, cognition, and behavior.
>
> —*Sara S. Sparrow, Alice S. Carter, Gary Racusin, and R. Morris, 1995*

> Negative appraisal by agemates in childhood is a strong predictor of such
> important long-term outcomes as school dropout, delinquency, and global
> indices of psychopathology.
>
> —*Stephen Hinshaw, 1994*

In the past few decades, research on children's peer relationships has exploded. But for the most part, this resurgence of interest in peers has been limited to normal children or children under various types of psychosocial distress. In contrast, relatively few studies have examined how children with neuropsychiatric disorders make friends, get along with peers, and meet the demands of everyday life. This neglect is particularly true in the case of Tourette's syndrome, where just a few studies hint at peer and socialization difficulties. Ironically, as research expands exponentially on the genetic and neurologic intricacies of Tourette's syndrome, some of life's more basic questions are left unanswered: How do children with Tourette's syndrome make friends and get along with others? Which children with Tourette's are at greatest risk for peer and adaptive difficulties? How do ways of socializing with others help or hurt Tourette's syndrome children as they develop and ultimately chart their life course? As discussed in Chapter 1, these are crucial issues in the development of resilience and the maintenance of normative developmental progress.

Our aim in this chapter is to review the scientific literature and to kindle excitement for future research that addresses these basic questions. Pivotal to all these questions is the need to determine exactly how widespread peer and adaptive difficulties are in children with Tourette's. Studies to date have relied on clinical samples; peer relations may be less problematic among nonreferred samples. Although the exact prevalence of peer difficulties in Tourette's syndrome is thus unknown, at least some children with Tourette's syndrome appear to experience peer and adaptive difficulties. This chapter outlines several etiologic avenues that might lead to these difficulties.

One possible road to peer difficulties is the stigmatizing effects of tics themselves. If tics are indeed stigmatizing, then we would expect the age of onset of tics, as well as their severity and course, to emerge as significant mediators of peer adjustment. Though the chapter addresses these hypotheses, we also take up the possibility that peer difficulties may be secondary to comorbid conditions associated with Tourette's, primarily attention-deficit/hyperactivity disorder (ADHD) and obsessive-compulsive disorder. Finally, peer problems may be associated with both of these possibilities, or these difficulties may have little to do with Tourette's syndrome per se and instead relate to other child or environmental factors.

In this chapter, then, we first review findings on friendships, peer relationships, and social-adaptive behavior in children with Tourette's. As data are sparse, we turn in some detail to a research agenda in each section that builds on these previous findings. We propose that Tourette's unique clinical features are particularly well-suited for studies on peer relationships. Some of these features include various comorbid conditions associated with Tourette's syndrome, and others relate to tics themselves. Research on how these and other aspects of this syndrome are associated with social adjustment may offer important clues to peer relationships among children in general. Such data could also guide new interventions to improve peer relations and social skills among Tourette's children who are at greatest risk for social dysfunction. This chapter thus shows how Tourette's syndrome provides as yet undiscovered opportunities for insights into peer relationships in children with or without this complex disorder.

FRIENDSHIPS AND PEER RELATIONS IN CHILDREN WITH TOURETTE'S SYNDROME

Friendships

Several parent surveys have been conducted that include questions on the friendships of children with Tourette's syndrome. Findings from these surveys are contradictory: some suggest few problems, whereas others point to substantial difficulties in the social arena.

Most children with Tourette's syndrome report having some friends. In one survey, parents of children and adolescents with Tourette's syndrome reported that 72% of their children age 5 to 12 years had a best friend (Jagger et al., 1982). Among older children sampled, age 12 to 18 years, 77% indicated they had a best friend, and about half had begun to date. Optimistic findings about friends were also reported by Nomura, Kita, and Segawa (1992), who sampled 53 adolescent Japanese boys with Tourette's syndrome. Approximately 70% of these boys reported that they had met with five or more different friends in the prior two weeks, socializing at least three times with them.

At the same time, however, parents and youngsters also indicate widespread teasing related to tic symptoms. Jagger et al. (1982) found that 75% of their older and 73% of their younger samples of Tourette's children experienced teasing by peers. Similarly, 62% of Nomura et al.'s (1992) sample of Japanese boys said that others pointed out their tic symptoms, and most (55%) admitted to feeling hurt when they did so. Reporting on over 200 6- to 18-year-old youngsters with Tourette's syndrome, Shady, Fulton, and Champion (1988) found that 68% had difficulties getting along with their classmates. Ridicule from peers and increased isolation from them have also been informally reported by others (Hagin et al., 1982; Lerer, 1987).

Although suggestive of peer difficulties, surveys are often limited in scope and do not necessarily pinpoint why peer problems exist. Further, these data do not reflect more recent thinking on friendships and peers, including innovative new ways of measuring these constructs. This work can add much rigor to the study of peer relationships in Tourette's syndrome.

Next Steps

Accurate measurements of friendship need to include the element of reciprocity between children, of their mutual liking or affection. Both children in a friendship dyad need to be assessed and to view one another as a friend. Without this, one runs the risk of simply measuring a child's degree of attraction to others or his or her desire to have friends (Hays, 1988).

Unlike children's casual acquaintances (e.g., other members of their sports team or school band), children's friendships provide several supportive functions (Adler & Furman, 1988). These include improved esteem and self-image, feelings of intimacy with others, emotional security, help or advice with challenging tasks, companionship, and stimulation (for a review, see Parker, Rubin, Price, & DeRosier, 1995). Most researchers agree that these properties of friendships are crucial to children's social, emotional, and cognitive development. Indeed, some of the renewed interest in peer research stems from emerging evidence for the importance of peers as a major socializing agent, above and beyond the role of parents and family.

Measures of friendships, then, needs to reflect these key components: intimacy, help with tasks, and emotional security. Several tools now do so. One measure, for example, asks children to rate 40 items about a specific friend; the items tap four supportive dimensions of friendship (companionship and recreation, validation and caring, help and guidance, intimate exchange), as well as conflicts and conflict resolution (Parker & Asher, 1993). This tool, the Friendship Quality Questionnaire, has promising psychometric properties and is easily administered in a classroom setting. Other measures depend less on children's self-reports and more on direct observations of how dyads of children play and interact (e.g., Youngblade, Park, & Belsky, 1993). Future research on friendships in Tourette's syndrome children could thus benefit from these more sophisticated concepts and measures that examine the reciprocal and supportive elements of friends.

Peer Relations

Whereas studies of friendships emphasize reciprocity between dyads of children, studies of peer relations evaluate how children fare in an aggregate or their social status relative to others. Although the two are related, friendships and peer relations are generally viewed as different means to understanding a common end: children's social and peer adjustment (Parker & Asher, 1993).

To date, just one study has been conducted on the peer relations of children with Tourette's syndrome. Stokes and colleagues (1991) examined 29 children with Tourette's, age 8 to 15 years, using the Pupil Evaluation Inventory (PEI; Pekarik, Prinz, Leibert, Weintraub, & Neale, 1976) as well as standard neuropsychological, familial, and behavioral assessments. The PEI assesses three dimensions of peer relations: likability, aggression, and withdrawal. Both children and teachers were asked to complete the inventory.

Relative to same-sex peers, children with Tourette's syndrome in the Stokes et al. (1991) study emerged as significantly more withdrawn and less popular or well liked. A full 35% of the Tourette's syndrome sample obtained the lowest peer nomination ratings on one or more of the PEI dimensions. Teachers rated students with Tourette's syndrome as significantly more withdrawn and also as more aggressive than other students in their class. Indeed, no Tourette's syndrome subjects were rated by their teachers as being less aggressive or withdrawn than their classmates.

Findings from this study suggest that Tourette's syndrome children are at increased risk for peer problems. Importantly, however, children in the Stokes et al. (1991) study were drawn from a clinic sample, and peer difficulties may be more common in clinic patients or hard-to-manage Tourette's syndrome cases than in children with milder symptom expression.

Next Steps

Research on peer relations has rapidly expanded over the past decades, in part because of advances in measuring peer relations. Yet aside from the Stokes et al. (1991) study, few of these advances have been incorporated into research on the peer adjustment of children with Tourette's syndrome.

Most studies on peer relations now rely on sociometric, or nomination, techniques. Although sociometric tasks often differ from study to study, in general they ask children for the names of classmates that they particularly like; either a finite or unlimited number of nominations may be sought. Tallies and rank orderings of youngsters are then produced. In contrast to early sociometric work, these techniques now include so-called negative nominations, asking children for the names of peers that they dislike the most or don't like to play with.

A related set of techniques involves a roster-and-rating approach, in which each child rates every classmate on a Likert-type scale, typically answering how much they would or would not like to play with a given peer. Pictures of classmates are sometimes used as aids for younger children. An average score, based on multiple ratings, is then obtained for every student in the class.

Using these innovative sets of techniques, considerable progress has been made classifying children into various categories. The most widespread schemes designate children as belonging to one of five categories (Coie, Dodge, & Coppotelli, 1982; Newcomb & Bukowski, 1983). *Popular* children receive many nominations and also have more positive than negative designations; *rejected* children also receive many nominations, but more negative than positive ratings; *neglected* children obtain very few positive or negative nominations; *controversial* children have a mixture of many positive and negative nominations; and *average* children do not fall into any of these four extreme categories. Most children are classified as average, and between 7% and 13% fall into the popular, rejected, or neglected categories; controversial children are less routinely found (Terry & Coie, 1991).

Studies have yet to use these approaches to describe peer relations in children with Tourette's syndrome. Based on Stokes et al.'s (1991) preliminary findings, children with Tourette's syndrome appear at increased risk for being rejected by their peers. Yet, as detailed in later sections, peer relations may differ across the range of symptomatic expression in Tourette's syndrome. If so, these findings have important implications for adaptive behavior, how children and adults with Tourette's adapt to the social demands of everyday life.

ADAPTIVE BEHAVIOR

Although friendships and peer relationships are critical to adaptive behavior, they are just one part of a larger, complex picture. Equally important to adaptive behavior is how one fulfills family, job, or school expectations and tasks; relaxes; copes with frustrations; communicates with others; takes care of oneself; performs chores; and participates in community life. In short, adaptive behavior is both practical and social and embodies the performance of those behaviors required for personal and social suffi-ciency (Sparrow, Balla, & Cicchetti, 1984).

Furthermore, adaptive behavior is an inherently developmental and social construct, changing as children grow into adolescence, and from adoles-cence into adulthood. Adaptive demands are also defined by expectations from others—from one's family, society, and culture. Adaptive skills typi-cally change across various settings; one's adaptive performance on the job or at school may differ from one's performance with friends or at home. Measurements of adaptive behavior, then, need to have a developmental ori-entation, to be socially and culturally sensitive, and to represent the many settings in which people live, work, and play.

Few Tourette's syndrome studies have used measures of adaptive behav-ior that meet these multiple requirements. Based on surveys, Nomura et al. (1992) found that approximately 85% of Japanese adolescents with Tourette's syndrome had hobbies that they regularly pursued, and 83% of adolescents in the Jagger et al. (1982) survey participated in sports. In a similar vein, Stokes et al. (1991) found that many children in their Tourette's syndrome sample engaged in age-appropriate levels of activities such as hobbies, games, and chores, as measured by the Activity Compe-tence domain of the Child Behavior Checklist (CBCL; Achenbach, 1991b). On average, however, these same children showed CBCL Social Compe-tence domain scores that fell below the normative sample, suggesting more limited involvements with clubs, organizations, and friends.

These studies provide some clues about adaptive behavior, but they do not take advantage of more sophisticated measures of social adaptation. Using a more rigorous measure, Dykens et al. (1990) administered the Vineland Adaptive Behavior Scales (Sparrow et al., 1984) to parents of 30 children with Tourette's syndrome. The Vineland Scales assess adaptive functioning in three domains (communication, daily living skills, social-ization) and nine subdomains. Tourette's syndrome children manifested significant weaknesses in the socialization domain relative to the commu-nication or daily living skills domains; their personal grooming was a rela-tive strength (Dykens et al., 1990). Among these children, then, social skills seem more compromised than other adaptive activities.

Less work has been done on the adaptive concerns of older adolescents or adults with Tourette's syndrome. Among 27 adults surveyed by Jagger et al. (1982), 67% reported that their Tourette's syndrome symptoms did not particularly interfere with their job performance; moderate interfer-ence was noted by 36%, and only 7% noted severe levels of Tourette's syndrome-related job concerns. These encouraging findings may reflect general improvements in tic symptoms that are often observed among older adolescents and young adults (see Chapter 2 and Leckman, Zhang, et al., 1998). Reasons for these improvements are unknown, and often in-clude relative decrements in the number or severity of tics and other asso-ciated symptoms, as well as less marked social impairment (Cohen &

Leckman, 1994). For some, then, young adulthood may bring about symptom reduction and new ways of interacting and coping. For others, symptoms do not remit, and these young adults may struggle to assimilate their tics, especially socially inappropriate or aggressive ones, with their emerging adult identity.

How adults or children with Tourette's syndrome fare at school, on the job, and in friendships is likely to be mediated by a host of variables in the Tourette's syndrome individual, as well as in the environment, particularly the family and school. We now turn to a discussion of those mediating variables that hold particular promise for future research on friendships, peers, and adaptive behavior in persons with Tourette's syndrome.

MEDIATING VARIABLES

Child Variables

Comorbid Conditions

As described in Chapter 4, up to 50% of children with Tourette's present in the clinical setting with attention deficits, overactivity, impulsivity, and poor frustration tolerance (Cohen & Leckman, 1994; Walkup et al., 1995). These difficulties typically precede the onset of tics, yet they may also appear or worsen as tics begin (Cohen, Friedhoff, et al., 1992). Further, Tourette's syndrome is associated with obsessive thoughts and compulsive behaviors. Indeed, considerable work now documents genetic, phenomenologic, and neurologic associations between Tourette's syndrome and obsessive-compulsive disorder or obsessive-compulsive symptoms (Leckman, Walker, et al., 1994; Pauls, Raymond, Stevenson, & Leckman, 1991).

More often than not, impulsivity, ADHD, and compulsive behaviors are viewed as more impairing to adaptive and social functioning than tics per se (Cohen & Leckman, 1994; Jagger et al., 1982). Although diagnostic criteria for obsessive-compulsive disorder include impairments in social-adaptive functioning, research has yet to carefully describe the peer relations of obsessive-compulsive disorder children with or without Tourette's syndrome.

Stokes et al. (1991) examined Tourette's syndrome children with a mixture of psychiatric diagnoses, including obsessive-compulsive disorder, oppositional defiant disorder, overanxious disorder, and ADHD, and found no differences in peer relations between Tourette's syndrome children with and those without these additional diagnoses. When seven subjects with ADHD were separately analyzed, however, they were rated by their peers as significantly more aggressive than the rest of the sample. Although based on small numbers, these findings are consistent with data on the peer relations of ADHD children without Tourette's syndrome. Children with ADHD are generally viewed by their peers as loud, annoying, intrusive, impulsive, and aggressive (e.g., Barkley, 1981; Landau & Moore, 1990).

Not surprisingly, these youngsters often show social skill deficits and negative social reasoning (Whalen, Heneker, & Granger, 1990). Further, a robust association has been observed between peer rejection and aggressive behavior among children in general (e.g., Rubin, Chen, & Hymel, 1993).

Studies are needed to sort out the differential impact of various comorbid conditions on peer relations in children with Tourette's syndrome. Given the natural history of Tourette's syndrome, symptoms of ADHD often show before the onset of tics, whereas obsessive-compulsive disorder or obsessive-compulsive symptoms typically emerge after tics begin. These observations lend themselves to two types of prospective approaches: peer relations of ADHD children at risk for Tourette's could be assessed before and after the onset of tics; for obsessive-compulsive disorder, peer relations could be assessed in Tourette's syndrome children before and after the onset of obsessive-compulsive disorder or obsessive-compulsive symptoms. This line of work could also shed light on treatment priorities. In the context of peers, for example, is it best for interventions to target tics or co-occurring behavioral dysfunction? Clinical observations suggest the latter, yet as described below, very little is known about the impact of tics themselves on friendships and peer relationships.

Age of Onset of Tics

As discussed in Chapter 2 (Figure 2.4), the modal age of onset of tics in Tourette's syndrome is approximately 6 to 7 years; rarely, tics are first seen in children as young as 2 years or in youngsters in their late adolescence (Cohen & Leckman, 1994). Middle to late childhood (6 to 12 years) is thus a common time for tics to begin, a period that also marks an important transition in peer relations for children in general. Unlike the preschool years, school-age children are exposed to increased numbers of peers both in and out of school, as well as to increased diversity in the personalities and cultural backgrounds of the peer group.

Major shifts are also seen in children's games and play activities. Whereas the preschool years are marked by elaborate pretend play, games among school-age children show more divisions based on social status, leadership, roles, and teamwork. A rule-bound orientation dominates in both formal games (e.g., softball, board games), and informal games (e.g., tag, hide-and-seek). Not surprisingly, relative to younger children, school-age youngsters express considerable insecurity about their social acceptance and position among peers (e.g., Parker & Gottman, 1989). Further, alliances among friends, or who is "in" or "out," undergo rapid shifts. Verbal aggression is increasingly common, with hostilities aimed directly at peers instead of instrumental struggles over toys or space.

Against this developmental backdrop, the Tourette's child seems particularly vulnerable. For most children with Tourette's syndrome, their tics begin just when they are exposed to a larger, more diverse peer group and when they must negotiate peer interactions dominated by social status, shifting loyalties, and hostile verbal aggression. These features differ from the peer dynamics of the preschool years and from the demands for increased intimacy in later adolescence. Peer dynamics change across development, and so too may children's responses to their classmates' tics. Although speculative, conditions seem ripest for peer teasing and rejection of the Tourette's syndrome child during the school-age years. Future studies could test this hypothesis by examining peer relations in children whose tics begin in this period, and by comparing them to children showing earlier versus later tic onset.

Severity of Tics

Most ratings of tic severity emphasize the number, frequency, intensity, and complexity of tics, as well as the degree to which tics impede adaptive activities or speech (Leckman et al., 1989). Using one such scale, Stokes et al. (1991) found no significant relations between tic severity and peer adjustment.

Instead of tics per se, peer difficulties or poor social adjustment in children with Tourette's syndrome may be more strongly associated with one or more comorbid conditions. Yet before tic severity is dismissed as nonsignificant to peer relations, more detailed work is needed that describes how peers themselves view their classmates' tics. In the context of peer relations, tic severity ratings perhaps need to go beyond the judgment of clinicians to include assessments of how tics are understood or accepted by children. Children may have their own way of judging tic severity, or they may make judgments very similar to adults'. A tic that is rated by a clinician as mild because it is neither frequent nor forceful may actually stand out among peers as weird or odd, prompting much teasing (e.g., an infrequent yelp or bark). In contrast, other tics, even those that are frequent or forceful, may not stand out among peers (e.g., certain motor tics). Future work on peer relationships might thus assess tic severity through the eyes of both the clinician and the peer group.

Waxing and Waning of Tics

Tics show a variable course, waxing and waning in severity over time in any particular individual. Anxiety, fatigue, excitement, and psychosocial stresses have all been associated with increased symptom expression. But tics also worsen and remit without apparent provocation. Variability in tic expression poses interesting twists to the study of peer relationships.

It is unclear if the risk of peer rejection in Tourette's syndrome children changes with tic expression. On the one hand, research points to remarkable stability in children designated as popular or rejected; rejected children generally stay rejected and rarely become popular (e.g., Coie & Dodge, 1983; Newcomb & Bukowski, 1983). Such findings do not bode well for Tourette's syndrome children rejected by their peers.

On the other hand, children who receive transient as opposed to chronic ostracism from peers generally fare better in terms of behavioral outcome (DeRosier et al., 1994). If peer teasing of the Tourette's syndrome child is more intermittent, perhaps easing up as tics decline, then the outcome may be more favorable. On the down side, peer teasing may also serve as a stressor that exacerbates tic expression.

Although studies are needed, it may well be the case that peer responses to the Tourette's syndrome child change as the child's tics change, underscoring the need for effective interventions that reduce tics and comorbid conditions. Variable tic expression in Tourette's syndrome is also an ideal, naturally occurring laboratory to better understand how and why peer status does or does not change among children in general.

Family Variables

As with families in general, families of children with Tourette's are an important mediating agent for offspring's friendships and social adjustment. Certain parenting styles, for example, lend themselves to favorable peer outcomes. Rejected children have a greater likelihood of having parents who show ineffective, negative, and power-oriented discipline, and who also engage in poorly regulated, overstimulating interactions with their offspring. In contrast, socially accepted children tend to have parents who are more feelings-oriented and who use more positive disciplinary skills and inductive reasoning with their offspring (see Parker et al., 1995 for a review).

It is unclear how these or other factors operate in families with a Tourette's syndrome child. Children with Tourette's syndrome generally fare better when their parents accept their disorder and do not blame or punish them for their tic symptomatology. Supporting these clinical observations, Carter et al. (1994) examined children either with Tourette's syndrome or at risk for Tourette's syndrome. They found positive correlations between children's views of maternal acceptance and Vineland socialization skills. Relationships may also exist between Tourette's syndrome children's perceptions of parental efficacy or competence and diminished peer ratings of aggression (Stokes et al., 1991). Although additional work is needed, it appears that Tourette's syndrome children fare better in the social arena when they perceive their parents as being supportive, accepting, effective, and tolerant.

School Variables

Teachers and other school personnel play a critical role in how children with Tourette's syndrome fare both academically and socially (Scahill, Lynch, & Ort, 1995; Scahill, Ort, & Hardin, 1993a, 1993b). Parents, teachers, and clinicians all agree that the Tourette's syndrome child adapts better to the classroom when school staff are knowledgeable about Tourette's syndrome and are well versed in the syndrome's wide range of expression. With such knowledge, teachers often provide a supportive classroom environment for their Tourette's syndrome students.

Yet many teachers and schools remain uninformed about Tourette's syndrome. Shady et al. (1988) found that 70% of teachers surveyed were "not at all" knowledgeable about Tourette's. Close to half of these noted their need for information about the syndrome, including specific behavioral or teaching strategies for the Tourette's syndrome student. Remaining respondents felt that nothing could be done to improve the Tourette's syndrome student's school situation. Not surprisingly, then, approximately half of Tourette's syndrome students in both Shady et al.'s and Jagger et al.'s (1982) surveys admitted to difficulties getting along with their teachers. Sadly, Jagger et al. reported that almost a quarter of their adolescent sample had teachers who had teased or ridiculed them about their Tourette's syndrome symptoms. These studies were conducted over 10 year ago, and may not reflect more recent efforts from Tourette's syndrome organizations to educate teachers and the general public about Tourette's syndrome. Up-to-date research is needed, then, on what teachers understand about Tourette's syndrome, how they perceive their students with Tourette's syndrome, and how their perceptions facilitate or impede the social adjustment and peer relations of Tourette's syndrome students.

FUTURE DIRECTIONS

Relative to other aspects of Tourette's syndrome, research on friendships, peers, and social adaptation is in its beginning stages. As discussed in Chapter 1, many research questions are of key concern to parents and clinicians alike: What factors are associated with optimal peer relations and social-adaptive functioning? Which children are at greatest risk for social maladjustment in adulthood, and why? There are no easy answers, but as this chapter highlights, progress can be made by borrowing insights from peer research in children in general, and by building on rich clinical observations about the course of this syndrome.

Although it remains sketchy, a picture is slowly emerging of the relations between Tourette's syndrome and ultimate peer and adaptive functioning. Clinically, we (Cohen & Leckman, 1992) observe that people with Tourette's syndrome do best when they feel relatively good about themselves, are warmly engaged with their families, have capacities for friendship and humor, and are less burdened by attentional and other problems, especially aggression.

Such observations speak to a transactional model of peer relations and social adaptation (e.g., Samaroff, 1987). In this model, factors within the child (e.g., tics, ADHD, obsessive-compulsive disorder, esteem, personality), as well as in the environment (e.g., family, school) undergo continual change, influencing one another over the course of time. How children with Tourette's syndrome view themselves and their disorder, for example, is shaped by information derived from others: parents, teachers, and classmates. Their self-concept, in turn, influences their interactions with family, friends, and peers, and all this occurs in a never-ending cycle across development.

It is thus an oversimplification of complex interactions to say that Tourette's syndrome in and of itself causes or predicts poor social-adaptive outcomes, or that peer rejection (regardless of the cause) should take the sole blame for later maladjustment. Instead, as emphasized in our evolving model of pathogenesis (Chapter 9), treatment needs to take into account the multiple factors in the child, family, and school that influence one another over time.

It is not always clear, then, which children are at greatest risk for social maladjustment in adulthood—for difficulties on the job or in their marriages. The Tourette's syndrome child who does well with friends in the school years may flounder with the increased demands for friendship and intimacy in adolescence and young adulthood. Conversely, those Tourette's syndrome children who are rejected by classmates may take advantage of new social opportunities afforded by symptom declines in later adolescence and ultimately do quite well. Determining how best to foster such resiliency in a particular child is a recurrent challenge for clinicians.

As discussed in Chapters 1, 8, 15, and 18, our anecdotal experience is that many children with Tourette's syndrome show immediate benefits from interventions aimed at improving their symptomatology and social skills. Although pharmacotherapy is one type of intervention, and peer acceptance may indeed be better among Tourette's syndrome children receiving medication for their symptomatology (Stokes et al., 1991), other interventions have also increased peer acceptance among children with or without Tourette's. Some interventions provide informal opportunities for increased peer interaction in positive, goal-oriented ways; examples include joining a sports team, band, or Scout troop. Other interventions are more formal and intensive, such as therapy groups or specialized curricula that teach social skills. These therapy programs are likely to meet with more success and improved peer acceptance when they simultaneously decrease aggressive behavior and teach positive social skills (Bierman, 1986).

Of note, however, is that not all children with Tourette's syndrome need special intervention or even show peer or socialization difficulties. As most research relies on clinic samples, epidemiologic studies are needed to identify the extent to which peer problems are seen in the nonreferred population of people with Tourette's syndrome. A recent population-based study found that although chronic tics were common in children (4%), as many as two-thirds of these children showed no functional impairment (Costello, Angold, Burns, Stangl, Tweed, & Erkanli, 1996). Although peer adjustment was not specifically examined, Costello and colleagues' findings suggest that if peer problems are present, they are more likely to be associated with comorbid conditions rather than with tics per se.

Other research approaches can also help identify the range and causes of peer difficulties in children with Tourette's syndrome. These include following children at risk for Tourette's over time and observing peer functioning relative to tic onset, as well as comparing peer relationships in at-risk children who do or do not develop tics. Preliminary findings from one study of at-risk children suggest that family relations are important mediators of child psychiatric disorders but not of tic disorders (Carter et al., 1994). Findings again implicate comorbid conditions as important mediators of the child's response to having tics. Finally, family genetic studies could also shed light on social-adaptive and peer functioning. It may be, for example, that the inheritance risks for socialization problems in children with tics vary across families, with some families showing a greater inheritance risk for co-occurring tics and peer difficulties than others.

With improved research methodologies and measures, many unanswered questions about peer relationships in children with Tourette's syndrome may soon be answered, including the long-term adaptive adjustment of these children. Indeed, the time is ripe to link the remarkable genetic and neurologic advances in Tourette's syndrome to social and adaptive functioning. Such work adopts a *whole person* approach, examining ties between specific Tourette's syndrome symptoms, tics, and comorbidity, and functioning in everyday life. Until such future research can better inform us, all children with Tourette's syndrome should be evaluated with an eye toward informal or formal interventions that can improve and sustain their friendships, peer relations, and social-adaptive adjustment.

SUMMARY OF CHAPTER 6

Peer relationships are a crucial aspect of growing up. Tourette's syndrome patients can face formidable obstacles from their peers: prejudice, stigmatization, and teasing. Many Tourette's patients show marked delays in their social-emotional development. Are these difficulties solely the consequence of the tics and Tourettic displays, or do they form some deeper part of the Tourette's syndrome phenotype? With some exceptions, we see these delays in social development as reactive to an ignorant and disapproving culture. Certain personality traits and the presence of a concerned circle of friends, on the other hand, can do much to buffer these adversities. Although we know little about how best to encourage resiliency and to protect the child from these assaults, many of our therapeutic interventions are directed at this end. We will return to this topic in Section Three.

PREVIEW OF CHAPTER 7

Does this child really have Tourette's syndrome or some related form of illness, or is it some other neurological or psychiatric disturbance? On rare occasions, this is a life-and-death question. We next review features of the extended Tourette's syndrome phenotype and consider formally the question of differential diagnosis.

CHAPTER 7

Differential Diagnosis

KENNETH E. TOWBIN, BRADLEY S. PETERSON, DONALD J. COHEN,
and JAMES F. LECKMAN

> Everything should be made as simple as possible, but not simpler.
>
> *—Albert Einstein*

> There are no whole truths; all truths are half-truths. It is trying to treat
> them as whole truths that plays the devil.
>
> *—Alfred North Whitehead, 1954*

Psychiatric diagnosis is an uncertain art. In creating a diagnostic system, clinicians and researchers have evolved a common language that is based on behaviors, observable features, and the reports patients have offered about distressing mental experiences. With each new version of the diagnostic system, there has been an attempt to produce increasingly refined categories. This process aims to forge categories or labels that correspond exactly to disease entities—entities that possess discrete diagnostic boundaries, a definite pathophysiology, specific symptoms, and characteristic natural histories. Despite these valuable efforts, we have yet to achieve diagnoses that are congruent to diseases. The promise of sensitive and specific biologically based diagnostic tests has been realized for some neurological syndromes, but for most conditions the boundaries dividing one disorder from another remain much more nebulous.

A problem that follows from this uncertainty is the complication generated by acting as if we can discover the exact diagnosis when the boundaries between diagnoses are so vague. Under these conditions, does the pursuit of *the* diagnosis help in the care of patients and their families? Ideally, making the right diagnosis will aid clinicians in advising patients and families on what to expect and how best to intervene. But under suboptimal conditions, does this perspective hold out the same promise?

118

In this chapter, we address this complexity. Building on the contents of earlier chapters we present a brief reprise of the distinctive features of tic disorders, obsessive compulsive disorder, and attention deficit hyperactivity disorder in an effort to distinguish them from each other and from neighboring hyperkinetic and psychopathological disorders. We then offer a modest compendium of case histories selected to illustrate several key features and to acknowledge the conundrums and vagaries of the diagnostic process. The chapter concludes with a consideration of the differences between diagnoses and disorders and points to the unity that may underlie these conditions when viewed through genetics and neurobiology as opposed to diagnoses.

THE DIAGNOSTIC LANDSCAPE

At one time tic disorders and Tourette's syndrome were regarded as unusual "boutique" conditions. The treatment and care of persons with tic disorders were entrusted to those with specific interest and experience or investigators who were particularly attentive to the pharmacotherapy and etiology of movement disorders. Over the past three decades, Tourette's syndrome and tic disorders have emerged from relative obscurity to assume importance for generalist clinicians in pediatrics, child psychiatry, and neurology. Several developments account for this change. First, there has been a heightened awareness that tics are common in children. Second, there is mounting data suggesting that the presence of tics is relevant to treatment choice and prognosis for a variety of symptoms. Finally, the foremost development is the consensus that the presence management of tics, and their associated features, enhances the adaptation, development, and prognosis of children with these conditions.

Consequently, it is more important than ever for clinicians to know the characteristics of tics and other hyperkinetic movement disorders, the diverse manifestations of tic disorders, and other symptoms that are commonly associated with tics. It is evident that children with tic disorders display a variety of other symptoms, some of which also are impairing and affect daily living. Over time, it has become increasingly recognizable that tic disorders encompass a wider array of symptoms than simple movements.

There has been a long-standing interest in identifying features associated with Tourette's syndrome. A major question was the extent to which such associated features are truly core symptoms of Tourette's syndrome or comorbid findings. A description of associated features of Tourette's syndrome was advanced by Gilles de la Tourette himself (Goetz & Klawans, 1992). This was given further support as investigators sampled clinic populations. Early studies reported high rates of comorbidity and associated symptoms in patients who presented for treatment (Fernando, 1967; Morphew & Sim, 1969; Nee et al., 1980).

Yet these findings were dubious. Researchers had long been aware that samples drawn from clinics represented a select group. *Compound* disorders are more common in patients who seek treatment. It is possible that those in the clinic seek care precisely because they suffer multiple disorders. Consequently, their clinical presentation does not reflect accurately the frequency of many symptoms in the general population of persons with tics or Tourette's syndrome. Concern about the artifact of what is known as Berkson's Bias (Berkson, 1946) steadily declined as longitudinal studies and better community surveys followed. However, it was also apparent that those with multiple conditions were more likely to seek treatment (Caine et al., 1988) and that clinic samples do overestimate the frequency of these comorbid conditions.

Later studies suggested that in persons with Tourette's syndrome, the early course displayed frequent problems with inattention, distractibility, and impulsivity resembling attention-deficit/hyperactivity disorder (ADHD; Bornstein et al., 1990; Comings & Comings, 1987a). During the course of their disorder, they reported excessive rates of obsessive-compulsive symptoms sufficient to meet criteria for disorder (Bornstein et al., 1990; Frankel et al., 1986). Soon, many thought there was a connection among obsessive-compulsive disorder, ADHD, and Tourette's syndrome. Did Tourette's syndrome produce obsessive-compulsive disorder and symptoms of ADHD, or was this comorbidity?

As discussed in Chapter 11, genetic studies also had a role in clarifying what belongs to Tourette's syndrome and what might be an artifact of sampling methods. Family genetic studies of Tourette's syndrome probands reported high rates of both obsessive-compulsive disorder and ADHD. Yet, in first-degree relatives, the findings for obsessive-compulsive disorder and ADHD diverged. Among first-degree relatives who did not exhibit tics or Tourette's syndrome, highly elevated rates of obsessive-compulsive disorder were discovered whether the proband had obsessive-compulsive disorder or not (Pauls, Towbin, et al., 1986). But rates of ADHD were only elevated if the proband had Tourette's syndrome and ADHD (Pauls, Hurst, et al., 1986; Pauls et al., 1993). Evidence that first-degree relatives who did not have tics displayed obsessive-compulsive disorder implied that obsessive-compulsive disorder might be an alternative expression of the same genetic cause of Tourette's syndrome (Pauls & Leckman, 1986; Pauls, Towbin, et al., 1986). Subsequently, models based on patterns of inheritance that used obsessive-compulsive disorder and chronic motor tics (CMT) as alternative manifestations of a Tourette's syndrome gene provided the closest fit to family study data (Pauls & Leckman). Models that relied solely on inheritance of Tourette's syndrome or Tourette's syndrome and ADHD or combinations of Tourette's syndrome, CMT, obsessive-compulsive disorder, and ADHD did not fit the data well (Pauls & Leckman, 1986; Pauls et al., 1993). In a reciprocal way, investigation of tics and Tourette's syndrome in populations ascertained for obsessive-compulsive disorder (Riddle et al., 1990; Swedo, Rapoport, Leonard, Lenane, & Cheslow, 1989) or ADHD (Biederman et al.,

1992, 1996) also demonstrated much higher than expected rates of tics and Tourette's syndrome. Longitudinal studies of these subjects following initial evaluation revealed subsequent development of very high rates of Tourette's syndrome or tics (Biederman et al., 1996; Leonard et al., 1992).

It thus seems that tic disorders may be closely associated with obsessive-compulsive disorder and that ADHD symptoms commonly arise early in the course of those with Tourette's syndrome and CMT disorders. Acknowledgment that tics, obsessions, compulsions, and symptoms of fidgetiness, impulsivity, and distractibility can co-occur has now found its way into the diagnostic characterization of ADHD and obsessive-compulsive disorder (*DSM-IV*, APA, 1994). The close association among these syndromes means that a comprehensive review of tic disorders should include a discussion of obsessive-compulsive disorder and ADHD as well.

DIFFERENTIAL DIAGNOSTIC CONSIDERATIONS

Differential Diagnosis of Tics

Distinguishing tics from other movement disorders that have an onset in childhood can usually be readily accomplished by obtaining a careful history and direct observations. Although there are no definitive laboratory tests or pathognomonic signs, the movements themselves do exhibit characteristics that are uncommon in other movement disorders. Tics are rapid, periodic, stereotyped muscle contractions. They may affect any part of the body but characteristically begin in the face and, over time, involve other muscle groups, spreading to the neck, shoulders, trunk, legs, and feet in a rostral to caudal migration. Involvement of the entire body in this migratory pattern does not always occur; it is common that the face and upper areas develop symptoms before the trunk and lower extremities. In addition, tics are temporarily suppressible, variable in frequency, location, and intensity, and diminish during sleep. More recently, it has been reported that they are accompanied by mental components of anticipation or a vague awareness.

The suppressibility of tics often is puzzling to patients and parents. If tics may be postponed for some interval, then the presumption is made that they ought to be suppressible for longer periods and at critical moments. Occasionally, this level of control can be achieved but it is rare, and even more rare that such control can be applied dependably. The ability to suppress movements for short periods is characteristic in tic disorders and can distinguish them from other childhood-onset repetitive movements such as chorea or dystonia.

As reviewed in Chapter 2, tics are highly variable in their location. On any day or across weeks, the movements of a part of the body appear highly stereotyped, but over weeks to months it is common for the location and type of movement to change. Additional regions may become affected.

Similarly, parts of the body that have been affected may become quiet; tics may return later or move on to involve yet another site. This kind of migration is not exhibited in dystonias, myoclonus, and athetosis. In addition, tics are typically variable in their intensity and frequency. Like many other movement disorders, emotion and intention may influence tics; emotional arousal may produce increasing frequency and intensity of tics in some persons. Changes may occur in reaction to any intense emotion, not only stress; increasing frequency or severity may be seen in association with emotions as diverse as anxiety, eager anticipation, and the thrill of success.

Tics typically diminish with sleep, but they may not disappear entirely (Glaze, Frost, & Jankovic, 1983). This contrasts with the complete disappearance of chorea and the dystonias during sleep. Another distinguishing feature of tics is the decrease in movements with intention. Carrying out purposeful acts such as pointing reduces the frequency and intensity of tics. This is the opposite of what occurs with other movements disorders, particularly chorea.

One of the most intriguing features of tics is the emergence of premonitory urges (Leckman, Walker, et al., 1993). This term denotes somatic, sensory, or ideational symptoms that precede tics. Persons report diverse experiences such as needs, urges, prickly feelings, and tension that build prior to and are relieved by tic movements. Studies of persons with Tourette's syndrome suggest that premonitory urges are common—reported by 75–90% of adults—and first occur on average, several years after the tics themselves (Kurlan, Lichter, & Hewitt, 1989; Leckman, Walker, et al., 1993). Premonitory urges do not occur in other movement disorders and can be an important differential diagnostic clue. In addition, they link cognitive, motor, and sensory functions. Their existence is considered an important sign of the involvement of a cortico-striao-thalamo-cortical circuit in the production and maintenance of symptoms.

Tics may be categorized as simple or complex, distinctions that may be applied to both motor and phonic symptoms. The discrimination may be useful in determining the severity and extent of the disorder. Simple tics are rapid and involve only a small number of muscle groups or confined areas. Complex tics tend to be longer lasting and involve combinations or a number of groups in orchestrated bouts or a stereotyped series of actions. Examples of a simple motor tic are a wink, a quick puckering movement of the lips, a shoulder jerk, and a quick kicking-out movement of a leg. Examples of complex motor tics are copying of another person's movements (echopraxia), pushing against one's own stomach, repetive tapping on a desk or one's face, and repeated turning in pirouettes while walking. Simple phonic tics are rapid, short sounds such as "hawks," grunts, and short coughs. Complex phonic tics are longer, more formed utterances such as protracted throat clearing, repeating others' words or phrases (echolalia), or repeating one's own words or phrases (palilalia). In general, simple motor or phonic tics are the first symptoms to emerge. Simple tics may occur without complex tics, but it is unusual to see only complex tics; such a presentation should inspire the clinician to investigate the differential diagnosis with care.

Blocking is a symptom that occurs in some individuals with tics and Tourette's syndrome (Fahn, 1993), but is highly unusual in other movement disorders. At a surface level, blocking resembles the akinesia of Parkinson's disease, in that there is a sense of being unable to initiate or implement a movement. However, blocking has a much shorter duration when compared to akinesia. In general, Parkinsonian patients report difficulty initiating movement that diminishes as the movement progresses and can be overcome with sustained effort. Persons with Tourette's syndrome report that they cannot initiate movements even with effort. The overall pattern of symptoms, their duration, and the presence of premonitory urges or sensory experiences that accompany tics facilitate differentiating them from other conditions such as dystonia, akinesia, or myoclonus that also can impede initiating movement.

In summary, tics are rapid movements that may be phonic or motor and over time show considerable variability in their intensity, location, and type. Tics are paradoxical; they are stereotyped and at the same time characteristically changeable. Features of premonitory urges, suppressibility, intention reactivity, and continuation during sleep are highly distinctive of tics and should be borne in mind when considering the diagnosis of other movement disorders.

The primary differential diagnostic considerations stem from the morphology, rhythm, and influences on movements. Movement disorders may be divided into continuous and paroxysmal types (Fahn, 1993). Continuous movements are athetosis, chorea, tremor, myoclonus, dyskinesia, and the dystonias. Paroxysmal disorders are tics, the hyperekplexias (paroxysmal kinesiogenic choreoathetosis and paroxysmal dystonic choreoathetosis), paroxysmal ataxia, and paroxysmal tremor. Stereotypies may also be considered to be paroxysmal movement disorders. Differentiating tics from other movements may be difficult when there are unusual presentations of typical movements, such as when tics are so frequent as to be nearly continuous, or when a movement is seen without sufficient information about its history and progression. However, when the movements are typical and their broader context is gathered, the predicament of diagnosis usually is eased. Table 7.1 offers several features that may be helpful in differentiating tics from other forms of childhood-onset movement disorder (Fahn & Erenberg, 1988).

There has been recent interest in tics that arise subsequent to streptococcal or viral infection. Morphologically, these tics may be indistinguishable from tics that are not postinfectious in origin. The concept of tics or Tourette's syndrome, as opposed to chorea, arising following infection is still new and much remains to be learned about it (Swedo, Leonard, & Kiessling, 1994). Researchers in this area emphasize that history and laboratory verification are critical to confirming the association (A. Allen, Leonard, & Swedo, 1995; Swedo et al., 1998). Some features of Sydenham's

TABLE 7.1   Differential Diagnostic Considerations of Stereotyped Movements

	Simple Clonic Movement	Complex Clonic Movement	Abrupt	Suppressible	Effect of Distraction[f]
Tics	++	++	++	++	↓
Chorea	+	—	+[c]	±	↑
Dystonia	+[a]	±[b]	—	—	↓↑
Myoclonus	+	—	+[d]	—	↓↑
Dyskinesias	—	—	+[e]	—	↑↑
Restless legs	—	—	—	—	—
Akathisia	—	+	—	+	↓
Stereotypy	—	+	—	+	↓

Key:

— Not characteristic	E-↑ Increases w. effort
R-↓ Decreases w. relaxed	R-↑ Increases w. relaxed
↓ Decreases	↑↑ Marked increase
↑ Increases	++ Highly characteristic
+ Typical or characteristic	E-↓ Decreases w. effort
± Seen uncommonly	↓↑ Variable response

[a] Myoclonic dystonia may be a brief, clonic movement; other forms are slower, more protracted.
[b] Complex clonic movements are rare in dystonia, but do occur (Stone & Jankovic, 1991).

chorea (SC) may be confused with tics, particularly when movements are simple and rapid. However, in general, the choreiform movements of SC are continuous, not stereotyped, and obey the morphological characteristics of chorea. SC movements increase with intention and prevent an individual from maintaining sustained contractions (e.g., "milkmaid's grasp"). The rapid onset or exacerbation of symptoms should suggest the possibility of a postinfectious influence or etiology.

Differential Diagnosis of Obsessive-Compulsive Disorder

The clinical meanings of obsession and compulsion are narrower and more specific than their familiar or public connotations. In popular use, compulsion suggests a range of behaviors from cleanliness to excessive fastidiousness, punctuality, rigidity, or an unreasonable pursuit of accuracy. Similarly, the common implication of obsession suggests a voluntary preoccupation, a consuming mental undertaking, or a romantic infatuation. The widespread use of these words in popular culture has influenced their clinical application and blurred their meaning. As a result, there has been an erosion of the concepts originally conveyed by these terms and so it is worthwhile to review their explicit clinical connotations.

As discussed in Chapter 3, obsessions and compulsions are precise terms for psychiatric symptoms that exhibit specific characteristics. *Obsessions* are mental events such as thoughts, images, or urges; however,

Movement Relieves Tension	Effects of Relaxation or Effort[f]	Present during Sleep	Associated w. Inattention or Impulsivity-Hyperactivity	Associated w. Obsessions or Compulsions
+	R-↑, E-↓	+	±	+
—	E-↑[g]	—	±	±
—	E-↑	—	—	—
—	E-↑	+	—	—
—	E-↑ (mild)	—	—	—
++	0	++	—	—
++	↓↑	—	—	—
±	R-↑, E-↓	—	—	+

[c] Mild chorea can lead to confusion. Usually chorea presents as a continuous flow of *nonstereotyped* movements.

[d] If arrhythmic type; movements often described as "shocklike" and "stimulus sensitive" (P. Brown & Marsden, 1992).

[e] Brief paroxysmal type is rare, can be abrupt, occur in bouts, and is often preceded by a sensory aura. Hyperekplexias are a subtype. Typically related to another disorder, or familial. Movements are dystoniclike (Goetz & Bennett, 1992).

[f] *Adapted from* Lang (1992) and Fahn and Erenberg (1988).

[g] "Motor impersistence" or inability to maintain a sustained contraction is highly characteristic.

these events are excessive and go far beyond typical worries or concerns. In fact, the most recent diagnostic criteria *(DSM-IV)* underscore the difference between worries that arise in reaction to actual life stressors and the excess, irrationality, and relative groundlessness of obsessions. Obsessions exhibit definite characteristics; they are incessant, taxing, and difficult (or impossible) to suppress. They impede ordinary mental activity and commonly have a subjectively revolting content. Obsessions force themselves on a person and distract him or her from volitional thinking. As a result, obsessions usually produce significant anxiety and distress. Despite this distress, embarrassment over the content and shame about the impairment may prevent a person from disclosing the obsession to anyone.

In many ways, *compulsions* are a behavioral parallel to obsessions. Compulsions, too, exhibit recurrence, intractability, intrusiveness, and pointless excess. However, compulsions are repetitive behaviors or mental acts that a person feels he or she must carry out *(DSM-IV)*. This demand may arise in reaction to an obsession or according to exacting idiosyncratic rules. Often, compulsions are attempts to fend off a dreaded event or reduce the distress produced by an obsession. Like obsessions, compulsions are strikingly excessive. Although they are responses to obsessional fears, compulsive behaviors may be logically remote from the event they are intended to avert. Like obsessions, they produce significant subjective distress, are time-consuming, and interfere in the person's life.

Under stringent *DSM-IV* criteria, the threshold of time that is necessary to reach clinical levels of impairment is at least one hour each day; however, even less time may be needed if there is definite impairment in social, occupational, family, or academic functioning.

People with obsessions or compulsions often display characteristic responses to their symptoms. "Resistance" is the term applied to describe a person's attempts to overlook, subdue, or neutralize obsessions or compulsions. In addition, he or she may well avoid situations that would provoke such thoughts or acts. Also, it is typical that a person with obsessions or compulsions recognizes that these thoughts, images, or urges are a product of the person's own mind. This insight may deteriorate or fluctuate over time or during periods of extreme intensity, but it should be manifest at some time during the course of the disorder.

Obsessive compulsive *personality disorder* may be confused with obsessive compulsive disorder. This misunderstanding may be a product of generalizing about perfectionism, fastidiousness, and compulsions. Although persons with obsessive compulsive disorder and obsessive compulsive personality disorder may display fastidiousness, the source and objects of these behaviors are quite different. Persons with obsessive compulsive disorder typically are themselves anxious and distressed about their symptoms and are making (or have made) earnest, even desperate efforts to suppress or re-direct their anxieties. When these efforts fail they may resort to avoidance and increasing isolation. In contrast, persons with obsessive compulsive *personality disorder* do not exhibit compulsions, as just described. Persons with obsessive compulsive personality are distressing to those around them more than they themselves are distressed by their strivings for control, efficiency, orderliness, and punctuality. The desire for orderliness and efficiency in persons with obsessive compulsive personality disorder can supersede all other values and assume an importance that leaves the person devoid of warmth or attachment to others. Persons with obsessive compulsive disorder commonly are trapped by their symptoms and anxious, but interpersonally sensitive and capable of empathy. Persons with obsessive compulsive personality more commonly are aloof, rigid, self-righteous individuals who are socially and occupationally impaired as a result of the burden their self-centered demands produce for others. Persons with obsessive compulsive disorder most wish they could control themselves and their symptoms; persons with obsessive compulsive personality wish to control others so that they can achieve perfection, more efficiency, or order.

The differential diagnostic considerations in obsessive-compulsive disorder are more complex than has been generally appreciated (Towbin, 1987). This is a product, in part, of the many conditions that also display symptoms of obsessions or compulsions but are not obsessive-compulsive disorder. In addition, obsessive-compulsive disorder itself also shows high rates of comorbidity. This creates confusion and risks errors of omission. For clinicians and researchers who do not characterize their patients completely, comorbid or primary conditions may be overlooked. This stems from the tendency to identify obsessions or compulsions in isolation without sufficient recognition of the background or context whence they come. As a result, clinicians may jump too quickly to a final diagnosis of obsessive-compulsive disorder or stop the differential diagnostic engine once obsessions or compulsions are discovered. When a clinician tries only to confirm the presence of obsessions or compulsions and then goes on to equate this with the diagnosis of obsessive-compulsive disorder, he or she risks missing other conditions within which obsessions or compulsions may arise, but are not obsessive-compulsive disorder.

Some of this confusion arose with revisions in the diagnostic criteria. *DSM-III* (APA, 1980) ignored the distinction between obsessive-compulsive disorder and other disorders that might display obsessions or compulsions as a part of the symptom picture. Prior to *DSM-III-R* (APA, 1987), for example, anorexia nervosa patients who had frequent, intrusive, reproachful thoughts about how much they had eaten were considered to have two diagnoses: obsessive-compulsive disorder and anorexia nervosa. Experienced clinicians did not believe this was a reliable way to group obsessive-compulsive disorder patients and, for *DSM-IV,* both obsessive and compulsive symptoms of obsessive-compulsive disorder had to be independent of another disorder if a comorbid condition existed.

Another part of the confusion is the difficulty in recognizing the features of preoccupations or intrusive thoughts that are a part of other disorders. Table 7.2 provides a list of conditions that commonly display obsessions or compulsions as a part of the presentation. Consideration of these other possible conditions is critical in the care of a patient whether they are primary or comorbid with obsessive-compulsive disorder. An appreciation of the context of the symptoms is critical in approaching treatment and choosing treatment modalities. It also has significant ramifications for treatment management and prognosis once the modalities have been selected (Towbin, 1995).

Differential Diagnosis of ADHD

Attention-deficit/hyperactivity disorder (ADHD) is a syndromic collection of symptoms that originate from excessive motor activity, distractibility, inattention, poor concentration, and impulsivity. This constellation of symptoms has been recognized, under assorted labels, for over 40 years. It is certainly one of the most common diagnoses of children and adolescents (Szatmari, 1992), and some of these symptoms are among the most frequent complaints that parents bring about their children when seeking an evaluation (Costello et al., 1988). It is a widespread practice in the United States to propose this disorder as an explanation for academic difficulties.

The prevalence and morbidity of this condition have generated a great deal of interest and research effort. Much of it has focused on verifying that the disorder qualifies as a discrete diagnostic entity. Consequently,

TABLE 7.2   Conditions in Which Obsessions or Compulsions May Be Evident

Anorexia nervosa (including bulimia nervosa)
Body dysmorphic disorder
Delusional disorder (all types)
Depression
Generalized anxiety disorder
Hypochondriasis
Obsessive compulsive disorder
Obsessive-compulsive personality disorder
Schizotypal personality
Schizophrenia
Separation anxiety disorder
Somatization disorder
Somatoform disorders
Trichotillomania
Tourette's syndrome
"Fear of AIDS"
Organic mental disorder (or obsessions or compulsions due to a medical disorder)
Panic disorder
Pervasive developmental disorder (including autism and Asperger's syndrome)
Phobias
Post-traumatic stress disorder (PTSD)

there are many studies pointing to the presence of biological (McCracken, 1991; Zametkin et al., 1990, 1993), genetic (Biederman et al., 1992; Pauls, Hurst, et al., 1986), cognitive (Barkley et al., 1992; Benson, 1991), and prognostic (Barkley, DuPaul, & McMurray, 1990; Hechtman, Weiss, Perlman, & Amsel, 1984; Mannuzza, Klein, Bessler, Malloy, & LaPadula, 1993) features that are particularly common to individuals with these symptoms. There has been an additional flurry of interest recently in residual symptoms that are believed to affect social and occupational adaptation in adults (L. Silver, 1992).

As presented in Chapter 4, the current diagnostic criteria are empirically based and begin with observable signs that can be perceived by parents and teachers. Children with ADHD have difficulties in school, in their homes, or in their peer group as a result of their inattention, restlessness, and impulsivity. Their inattention leads them to disregard comments and instructions; they forget things and cannot get organized. Their impetuousness engenders carelessness and impatience. High levels of distractibility with these other features hamper their effectiveness in completing things and keeping their belongings in order. *DSM-IV* has arranged symptoms in two separate categories—inattention and hyperactivity/impulsivity—based on their factor-analyzed association in persons with the disorder. The majority of criteria are framed in a manner that relates specifically to classroom behaviors, such as careless mistakes in schoolwork, inattention to work tasks, failure to follow through on instructions, difficulty in initiating school and homework, leaving one's classroom seat frequently, and precipitously blurting out answers to questions. Also, several of the criteria focus on symptoms that may be exhibited with peers or family apart from school.

However, the diagnosis is based on more than the manifestation of symptoms of inattention and hyperactivity or impulsivity. The behaviors must be more than merely present: they must be relatively pervasive, seen in more than one setting, and in relationship to a child's other traits. Any behavior must be considered in light of other conditions or adversities a child is facing. It is critical to view symptoms within the context of the child's age and developmental level and to consider his or her background. Elements of the child's life such as his or her medical health, caretaking climate, and exposure to psychosocial stress must be weighed. The criteria highlight that the age at which symptoms emerge is early, before age 7 for *DSM-IV*. In addition, it can be readily recognized that behaviors like inordinate activity and inattention are very common in children; quantitative judgments about how excessive such behaviors may be are subjective. As a result, an assessment is more credible when one obtains similar opinions from several adults who see the child in comparable settings.

As with obsessive-compulsive disorder, there is a high risk of overlooking other conditions or the contribution of hardships in life circumstances when one seeks to only verify the presence of symptoms of ADHD. The emergence in a variety of situations of symptoms such as impulsivity, poor concentration, and excessive activity imposes a responsibility on the clinician to consider other disorders ahead of ADHD. For this reason, the criteria stress that symptoms of ADHD cannot be a product of another disorder or developmental condition such as mood disorders, anxiety disorders, pervasive developmental disorders, personality disorders, or mental retardation. Table 7.3 identifies conditions that may produce symptoms like ADHD or are frequently comorbid with ADHD.

ATYPICAL CASES: THE CONFUSION OF COMPOUND SYMPTOMS

Despite the best attempts to categorize symptoms and unequivocally link them to discrete disorders, nature and biology provide endless examples that violate seemingly reliable guidelines and definitions. Atypical presentations are very common within the triad of ADHD, Tourette's syndrome, and obsessive-compulsive disorder. It is as if these symptoms perpetually display a kind of resistance to falling naturally into clear, organized, dependable patterns. For clinicians, this characteristic evokes uncertainty and apprehension as well as limitless fascination. By contrast, for the patients whom these clinicians treat, this disarray often produces disappointment, doubt, and anxiety.

TABLE 7.3   Conditions in Which Inattention, Distractibility, or Impulsivity Are Seen

ADHD
Autism (especially high functioning autism)
Bereavement
Communication disorders
Conduct disorder
Degenerative psychoses
Depression
Generalized anxiety disorder
Learning disorders
Mental retardation
Oppositional defiant disorder
Pervasive developmental disorders (Asperger's syndrome or PDDNOS)
Post-traumatic stress disorder (PTSD)
Separation anxiety disorder
Substance abuse disorders
Schizophrenia
Tourette's disorder

Obviously, it is not feasible to describe all situations or even generalize about the atypical presentations that produce this uncertainty and puzzlement. But there are circumstances that produce this confusion more commonly and warrant description. The more frequent atypical circumstances are when (a) tics and obsessions occur together, (b) inattention, impulsivity, and distractibility arise along with tics, and (c) obsessions are seen along with inattention and distractibility in the absence of hyperactivity. There is also uncertainty when compulsions are disclosed but exist at a level beneath any threshold of impairment; consequently, they do not warrant being deemed pathological, despite some symptoms being present. What follows is an example of patients with obsessive-compulsive disorder and Tourette's syndrome occurring simultaneously:

Case Example. Bill was diagnosed with diabetes mellitus at 3 years of age and a malabsorption disorder at 6. When he was 8 he developed obsessions. Doubts and ritualized mental events such as counting to himself, making mental lists, and needing to complete things in a certain sequence began to affect his academic performance. Bill worsened over the next two years; from classes for talented and gifted students, he became so impaired that he could no longer attend school. Racked by doubts and frustrated by his decline, he began to throw and break things with little provocation. He had been started on fluoxetine, and the doses increased to 120 mg per day. Partial benefit had been achieved but at the expense of substantial side effects—nervousness, sleep difficulties, and emotional blunting. Despite these doses, he continued to have severe obsessional symptoms and impairment. At age 12, he was noted to have a variety of simple motor tics. Infrequent vocal sounds—a kind of "hup"—were audible. He received the diagnosis of obsessive-compulsive disorder and Tourette's syndrome. The Tourette's syndrome diagnosis was mentioned vaguely during a last meeting with the departing clinician; according to Bill and his parents, its implication was insignificant. Over the next six years he remained on high doses of fluoxetine, and attempts to offer psychotherapy were thwarted by his inconsistent attendance. Bill was "too angry and frustrated" to listen, he lamented. Pharmacologic augmentation strategies with lithium and buspirone were attempted without effect. Attempts to provide psychotherapy throughout this time were not helpful. Upon transfer to another clinician, the Tourette's syndrome diagnosis was overlooked. Bill refused to attend psychodynamic psychotherapy treatment, although he remained on his medication. Several weeks on 2 mg of haloperidol per day plus fluoxetine resulted in profound sedation and was discontinued. Combining clomipramine with the fluoxetine produced terrible side effects. Sometime later, he sat mute through most sessions and attended erratically. He became quite hopeless and voiced passive wishes for death. As his functioning continued to deteriorate, he was referred for a second opinion, nearly ten years after the first appearance of his obsessions. During the review of Bill's history, subtle, multiple, simple motor tics were observed in Bill's father. This led to an account of conspicuous motor and phonic tics in Bill's paternal uncle that had never been disclosed. Bill himself exhibited small, unobtrusive motor tics, but complex tics were also evident. Neither Bill nor his parents comprehended what Tourette's syndrome was nor its implication for his symptoms or treatment. They reported that Bill's condition had been understood predominantly as a psychological disorder, particularly a response to his chronic medical illness accompanied by his "resistance"; there was acknowledgment of some contribution of a biological predisposition to obsessive-compulsive disorder, but this was not emphasized.

Bill's history is relevant for the appearance of obsessions before the onset of obvious tics and the incomplete formulation of his disorder. A thorough scrutiny of the family history and progression of Bill's disorder were vital even at this relatively advanced point in its course. The discovery of and emphasis on tics might have influenced both pharmacologic and psychotherapeutic strategies, affected his parents' perception of his condition, and changed something in the understanding among parents, patient, and mental health professionals.

Sometimes inattention, impulsivity, and distractibility accompany tics:

Case Example. Chris, age 8, presented for a second opinion for treatment of problems with inattention, distractibility, and hyperactivity. He had been treated over the previous year or two with a combination of methylphenidate, imipramine, and clonidine. Despite this, he continued to display symptoms and inferior academic performance. Classroom observations reported that throughout the day Chris displayed restlessness and fidgetiness, repetitive talking in class, inattention, poor organization when approaching tasks, and distractibility. He was viewed as an intelligent boy and achievement tests showed excellent potential and good knowledge and skills. His parents were highly educated and deeply devoted to Chris. They were concerned that Chris was having trouble with peer relationships and school adjustment and was making derogatory remarks about himself. There were conflicts at home over completion of homework, chores, and daily hygiene. These were particularly puzzling to his parents because even simple tasks that were not challenging to Chris, such as bathing or brushing his teeth, produced friction and protracted conflict. He would take "forever" getting started even after entering the bathroom. Recommendations for adding an additional agent—perhaps a selective serotonin-reuptake inhibitor—for depression had been offered by his psychiatrist. A behavioral psychologist who would focus on organizational and study skills had been urged. Yet Chris's parents worried that pharmacotherapy and academic counseling were insufficient for his needs.

In the first visit with Chris it was apparent that he had multiple motor and phonic tics. The evaluator worried that many of the complaints about his talking in class were complex vocal tics that Chris had suppressed to the point of whispering under his breath but still erupted at inopportune moments. Fidgetiness, restlessness, and impulsive utterances were displayed in the consulting room. Chris himself had no awareness of his motor movements. He admitted that other students had noticed and asked about his movements, but he had sloughed off their remarks. He was not being teased about his movements, although they appeared to be obvious.

In later meetings, Chris's parents were informed about his symptoms. They were instructed about his tics and reported that these had been present for over a year but they had never really paid attention to them. Observations over the next year confirmed the probability of Tourette's syndrome. Over this time, treatment entailed cessation of stimulants, specification of additional learning problems, discovery of symptoms of blocking, and revelations about obsessional intrusions. A number of sensory idiosyncrasies and constraints came to light. Opportunities to talk about his symptoms, classroom activities, and home life proved useful in making changes in routines and expectations. Work with his parents facilitated advocacy and insight into Chris's behavior. A course of a dopaminergic blocking agent proved useful for four or five months at a later point. Symptom control with the fewest side effects was achieved with clomipramine, which reduced intrusive thoughts, impulsivity, inattention, and distractibility. Increasing obsessions and anxieties responded to the addition of a selective serotonin-reuptake inhibitor.

Chris's history highlights the demand to review symptoms and continuously reconsider the implication of new symptoms. When Chris's syndrome was conceptualized as ADHD exclusively, its complexity was misjudged and an array of interventions—psychological and pharmacological—were overlooked. Furthermore, Chris's course features the concurrent onset of ADHD symptoms and tics that were apparent only subsequent to a detailed review.

It is a possibility that patients may experience symptoms of severe obsessions along with mild tics. A case of obsessions with inattention and distractibility but without hyperactivity follows:

Case Example. Don was first seen when he was 5 years old. At that time, Don did not display tics but was brought to the evaluation by his father, Mr. D., who had obvious tics and openly volunteered his own diagnosis of Tourette's syndrome. Mr. D. was familiar with the risk of tics or Tourette's syndrome in his children and wanted Don to be evaluated before the onset of any serious motor symptoms. A recent separation and divorce placed Don and his younger brother primarily with his father, coupled with frequent visiting with his mother, who lived nearby. Mr. D. wanted to be sure that Don received whatever support might be needed at this stressful time. Anxious thoughts were noted without somatic symptoms and there were movements that the evaluator thought might be simple motor tics.

A year later, Don returned as a result of symptoms of anxiety and troubles with inattention and distractibility. Teachers at school had begun to voice concerns that Don was not attentive in class and kept looking out the window and that his thoughts seemed far away. They raised the hope that giving stimulant medication might be helpful, but Mr. D. thought that stimulants might provoke tics in Don. Upon closer examination, it appeared that Don had one complex tic and several mild simple tics. Don and Mr. D reported that the symptoms of anxiety occurred at particular times. When Don was on the way to school, he repeatedly asked his father about the plans for his being picked up; they might have to review who, where, and when four or five times during the 30-minute car trip to school. This repetition was needed despite a highly consistent plan; Don was always picked up by his baby-sitter and taken home, except on Wednesdays, when his grandmother retrieved him and his brother and sat with them at her house. The morning repetitions irritated Mr. D., who went along with them unwillingly. A second feature was that Don had much more difficulty with inattention as the afternoon wore on, according to his teachers. Don himself disclosed that he was beset with worries about the pickup during the afternoon. Despite earnest attempts to reassure himself and focus on schoolwork, he could not keep his doubts and fears away. He was bombarded by worries that he would not be picked up and not make it home. This was all the more curious because there were no incidents of a break in the pattern or mistakes in fulfilling the arrangements. Don agreed that his worries were not sensible or fitting for the situation, but this did not help him stop asking his father in the morning or worrying in the afternoon.

After thorough discussion, it was decided that behavioral strategies would be tried. There were modest results. Sometime later, pharmacotherapy with a selective serotonin-reuptake inhibitor was added and produced robust improvement without side effects. Don has since developed other simple and complex motor tics that are mild. He has continued to be free of anxiety and obsessional symptoms while receiving low doses of medication and a periodic review of behavioral strategies. There was an attempt to taper and discontinue medication during a one-week vacation; this produced a rapid return of anxiety and intrusive worries.

Don's symptoms had been formulated as obsessions and perhaps some compulsive rituals in the context of vulnerability or predisposition to Tourette's syndrome. A careful review of the timing, subjective experience, and quality of symptoms as well as the family history was critical to this formulation. Don's history underscores that severe obsessions can occur with mild tics, mimic symptoms of ADHD by producing distractibility and inattention, and present early in the course of the disorder. There were invitations to consider Don's symptoms as an adjustment reaction with anxiety, ADHD, depression, or passive-aggressive defiance.

COMORBIDITY AND TOURETTE'S SYNDROME

The problem of comorbidity, whether symptoms are a part of the core syndrome or the comorbid occurrence of a separate condition, has scientific and clinical relevance; it affects the investigator and the treater. In research, demarcating the core syndrome is critical for studies of the etiology, pathophysiology, neuroanatomy, treatment, and natural history. Multiple diagnoses create uncertainty and obscure the implications of findings.

In clinical work, conceptualizing a patient's condition as a product of three or more separate diseases creates confusion, impedes comprehension, complicates prescribing treatments, and hinders accurate prognostication. For example, when patients are told they have several diseases and are given information generated from studies of patients in which only one disorder was present, those conclusions may not be applicable. Patients with only one disorder and patients who suffer from multiple disorders are likely to be different, and it is questionable whether one can extrapolate from findings from one group to make predictions about or explain the other. Comorbid, multiple-diagnosis conditions may be the expression of different disorders compared to single-diagnosis conditions, even when they exhibit some of the same symptoms (Zeitlin, 1986). Consequently, when comorbidity is present, the clinician may be confused about what entity accounts for which symptoms, which treatments to advance, or how to offer an overarching formulation of a patient's condition. He or she may be unable to provide accurate answers about the course and future of the patient's condition. Such complexity is difficult for the clinician and patient to assimilate and an emotional burden for the patient.

If we leave aside for a moment the chance that a diagnostic error has occurred, there appear to be three possible relationships that may exist between two disorders when they are observed in one person. One is that the disorders are entirely separate entities, each of which are running its course independently: true comorbidity. An example is an attack of the flu in someone with a leg fracture. A second relationship is when one disorder sets the stage for the appearance of the second, but the two are caused independently. Examples are cerebral infarction in someone with heart valve lesions from rheumatic fever, and an opportunistic fungal infection in someone whose immune system is compromised; rheumatic fever did not cause the cerebral infarct, nor did the deficit in immunity produce the fungal infection directly. In this second relationship, one disorder fosters the development or boosts the chances of developing the second, although the two conditions are not etiologically related. Nevertheless, the two disorders do not share the same pathophysiology. A third relationship is when the two are related etiologically and are alternate expressions of some underlying pathophysiology. In this relationship, a single pathological entity produces both disorders. Examples are retinal hemorrhages and peripheral neuropathy in persons with diabetes millitus, and dermatologic changes and depression in hypothyroidism. Without knowledge of the underlying pathophysiology, disorders that are linked might be thought, erroneously, to be separate. This third relationship may be particularly inscrutable if one has only signs and symptoms.

What are the relationships among ADHD, obsessive-compulsive disorder, and Tourette's syndrome? Are they three separate disorders, one disorder with three different presentations, or some combination? It is premature to declare an answer, but it appears probable that some cases of ADHD (Biederman et al., 1996; Pauls, Leckman, Cohen, et al., 1993) and certainly some of obsessive-compulsive disorder (Leonard et al., 1992; Pauls, Towbin, et al., 1986) are expressions of the same etiology (or etiologies) that produces (or produce) Tourette's syndrome. The contemporary answer is that sometimes these symptoms are reflections of separate disorders and sometimes the expression of one disorder. Symptoms of ADHD can be the leading edge of a condition that will produce Tourette's syndrome (Biederman et al., 1996), although most cases of ADHD are not related to Tourette's syndrome. What is even more striking is that some cases of obsessive-compulsive disorder may be the product of the same etiology as Tourette's syndrome, even in the absence of tics (Pauls & Leckman, 1986).

Misinterpreting the systems of classification may contribute to this puzzlement. Current classification schemes cluster conditions that are considered to be linked in some way (*DSM-IV, ICD-10*). The connotation is that disorders in different clusters will not be related to each other. Based on the classification systems, there would be no reason to think that Tourette's syndrome (a movement disorder), ADHD (a disruptive disorder), and obsessive-compulsive disorder (an anxiety disorder) would be related. By contrast, placing obsessive-compulsive disorder and panic disorder together under the anxiety disorders, or transient tic disorder and Tourette's disorder under movement disorders, implies some similarity, connection, or parallel.

There is a discrepancy between the view that Tourette's syndrome, obsessive-compulsive disorder, and ADHD are quite separate disorders (in separate clusters) and new hypotheses about their pathophysiology and neurophysiology. As discussed in Chapters 8 and 12, recent work suggests that these disorders may have overlapping mechanisms and evolve from impairment at related anatomical sites, particularly the cortico-striato-thalamo-cortical (CSTC). A malfunction of the CSTC circuit has been proposed to underlie the pathophysiology of ADHD (Barkley et al., 1992; Castellanos et al., 1996; Lou et al., 1989; Zametkin et al., 1993), Tourette's syndrome (D. Cohen & Leckman, 1994; Leckman et al., 1992; Witelson, 1993), and obsessive-compulsive disorder (Insel, 1992b). Abnormalities in frontal lobes, striatum, basal ganglia, and thalamus have been reported in Tourette's syndrome (Chappell, Leckman, Pauls, & Cohen, 1990; B. Peterson, Riddle, Cohen, Katz, Smith, Hardin, et al., 1993; Singer et al., 1993), obsessive-compulsive disorder (Baxter et al., 1992; Laplane et al., 1989; Modell, Mountz, Curtis, & Green, 1989; Swedo, Schapiro, et al., 1989), and ADHD (Barkley et al., 1992; Lou et al., 1989; Zametkin et al., 1993). Thus, each of these syndromic entities may be a product of problems in the CSTC circuit. If this is true, then these conditions possess a closer pathophysiologic relationship than is indicated by the current classification schemes. In other words, the phenomenology or overt morphology alone does not permit one to conclude whether a patient possesses one disorder or more. What is a clinician to do in the face of this ambiguity?

In most respects, the ambiguity is the result of something we created. The predicament is a product of our attempt to impose a system of classification on the real world. After we impose this system, we presume that it is real—an accurate road map reflecting nature. The root of the problem resides in thinking that *diagnoses,* which we created, are equivalent to *diseases,* entities in the real world. Yet, we encounter individuals who display symptoms that bridge partitions erected by the classification schemes. For example, a patient who presents symptoms of ADHD and tics, from the perspective of a classification scheme, would appear to have two disorders, each from very different clusters. Yet in reality, there is the potential that he or she is displaying symptoms of one condition that crosses two *apparently* distinct diagnoses. The classification system may not yet have reached the point of recognizing the single entity that exhibits symptoms of two diagnoses as they are defined in the system. It is also true that symptoms may have more predictability than diagnoses (Zeitlin, 1986).

A constructive alternative to this disarray returns to the view that diagnoses are only hypotheses (Popper, 1959), not the unique manifestation of the disease. If diagnoses are not equivalent to diseases, then comorbidity might not be present, even when criteria are met for two diagnoses. Comorbidity usually presumes that the patient has two or more independent diseases that are running their courses simultaneously. However, for these conditions, this presumption may be false. It is more accurate to say that the condition the patient possesses displays features of two different diagnoses (as described in the classification scheme). This reflects the task of diagnosis more clearly, to describe the patient's symptoms with reference to the classification system. But it does not presume that the patient has two *diseases*.

Equating diagnoses and disorders creates a variety of difficulties. Foremost among these are (a) efforts to make signs and symptoms fit the menu in the classification scheme, and (b) thinking in a narrow way about the patient's condition and treatment. Efforts to justify or shoehorn the patient's symptoms into a diagnosis can be detrimental. It is vital to remember that classification is an ordering of conditions, not individuals (Rutter & Gould, 1985). Clinicians may inadvertently color their perceptions to fit the classification scheme, either by minimizing unimportant or highlighting salient symptoms in an effort to coerce diagnostic clarity out of ambiguous data. This approach can produce reversals and confusion, and a desperate compounding of logical errors may result. Sometimes grasping for confirmation of the diagnosis leads to irrational conclusions, such as when a positive response to a medicine is used as evidence to support a diagnosis (e.g., "The patient's symptoms decreased during fluoxetine treatment, suggesting that he was suffering from obsessive-compulsive disorder."). If diagnoses are no longer equivalent to real phenomena, then the clinician does not have to continually justify which *one* diagnosis is being used. If the clinical picture changes, such as when a patient previously thought to have ADHD develops tics, the first set of symptoms can be understood as a syndrome that evolved from the same condition that produced the tics, not necessarily the acquisition of a new disorder.

Separating the concepts of diagnoses and disorders can open the way to thinking more flexibly. The formulation of the patient's condition can be disentangled from generalizations about the treatment, course, and prognosis of dissimilar entities. For example, the course and treatment of obsessive-compulsive disorder with Tourette's syndrome may be different than that of obsessive-compulsive disorder alone, and the prognosis may be different as well. The clinician avoids making assumptions from a certain diagnostic vantage point and generalizing from them. In addition, the clinician's doubts are set aside and attention can be devoted to observing and monitoring the unfolding of the phenomenology. As a result, the clinician can observe the patient's progress without being preoccupied or confused by nagging questions about the diagnosis. This approach is likely to enhance the clinician's ability to detect additional or new symptoms.

The system of classification facilitates thinking in an organized way about diagnoses, but it should not be regarded as a reliable manual of pathophysiology. If this is kept in mind, one can avoid the thinking that clusters of syndromes in the diagnostic scheme are actually separate. Patients will not be presumed to have multilayered complexes of distinct conditions with separate etiologies, treatments, and courses. Changes in the course need not throw the formulation and treatment into confusion. Instead, the patient's clinical course can be followed in an astute, thoughtful, calm manner. Although there may be less certainty in such an approach, it reflects a closer approximation to the current state of understanding.

NOSOLOGICAL PERSPECTIVES

Neuropsychiatry has made substantial gains in identifying and clarifying the critical features of Tourette's syndrome, obsessive-compulsive disorder, and ADHD. As a result, we have a better understanding of the pathophysiology and neuroanatomical loci of these intricate phenomena. This deeper comprehension has extended our knowledge of the complicated relationships among these conditions beyond empirical observations of their comorbid occurrence. Investigation has shown that symptoms of these disorders are not uniquely related to one diagnosis, but may suggest the presence of one or another of these conditions. In the clinical setting, observation over time can reveal that a symptom that was first thought to be a manifestation of one diagnosis actually is more consistent with another.

Beyond its immediate clinical relevance, this new knowledge has forced investigators and clinicians to reassess conventional boundaries and relationships among diagnoses. Knowledge of the common neural circuits and neuroanatomical overlays of these diagnoses casts a different light on the system of classification. Diagnostic systems invite the clinician to view diagnoses as embodiments of real, discrete, unique entities. Study of this trio of conditions suggests that this view may be flawed; symptoms can have multiple origins.

Clinical care (and research) can be advanced by resisting the temptation to reify the *hypothetical* constructs of nosology. Thinking of diagnoses as equivalent to diseases runs the risk of making a systematic error or missing the big picture by closing off opportunities to observe new symptoms. Yielding to this invitation runs counter to the commitment to acknowledge new symptoms and reformulate a presentation that has changed. The appearance of comorbidity can be less confusing by regarding classification and diagnoses as hypothetical constructs or as descriptive terms that do not adequately capture actual diseases. This perspective benefits patient care by promoting a flexible way of thinking about symptoms and accommodating complex presentations. It promotes careful observation and avoids the temptation to use simplistic formulations and treatments. In this way, it gives patients the greatest opportunity for the highest quality care.

SUMMARY OF CHAPTER 7

An appreciation of the range of other disorders that can resemble Tourette's syndrome is crucial for clinicians treating this disorder. Although the boundaries are far from distinct, a number of features, including premonitory urges, suppressibility, and some persistence during sleep, when considered in aggregate, can provide a useful guide to the presence of tics. No current diagnostic system does justice to the complexities of Tourette's syndrome and its attendant comorbidities. In resisting our best efforts at classification, nature teaches us to be suspicious of diagnostic systems that invite the clinician to consider diagnostic categories as real, discrete entities.

PREVIEW OF CHAPTER 8

Section Two closes with a look beyond traditional diagnostic categories. What matters most is not what nosological category is most appropriate, but how, given an individual's unique set of strengths and weaknesses, he or she is able to adapt in the struggles of life. Echoing themes first presented in Chapter 1 and later explicated in terms of clinical practice in Section Three, Chapter 8 explores areas of strength and resilience and asks the Darwinian question: What, if anything, is "good" about having the vulnerability to develop Tourette's syndrome?

CHAPTER 8

Beyond the Diagnosis—Darwinian Perspectives on Pathways to Successful Adaptation

JAMES F. LECKMAN and DONALD J. COHEN

It's part of my nature.

—*Jim Eisenreich, 1996*

If variations useful to any organic being do occur, assuredly individuals thus characterized will have the best chance of being preserved in the struggle for life.

—*Charles Darwin, 1859*

Knowledge of the ways in which each of the evolutionarily conserved core processes are used in humans, and the many ways their perturbations can lead to disease, will only come from the study of humans themselves.

—*George L. Gabor Miklos and Gerald M. Rubin, 1996*

In the usual practice of medicine, clinicians focus their diagnostic skills on identifying problems, quantifying symptoms, and labeling syndromes. Pragmatically, the diagnostic emphasis on dysfunction is understandable when a diagnosis can lead to a specific treatment or cure. Yet, for children and adolescents with persistent difficulties, such as Tourette's syndrome, the emphasis on impairment also has the potential to deform self-perceptions—to promote the individual's view of himself or herself as defective or victimized (D. Cohen, 1980). For Tourette's syndrome and similar, long-term disorders for which there is no cure, the selective focus on the potentially disabling aspects of the syndrome is usefully balanced with an alternative approach that is more conducive to promoting healthy personal development. In this chapter, we look beyond the formal diagnosis and consider what is the most fruitful perspective from which to view Tourette's in order to enhance strengths and adaptation in the face of a major developmental challenge. As part of this endeavor, we adopt a Darwinian perspective and consider the possibility that some of the etiological factors that contribute to a person's vulnerability to develop Tourette's may confer certain advantages as well. If in Tourette's syndrome the self is chronically under siege, then this chapter focuses on the defenses available to the self and the positions of strength that will minimize the adverse impact of this disorder.

WHAT IS THE MOST FRUITFUL PERSPECTIVE ONCE A DIAGNOSIS HAS BEEN MADE?

As a complement to the formal diagnostic assessment, it is crucial to undertake a holistic appraisal of a person's strengths, as well as weaknesses, within specific environmental contexts. The goal of assessment of this type is to define the dynamic interplay between the individual's gifts and vulnerabilities and the psychological, social, physical, and microbiological environments in which he or she lives. What special abilities or strengths does this individual manifest, and how can clinicians and others build on these strengths to promote a positive self-image and a more supportive set of responses from the people who matter most?

Patients with Tourette's syndrome, other tic disorders, and obsessive-compulsive disorder differ dramatically in their personal adaptation and the level of impairment. The nature and degree of their impairment is, to a certain degree, a function of the severity of the tic and obsessional symptoms, as such. However, as clinicians we have often been impressed that frequency, forcefulness, range, other features of the tics, and other symptoms do not account fully for the degree of impairment or social and emotional dysfunction. Rather, impairment is a resultant of the interaction of various positive as well as negative factors. How does an individual respond to being besieged by distracting internal cues and a hyperawareness of one's surroundings? Table 8.1 provides an overview of the strengths that are found, in varying combinations and degrees, among individuals who appear to be more resilient in the face of the chronic demands that a tic disorder places on the psyche. Assessing these domains is every bit as important as doing a thorough differential diagnosis.

Neurophysiological Stability

Children and adults with Tourette's syndrome and related forms of obsessive-compulsive disorder and attention-deficit/hyperactivity disorder (ADHD) tend to do better if their lifestyle (apart from the capricious demands of the tics and obsessions) is predictable. Perhaps more than others,

Table 8.1   Domains of Potential Strength That May Foster an Adaptive Response to Tourette's Syndrome and Related Conditions over the Course of Development

Domain	Potential Strengths
Neurophysiological stability	Maintenance of normal circadian rhythms, regular exercise regimens, and balanced diet.
Intrapsychic resilience	Resilient to stressful situations, optimistic outlook, ability to enjoy life and maintain a positive sense of self, humor, imagination, and absence of psychopathological states (chronic anxiety, depression, thought disorder).
Interpersonal and social skills	Ability to form and sustain friendships, sensitivity to the needs of others.
Other psychological gifts and talents	Academic gifts, strong problem-solving abilities, sustained areas of interest, musical, or other artistic talents.
Physical appearance and psychomotor talents	Attractive physical appearance and athletic skills.
Family strengths	Optimistic outlook, acceptance of symptoms with minimal anxiety and distress, ability to overlook the symptoms, ability to help the patient find a way of talking about the symptoms with a minimum of embarrassment, ability to idealize the patient and focus on the patient's strengths, cohesive family structure, absence of marital discord, and strong parental support network.
Social supports	Absence of teasing, supportive peer group, understanding teachers and/or supervisors and coworkers.
Physical and socioeconomic advantages	Secure home, school, and/or occupational environment; educational and/or occupational success, minimal stress due to socioeconomic disadvantage.

they need and benefit from well-established rhythms of rest and activity. In her 1946 follow-up study of 10 patients with Tourette's syndrome diagnosed in childhood, Margaret Mahler was the first to note the benefits of "outdoor activity" (Mahler & Luke, 1946). Clinical experience clearly supports the hypothesis of a beneficial effect of a steady habit of rest and physical activity:

> **Case Example.** Ben was a 22-year-old medical student who had Tourette's syndrome since childhood; he coped well with his symptoms and had a range of friends and activities. Because of his own experience, he was interested in promoting the adaptation of other youngsters with Tourette's. For him, a central aspect of adaptation was engagement in sports and a structured, "clean" lifestyle. He thought children with Tourette's needed a summer program with several key goals: to establish stable circadian rhythms, develop athletic skills through a sports and exercise program, and to encourage children to eat nutritionally balanced meals at regularly

scheduled times. In part, the rigid structure of the envisioned curriculum might reflect Ben's own vulnerability to obsessive-compulsive behaviors, of which he was aware, but it was also based on the efficacy of this approach for him and others.

For Ben and other patients, disabling tic symptoms often diminish during a period of rigorous self-discipline and engagement in sports. They exacerbate with over-excitement, exhaustion, and unpredictability, such as during final examination weeks, tax season, and visits to distant theme parks with their long lines and thrilling rides.

As noted by Ben and other patients with Tourette's syndrome, emotional upset disrupts sleep regulation and circadian rhythms (Cartwright & Wood, 1991); this disruption, in turn, leads to increased anxiety and the onset and worsening of tic and obsessive-compulsive symptoms. A vicious cycle thus becomes established, in which stress leads to symptoms that then become traumatic in their own right. A similar cascade follows traumatic losses, as well as in psychopathological conditions characterized by depression and anxiety. Therapeutically, it generally seems necessary to try to ameliorate the depression and anxiety before helping the patient to resume stable sleep-activity cycles; however, the two constellations of difficulties may best be considered as reflecting the emergent dysfunctions in self regulation. Individuals with Tourette's syndrome and obsessive-compulsive disorder often have troubles falling asleep or have night awakenings (Allen, Singer, Brown, & Salam, 1992; Glaze, Frost, & Jankovic, 1983; Insel et al., 1982; Mendelson, Caine, Goyer, Ebert, & Gillin, 1980), perhaps as a manifestation of their underlying diathesis in arousal as well as a result of the emotional distress elicited by the symptoms. As part of their full care, it is useful to consider ways of stabilizing the circadian rhythms of rest and activity by helping patients plan their schedules, as well as by the judicious use of medication, when needed. The creation of summer camping programs for individuals with Tourette's syndrome offers an opportunity for a rigorous investigation of Ben's hypothesis. Research on sleep-wakefulness and the regulation of arousal may help clarify other aspects of Tourette's, such as the marked diminution of tics during sleep (Jagger et al., 1982; A. Shapiro, Shapiro, Young, & Feinberg, 1988).

Resilience and Interpersonal Style

There are enormous individual differences in the ability to handle stressful or emotionally laden situations. Such differences appear early in life and are apparent at each phase of development. Faced with an external threat, some individuals focus their attention on the problems at hand, devise a strategy, and proceed systematically. For them, stressful events are organizing. At the other pole are individuals who become immobilized with anxiety—their minds flood, they sweat and feel cold, and they look to others for support, or they flee. There is every gradation in-between. Studies of animal behavior and human development have provided useful clues to understanding the constitutional and experiential origins of resilience and adaptability in the face of environmental or physiological stress, threat or trauma (Cicchetti & Cohen, 1995; Cicchetti & Tucker, 1994; Waddington, 1977).

Patients with Tourette's syndrome and associated disorders also show an enormous range of resilience and adaptability over the course of their childhood and early adulthood. Those who have been the most successful have been able to maintain an optimistic outlook and a positive sense of themselves in the world. These individuals continue to enjoy their lives regardless of the demands of their symptoms. Many of these patients have an engaging and affectionate personal style, a lively imagination, and an ability to use humor to deflect the pain caused to them and others by their chronic vulnerability and symptoms:

> **Case Example.** We have cared for and known Dennis for almost 20 years. In his childhood, when he first came for treatment, his forceful, nonstop tics were punctuated by bouts of colorful, coprolalic swearing and dramatic, copropraxic, lewd gestures. His family and teachers were deeply distressed by Dennis's symptoms, but they were able to remain warmly supportive and engaged, and to appreciate Dennis' charm and wit. Indeed, Dennis was able to maintain a sweet humor and an easygoing, friendliness that attracted people, including his clinicians. While many children with vocal tics are banished from school, Dennis's teachers and classmates were welcoming and tolerated his symptoms to an amazing degree. Dennis's older brother was a professional comedian, and we saw bits of a comedian in Dennis, with his ready wit and self-deprecating style. Still, we all worried about Dennis's adult life if his tics continued at such a level of intensity. As a young adult, Dennis remains severely affected with tics. His vocal tics disrupt conversation and his motor tics erupt in sudden, forceful displays. Despite these quite odd symptoms, Dennis continues to maintain his sense of humor and self-acceptance. He owns a small, successful business, has married a fine young woman, and has become a proud father. The Tourette Syndrome Association's *Newsletter* has a sidebar in each issue under the heading "Victory," in which the accomplishments of an individual with Tourette's syndrome are recounted. Dennis is one such victor.

Many factors appear to contribute to the vast range of individual differences in outcome. For those children and adolescents who do the best, does their positive outlook on life and good humor make them more attractive to others so that they can more readily maintain their developmental progress? Or, do these traits carry some other intrinsic benefit? Whatever their roots, the capacity to form relationships and to maintain a positive regard in the eyes of others is a powerful source of resiliency and defense. Stress resilience and interpersonal competence go hand-in-hand; the therapeutic process and the relationship with a clinician, may be a compensatory or intermediate structure that may help patients to improve or make full use of their interpersonal abilities.

The Role of Family and Friends

Another important protective factor is the understanding of the disorder by the patient, family, peers, and colleagues. Individuals with Tourette's syndrome can be frightened and frightening, bewildered and confusing. As reviewed in Chapter 6, they often have trouble establishing and sustaining friendships (Dykens et al., 1990) and are frequently viewed by their peers as aggressive and socially unappealing (Stokes, Bawden, Camfield, Backman, & Dooley, 1991). A patient's own shame about his behavior, his fears about what is taking place inside of his mind, and his confusion about the source and nature of his ever-changing symptoms can lead to retreat from the social world. Well-meaning parents, too, may reinforce this shame by enabling or encouraging the patient to avoid the dangers of the outside world, where his symptoms will attract attention, curiosity, and ostracism. For both parents and children, the outside world may become increasingly dangerous just as their inner worlds are in turmoil.

A patient's withdrawal from social contacts, however, can herald a downward spiral in which the patient's and family's negative feelings and cognitions lead to an increasing sense of being damaged and unacceptable. It has appeared to us that the children who do best in overall, long-term adjustment are those from families that do not allow the child to take a sick role or to be treated as too delicate or vulnerable to stand up for himself. In such families, parents insist that the child will remain in the mainstream, as much as possible. For the most fortunate, the child or adolescent has the capacity to maintain a sense of humor and feeling that he has a right to be accepted among others. Everything being equal, it is better for a child and family to be angry and assertive when the symptoms elicit negative responses from others than to feel ashamed. It is best when the child and parent are able to help others relate positively, in spite of symptoms.

Being socially adept can be a powerful mitigating force. We have seen friends and family rally during periods when the tics are at their worst. Their steadfast friendship and their empathic understanding of the patient's predicament, even when not spoken, are powerful antidotes against the pains of being stared at, teased, or shunned.

The Clinician's Attitude

A major goal of the therapeutic process with patients with Tourette's and families is to encourage patterns of behavior that will increase coping and adaptation, even when the symptoms persist. The clinician's positive regard and acceptance of the patient and family, his ability to recognize and modulate anxiety, and his interest in the child as a whole person and not only as a collection of symptoms can serve as an important model for both the child and family. Children know when they are listened to and respected, and they appreciate the availability and the human interest of the clinician. Through the clinician's attitude, the parents can sometimes again begin to see their child as a person and not only as a case. Although we do not know how to give a child resilience, we believe that it is possible to help teach skills and encourage compensatory behaviors that help children deal with their adversity. This includes the clinician's role as an advocate in schools and other settings, and his guidance to help these children find areas in which they can achieve and experience success. The physician's model of positive regard and friendly acceptance of the patient and family increasingly can become internalized within the family, and help move their development back on course.

Other Cognitive, Psychomotor, and Physical Gifts and Talents

Sometimes, discussions of protective factors appear to be banal. It is almost self-evident that being bright, athletic, and handsome helps a child navigate life's obstacles or, at least, buffers some of life's grief. And while money is not everything, it is just as well to be rich than poor, given the choice. Yet, it is important to recognize that outcome in Tourette's syndrome is very much related to nonspecific factors—such as intelligence and good looks—and that these other factors are often the major determinants of adult status.

Over the decades, we have had the pleasure of knowing a succession of talented and successful business executives, professionals, professors, entrepreneurs, and athletes with Tourette's. Although they were burdened, to varying degrees, by their symptoms, they were able to make full use of their potentialities and achieve remarkable goals. Often, they showed their skills and motivations in childhood, and were not willing to accept a second-class role. Their adult status was very much related to their accomplishments, and their tics were either not noticed or commented upon.

For some of these individuals, the development of tics and associated problems in their children posed a special burden. They felt guilty and either became overly permissive or overly distant. The children of these very successful individuals were sometimes at a disadvantage compared with their parents, especially when the children did not have the drive, talent, or luck that they had. In reflecting on this, it has sometimes seemed that early in the parent's life, he or she showed the determination not to let the tics get in the way of achievement. He (or she) developed a stubbornly tough and assertive approach to life, refused to feel sorry for himself, and rejected the possibility of being second class or second best. This tough-mindedness was a major determinant of his remarkable determination to achieve. The children of such parents, however, were often provided with a safety net of parental concern and indulgence, fueled at least in part by parental guilt as well as by over-identification and empathy. Because of this parental response and ambivalent indulgence, the children were deprived of the need and full opportunity to become autonomous, assertive, tough, and effective. In these situations, fathers were often both disappointed in their children as well as self-punitive and remorseful. The fathers' achievements and the sons' difficulties illuminate similar phenomena about adaptation in the face of adversity:

> **Case Example.** Professor T. is a distinguished law professor at a prestigious university. His tics have been with him for as long as he can remember. He had tics throughout law school and he has recurrences during periods of stress and physical fatigue. At present, the sensory urges that prompt the tics are the most troublesome feature of the condition. They are a source of distraction as he reads or prepares his articles for law review journals, but he has not compromised his career. He has used his intelligence with special determination, as if working against a resistance has toughened and strengthened his mental musculature.

> **Case Example.** Mr. Harvey K. is a middle-aged entrepreneur whom we first met when he brought his son to be evaluated for Tourette's syndrome eight or nine years ago. A remarkably successful international investor, Mr. K. was furious at the prospect of his son having Tourette's. Although he was himself never diagnosed, Mr. K. had many tics and he recalled the distress of his youth and his struggle to contain the tics. Now, he claimed, he was oblivious to these tics, but he could barely contain his fury at his son's "unwillingness" to control his facial grimaces and frequent throat clearing. Over the course of years, we came to learn that Mr. K.'s response to his son's tics echoed his own mother's forceful efforts to encourage him to suppress his tics and his own rage at her and at the tics. In one way, Mr. K.'s success exemplified the possibility of achievement in spite of emotional turmoil. However, from another perspective, perhaps his business savvy, grit, denial, and ability to make tough deals were also a reflection of a mode of defensive adaptation, a way of avoiding the emotional distress and distancing himself from the image of being a passive, shameful boy who could not control his own body. Through his hard work and brilliance, Mr. K. became a prominent and wealthy member of his community, as well as a committed father.

Although one might expect that tics, obsessions, and compulsions would be insurmountable barriers to participating in sports, many children and adolescents with Tourette's are actually surprisingly good athletes. We are always pleased to meet a child with Tourette's who is interested in competitive sports, and who already has some skills. Some individuals with Tourette's syndrome have become successful professional athletes, in spite of very impairing obsessions, compulsions, and motor tics. Athletic competence is important in helping to establish a positive self-perception. Building on these strengths often helps define a successful developmental trajectory for individuals with Tourette's as they cope with the burdens of the syndrome:

> **Case Example.** Tommy, age 11 years, has a disfiguring mouth stretching tic and he emits bouts of high-pitched squeaks. Yet, he is bright and outspoken, and he has a compelling interest in the reigning NBA team and its star player, whose salary is in the millions. When Tommy started a new

school, his mother was anxious that he get off to a good start and she and his new teacher encouraged him to take the sign of his competence, a basketball, with him to school. Soon, he put the basketball aside to enter the football games that brought the boys together in the new school. Through his self-identification as an athlete and his acceptance by the others in this role, he was able to present himself as competent rather than as odd.

However, for some adolescents with Tourette's syndrome and obsessive-compulsive disorder, participation in sports has become a preoccupation. In these cases, the adolescent or young adult might spend hours in body-building and weight lifting, sometimes causing injuries by pushing themselves too long and too far. In these situations, the underlying dysfunction takes over, and the athletic activity becomes as much a symptom as a mode of adaptation.

Children with Tourette's syndrome will often see their bodies as their enemies, rather than being a source of narcissistic pride. Their engagement in sports helps to counterbalance this attitude with a feeling that their bodies can be brought under control. Sports can bring children with Tourette's syndrome into the mainstream and closer to other children. In the running and kicking of soccer, while swimming in a race, lifting weights, or performing gymnastics, tics are camouflaged or marginal. Indeed, the focused actions associated with participating in sports can also provide real relief from the onslaught of premonitory urges and intrusive thoughts that characterize Tourette's and obsessive-compulsive disorder.

From a Darwinian Point of View: Are There Any Advantages Associated with Having the Vulnerability to Develop Tourette's Syndrome and Related Conditions?

Over 2000 years ago in communities near Cappadocia, Turkey, Aretaeus described individuals who barked, twitched, grimaced, and gestured strangely (Sacks, 1992). Why have the genetic and neurobiological substrates for such traits persisted for such a long period in the human behavioral and biological repertoire? Is there an advantage or usefulness, however slight, in having the vulnerability to develop Tourette's or obsessive-compulsive disorder? To begin the consideration of this issue, it is important to look beyond the tics and other symptoms. Instead, we need to consider other closely related behaviors that may share fundamental features with tics and other symptoms and yet have adaptive value.

In the Autumn of 1993, we convened a small meeting one afternoon at the Yale Child Study Center. We invited several members of the local chapter of the Tourette's Syndrome Association to meet with us and with Oliver Sacks, to consider the question "What's good about having Tourette's?" For most diseases, this would be a very odd question. Yet, for Tourette's syndrome, this is a question we have been asking ourselves and our patients for some time. The discussion was lively and focused mostly on the mutative effects on one's personality of having a chronic stigmatizing disorder. One point of consensus reached by the group was their awareness of—their sensitivity to—the plight of people who were disabled. We wondered aloud whether that was a unique trait or one that might be frequently encountered among any group of individuals with chronic symptoms of whatever sort who have had to struggle mightily against the ignorance and prejudices of society. The participants felt there was something special about the way individuals with Tourette's syndrome perceived others, including those with other types of handicaps. In a special way, individuals with Tourette's are sensitive to the feelings and experiences of others, and have a thinner barrier to stimulation. They may feel the feelings of others more strongly, just as they feel their own, and they are thus more aware of the pains of others and more empathic. This is not always a blessing, but it is a special gift.

More specifically, individuals with Tourette's syndrome have a heightened awareness of both the internal sensations from within their body and selected stimuli from the external environment. Michael Kane (1994), a graduate student with Tourette's, has suggested that the syndrome reflects failed attentional inhibition—that the tics arise from a somatosensory "hyper-awareness." Could this hyper-awareness be useful or adaptive, in some circumstances, and might this increased sensitivity extend to other neuropsychological domains? Being aware of dangers, from the internal or external milieu, can be life saving, and protect both the individual and those with whom he is bonded.

Being fearful is adaptive, when the fears orient an individual to potential dangers and mobilize suitable protective or preventive behaviors. When things go normally, the fears are attenuated by experience of safety, and are aroused only when there are hints of a new threat that lead to foreboding. Thus, it is natural to be concerned about the safety of one's home, the security of one's children, the cleanliness of the dishes and silverware that we use. It is also sensible to be aware, at some level, when the environment is not "just right," when something is out of kilter. Hypothetically, the obsessive-compulsive symptoms associated with Tourette's syndrome may, thus, reflect a failure to inhibit these rational, almost innate fears (Mayes & Leckman, in press-a, in press-b). In this circumstance, the experience of safety does not mute the preoccupation that something bad will, or already has, happened, and no amount of cleaning can reassure the individual that there are no more germs.

Indeed, individuals with Tourette's and obsessive-compulsive disorder are remarkably attuned to their internal and external environments. Perhaps there was a time when this selective hyper-awareness of the environment made a difference in survival and reproductive success. Examples might include identifying in a fleeting glance a possible predator, or being acutely aware of some insect on the skin. Alternatively, compulsively checking to make certain that the home is safe and the bedroom "just right" before falling asleep, in whatever shelter is available, could make the difference between life and death. In this formulation, then, some of the traits associated with Tourette's, obsessive-compulsive disorder, and ADHD may have been adaptive in the distant past. They are less adaptive today, in our current relatively more secure environments, where there is so much information, so many distractions, and so many choices. What is adaptive in these traits may also be a matter of degree, conferring a selective advantage only when present in smaller doses in particularly life-threatening situations.

Another possible area of strength for Tourette's patients emerged as part of a series of neuropsychological studies (see Chapter 5). We found that patients with Tourette's, on average, do better at certain neuropsychological tasks such as a simple one that requires them to divide a straight line at its midpoint. Normal individuals tend to displace the midline slightly to one side, while those with Tourette's are more accurate in bisecting the line (Yazgan et al., 1995). Although individuals with Tourette's tend to have more difficulties in constructing objects in three-dimensional space, it seems fair to ask how this attention to symmetry might have certain advantages:

> **Case Example.** When asked if there was anything distinctive in the way he thought, Professor T. replied after some deliberation, that several of his colleagues were surprised by the novelty of the legal questions he pursued. In one study, he was interested in whether the implicit rules that govern the assignment of blame and guilt were the same as those that implicitly govern the conferring of praise and credit.

Professor T.'s account of the search for novel cognitive symmetries was reminiscent of other patients and their preoccupations with symmetry and balance (see Abe's account in Chapter 1).

Molecular geneticists and clinical researchers are working together to identify susceptibility genes of major and minor effect. This is an area that exemplifies the triumphs of biomedical research. The identification and eventual characterization of these genetic loci has the potential to identify individuals at increased risk, to improve diagnosis, to develop animal models, to understand the normal adaptive role of the gene products in brain development in diverse environments, and to point the way to advances in treatment. Yet, we would not be surprised to discover that one or more of the long sought after "vulnerability genes" associated with Tourette's are also genes associated with certain positive adaptive potentials. Although these potentials likely remain despite the emergence tics and other symptoms, their benefits may be most clearly seen in close relatives whose early developmental histories have not been compromised by untoward epigenetic events. This perspective also emphasizes the often neglected, role of the genetic background in influencing the presentation and course of the disorder. Depending on this background, the syndrome may be more or less severe. Similarly, the individual's ability to cope successfully with the adversities of Tourette's are likely to be mediated in part by genes that are not directly involved in the pathogenesis of the disorder.

Another view from this Darwinian perspective emphasizes the dimensional character of basic neurobiological core systems that are crucially important for the emergence of normal adaptive functioning. From this perspective, tics are viewed as selectively disinhibited fragments of normal behavior that on themselves serve as the basic building blocks of motor action and cognition. It may even be possible to identify the earliest developmental precursors of tics as psychomotor ensembles begin to emerge in the first months of life (Thelen & Smith, 1994). Similarly, the dimensional traits encountered in obsessive-compulsive disorder may be disinhibited pieces of complex action plans that also had their earliest normal expression in the first years of life (Evans et al., 1997). This viewpoint encourages patients to think about their symptoms as being, in some sense "normal" and not something to be ashamed of. This approach may also provide our best opportunity to destigmatize the syndrome by firmly placing it on the continuum of normal variation and expectable developmental outcomes.

A COMBINED APPROACH

It is our sense that this focus on strengths and resilience usefully complements the detailed biomedical diagnostic assessment and is fundamental to determining the right treatment for patients. Most often, clinical interventions and research focus on the so-called "deficit model" of psychopathology. While this standard biomedical approach in Tourette's syndrome has led to incremental progress in defining the disease phenotype, identifying environmental risk factors, charting the natural history of the disorder, and offering a range of interventions, it has the potential to distort self-perceptions by emphasizing what is wrong with the patient. A combined approach invites patients and families to focus on the whole person with Tourette's syndrome. Crucial to this undertaking is a recognition of the individual's strengths. These competencies may serve as valuable defenses against the developmental and emotional threats of tics and related symptoms.

SUMMARY OF CHAPTER 8

Application of the biomedical models of disorder and the assignment of diagnostic labels may have unforeseen negative effects. A goodness-of-fit approach is introduced that directs the clinician's attention to the long-term goal of improved adaptive function. It may be more important to identify an individual's strengths than to focus exclusively on areas of weakness and disability. This analysis leads to a consideration of Darwinian principles and an initial effort to answer the question, "What, if any anything, is good about having the vulnerability to develop Tourette's syndrome?" The chapter and Section One concludes with an appeal to pursue a combined approach, refining and extending models of pathogenesis without losing sight of the individual's unique strengths and talents.

PREVIEW OF CHAPTER 9

Section Two begins with a presentation of a general model of pathogenesis that attempts to integrate genetic, epigenetic, and neurobiological findings with complex phenotypic features encountered in Tourette's syndrome, obsessive-compulsive disorder, and related conditions. This general model, in elaborated form, has served as a guide for research for more than a decade. We anticipate that major therapeutic gains will follow from scientific advances that further refine and extend specific models of pathogenesis.

SECTION TWO

Causes and Determinants

Just as an area is a product of length multiplied by width so every biological character, whether it be morphological, physiological, or behavioural, is a product of the interaction of genetic endowment and environment.

—John Bowlby, 1969

The pathways of induction and determination involve a historical series of milieu-gene expressions that are coupled to those mechanical and mechano-chemical events that actually govern the achievement of form and pattern. At any one time there is an interplay between the place, scale and size of bordering collectives, and various inductive molecular signs not only maintain the pattern so far established but also transform it into a new pattern.

—Gerald M. Edelman, 1987

CHAPTER 9

Evolving Models of Pathogenesis

JAMES F. LECKMAN and DONALD J. COHEN

> The extraordinary intricacy of all of the factors to be taken into considera-
> tion leaves only one way of presenting them open to us. We must select first
> one and then another point of view, and follow it up through the material as
> long as the application of it seems to yield results.
>
> —*Sigmund Freud, 1915*

Our long-term goal has been to understand the vulnerabilities that can
lead to Tourette's syndrome, obsessive-compulsive disorder, ADHD, and
related difficulties in hopes of mitigating risk, preventing disabling outcomes, and doing our best to help affected individuals and families. One
approach has been to challenge our growing scientific knowledge base.
Which facts encountered in the literature are supported by sound research and which are not? How does yesterday's formulation fit today's
data? Is there some way to better integrate what we know to develop better interventions?

In this chapter, we present an overview of an evolving and increasingly
explicit model of pathogenesis. It is instructive to consider our earliest formulation of this model more than a decade ago (Leckman, Price, Riddle,
Minderaa, Anderson, & Pauls, 1986). The same elements are present—an
underlying genetic diathesis combined with a variable set of epigenetic
stressors that constrain the potentialities of the developing brain. What has
changed, thanks to advances in molecular neurobiology, genetics, and in
vivo neuroimaging, is our ability to identify specific mechanisms. This
chapter summarizes material that is explored in greater depth in the subsequent chapters of Section Two.

The construction of this model serves many functions—to integrate our
current knowledge base, to serve as a scaffold for future research, and to
focus our attention on potential preventive and therapeutic interventions.

However, as with any model it is an oversimplification—incomplete and, doubtless, at times mistaken.

We believe this is an ideal time to advance our knowledge. Recent advances in the fields of genetics and the developmental neurosciences have led to optimism that the vulnerability genes that underlie these conditions can be characterized and their role in normal development understood. Advances in this area will improve the accuracy of diagnoses and permit the identification of vulnerable individuals prior to the onset of disease. A number of other nongenetic risk and protective factors have already been identified that appear to mediate the course and outcome of these diseases in vulnerable individuals. A more complete understanding of these factors should lead the way to the development of successful preventive interventions.

Recent progress in neuroanatomy, systems neuroscience (an approach that considers the brain at the level of integrated systems, wherein different components of circuits contribute unique computational activity), and functional in vivo neuroimaging are setting the stage for deeper insights into these disorders and the neurobiological substrates that underlie them. Success in this area will lead to the targeting of specific brain circuits for more intensive study. Diagnostic and prognostic advances can be anticipated, for example, determining which circuits are involved and to what degree. There is even hope for circuitry-based therapeutic approaches using transcranial magnetic stimulation, briefly discussed in Chapter 20.

Tourette's syndrome and obsessive-compulsive disorder can be considered model disorders to study the interplay of genetic, neurobiological, and environmental factors during evolution and development (D. Cohen & Leckman, 1994; Leckman & Peterson, 1993; Leckman, Peterson, et al., 1997; B. Peterson, Leckman, & Cohen, 1995). Two decades ago, we naïvely thought that these disorders and their manifest phenotypic complexity were the consequence of a single autosomal gene and its interaction with a limited number of environmental risk and protective factors. In light of our failure to identify this genetic locus, we now consider it probable that multiple genes of both major and minor effect are involved. It is likely that the research paradigms developed in these studies, and many of the empirical findings resulting from them, will be relevant to other disorders of childhood onset and to our understanding of normal development.

A WORKING MODEL OF PATHOGENESIS

A schematic presentation of the general model of pathogenesis is presented in Figure 9.1. Our model involves the reciprocal interaction of a set of interrelated genes and their microscopic and macroscopic environments. The normal copies of these specific vulnerability genes are presumed to be turned on and off at specific points in development. Abnormal copies of these genes constrain the course of development by changing the timing or

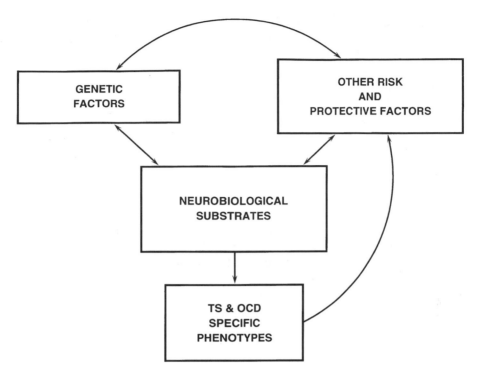

Figure 9.1   General model of pathogenesis. This figure depicts the interactions among genetic factors, neurobiological substrates, and environmental factors in the production of the clinical phenotypes. The genetic vulnerability factor(s) that underlie Tourette's syndrome and related disorders undoubtably influence the structure and function of the brain, which in turn produces clinical symptoms. Available evidence (see text) also indicates that a range of epigenetic or environmental factors are also critically involved in the pathogenesis of these disorders. In addition, symptoms of the disorder can affect and alter aspects of the microenvironment of the brain, which in turn may alter the expression of the genetic factor(s).

degree of expression of specific gene products. A number of other risk and protective factors are also likely to be involved that may influence gene expression directly. Some of these influences are likely to occur early in brain development. In other cases, gene expression may be affected indirectly when aspects of the macroenvironment of the individual alter the microenvironment of neural systems through a variety of signal transduction and second-messenger systems. Conversely, these vulnerability genes influence directly their microenvironment by facilitating or repressing the production of specific proteins. This general model also presumes that these vulnerability genes acting in concert with specific environmental factors play a crucial role in the formation and/or activity of specific neural circuits that provide the neurobiological substrate for symptoms associated with these disorders. Indeed, we hypothesize that some of these gene-environment interactions may occur early in CNS development and set the stage for the later expression of the disorder. We will present data that support the conclusion that events during pregnancy and delivery can dramatically influence the nature and severity of symptoms encountered decades later.

Other gene-environment interactions may occur at later points during development. For example, exposure to certain bacterial antigens may lead to autoimmune reactions and injury in certain brain regions—a response that may well depend on genetically determined host susceptibility factors. At the level of the macroenvironment, this general model predicts the possibility of vicious cycles where increasing tic or obsessive-compulsive symptoms create secondary problems of peer rejection that lead to a further stress-induced exacerbation of these symptoms.

This model of pathogenesis should also be seen as being consistent with dynamical theories of development in which epigenetic factors play a crucial role in the structuring of a nervous system (Edelman, 1987; Thelen & Smith, 1994; Waddington, 1966). At any moment in time, there is an interplay of activation and inhibition between adjacent collectives located within these circuits that is remarkably attuned to selected aspects of the internal milieu of the body and the external world of sensory perception. These collectives are also governed to a large extent by their own immediate past history of activation or inhibition. Indeed, the timing of intertic or interobsession intervals may well reflect the dynamical properties of these reciprocally connected cellular collectives (König & Enge, 1995).

We begin with a brief reprise of the phenomenology and natural history of Tourette's syndrome and obsessive-compulsive disorder (summarized in Table 9.1 and presented in more detail in Chapters 2 and 3) as well as a brief consideration of ADHD (see Chapter 4) and other comorbid conditions.

Phenomenology and Natural History

At a conceptual level, we view Tourette's syndrome and obsessive-compulsive disorder phenotypes as products of a heightened, but selective, sensitivity to alterations in both the internal milieu of the body (a kind of somatic hyperawareness) and the external psychosocial environment of the individual. This heightened sensitivity can in turn lead to the exaggerated, disinhibited expression of fragments of cognition and behavior that are normally assembled into voluntary action repertoires.

Descriptively, Tourette's syndrome (Table 9.1) is a chronic neuropsychiatric disorder of childhood onset that is characterized by tics that wax and wane in severity and an array of behavioral problems that include some forms of obsessive-compulsive disorder (D. Cohen & Leckman, 1994). The range of symptoms in Tourette's syndrome is enormous and includes motor and phonic tics (sudden repetitive movements, gestures, or utterances) that typically mimic some aspect of normal behavior, and obsessions and compulsions (sudden repetitive thoughts, images, urges, and actions that are intrusive and difficult to resist). Less well appreciated are the sensorimotor phenomena that frequently accompany tics and

TABLE 9.1   Clinical Phenotypes

Phenotype	Description of Latent Variable	Operational Measures
Tourette's syndrome	A chronic neuropsychiatric disorder of childhood onset characterized by tics that wax and wane in severity and an array of behavioral problems that include some forms of obsessive-compulsive disorder and attention-deficit/ hyperactivity disorder (ADHD).	History and presenting tic symptoms based on information from multiple informants; ratings of symptom severity; treatment response; performance on neuropsychological battery; subtypes of Tourette's syndrome will be distinguished on the basis of family study data from first-degree relatives.
Obsessive-compulsive disorder	A chronic neuropsychiatric disorder characterized by the frequent and sudden intrusion into consciousness of unwanted worries or unpleasant images and/or urges to perform repeatedly seemingly senseless acts.	History and presenting obsessive-compulsive symptoms based on information from multiple informants; ratings of symptom severity; treatment response; performance on neuropsychological battery; subtypes of obsessive-compulsive disorder will be distinguished on the basis of family study data from first-degree relatives.

obsessive-compulsive behavior (Kurlan et al., 1989). These experiences include premonitory feelings or urges that are relieved with the performance of tics (A. Cohen & Leckman, 1992; Leckman, Walker, et al., 1993) and a need to perform tics or compulsions until they are felt to be just right (Leckman, Grice, et al., 1995; Leckman, Walker, et al., 1994). A significant proportion of individuals with Tourette's syndrome within clinic populations also present with attentional difficulties, impulsivity, and disruptive behaviors that often overshadow the tic symptoms as sources of impairment for the child and distress for the family (D. Cohen & Leckman, 1994; Comings & Comings, 1987a; Nolan et al., 1996). Regrettably, many patients suffer from all three disorders: Tourette's syndrome, obsessive-compulsive disorder, and ADHD. The expression of these symptoms alters over the course of development. For example, tics typically have their onset during the first decade of life. Paradoxically, although tics usually diminish in frequency and intensity by early adulthood, the most severely affected individuals are adults whose symptoms may include self-injurious motor tics (e.g., being blinded by a detached retina secondary to hitting tics), coprolalia (shouting obscenities), and markedly disinhibited speech and behavior.

Once thought to be a rare condition, the prevalence of Tourette's syndrome is currently estimated to be between 1 and 8 cases per 1,000 boys, and between 0.1 and 4 cases per 1,000 girls (see Chapter 10; Apter et al., 1993; Burd, Kerbeshian, Wiknheiser, & Fisher, 1986b; Comings et al., 1990; Costello, Angold, Burns, Stangl, Tweed, & Erkanli, 1996; Costello, Angold, Burns, Stangl, Tweed, Erkanli, & Worthman, 1996). Community surveys indicate that chronic tics are frequently observed and may affect as many as 4–5% of school-age children (Costello, Angold, Burns, Stangl, Tweed, & Erkanli, 1996; Costello, Angold, Burns, Stangl, Tweed, Erkanli, & Worthman, 1996; Zahner, Clubb, Leckman, & Pauls, 1988). Although the etiological relationship between these chronic tics and Tourette's syndrome has not been generally established, studies of monozygotic twins indicate that in some instances, chronic tics are simply lesser variants (Price, Kidd, Cohen, Pauls, & Leckman, 1985).

Two putative forms of Tourette's syndrome are discussed in this volume: familial Tourette's syndrome and sporadic, nonfamilial Tourette's syndrome. The first category includes a majority of Tourette's syndrome patients who have a positive family history of chronic tics or Tourette's syndrome (Pauls, Raymond, et al., 1991). A familial form of obsessive-compulsive disorder (so-called tic-related obsessive-compulsive disorder) also appears in these families (Pauls, Alsobrook, Goodman, Rasmussen, & Leckman, 1995; Pauls & Leckman, 1986; Pauls, Raymond, et al., 1991). A form of ADHD may also be present in these families that appears to be unrelated to other familial forms of ADHD (Pauls et al., 1993). We will present evidence that suggests that these conditions— Tourette's syndrome, chronic multiple tics, tic-related obsessive-compulsive disorder, and tic-related ADHD—share a common genetic diathesis and are distinguishable from other phenotypically similar conditions on the basis of clinical phenotype, neurobiology, and treatment response (see Chapter 10; Leckman, Goodman, et al., 1994a; Leckman, Goodman, et al., 1995; Leckman, Grice, et al., 1995; Leckman, Walker, et al., 1994; McDougle, Goodman, Leckman, Barr, et al., 1993; McDougle et al., 1994; McDougle, Goodman, Leckman, & Price, 1993; Pauls, Raymond, et al., 1991; Randolph et al., 1993). The second category, sporadic, nonfamilial Tourette's syndrome, at present is a residual category. A variety of factors have been implicated in the appearance of these sporadic cases, including trauma and chronic exposure to neuroleptic agents. Putative postinfectious autoimmune forms of Tourette's syndrome and obsessive-compulsive disorder may also fall into this residual category (A. Allen, Leonard, & Swedo, 1995; Kiessling, Marcotte, & Culpepper, 1993a, 1993b; Swedo et al., 1994; Tucker et al., 1996). However, it is also possible that neuroimmunological factors, including genetically mediated host susceptibility, may play a prominent role in the pathogenesis in a large proportion of Tourette's syndrome cases, including those with a positive family history.

Obsessive-compulsive disorder (Table 9.1) is a chronic, disabling condition in which the individual repeatedly experiences the sudden intrusion into consciousness of unwanted worries or unpleasant images and repeated urges to perform seeningly senseless acts. The intrusive mental images that besiege the consciousness often involve aggressive or sexual content that the individual regards as repugnant and morally reprehensible. Other obsessive thoughts include a need for symmetry or exactness in how things look, feel, or sound. Compulsions are repetitive acts, typically performed a certain number of times or according to certain private rules, that the individual is driven to complete, even though the acts are perceived as excessive and/or senseless. Compulsions are often preceded by an urge that is recognized to be of internal origin and that bears some relationship to obsessional worries (Rachman & Hodgson, 1980). The most common compulsions are concerned either with fears of contamination that lead to hand washing or other grooming behaviors or with "pathological" doubting that leads to repetitive checking to prevent some catastrophe, for example, repeatedly checking the stove to ensure that a fire does not start inadvertently. Despite potential embarrassment, performance of compulsive washing and checking is frequently associated with a measurable reduction in the subjective discomfort generated by the obsessional worries (Rachman, de Silva, & Röper, 1976; Röper & Rachman, 1976; Röper, Rachman, & Hodgson, 1973). Patients frequently report their mental efforts to resist these unwanted ideas, images, and urges to act. As noted above, some individuals with obsessive-compulsive disorder experience problems with tics and/or Tourette's syndrome.

Recently, childhood obsessive-compulsive disorder has been recognized as being much more common (in the range of 1–5%) than previously believed (Costello, Angold, Burns, Stangl, Tweed, & Erkanli, 1996; Costello, Angold, Burns, Stangl, Tweed, Erkanli, & Worthman, 1996; Flament et al., 1988; Valleni-Basile et al., 1994; A. Zohar et al., 1992). These figures are largely consistent with those of Karno, Golding, Sorenson, and Burnam (1988), who reported that 3% of the adult population suffers from diagnosable obsessive-compulsive disorder (see Chapter 10 for a review).

Three putative forms of obsessive-compulsive disorder are considered in this volume: familial tic-related obsessive-compulsive disorder, familial non-tic-related obsessive-compulsive disorder, and sporadic, nonfamilial obsessive-compulsive disorder. As noted above, a familial form of obsessive-compulsive disorder (so-called tic-related obsessive-compulsive disorder) appears in Tourette's syndrome families (Pauls & Leckman, 1986; Pauls, Raymond, et al., 1991). In addition, approximately 30–40% of obsessive-compulsive disorder families have a positive family history of obsessive-compulsive disorder or subclinical obsessive-compulsive disorder in the absence of any history of tics in the proband's family members (Pauls et al., 1995; Rasmussen, 1994). Evidence exists to suggest that familial, non-tic-related obsessive-compulsive disorder is distinguishable from tic-related obsessive-compulsive disorder on the basis of clinical phenotype, neurobiology, and treatment response (Leckman, Goodman, et al., 1994a; Leckman, Walker, et al., 1994; McDougle, Goodman, Leckman, Barr, et al., 1993; McDougle, et al., 1994; McDougle, Goodman, Leckman,

& Price, 1993; Pauls, Raymond, et al., 1991). The third obsessive-compulsive disorder category, sporadic, nonfamilial obsessive-compulsive disorder, at present is a residual category that is usually associated with specific brain injury or damage.

Although the division of Tourette's syndrome and obsessive-compulsive disorder into discrete etiological subtypes has been heuristically useful, it doubtless is an oversimplification. A complementary approach has been to examine the symptom dimensions within each of these phenotypes. This effort is best exemplified by our recent work on the symptoms of obsessive-compulsive disorder (Leckman, Grice, et al., 1997), in which four symptom domains emerged from two independent data sets. In this study, obsessions of symmetry and exactness usually co-occurred with compulsions of ordering and arranging, doing and redoing, and counting. These symptoms, however, did not as frequently co-occur with other symptom dimensions, for example, contamination worries and cleaning rituals that form their own separate dimension. Using this approach, we hope to discover vulnerability genes and other risk factors that are specific to particular symptom dimensions.

Although not the principal focus of this volume, the clinical phenotype and pathogenetic mechanisms that underlie ADHD are also considered in this overview, given its importance as a major and frequent source of comorbidity. Briefly, ADHD is a clinically heterogeneous syndrome of childhood onset characterized by problems of inattention, distractibility, impulsivity, and motoric hyperactivity. The symptoms of ADHD usually manifest themselves in loosely structured academic, social, or occupational settings where there are many distractions as well as a clear need to be attentive to succeed. In highly structured one-on-one situations, the symptoms of ADHD may not be noticeable. Extensive studies of comorbidity among children and adults with ADHD have been undertaken (Biederman, Faraone, Keenan, Steingard, & Tsuang, 1991; Biederman, Faraone, Keenan, & Tsuang, 1991; Biederman, Newcorn, & Sprich, 1991a; Faraone et al., 1992; Faraone, Biederman, Keenan, & Tsuang, 1991; Faraone, Biederman, Krifcher, et al., 1993; Lahey et al., 1988; Semrud-Clikeman et al., 1992; Szatmari, Offord, & Boyle, 1989). Comorbid chronic tic disorders and/or obsessive-compulsive disorder are known to occur. But the more common comorbid conditions are conduct disorder, oppositional defiant disorder, major depression, anxiety disorders other than obsessive-compulsive disorder, and learning disabilities. Some of these data suggest that some forms of ADHD, ADHD plus oppositional defiant disorder, and ADHD plus conduct disorder exist along a continuum of vertically transmitted familial factors (Faraone et al., 1991). In the case of the other comorbid syndromes, the preponderance of evidence suggests that the genetic vulnerability to ADHD segregates independently from these other traits or conditions.

The prevalence of ADHD in community surveys of children and adolescents usually ranges from 2% (Costello et al., 1988; Costello, Angold,

Burns, Stangl, Tweed, & Erkanli, 1996; Costello, Angold, Burns, Stangl, Tweed, Erkanli, & Worthman, 1996) to 9% (Bird et al., 1988). Most studies report that boys are 2 to 9 times more likely to manifest ADHD than are girls.

Empirically, we have sought to characterize the ADHD specifically associated with Tourette's syndrome and obsessive-compulsive disorder (Pauls et al., 1993). However, it is clear that there are multiple and potentially overlapping forms of ADHD. Once again, a dimensional approach may be the most promising. In this regard, the current *DSM-IV* distinction between predominantly hyperactive-impulsive and predominantly inattentive forms of ADHD may be a step in the right direction.

Genetic Factors

Genetic factors play an important role in the transmission and expression of these disorders, as reviewed in detail in Chapter 11. Twin and family studies support the view that Tourette's syndrome is a genetically mediated disorder (Hyde, Aaronson, Randolph, Rickler, & Weinberger, 1992; Pauls & Leckman, 1986; Pauls et al., 1993; Price, Leckman, & Pauls, 1986; Walkup et al., 1996). Although the initial segregation analyses were compatible with a single major autosomal gene, subsequent linkage studies have thus far failed to detect a genomic region linked to the Tourette's syndrome phenotype in large multigenerational families (Pakstis et al., 1991). As part of this effort, a number of candidate genes have been evaluated in Tourette's syndrome (Comings et al., 1991, 1996; Gelernter et al., 1990, 1993; Gelernter, Pauls, Leckman, Kidd, & Kurlan, 1994). To date, one of the most promising of these results concerns an allelic variant of the dopamine 4 receptor (DRD4) gene (Grice et al., 1996). However, this variant appears to contribute only modestly to the Tourette's disorder phenotype in just a few families.

As described in Chapter 11, we and others are continuing the search for the Tourette's syndrome vulnerability genes using both nonparametric (sib-pair design) and parametric approaches to linkage, as well as candidate gene and haplotype relative risk and transmission disequilibrium test association studies. We anticipate that a small number of genetic loci will eventually be detected that have a measurable effect on an individual's vulnerability to develop Tourette's syndrome or a related form of illness (Table 9.2 and Figure 9.2a).

Twin and family studies also suggest that genetic factors are likely to play an important role in the transmission and expression of obsessive-compulsive disorder (Pauls et al., 1995; Rasmussen, 1994). A small number of candidate genes have been evaluated in obsessive-compulsive disorder with negative results (Catalano et al., 1994; Novelli, Nobile, Diferia, Sciuto, & Catalano, 1994). However, with a few exceptions, neither segregation analyses nor classical genetic linkage studies have yet been performed. As indicated in Table 9.2, we hypothesize that there is a specific set of genes

TABLE 9.2   Genetic Factors

Factor	Description of Latent Variable	Operational Measures
Tourette vulnerability genes	Genes of major and minor effect that underlie the vulnerability to develop familial Tourette's syndrome and tic-related forms of obsessive-compulsive disorder and ADHD.	Positive family history of Tourette's syndrome or chronic motor or vocal tic disorder in first-degree family members; candidate genes involved with the development and activity of cortico-striato-thalamo-cortical (CSTC) circuits implicated in Tourette's syndrome.
Obsessive-compulsive vulnerability genes	Genes of major and minor effect that underlie the vulnerability to develop familial, non-tic-related forms of obsessive-compulsive disorder.	Positive family history of obsessive-compulsive disorder in the absence of Tourette syndrome or chronic motor or vocal tic disorder in first-degree family members; candidate genes involved with the development and activity of the CSTC circuits implicated in obsessive-compulsive disorder.
Other vulnerability genes	Other genes that can modify the expression and clinical severity of Tourette's syndrome, obsessive-compulsive disorder, and/or ADHD including the genetic factors associated with comorbid conditions including ADHD, depression, bipolar disorder, anxiety disorders, learning disabilities, and Sydenham's chorea.	Positive family history for comorbid psychiatric conditions and genes linked to these comorbid disorders; positive family history for possibly related autoimmune disorders, including rheumatic fever, in first-degree family members; candidate genes implicated in ADHD; candidate genes relevant to the immunological processing of streptococcal antigens.

that confer vulnerability to familial, non-tic-related obsessive-compulsive disorder (Table 9.2 and Figure 9.2b; Pauls et al., 1995).

Twin, family genetic, and adoption studies also provide consistent evidence that genetic factors contribute to the transmission and expression of ADHD (Biederman et al., 1986, 1992; Cantwell, 1975; Faraone & Biederman, 1994; R. Goodman & Stevenson, 1989; Hudizak & Todd, 1993; Lopez, 1965; Morrison & Stewart, 1973). Segregation analyses are consistent with the effect of a single major gene, but the differences in fit among the genetic models are small, suggesting an indeterminant result (Deutsch, Matthysse, Swanson, & Farkas, 1990; Eaves et al., 1993; Faraone et al., 1992). Yet to be replicated, candidate gene studies have reported associations between an allelic variant at DRD4 (James Kennedy, personal communication, 1997) and at dopamine transporter (DAT) locus and the transmission of ADHD (Cook et al., 1995). As with obsessive-compulsive disorder, classical genetic linkage studies and affected sib-pair methods have not yet been performed in ADHD. We hypothesize that the vulnerability to develop ADHD and/or other comorbid conditions will be associated with a third set of genes (Table 9.2). This set of genes may partially overlap with the vulnerability genes associated with Tourette's syndrome and obsessive-compulsive disorder. Alternatively, the presence of these genetic vulnerabilities in individuals susceptible to Tourette's syndrome or obsessive-compulsive disorder may influence their clinical presentation and course.

Vulnerability genes associated with a range of other important comorbid conditions, including depression, bipolar disorder, other anxiety disorders, conduct disorder, and learning disabilities, are also included in this category. Although the available evidence suggests that these disorders do not cosegregate with Tourette's syndrome or obsessive-compulsive disorder in family studies (Pauls et al., 1994, 1995), their presence has the potential to alter the severity and course of these disorders.

One last set of genes to consider are those that may influence some aspect of the body's immunological system that may make some individuals more susceptible to conditions such as Sydenham's chorea or related post-streptococcal autoimmune tic and/or obsessive-compulsive phenomena.

Historically, many of the disease-susceptibility genes identified through genetic linkage studies are novel genes whose function under normal circumstances was previously unknown. Although this is likely to be the case for Tourette's syndrome and obsessive-compulsive disorder, the apparent involvement of multiple, or at least a few, genes lends encouragement to speculations concerning possible classes of candidate genes. What, then, are some of the important features that these genes might possess? A consideration of the known environment risk factors and the neurobiology of these disorders provides some clues.

Other Risk and Protective Factors

The prevailing models of Tourette's syndrome and obsessive-compulsive disorder pathogenesis emphasize the importance of the interaction between genes and epigenetic or environmental factors over the course of CNS development (Leckman, Peterson, et al., 1997). In contrast to the relatively slow progress in identifying specific vulnerability genes, efforts to identify risk and protective factors that mediate the expression of Tourette's syndrome and obsessive-compulsive disorder have been more successful (see Chapter 12 and Leckman & Peterson, 1993).

Events during the perinatal period (Table 9.3 and Figures 9.2a and 9.2b) have been consistently implicated in both Tourette's syndrome and obsessive-compulsive disorder (Capstick & Seldrup, 1977; Hyde et al., 1992; Leckman et al., 1990; Pasamanick & Kawi, 1956; Santangelo et al., 1994;

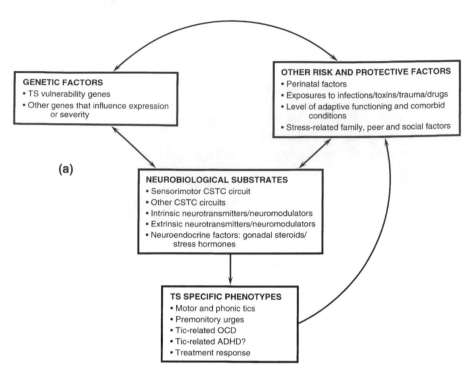

Figures 9.2a and 9.2b   Hueristic models of pathogenesis for Tourette's syndrome and obsessive-compulsive disorder. These figures provide a more detailed summary of putative contributors to the pathogenesis of Tourette's syndrome (a) and obsessive-compulsive disorder (b). These figures correspond to the descriptions provided in Tables 9.1, 9.2, 9.3, and 9.4. In addition, each of these areas is the subject of subsequent

Sprich-Buckminster, Biederman, Milberger, Faraone, & Lehman, 1993; Whitaker et al., 1997). We hypothesize that perinatal risk and protective factors influence the development and function of specific brain circuits that in turn influence the subsequent natural history of Tourette's syndrome, obsessive-compulsive disorder, and ADHD (Leckman & Peterson, 1993).

A second set of environmental risk and protective factors (Table 9.3) concerns the possible role of accidents of nature (infections, trauma, toxins, and drugs). For example, in the aftermath of the epidemic of encephalitis lethargica (1916–1926), tic, obsessive-compulsive, and attentional problems were commonplace. Recent attention has focused on the role of poststreptococcal autoimmune phenomena in the development of Sydenham's chorea, obsessive-compulsive disorder, Tourette's syndrome, and ADHD (A. Allen et al., 1995; Husby, van de Rijn, Zabriskie, Abdin, & William, 1976; Kiessling, Marcotte, & Culpepper, 1993a, 1993b; Swedo et al., 1994). We hypothesize that infectious agents and autoimmune phenomena can influence the development and function of specific

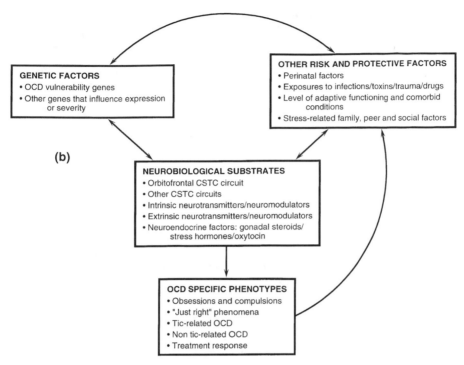

chapters in this volume. The phenomenology and natural history of Tourette's syndrome and obsessive-compulsive disorder are covered in Chapters 4 and 5, respectively. Chapter 11 describes our knowledge of genetic factors, and Chapter 12 addresses our emergent knowledge of environmental risk factors that likely shape the expression of these complex phenotypes. The neurobiological substrates are described in Chapters 13 and 14.

brain circuits and that these effects result in a range of phenotypic outcomes with regard to tics and obsessive-compulsive symptoms.

A third set of risk factors (Table 9.3 and Figures 9.2a and 9.2b) concerns an individual's level of adaptive functioning and the presence of comorbid medical and psychiatric disorders (particularly ADHD, depression, other anxiety disorders, conduct disorder, and specific developmental and learning disabilities; Coffey, Frazier, & Chen, 1992; Pauls et al., 1993, 1994). The presence of these difficulties may further burden the individual and limit his or her capacity to remain on track. As discussed in Chapter 8, the absence of these risk factors combined with hard-to-define personality traits associated with a determination to succeed likely contributes to resilience.

A fourth set of nongenetic risk factors (Table 9.3 and Figures 9.2a and 9.2b) includes aspects of the interpersonal and social environment. Tourette's syndrome and obsessive-compulsive disorder are to some extent stress-sensitive conditions, so that events experienced as emotionally

TABLE 9.3   Other Risk and Protective Factors

Factor	Description of Latent Variable	Operational Measures
Perinatal	Early perinatal factors that influence the development and age-related activity of cortico-striato-thalamo-cortical (CSTC) circuits and related structures implicated in Tourette's syndrome and obsessive-compulsive disorder.	History of events and exposures occurring during the perinatal period. Prime candidates include chronic or acute hypoxic insults (maternal smoking, placenta insufficiency, prolonged labor); maternal emotional stress during pregnancy, severe nausea and vomiting in the first trimester, and exposure of the male fetus to high levels of androgens in utero.
Microenvironment	Other microenvironmental factors that may influence the activity of CSTC circuits as well as the severity and course of Tourette's syndrome and obsessive-compulsive disorder.	History of exposures to infectious agents, trauma, and/or medications that may contribute to a worsening of Tourette's syndrome and obsessive-compulsive disorder; serum titers for streptococcal related antigens.
Adaptive function/strengths	Level of adaptive functioning and the presence of comorbid conditions that may influence the course and outcome of Tourette's syndrome and obsessive-compulsive disorder.	Level of adaptive behavior; presence of comorbid medical, neurological and/or psychiatric disorders (particularly depression, bipolar disorder, other anxiety disorders, conduct disorders, and learning disabilities).
Support systems—stress	Stressful and/or supportive external events, interpersonal and social factors that may influence the course and outcome of Tourette's syndrome and obsessive-compulsive disorder.	Socioeconomic status; familial, peer and social supports; history of stressful events including limited peer and family acceptance, punitive parenting styles, marital discord.

arousing by the individual (exciting holidays, marital discord, punitive parenting styles, and limited peer and family acceptance) may contribute to a worsening of the syndrome (Bornstein et al., 1990; Silva et al., 1995; Surwillo et al., 1978). The effects of supportive family, peer, and social environments have not been systematically evaluated, but are likely to have a beneficial influence.

In each instance, we anticipate that the impact of these nongenetic risk factors is translated through established neurobiological pathways that selectively translate aspects of the external world into cellular realities.

Neurobiological Substrates

Based on available neuroanatomical and neurobiological data, there is convincing evidence for the involvement of specific cortico-striato-thalamo-cortical (CSTC) circuits in the expression of these disorders (see Chapter 13, Table 9.4, and Figures 9.2a and 9.2b). These circuits contain multiple modular units (cellular collectives) that are distributed according to highly ordered repetitive patterns. These anatomic arrangements are well suited to convey cortical information in a highly specific manner throughout the basal ganglia and to modulate precisely the neuronal activity of several functional brain systems that are intimately related to the control (initiation and monitoring vs. inhibition) of different aspects of psychomotor behavior (Alexander et al., 1986; Parent & Hazrati, 1995a, 1995b). We hypothesize that some of these circuits are selectively disinhibited in Tourette's syndrome and obsessive-compulsive disorder, making these circuits unusually sensitive to alterations in the internal milieu of the body or the larger psychosocial environment (Leckman, Peterson, et al., 1997).

The sensorimotor CSTC circuit includes projections from the sensorimotor, primary motor, and supplementary motor cortices to matrisomal portions of the putamen and the head of the caudate nucleus. These striatal sites in turn project to portions of the globus pallidus and the pars reticulata of the substantia nigra. These output neurons of the basal ganglia then project to ventral-lateral and midline nuclei in the thalamus that in turn project to the cortex. Based on extensive pilot data (B. Peterson, Leckman, Duncan, et al., 1994; B. Peterson, Riddle, Cohen, Katz, Smith, Hardin, et al., 1993) and the work of other investigators (Braun et al., 1993; Singer et al., 1993), we anticipate that the development and functional activity of this circuit and its commissural connections are intimately involved in the initiation and performance of tics and compulsions (Peterson, Skudlarski, Anderson, Zhang, Gatenby, Lacadie, Leckman, & Gore, 1998).

A second CSTC circuit, labeled orbitofrontal (OF) by Alexander et al. (1986), includes projections from the orbital-frontal, cingulate, and temporal cortices to striosomal portions of the head of the caudate nucleus. These striatal neurons in turn project to portions of the globus pallidus, the pars reticulata of the substantia nigra, and the ventral pallidum. These output neurons then project to portions of the ventral-anterior and medial-dorsal nuclei in the thalamus that in turn project back to the cortex. As reviewed in Chapter 13, we and others hypothesize that the development and functional activity of this circuit and its commissural connections are critically involved in our brain-based error detection and harm-avoidance systems and as such play a key role in the pathobiology of some symptoms encountered in obsessive-compulsive disorder (Baxter et al., 1992; Graybiel, 1995; Insel, 1992b; Schwartz, 1996).

We presume that the OF circuits are to some degree anatomically and functionally distinct from the remaining other association (AS) circuits described by Parent and Hazrati (1995a, 1995b). These AS circuits include

TABLE 9.4   Neurobiological Substrates

Substrate	Description of Latent Variable	Operational Measures
CSTC	Cortico-striato-thalamo-cortical circuits that contain multiple modular units that are distributed according to highly ordered repetitive patterns. The anatomic arrangements are well suited to convey cortical information in a highly specific manner throughout the basal ganglia and to modulate in a precise manner the neuronal activity of several functional brain systems that are intimately related to the control of different aspects of psychomotor behavior. Specific CSTC circuits have been implicated in Tourette's syndrome and obsessive-compulsive disorder.	Structural and functional in vivo MRI measures of specific subcortical nuclei and cortical areas associated with the CSTC circuits and positron emission tomography (PET) studies of metabolic activity; morphometric and stereological measures using postmortem brain material.
Intrinsic neurotransmitters- neuromodulators	Neurotransmitters and neuromodulators intrinsic to the CSTC circuits, principally the classical excitatory neurotransmitter glutamate and inhibitory neurotransmitter gamma-aminobutyric acid (GABA).	In vivo magnetic resonance spectroscopy studies as well as neurochemical, immunohisto- chemical, in situ studies of specific subcortical nuclei and cortical areas associated with the CSTC circuits using postmortem brain material.
Extrinsic neurotransmitters- neuromodulators	Neurotransmitters and neuromodulators extrinsic to the CSTC circuits and that regulate their activity, principally dopamine, serotonin, and norepinephrine that have been implicated in Tourette's syndrome and obsessive- compulsive disorder or a comorbid condition.	Neurochemical, immunohistochemical, in situ studies of specific systems using postmortem brain material; in vivo single photon emission computed tomography (SPECT) studies; and cerebrospinal fluid (CSF) assays; clinical response to selective psychopharmacological agents.
Other neurotransmitters- neuromodulators	Other neurotransmitters and neuromodulators outside of the classical neurotransmitter and neuromodulator systems that have been implicated in the pathobiology of Tourette's syndrome and obsessive- compulsive disorder, and/or a comorbid condition: principally gonadal steroids and other centrally active hormones including oxytocin.	Neurochemical, immunohistochemical, in situ studies of specific neurotransmitter systems using postmortem brain material; cerebrospinal fluid assays; clinical response to selective psychopharmacological agents; clinical response to selective psychopharmacological agents.

projections from various AS cortices in the frontal, temporal, and parietal lobes to the matrisomal compartments of the striatum (most of the head, body, and tail of the caudate, and portions of the putamen). These striatal neurons then project to portions of the globus pallidus and the pars reticulata of the substantia nigra. These output neurons then project to portions of the parvicellular areas of the ventral-anterior and medial-dorsal nuclei in the thalamus that in turn project to the cortex. We hypothesize that the development and functional activity of these circuits and their commissural connections are involved in compensatory cognitive efforts to regulate or inhibit maladaptive psychomotor behaviors such as the tics and compulsions seen in Tourette's syndrome.

A fourth CSTC circuit, labeled limbic (LI) by Parent and Hazrati (1995a, 1995b) includes projections from anterior cingulate, hippocampal, entorhinal, and temporal cortices and amygdala to the ventral striatum (ventral-most putamen and caudate nuclei, nucleus accumbens, and portions of the olfactory tubercle). These ventral-striatal neurons then project to the ventral pallidum and to portions of the globus pallidus and the pars reticulata of the substantia nigra. These output neurons then project to portions of the parvicellular areas of the ventral-medial-dorsal nuclei in the thalamus that in turn project back to various cortical regions. This circuit is thought to process emotionally laden LI information. There is clear evidence for its involvement in obsessive-compulsive disorder and other anxiety disorders (Baxter et al., 1992; Rauch et al., 1994). These circuits may well contribute to aspects of the Tourette's syndrome phenotype that are involved in heightened responsiveness to emotional stimuli (Peterson, Skudlarski, Anderson, Zhang, Gatenby, Lacadie, Leckman, & Gore, 1998).

As detailed in Chapter 14, the intrinsic neurotransmitters and neuromodulators (Table 9.4 and Figures 9.2a and 9.2b) involved in these circuits include excitatory amino acids, such as glutamate, in the cortico-striatal and thalamo-cortical projections, and inhibitory amino acids, such as gamma-aminobutyric acid (GABA) in the striato-pallidal and pallido-thalamic projections (Graybiel, 1990). The arrangement of projections in these CSTC loops (cortico-striatal, excitatory; striato-pallidal, inhibitory; pallido-thalamic, inhibitory; and thalamo-cortical, excitatory) suggests that cortical sites could be disinhibited by a number of mechanisms, including abnormalities in the thalamus and a reduction in the tonic inhibition of thalamo-cortical projections due to either underactivity of the pallido-thalamic projections or overactivity of the striato-pallidal projections.

As noted above, we hypothesize that Tourette's syndrome, obsessive-compulsive disorder, and ADHD can be usefully viewed as syndromes of disinhibition that directly involve these particular CSTC circuits (Peterson, Skudlarski, et al., 1998). As part of this conceptualization, Tourette's syndrome is seen as a disorder in which individuals are unable to inhibit premonitory sensory urges, leading to the emergence of small, prewired bits of motor and phonic behavior. In obsessive-compulsive disorder, individuals are unable to inhibit specific, perhaps evolutionarily conserved, innate worries leading to the emergence of intense ego-dystonic obsessions and compulsions.

Based on data from highly sensitive anterograde tract-tracing methods, attention has recently focused on the modulatory role of the external segment of the globus pallidus and the subthalamic nucleus on the output of the basal ganglia (Parent & Hazrati, 1995a, 1995b). These structures can markedly influence the neuronal computation that occurs at the level of the internal segment of the globus pallidus and the pars reticulata of the substantia nigra. Specifically, there is evidence from pilot postmortem brain studies that levels of the excitatory amino acid transmitter glutamate is altered in the brains of Tourette's syndrome patients in both the internal and external segments of the globus pallidus as well as the pars reticulata of the substantia nigra (G. Anderson et al., 1992a, 1992b). These data, together with the evidence of reduced globus pallidal volumes in Tourette's syndrome subjects (B. Peterson, Riddle, Cohen, Katz, Smith, Hardin, et al., 1993; Singer et al., 1993) and the key regulatory position of these nuclei in the CSTC circuits, support the hypothesis that developmentally sensitive alterations of the structure and function of these nuclei may be important determinants of tic-related behavioral outcomes.

Some of the extrinsic neurotransmitter and neuromodulator systems (Table 9.4 and Figures 9.2a and 9.2b) that regulate the activity of these CSTC circuits include dopamine, serotonin, and norepinephrine. Serotonergic projections from midbrain, pontine, and medullary sites innervate cortical, striatal, pallidal, and thalamic structures. Norepinephrine projections arise from pontine and medullary tegmental regions and project throughout the neural axis, including the entire neocortex. Each of these systems is stress-sensitive. We hypothesize that the developmental course and functional activity of these modulatory systems critically influence the severity of the behavioral dysfunction seen in Tourette's syndrome (motor and phonic tics and other, more complex disinhibited behaviors) and obsessive-compulsive disorder (Leckman, Goodman, et al., 1995; Leckman, Grice, et al., 1995).

Dopamine projections from the midbrain merit special attention. Dopaminergic projections from the substantia nigra and ventral-tegmental area innervate cortical projection neurons and the medium spiny projection neurons in the striatum, among others. These dopaminergic fibers play a crucial role in the formation and coordination of behavioral repertoires through their innervation of tonically active neurons that are frequently positioned at the boundaries of matrisomal and striosomal compartments in the striatum (Graybiel, 1995). These dopaminergic along with other monoaminergic systems are likely to fire in response to salient (potentially rewarding) stimuli in the environment (W. Schultz, Dayan, & Montague, 1997).

Available evidence suggests that there may be a dopaminergic hyperinnervation of the striatum in some Tourette's syndrome patients (Malison et al., 1995; Singer, Hahn, & Moran, 1991); other studies have indicated the presence of hypersensitive dopamine D2 receptors in the striatum of

Tourette's syndrome patients (Wolf et al., 1996). Either of these conditions, alone or in combination, could significantly contribute to the disinhibition of thalamo-cortical projections and the appearance of motor and vocal tics (Leckman, Peterson, et al., 1997).

Other neuromodulatory systems also need to be considered in these models of pathogenesis (Table 9.4 and Figures 9.2a and 9.2b). For example, given the high prevalence of Tourette's syndrome, ADHD, and some forms of childhood obsessive-compulsive disorder in males, it is likely that gonadal steroids acting via sexually dimorphic brain systems, including the hypothalamus and other limbic structures, modulate the activity of these CSTC circuits and are important determinants of the natural history of these disorders (Leckman et al., 1992; B. Peterson et al., 1992). Similarly, based on research findings, we hypothesize that other neurobiological systems involved with the control of grooming, sexual, and affiliative behaviors, such as the oxytocin projections from the hypothalamus, can influence the CSTC circuits involved in obsessive-compulsive disorder (Leckman, Goodman, et al., 1994b).

Heuristic Models of Pathogenesis

In the spirit of offering a more integrated view of the pathogenic mechanisms and their involvement in particular outcomes, we present a schematic model of the pathogenesis of Tourette's syndrome and obsessive-compulsive disorder (Figures 9.2a and 9.2b). We recognize the hazards inherent in such reductionistic formulations: the categories are not necessarily mutually exclusive, nor are they necessarily internally homogeneous.

Figure 9.2a depicts a simplified version of our model of Tourette's syndrome pathogenesis. Unique features of this model include the role of the Tourette's syndrome–specific genes and their putative interrelationship with the environmental factors that are active early in CNS development. A crucial question remains: Do the Tourette's syndrome genes in any way set the stage for any of the perinatal risk factors, or are they separate and independent mechanisms? Heuristically, we entertain the view that some of the specific Tourette's syndrome genes are themselves involved in the development of the CSTC circuits, hence our interest in homeobox genes involved in the formation of the basal ganglia (Lin et al., 1996). We also are exploring the possible relationship between environmental risk factors active early in development and the range of phenotypic outcomes seen in tic-related disorders, given the hints that are already available (Hyde et al., 1992; Leckman, Dolnansky, et al., 1990; Santangelo et al., 1994). The potential involvement of all of the CSTC circuits and the preliminary volumetric and neuropathological findings have focused our attention on the role of the basal ganglia, particularly the globus pallidus and the subthalamic nuclei (Leckman, Peterson, et al., 1997; Peterson, Skudlarksi, et al., 1998).

Figure 9.2b depicts a simplified version of our model for obsessive-compulsive disorder pathogenesis. Unique features of this model include the role of obsessive-compulsive disorder-specific genes in the development and functional activity of the OF CSTC circuit. Although the most striking functional changes have been documented in the head of the caudate nucleus (Baxter et al., 1992), we are particularly interested in the role of the OF and LI cortices and the amygdala in activating the caudate. This interest is based in part on the finding of elevated levels of CSF oxytocin (OT) almost exclusively in this group of obsessive-compulsive disorder patients and that early in CNS development, OT receptors in rodents are found in high concentration in caudoputamen regions and in the cingulate cortex (see review by Leckman, Goodman, et al., 1994b). Corollaries to this interest in OT mechanisms include our ongoing haplotype relative-risk candidate gene studies with the OT receptor gene and examination of postmortem brain material from non-tic-related obsessive-compulsive disorder patients for evidence of OT receptors in the cingulate and caudate nuclei. On the treatment front, we plan to study the effects of nonpeptidyl OT agonists and antagonists in this form of obsessive-compulsive disorder as they become available. In addition, based on our pharmacological data (McDougle et al., 1994; McDougle, Goodman, Leckman, & Price, 1993; McDougle, Goodman, & Price, 1993), we consider it likely that dopaminergic mechanisms play less of a role in this condition than in tic-related forms of obsessive-compulsive disorder.

Nonfamilial, sporadic forms of Tourette's syndrome and obsessive-compulsive disorder may involve a different mix of genetic and environmental factors than the familial forms of these disorders. Although these are clearly residual categories at present, the Sydenham's story and a remarkable case that we have followed in our clinic (Tucker et al., 1996) have persuaded us that this is a potentially important avenue to follow.

FUTURE DIRECTIONS

During the past two decades, we have had the privilege of leading a multidisciplinary team of clinicians and researchers focused on the systematic study of Tourette's syndrome, obsessive-compulsive disorder, and related forms of psychopathology. In this endeavor, these disorders have emerged as model neuropsychiatric disorders. Based on our research and that of other investigators, we have formulated increasingly explicit models of pathogenesis that emphasize the role of identifiable genetic and epigenetic factors that shape the development and activity of specific brain circuits, circuits that in turn are crucially involved in the creation, maintenance, and facilitation of cognitive, emotive, and action repertoires. These model are provisional, but as working models, they lend structure to our knowledge and direction to our current hypotheses.

We can anticipate the further elaboration of these models with fresh details from basic research on the development of action repertoires in the CNS and how they are constrained by specific vulnerability genes and altered by particular epigenetic events. Clinical studies using in vivo imaging techniques will permit us to glimpse in a crude fashion the neurobiological correlates of these disorders as they develop in the first decade of life. Stereological studies of postmortem brain specimens will complement the imaging studies and for the first time allow accurate estimates of the number of neurons and glia in key brain nuclei. Application of nonlinear dynamical models may elucidate the temporal occurrence of symptoms and may allow us to gain deeper insight into the multicomponent neurobiological processes from which they derive. With the development of increasingly accurate and sophisticated models of neural networks, it may be possible to model the consequences of genetic and epigenetic constraints in simulation studies of sensorimotor processing. Finally, with the development of various transgenic methods, it may be possible to construct animal models that incorporate the human allelic variants associated with vulnerability. These animals could then be used experimentally to study the impact of various epigenetic factors in a dose-response fashion. Such animals would likely become valuable allies in our search for safe and effective treatments or, better still, preventive interventions.

SUMMARY OF CHAPTER 9

Over the course of the past twenty years, the Yale Child Study Center has provided care and pursued an interdisciplinary program of research focused on Tourette's syndrome, related forms of obsessive-compulsive disorder, and ADHD. Working models of pathogenesis are presented that emphasize the role of cortico-striato-thalamo-cortical circuits and the genetic and environmental factors that shape their development and activity. These models of pathogenesis, with their identification of risk and protective factors, have usefully served as a scaffold for our research endeavors. Heuristically, we propose that maladaptive phenotypes associated with Tourette's syndrome and obsessive-compulsive disorder phenotypes are in part the product of a heightened, but selective, sensitivity to alterations in both the internal milieu of the body and external psychosocial environment of the individual. This heightened sensitivity can in turn lead to the exaggerated, disinhibited expression of fragments of cognition and emotion, behavior that are normally assembled into voluntary action repertoires

PREVIEW OF CHAPTER 10

A few rigorous population-based studies of Tourette's syndrome and related disorders have not been conducted. They cast new light on the interrelationship of symptoms of Tourette's syndrome, obsessive-compulsive disorder, and ADHD. Future epidemiological studies are likely to clarify the role of various risk and protective factors in the etiology of these disorders.

CHAPTER 10

Epidemiological Studies

ADA H. ZOHAR, ALAN APTER, ROBERT A. KING, DAVID L. PAULS,
JAMES F. LECKMAN, and DONALD J. COHEN

> It is no great wonder if in long process of time, while fortune takes her
> course hither and tither, numerous coincidences should spontaneously occur.
> If the number and variety of subjects to be wrought upon be infinite, it is all
> the more easy for fortune, with such an abundance of material, to effect this
> similarity of results.
>
> —*Plutarch*

EPIDEMIOLOGICAL STUDIES OF PSYCHIATRIC DISORDERS:
GENERAL METHODOLOGICAL CONSIDERATIONS

Epidemiological studies of psychiatric disorders serve several goals. The
relative prevalence of various disorders informs the clinician trying to
decide among possible diagnoses indicated by the patient's symptoms. The
planning of mental health services is aided by prevalence estimates of
psychopathology in the population. Epidemiological studies help in identifying environmental and personal risk factors for the disorder. In addition,
the calculation of morbid risk to relatives of probands in family studies depends on having a good estimate of the prevalence and peak age of onset of
the disorder in the general population. Thus, epidemiological studies have
important implications for clinical decision making, for shaping mental
health policies, and for understanding etiologies.

Studies sampling from clinical centers can rely on well-trained clinicians to establish diagnoses, but suffer from sampling bias attendant on
clinical populations. Berkson (1946) showed that, compared to community
samples, clinical samples were more likely to suffer from comorbid diagnoses and more likely to have severe forms of the disorder under scrutiny.
Thus, they tend to underestimate prevalence and to overestimate severity
and comorbidity. True population samples afford the advantage of showing

177

the full range of the disorder and of assessing true comorbidity. The main difficulty of the epidemiological design lies in engaging well-trained clinicians to take part in large-scale diagnoses of population samples, prejudicing the validity of the diagnoses.

When the disorders are relatively common and are expected to occur in 1% or more of the population (e.g., attention-deficit/hyperactivity disorder [ADHD] or obsessive-compulsive disorder [OCD]), sample sizes of several hundred subjects will suffice, making it relatively easy to obtain sophisticated diagnosticians. The design of a satisfactory epidemiological study of a rarer disorder, such as autism or Tourette's syndrome, in which the expected prevalence is 100 times smaller, requires screening of tens of thousands of subjects. When the required sample size is so large, it is much more difficult and expensive to provide high-level diagnosticians for direct screening of the individual subjects, and a variety of shortcuts are taken: screening through clinical facilities; screening through referral contacts such as school psychologists; or initial screening of large samples using self-administered screens or lay interviewers, with subsequent referral of screen-positive subjects to a second-level, expert diagnostic interviewer. Each of these methodologies has its own costs and benefits. The studies reviewed in this chapter employ the full range of methodologies described.

PREVALENCE ESTIMATES OF TOURETTE'S SYNDROME

As summarized in Table 10.1, epidemiological studies of Tourette's syndrome were first conducted through clinical centers. Lucas, Beard, Raiput, and Kurland (1982) found that between 1968 and 1979 three individuals from the Rochester, Minnesota, area were diagnosed with Tourette's syndrome by a clinical center in Rochester. Taking into account the population size of the Rochester area, they estimated a prevalence of 0.046/10,000, or 4.6/1,000,000, making Tourette's syndrome a very rare disorder.

Spreading the sampling net a little wider, Burd, Kerbeshian, Wiknheiser, and Fisher (1986a, 1986b) asked all practicing physicians in North Dakota to identify the patients diagnosed with Tourette's syndrome in their care. Using doctor reports to make *DSM-III-R* diagnoses, they estimated a rate of 0.77/10,000 for adult men and 0.22/10,000 for adult women (Burd et al., 1986a). The estimates were higher for children: 1/10,000 in girls and 9.3/10,000 in boys (Burd et al., 1986b).

Using a similar methodology, Robertson, Verrill, Mercer, James, and Pauls (1994) conducted a postal survey of doctors in New Zealand. Because the response rate was relatively low and the time window in which data collection was made was narrow, their estimated 0.7 per 10,000 prevalence rate, with a 4:1 boy-to-girl ratio, is probably an underestimate.

Sampling from school populations, Caine et al. (1988) and Comings et al. (1990) used well-defined geographic areas. They alerted school personnel and parents by advertising in the media and by educating school staff and attempted to ascertain all the children in the school district meeting criteria for Tourette's syndrome. For children in Monroe County, New York, ages 5 to 18, Caine et al. found rates of 5.2/10,000 for boys and 0.6/10,000 for girls. In a school district in California, Comings et al. found much higher rates, 105/10,000 for boys and 13.1/10,000 for girls, probably due to a more liberal diagnostic scheme.

In a random population sample of 17-year-old adolescents, over 28,000 consecutive subjects undergoing physical examination by the military in preparation for military service were screened individually by specially trained physicians for Tourette's syndrome, chronic multiple tics (CMT), and transient tics (Apter et al., 1993). A second-level semistructured interview schedule was administered by child psychiatrists to all screen-positive subjects and, in random order, 500 screen-negative subjects. The resulting prevalence estimates were 4.9/10,000 for boys and 3.1/10,000 for girls. This research paradigm, screening a large random population sample with highly trained clinicians making the diagnoses, is both work-intensive and expensive, but is probably the most reliable and valid method of reaching prevalence estimates of psychiatric disorders.

Using a similar design, Costello, Angold, Burns, Stangl, Tweed, Erkanli, and Worthman (1996) examined 4,500 children 9, 11, and 13 years of age in rural North Carolina. The children were directly examined, as was one parent; both were asked questions about the previous three months. Altogether, 10/10,000 children met criteria for Tourette's syndrome: 13/10,000 for boys and 7/10,000 for girls.

Although the studies used different sampling strategies and different diagnostic procedures, a rate of 5–10 in 10,000 appears in most epidemiological studies based on population samples, excepting the much higher estimate from the Comings et al. (1990) study. This range of 5–10/10,000 is at least two orders of magnitude higher than that estimated from clinical samples, and suggests that a sizable proportion of individuals who meet criteria for Tourette's syndrome do not come to professional attention.

PREVALENCE OF TICS

There is evidence from family studies that CMTs are part of the phenotypic range of the vulnerability for Tourette's syndrome (see Chapter 11). Even so, there are no prospective longitudinal studies of epidemiological samples of children with tics. There are, however, several epidemiological studies of childhood tics. Lapouse and Monk (1964) obtained parental reports on 482 school-age children in the western United States, and estimated the prevalence of all tics—transient and chronic—to be 18% for boys and 11% for girls. Similar estimates using the same methodology were found for children in Buffalo, New York, by Achenbach and Edelbrock (1981) and for Dutch children by Verhulst, Akkerhuis, and Althaus (1985). Slightly lower

TABLE 10.1   Lifetime Prevalence of Tourette's Syndrome as Reported in Major Epidemiological Studies

Study	Study Site	Ascertainment and Evaluation	Ratio of Boys to Girls	Rates per 10,000
Lucas et al. (1982)	Rochester, MN	All medical records of the Mayo Clinic between 1968 and 1979; patients were mailed questionnaires, no direct examination.	3:0	0.46
Burd et al. (1986a, 1986b)	North Dakota	All physicians in North Dakota; questionnaires mailed to physicians, no direct examination.	9.3:1	0.77 for men 0.22 for women 1.0 for girls 9.3 for boys 5.2 total
Caine et al. (1988)	Monroe County, NY	Advertisement in the news media and referral by the school system. The potential sample was 142,636 children 5–18. Referred subjects were examined by study physicians using semi-structured interview schedules.	3.8:1	5.2 for boys 0.6 for girls 2.28 total
Comings et al. (1990)	Los Angeles, CA	All 3,034 children in a school district ages 5–13 were monitored over a 2-year period by clinicians. Referrals were made by parents or school personnel.	8:1	105 for boys 13.1 for girls 36.2 total
Apter et al. (1993)	Tel-Aviv area, Israel	28,037 17-year-old adolescents completed a screening questionnaire, which was verified by a physician; screen positives and 500 screen negatives were examined by psychiatrists using semistructured interview schedules.	1.6:1	4.9 for boys 3.1 for girls 4.1 total
Costello, Angold, Burns, Stangl, Tweed, Erkanli, & Worthman (1996)	Great Smokey Mountains, NC	4,500 children 9- to 13-years-old, a representative sample of the county's children, completed screening; all screen positives and every tenth screen negative were interviewed in person.	1.9:1	13.0 for boys 7.0 for girls 10 total

estimates were found for children in the Isle of Wight by Rutter, Cox, Tupling, Berger, and Yule (1975). Still lower estimates were found for Israeli adolescents, who were interviewed directly (A. Zohar et al., 1992); these lower estimates are probably due to the fact that many adolescents did not remember transient childhood tics. The study of Zohar et al. found a lifetime prevalence of 1.8% for transient tics and 1.6% for chronic tics. Costello, Angold, Burns, Stangl, Tweed, Erkanli, and Worthman (1996) directly interviewed 4,500 children 9, 11, and 13 years of age as well as interviewing one parent for all psychopathology over the prior three months. They found a three-month prevalence of motor tics of 3.5% and 0.75% for vocal tics. Overall, boys have prevalence estimates of 3–18% and girls of 0%–11%. All studies report a higher prevalence of tics in boys than in girls, as is found for Tourette's syndrome. The studies summarized in Table 10.2 relied on parental report of prepubertal children, except for the Zohar et al. study, which used retrospective report of adolescents, who were also individually assessed by a trained physician, and the Costello and colleagues' study, which interviewed both the child and a parent.

TABLE 10.2   Prevalence Estimates of Motor Tics as Reported in Epidemiological Studies

Study	Study Site	Ascertainment	Ratio of Boys to Girls	Rates per 100
Lapouse & Monk (1964)	Buffalo, NY	482 children 6 to 12 years of age ascertained through a probability sample of households.	1.6	18 for boys 11 for girls
Rutter et al. (1970)	Isle of Wight, United Kingdom	3,316 children, 10 to 11 years old.	2:1	5.9 for boys 2.9 for girls
Achenbach & Edelbrock (1981)	Western United States	1,300 children 6 to 18 years of age, a representative sample of the district schoolchildren.	1.2	13 for boys 11 for girls
Verhulst et al. (1985)	Zuid, The Netherlands	2,600 children 4 to 16 years of age, a representative sample of the county.	1.1	10 for boys 9 for girls
A. Zohar et al. (1992)	Tel-Aviv area, Israel	562 adolescents, 16 to 17 years of age, a random sample of their cohort.	not calculable	3.4 for boys 0 for girls
Costello, Angold, Burns, Stangl, Tweed, Erkanli, & Worthman (1996a)	Great Smokey Mountains, NC	4,500 children 9, 11, and 13 years of age sampled through the school system.	1.6:1	4.3 for boys 2.7 for girls 3.5 total

Although tics are generally accepted as important indicators of vulnerability to Tourette's syndrome, the epidemiological work has not systematically included the study of comorbid tics in disorders such as obsessive-compulsive disorder and ADHD. Thus, the following sections do not present figures for tics separately from Tourette's syndrome.

COMORBIDITY OF TOURETTE'S, OCD, AND ADHD AS ESTIMATED IN EPIDEMIOLOGICAL STUDIES OF TOURETTE'S SYNDROME

The association between Tourette's syndrome and obsessive-compulsive disorder was first noted in family studies of Tourette's (Pauls & Leckman, 1986). The elevation of OCD in first-degree relatives of Tourette's syndrome probands suggested that the two disorders may be alternate expressions of the same underlying genetic vulnerability. It was later noted that individuals diagnosed with Tourette's syndrome have high rates of comorbid OCD and ADHD. Calculation of morbid risk for OCD and ADHD in first-degree relatives of probands of Tourette's syndrome with and without comorbid OCD and ADHD (Pauls, Raymond, et al., 1991) suggested that OCD was in fact part of the same phenotypic range of Tourette's syndrome, whereas ADHD was not. Caine et al. (1988) found that out of 41 patients identified with Tourette's syndrome, 7.3% had OCD and over 48% had extensive obsessive-compulsive symptomatology; thus, more than half of the epidemiologically ascertained individuals with Tourette's syndrome also had extensive comorbid obsessive-compulsive behavior. Apter et al. (1993) found a significant elevation of OCD among 12 individuals identified with Tourette's syndrome, with over 40% meeting criteria for OCD, an order of magnitude elevation over the population rate for OCD of 2%–3%. Thus, both epidemiological studies provide support for joint etiology for Tourette's syndrome and OCD.

The implication of the observed comorbidity of Tourette's syndrome and ADHD remains a subect of controversy. At least three alternative explanations have been suggested (also see discussion in Chapter 7):

1. The comorbidity of Tourette's syndrome and ADHD is an instance of clinical referral bias (Berkson, 1946) and does not reflect the true comorbidity of the disorders, which is not elevated above chance.
2. The comorbidity is significant and is due to shared genetic variance (Comings et al., 1990).
3. The comorbidity is significant, but is not due to shared genetic variance. ADHD is secondary to Tourette's syndrome. Being vulnerable enough to meet criteria for one behavioral disorder (Tourette's syndrome) is a predisposing condition for developing another such disorder (ADHD).

Family and other studies are needed to decide between the second hypothesis and the alternative hypotheses. Epidemiological studies can help to decide between the first and the third hypotheses by estimating the comorbidity of the two disorders in an unreferred population. Unfortunately, most epidemiological studies of Tourette's syndrome did not diagnose additional disorders. Caine et al. (1988) found that out of 41 patients identified with Tourette's syndrome, 26.8% had comorbid ADHD and over 24% had learning disorders. Apter et al. (1993) found that 8.3% of epidemiologically ascertained individuals with Tourette's syndrome met criteria for ADHD; this was not a significant elevation over the rate of 3.9% observed in adolescents without Tourette's syndrome. A possible explanation for this disparity is that the study of Caine et al. used schools as a basis for ascertainment; thus, they were probably more sensitive to problems rated to school behavior and attention, increasing the probability of ascertaining children with ADHD. In contrast, the study of Apter et al. used a true population sample and screened all subjects directly. The age difference in the samples might also account for a lower overall rate of ADHD diagnosed among the 28,703 17-year-old adolescents examined by the Apter et al. study.

It is fair to conclude that epidemiological studies offer support for a significant comorbidity between Tourette's syndrome and obsessive-compulsive disorder, but are not conclusive for Tourette's syndrome and ADHD. This may be due to methodological limitations of the studies or may reflect real heterogeneity. Among first-degree relatives of Tourette's syndrome probands with and without ADHD, two subtypes of individuals with both Tourette's syndrome and ADHD were found: those in whom ADHD is independent of Tourette's syndrome, and those in whom ADHD is secondary to Tourette's syndrome (Pauls et al., 1993). The comorbidity as reported in the two relevant epidemiological studies is summarized in Table 10.3.

PREVALENCE OF OCD AND COMORBIDITY WITH TOURETTE'S SYNDROME AND ADHD AMONG INDIVIDUALS ASCERTAINED FOR OCD

Evaluating comorbid conditions with Tourette's syndrome depends on our understanding of the prevalence of these disorders in the population. The past 10 years have seen extensive study of the epidemiology of obsessive-compulsive disorder in adolescents. The various studies sampled unreferred adolescents through schools (Flament et al., 1988), geographically defined communities (Costello, Angold, Burns, Stangl, Tweed, Erkandi, & Worthman, 1996; Valleni-Basile et al., 1994, 1996), or random samples of adolescents at a military induction center (A. Zohar et al., 1992, 1993). Lifetime prevalence of obsessive-compulsive disorder in adolescence was

TABLE 10.3   Comorbid Obsessive-Compulsive Disorder and ADHD in
Individuals Diagnosed with Tourette's Syndrome

Study	N of TS Subjects Identified	Rate of OCD/OCS among TS Individuals	Rate of ADHD and LD among TS Individuals
Caine et al. (1988)	41	OCD 7.3% OCS 48.7%	26.8% ADHD 24.3% LD
Apter et al. (1993)	12	OCD 41.7% (population rate 3.6%)	8.3% ADHD (population rate 3.9%)

Notes: TS = Gilles de la Tourette's syndrome; OCD = obsessive-compulsive disorder; OCS = obsessive-compulsive symptoms; ADHD = attention-deficit/hyperactivity disorder; LD = learning disorders.

found to be 2%–5%, with no significant gender differences. Table 10.4 summarizes the prevalence estimates.

Not all studies report on comorbidity with ADHD and Tourette's syndrome. Flament et al. (1988) found that 10% of the adolescents with OCD also had ADHD; A. Zohar et al. (1992) also found 10% comorbidity, but it was not significantly higher than the rate of ADHD among individuals without OCD (3.9%). Only two of the studies looked for comorbid obsessive-compulsive disorder and tic disorders. In the study of Zohar et al., OCD and Tourette's syndrome were comorbid in 5% of the individuals diagnosed with OCD; counting individuals with tics, chronic or transient, multiple or single, vocal or motor, there was a comorbidity of 25% with OCD. In the second study, which employed a similar methodology on a larger sample (A. Zohar et al., 1993), 17.6% of individuals with OCD also had tics, and among individuals without OCD there was a significantly lower prevalence rate of 5.9% for all tics. If Tourette's syndrome and obsessive-compulsive disorder were independent, then the comorbidity observed when ascertaining individuals with OCD would be the product of the prevalence estimates, or about 1 per 100,000. The actual comorbidity observed was much higher.

This rate is identical to the comorbidity reported by Rasmussen and Eisen (1988) of 5 out of 100 clinically referred individuals with OCD who also had tics. Thus, epidemiological studies support joint etiology for obsessive-compulsive disorder and Tourette's syndrome. Figure 10.1 presents a Venn diagram that depicts the overlap between chronic tic disorders and OCD based on currently available data.

ADHD is the most common childhood-onset psychiatric disorder, with far-reaching developmental and educational implications. A variety of epidemiological studies on different populations are summarized in Table 10.5. The range of frequency is between 2% and 10%, making it a much more common disorder than Tourette's and more prevalent than OCD. Another way to evaluate the comorbidity between Tourette's and ADHD

TABLE 10.4   Lifetime Prevalence of Obsessive-Compulsive Disorder in Adolescence as Reported in Epidemiological Studies

Study	Study Site	Ascertainment and Evaluation	Mean Age of Onset	Rates per 100
Flament et al. (1988)	A semirural community, United States	5,596 high school students screened; all screen positive individually evaluated using semistructured interviews by clinical interviewers.	12.3	1.9 total
Honjo et al. (1989)	Nagoya, Japan	1,293 patients under 18 consecutively treated at the psychiatric clinic over a 2-year period. Children and parents were interviewed by staff psychiatrists.	11.6	5 total
A. Zohar et al. (1992)	Tel Aviv area, Israel	562 randomly sampled adolescents 16- to 17-years-old directly examined by child psychiatrists using a short semistructured interview.	Not reported	3.6 total
A. Zohar et al. (1993)	Tel Aviv area, Israel	861 randomly sampled adolescents screened by self-assessment and by child psychiatrists. All screen positives and 50 screen negatives administered a comprehensive semistructured interview by a child psychiatrist.	Not reported	2.3 total
Valleni-Basile et al. (1994)	Southeastern United States	3,283 adolescents from a community sample 12- to 15-years-old were administered a self-assessment for depression; 488 mothers and children pairs high on the screen were administered semistructured interviews by clinicians.	Not reported	3.3 males 2.6 females 2.9 total
Douglass et al. (1995)	Dunedin, New Zealand	930 adolescents 18-years-old, a population sample of their cohort.	Not reported	4.0 total

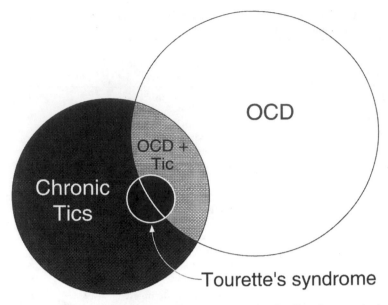

Figure 10.1   Overlap of Tourette's syndrome, chronic tic disorders, and obsessive-compulsive disorder. This Venn diagram depicts the overlap between chronic tic disorders and obsessive-compulsive disorder as seen in a series of population-based studies among Israeli adolescents (Apter et al., 1993; A. Zohar et al., 1992, 1993). Approximately 18% of individuals with a diagnosis of obsessive-compulsive disorder were also diagnosed with either Tourette's syndrome or another chronic disorder. In contrast, 40% and 27% of individuals diagnosed with Tourette's syndrome and chronic tic disorders, respectively, were also diagnosed with obsessive-compulsive disorder. This figure also roughly depicts the differences in the population prevalence of these disorders: 3.6% obsessive-compulsive disorder and 1.8% chronic tic disorders (including Tourette's syndrome).

would be to look for tics, Tourette's syndrome, and obsessive-compulsive disorder among children ascertained for ADHD in true population samples. However, so far, none of the epidemiological studies of ADHD have included evaluation of these disorders.

THE NATURAL COURSE OF TOURETTE'S SYNDROME, ADHD, AND OCD IN NONCLINICAL SAMPLES

There are no longitudinal studies of children diagnosed with Tourette's syndrome in population-based samples. Some research on clinically referred children suggests that a proportion of children who are diagnosed with Tourette's in childhood remit toward the end of adolescence (Leckman, Zhang, et al., 1998; Robertson, Trimble, & Lees, 1988a). One study of a birth-year cohort of Tourette's syndrome patients found that the peak

TABLE 10.5   Prevalence of ADHD in Nonreferred Populations of Children

Study	Study Site	Ascertainment and Evaluation	Rate per 100
J. Anderson et al. (1987)	Dunedin, New Zealand	792 11-year-old children, a representative sample of their cohort in the region, enrolled in a longitudinal developmental study, children assessed by semistructured interviews, additional information elicited from parents and teachers.	6.7 total boy to girl ratio 5.1 : 1
Bird et al. (1988)	Puerto Rico	A representative sample of 2,036 households. Parents and teachers completed the CBCL; all screen positives were examined by clinicians (semistructured interviews).	9.5 total
A. Zohar et al. (1992)	Tel Aviv, Israel	A random sample of 562 17-year-old adolescents, examined by clinicians using semistructured interviews.	3.9 total
August & Garfinkel (1993)	Minnesota, United States	1,490 school children grades 1–4 screened for attention and behavior problems; screen positives examined directly by semistructured interviews administered by clinicians.	7.5 total
Costello, Angold, Burns, Stangl, Tweed, & Erkanli (1996); Costello, Angold, Burns, Stangl, Tweed, Erkanli, & Worthman (1996)	Great Smokey Mountains, NC	4,500 children 9- to 13-years-old, a representative sample of the county's children completed screening, all children screen positive, and every tenth child who was not were interviewed in person.	1.9 total

tic severity occurred between 9 and 14 years of age (Leckman, Zhang, et al., 1998). The factors that influence the longitudinal course of Tourette's syndrome are not well understood. In particular, the identification of factors that lead to severe forms of this disorder in adulthood remains poorly characterized. Much more work has been done on the natural course of OCD and ADHD in childhood.

Berg, Rapoport, Whitaker, and Davies (1989) conducted a prospective study of epidemiologically ascertained adolescents with OCD, subclinical

OCD, and obsessive-compulsive personality disorder. They reassessed the subjects two years later, at ages 16 to 21 years. Of adolescents initially diagnosed with OCD, just under a third still fulfilled criteria for OCD; a quarter had partially remitted and met criteria for subclinical OCD. Only 12% no longer qualified for any obsessive-compulsive diagnosis. A. Zohar et al. (submitted) followed adolescents diagnosed in an epidemiological study with OCD and subclinical OCD. One year later, after being drafted into the army, put through basic training, and placed at their first posting, 11% no longer met criteria for any diagnosis. Complete remission was higher among those initially diagnosed with subclinical OCD than among those initially diagnosed with OCD. The rate of remission shown over adolescence in these community samples was lower than most of the remission rates reported for child clinical samples (Leonard et al., 1993). Valleni-Basile et al. (1996) examined a large community sample of adolescents and followed them for a year. At one-year follow-up, only 17% of those diagnosed with OCD retained their OCD diagnosis; 62% showed no psychopathology. Initial diagnosis of subclinical OCD was even less persistent than OCD, and was not predictive of having subclinical OCD a year later. This very high remission rate is not consistent with other findings. Because follow-up was a year after initial diagnosis, the rate may represent fluctuations in the course of OCD rather than complete remission. Follow-up studies of children diagnosed with early-onset OCD without tics show that OCD is a predictor for the development of tics and Tourette's syndrome (Berg et al., 1989; Flament et al., 1990; A. Zohar et al., 1997).

There is a wealth of work on the natural course of ADHD. By definition, it is diagnosed by the age of 7, and thus allows for prospective longitudinal studies spanning childhood and culminating in adulthood. In childhood, ADHD is associated with learning disorders and impairment of speech and language (Cantwell & Baker, 1991). In adolescence, ADHD is associated with impaired cognitive, school, family, and psychosocial functioning and with mood and anxiety disorders (Barkley, Fischer, Edelbrock, & Smallish, 1991; Biederman et al., 1996). In addition, adolescents who were diagnosed with ADHD in childhood have more oppositional defiant disorder and more numerous and intense family conflicts (Barkley, Fischer, et al., 1991). Children diagnosed with ADHD and with comorbid conduct disorder are at increased risk in adolescence of developing substance abuse disorders (Wilens, Biederman, Spencer, & Frances, 1994). As adults, these children are more likely to meet criteria for antisocial personality disorder and drug abuse disorders (Manuzza et al., 1993). They are also less likely to achieve educationally and occupationally, but are not at increased risk for anxiety and mood disorders. Most children diagnosed with ADHD may still exhibit symptoms but do not meet criteria for ADHD later in life. An analytic review of nine prospective studies showed an exponential decline of ADHD over development (Hill & Schoener, 1996). Although ADHD was present in 4% of school-age children, it declined by approximately 50% every five years, so that by the age of 40 only 0.05% still met ADHD criteria.

RISK AND PROTECTIVE FACTORS: EPIDEMIOLOGICAL PERSPECTIVES

One of the functions of epidemiological research is to identify environmental and personal variables that increase or decrease the probability of developing the disorder under scrutiny and affecting its prognosis. The most common approach is to focus on one or two probable risk factors and describe their association with the onset and/or the course of the disorder. This approach can be quite powerful if the risk factors are predictive. If the risk factors are such that they can be modified, then such research is helpful in improving interventions, for example, stress-reducing therapies for Tourette's syndrome and OCD. An alternative approach is to consider all possible risk factors as cumulatively contributing to the risk of the expression of the disorder in individuals. Gottesman (Gottesman & Shields, 1982) described this as the threshold model for the etiology of schizophrenia, suggesting that genetically vulnerable individuals, exposed to critical amounts of adversity (other genetic factors, intrauterine and postnatal environmental factors), would express the disorder. Rutter and his colleagues (1975) proposed a cumulative effect of psychosocial variables on the expression of childhood disorders. They listed six variables: severe marital discord, low social class, large family size, paternal criminality, maternal mental disorder, and foster placement. Although no single risk factor predicted childhood disorders, the presence of any two of these variables increased the risk by a factor of four. Unlike the Gottesman threshold model, the Rutter indicators-of-adversity approach does not attempt to separate environmental and genetic risk; instead, it lists all known risk factors together. In addition, most of the adversity indicators listed, although they may be powerful predictors, are not modifiable and thus cannot be used as guidelines in possible interventions. Most of the epidemiological studies reviewed in this chapter took the first approach, of attempting to single out major risk factors. Thus, we present the research according to variables singled out as risk factors. The reader is also referred to the presentation of our overall model of pathogenesis in Chapter 9, as well as Chapters 11 and 12, which address each of these factors in greater detail.

Genetic Predisposition

A wealth of twin, adoption, and family studies show that Tourette's syndrome, OCD, and ADHD run in families. There is also evidence for joint genetic etiology predisposing to Tourette's syndrome and obsessive-compulsive disorder or to Tourette's syndrome and ADHD.

Perinatal Risk Factors

As described in Chapter 12, a number of adverse perinatal events has been associated with the later expression of Tourette's syndrome, OCD, and ADHD. Briefly, there is evidence that hypoxic events, maternal emotional stress during pregnancy, and severe nausea and vomiting during the first trimester may affect tic severity (Leckman, Dolnansky, et al., 1990). Maternal smoking during pregnancy, as well as drug use, increase the probability of ADHD in the children (Milberger, Biederman, Faraone, Chen, & Jones, 1996) and the emergence of obsessive-compulsive disorder symptoms among individuals at risk of developing Tourette's syndrome (Santangelo et al., 1994).

Ethnicity

No racial differences have been reported for ADHD and Tourette's syndrome. For OCD, prospective longitudinal research on epidemiologically ascertained adolescents show that being African American increases the odds ratio for maintaining OCD or subclinical OCD diagnosis a year later (Valleni-Basile et al., 1996).

Intelligence

Individuals ascertained in epidemiological studies and diagnosed with Tourette's syndrome fall within the normal range of IQ (Apter et al., 1993). In clinical samples of children diagnosed with Tourette's syndrome, children test below average on IQ (Parraga & McDonald, 1996). This is probably due to comorbid attention and learning disorders (Burd et al., 1992; Dykens et al., 1990; Yeates & Bornstein, 1994). When clinical samples of children with Tourette's syndrome are screened negative for these comorbid conditions, no cognitive impairment is detected (Bornstein, 1991a). ADHD is associated with considerable impairment to IQ (Faraone, Biederman, Krifcher, et al., 1993). Children diagnosed with ADHD have lower IQ if they are exposed to a larger number of adversity indicators (Biederman, Milberger, et al., 1995). In epidemiological studies of obsessive-compulsive disorder, there is some cognitive impairment associated with the disorder, although the mean IQ of the individuals with obsessive-compulsive disorder is within the normal range (A. Zohar et al., 1992, 1993). This is true also of clinical samples of nondepressed individuals diagnosed with obsessive-compulsive disorder (Boone et al., 1991). Prospective samples of epidemiologically ascertained individuals have shown that for ADHD, normal IQ predicts better outcome in adolescence

and adulthood (Barkley, Fischer, et al., 1991). No such stu
Tourette's syndrome and obsessive-compulsive disorder.

Family Environment

In a prospective study of siblings and children of individuals with Tourette's syndrome (Carter et al., 1994), impaired family functioning was associated with attentional and anxiety problems, but was not associated with the onset of tics. However, it did affect prognosis; children diagnosed with Tourette's syndrome whose family environment was stressful suffered more from behavior problems and endured more anxiety symptoms.

Family studies of children clinically referred for obsessive-compulsive disorder show that parental hostility, criticism, and overinvolvement predict worse prognosis (Hibbs et al., 1991). Accommodation to the child with obsessive-compulsive disorder by family members is also associated with poor family functioning and family stress (Calvocoressi et al., 1995).

Familial stress and parental conflict are associated with increased risk for ADHD (Biederman, Milberger, et al., 1995; Johnston, 1996) and are associated with poor prognosis. Thus, for all three disorders, family stress and impaired family function predict worse outcome. An intriguing use of epidemiological research would be to examine the effect of family environment on children who meet criteria for a disorder but have not been diagnosed. Prospective longitudinal studies of probands identified epidemiologically are needed to show if the poor prognosis is the result of the interaction between the disorder and the family environment, or of the interaction between having a child identified as a patient and the family environment.

Life Events and Stress

Although individuals with Tourette's syndrome often report that change and stress exacerbate tics (Cohen, Friedhoff, et al., 1992), there is no firm evidence that environmental stress of any kind affects the onset of tics. Social gatherings, emotional trauma, and anxiety-causing events do tend to exacerbate tics in individuals with Tourette's syndrome (Silva et al., 1995; Surwillo et al., 1978). Case histories support extreme traumatic events as stressors affecting tics (Witzum, Bar-On, Dolberg, & Kotler, 1996). There is evidence from prospective studies of community samples of adolescents that negative life events increase the probability of maintaining an OCD or a subclinical OCD diagnosis, whereas positive life events decrease the probability (Valleni-Basile et al., 1996). There are some findings that extreme stress, for example, combat exposure, can precipitate OCD (Pitman, 1993). Similar reports link extreme stressors, such as life-threatening accidents and sexual abuse, to the onset of ADHD (Cuffe, McCullough, &

Pumariega, 1994; Merry & Andrews, 1994). Having a number of indicators of adversity increased the odds ratio for having ADHD in a large study comparing children diagnosed with ADHD to normal children (Biederman, Milberger, et al., 1995).

Socioeconomic Status

Socioeconomic status affects the likelihood of contracting ADHD (Biederman, Milberger, et al., 1995) or of maintaining an OCD or a subclinical OCD diagnosis over a one-year period (Valleni-Basile et al., 1996). No similar findings are available for Tourette's syndrome.

SUMMARY OF CHAPTER 10

Epidemiological studies sampling from the community find the prevalence of Tourette's syndrome to be 5–10/10,000 and more frequent in boys than in girls. Epidemiological studies find high rates of comorbidity of Tourette's syndrome and obsessive-compulsive disorder. Obsessive-compulsive disorder is found to be much more common, about 300–500/10,000. Thus, although there is evidence for some joint etiology, most of the obsessive-compulsive disorder encountered in population samples would not be due to this joint etiology. More epidemiological research is necessary to clarify the relationship among Tourette's syndrome, obsessive-compulsive disorder, and ADHD. Nongenetic perinatal risk factors identified for Tourette's syndrome also increase the probability for ADHD.

PREVIEW OF CHAPTER 11

Genetic factors have long been implicated in Tourette's syndrome. Despite years of effort, the nature of these genetic factors remains a mystery. Chapter 10 reviews the available evidence for genetic factors and outlines the current investigational strategies. It is likely that nonparametric gene-sharing studies will be successful in identifying chromosomal regions that contain genes of major and minor effect for Tourette's syndrome. The chapter closes with a discussion of genetic counseling and a restatement of the promise of genetic research.

CHAPTER 11

Genetic Vulnerability

DAVID L. PAULS, JOHN P. ALSOBROOK II, JOEL GELERNTER, and
JAMES F. LECKMAN

> One of the most difficult aspects of studying the genetics of complex disor-
> ders relates to phenotype definition.
>
> —*Neil Risch, 1990*

> Human genetics has sparked a revolution in medical science on the basis of
> the seemingly improbable notion that one can systematically discover the
> genes causing inherited diseases without any prior biological clue as to how
> they function.
>
> —*Eric S. Lander and Nicholas Schork, 1994*

> Thus the principal contribution of the model organisms to human biology
> over the next five years will be the reduction of most of the approximately
> 70,000 individual components encoded by the human genome into a much
> smaller number of multicomponent processes of known biochemical function.
>
> —*George L. Gabor Miklos and Gerald M. Rubin, 1996*

Tourette's syndrome and obsessive-compulsive disorder are complex neurobehavioral disorders that are familial and appear to share some common
etiological factors. It has been observed that a substantial number
(40–80%) of Tourette's syndrome individuals experience significant
obsessive-compulsive symptoms at some point in their life (Comings &
Comings, 1987a, 1987b, 1987c, 1987d, 1987e, 1987f; Nee, Polinsky, &
Ebert, 1982; Pauls, Raymond, et al., 1991). Furthermore, it has been estimated that approximately 20% of obsessive-compulsive disorder individuals either have a personal history or family history of tics (see Pauls et al.,
1995). As described in Chapter 9, Leckman, Peterson, et al. (1997) have
proposed a model of pathogenesis for Tourette's syndrome and obsessive-
compulsive disorder that consists of four interrelated areas: phenomenology
and natural history, genetic factors, nongenetic factors, and neurobiological

substrates. In this chapter, the evidence that genetic factors play a role in the pathogenesis of these conditions is reviewed. Specifically, (a) the data that suggest that genetic factors are important for the manifestation of each disorder separately is summarized; (b) the evidence that suggests that some genes may be important for the expression of both is reviewed; and (c) the evidence for a genetic relationship between Tourette's syndrome and other disorders is examined.

VERTICAL TRANSMISSION OF TOURETTE'S SYNDROME

The familial nature of Tourette's syndrome and chronic tics (CT) has been well documented (see Pauls, Raymond, et al., 1991), and twin studies have demonstrated that genetic factors are important for the manifestation of Tourette's syndrome (Price et al., 1985; Walkup et al., 1988). Historically, it was frequently reported that Tourette's syndrome showed a familial concentration, especially if CT was considered a minor manifestation of the syndrome. Early genetic analyses of family history data demonstrated that there was vertical transmission of Tourette's syndrome and CT and that simple genetic threshold models could explain the family history data (Kidd & Pauls, 1982). In addition, segregation analyses of family history data (Comings, Comings, Devor, & Cloninger, 1984; Devor, 1984; Price, Pauls, Kruger, & Caine, 1988) demonstrated that a single-major-locus hypothesis best explained the patterns of transmission observed in families of Tourette's syndrome individuals. Although a relatively simple mode of transmission was supported, the specific genetic model supported varied from study to study. Most results were consistent with an autosomal dominant mode of transmission; however, in the study reported by Devor, the autosomal dominant model could be rejected.

Subsequent genetic analyses undertaken using structured psychiatric interview data from all family members provided strong evidence that the mode of transmission is compatible with major gene inheritance (Eapen, Pauls, & Robertson, 1993; Hasstedt, Leppert, Filloux, van de Wetering, & McMahon, 1995; Pauls, Alsobrook, Almasy, Leckman, & Cohen, 1991; Pauls & Leckman, 1986; van de Wetering, 1993; Walkup et al., 1996). Although initial analyses suggested that the pattern of inheritance was consistent with an autosomal dominant mode of transmission (Eapen et al., 1993; Pauls & Leckman, 1986; van de Wetering, 1993), more recent analyses suggest that an additive model in which the penetrance of the heterozygote is lower than the penetrance for the at-risk homozygote best explains the familial transmission patterns. However, in one study (Pauls, Alsobrook, et al., 1991), when individuals with obsessive-compulsive disorder were included in the analyses, the most parsimonious model was still autosomal dominant. In contrast, results from recent studies reported by Hasstedt et al. and Walkup et al. suggest that an additive model may be more likely even when individuals with obsessive-compulsive disorder are included. Furthermore, Walkup and colleagues reported that there might also be a significant polygenic background important for the expression of Tourette's syndrome and related conditions. These recent studies suggest that the underlying genetic mechanism important for the expression of Tourette's syndrome and related conditions is likely to be more complex than was originally thought, although it still appears that there are major genes of significant effect. As discussed later, given these findings, it is important that different strategies, including ones that do not rely so heavily on understanding the correct mode of transmission, be employed in the search for susceptibility genes for Tourette's syndrome.

TRANSMISSION OF OBSESSIVE-COMPULSIVE DISORDER

The familial nature of obsessive-compulsive disorder has been observed since the 1930s and twin studies have provided limited evidence for the importance of genetic factors in its manifestation (see Alsobrook & Pauls, 1997, for a more thorough review). In several twin studies, the concordance rates ranged from 53% to 87% for monozygotic twins and from 22% to 47% for dizygotic twins, depending on the sample and the diagnostic criteria (Carey & Gottesman, 1981; Rasmussen & Tsuang, 1986). However, in two more recent twin studies (Andrews, Stewart, Allen, & Henderson, 1990; Torgerson, 1983), the evidence for the importance of genetic factors in the expression of obsessive-compulsive disorder alone was not compelling. These studies provided evidence that genetic factors were important for the manifestation of anxiety disorders, and the investigators concluded that, to the extent that obsessive-compulsive disorder is considered part of a spectrum of anxiety disorders, then genetic factors play some role in its manifestation.

Although a number of family studies on obsessive-compulsive disorder have been completed over the past 60 years, the area remains controversial. Some studies report rates as high as 35% (Lenane et al., 1990) among first-degree relatives, others report no increase (McKeon & Murray, 1987). Many of these studies are difficult to interpret because of differences in diagnostic criteria and assessment methodologies. Some of the shortcomings of earlier research were addressed in six recent studies of obsessive-compulsive disorder (Bellodi, Sciuto, Diaferia, Ronchi, & Smeraldi, 1992; Black, Noyes, Goldstein, & Blum, 1992; Lenane et al., 1990; Leonard et al., 1992; Pauls et al., 1995). Findings from these studies provide further support for the hypothesis that there is a familial component influencing the expression of some forms of obsessive-compulsive disorder. Lenane and co-workers studied families of 46 children and adolescents and found that 25% of fathers and 9% of mothers had obsessive-compulsive disorder. When subthreshold obsessive-compulsive disorder was included, the age-corrected morbid risks for all first-degree relatives was 35%. Another family study of childhood-onset obsessive-compulsive disorder (Leonard, Rao, Morton, &

Elston, 1992) found that 13% of all first-degree relatives met criteria for obsessive-compulsive disorder. Bellodi and colleagues reported that only 3.4% of the relatives in 92 families had obsessive-compulsive disorder. However, when probands were separated on the basis of age at onset, the morbid risk for obsessive-compulsive disorder among relatives of early-onset (before age 14) probands was 8.8%, compared to 3.4% among the relatives of later-onset probands. Black and colleagues studied families of 32 adult obsessive-compulsive disorder probands and found no evidence that the disorder was familial. However, the risk of a more broadly defined obsessive-compulsive disorder (i.e., subthreshold obsessive-compulsive disorder) was increased among the parents of obsessive-compulsive disorder probands. In addition, the rates of anxiety disorders were significantly increased among relatives of obsessional probands. Finally, in a family study of adult obsessive-compulsive disorder probands (Pauls et al., 1995), rates of obsessive-compulsive disorder (10.9%) and subthreshold obsessive-compulsive disorder (7.9%) were significantly increased among relatives of obsessive-compulsive disorder probands compared to control subjects. Furthermore, the age-corrected rate of broadly defined obsessive-compulsive disorder among relatives of early-onset (before age 12) probands was approximately 22%.

These recent studies provide additional evidence that some forms of obsessive-compulsive disorder are familial. However, family studies by themselves cannot demonstrate that genetic factors are necessary for the manifestation of the illness. Nevertheless, the data can be used to examine specific genetic hypotheses. If segregation analysis reveals that the patterns within families are consistent with a fairly simple mode of inheritance, the results can be taken as indirect evidence for the importance of genes in the etiology of the disorder.

Nicolini and colleagues (1991) performed segregation analyses on data collected from 24 obsessive-compulsive disorder families to examine whether transmission patterns were consistent with simple Mendelian models of inheritance. These investigators were unable to distinguish between an autosomal dominant and a recessive model; however, the dominant model was statistically more likely and most compatible with the observed patterns. In a more recent study, Alsobrook (1996) completed complex segregation analyses on the obsessive-compulsive disorder family study data of Pauls and colleagues (1995) using the computer program Pointer (Lalouel, Rao, Morton, & Elston, 1983). Three diagnostic schemes were analyzed separately: (a) obsessive-compulsive disorder and subclinical obsessive-compulsive disorder as affected; (b) obsessive-compulsive disorder, subclinical obsessive-compulsive disorder, and Tourette's syndrome as affected; and (c) obsessive-compulsive disorder, subclinical obsessive-compulsive disorder, Tourette's syndrome, and CT as affected. For each analysis, liability status was assigned based on gender and age at interview. The ascertainment probability was set at 0.01. The broadest affection category (which included obsessive-compulsive disorder, subclinical obsessive-compulsive disorder, Tourette's syndrome, and CT) allowed rejection of the polygenic and recessive models ($p <$ 0.05). An autosomal dominant model provided the best fit to the observed familial patterns. However, given that there was considerable heterogeneity in recurrence risks among families, it is likely that different etiological mechanisms are at work in different groups of obsessive-compulsive disorder individuals. Thus, although the autosomal dominant model was the most parsimonious for these data, the results should be interpreted with caution. It is safer to state that the results suggest that there are genes of major effect that play a role in the manifestation of obsessive-compulsive disorder and related conditions.

FAMILY GENETIC RELATIONSHIP BETWEEN TOURETTE'S SYNDROME AND OBSESSIVE-COMPULSIVE DISORDER

Data from several family genetic studies suggest a familial relationship between Tourette's syndrome and obsessive-compulsive disorder. In two family studies of Tourette's syndrome, the results suggested that some forms of obsessive-compulsive disorder are part of the phenotypic spectrum (Eapen et al., 1993; Pauls, Raymond, et al., 1991). This conclusion was reached because the rate of obsessive-compulsive disorder was higher among the biological relatives of Tourette's syndrome probands when compared to a control sample; and the rates of obsessive-compulsive disorder among first-degree relatives were not significantly different among relatives of Tourette's syndrome probands with obsessive-compulsive disorder and relatives of Tourette's syndrome probands without obsessive-compulsive disorder. In the study conducted by Pauls and colleagues, the age-corrected rate of obsessive-compulsive disorder was 0.104 ± 0.023 among relatives of probands with Tourette's syndrome but not obsessive-compulsive disorder and 0.136 ± 0.036 among relatives of Tourette's syndrome probands with obsessive-compulsive disorder; both rates were significantly higher than the rate of obsessive-compulsive disorder among controls.

Data from families of obsessive-compulsive disorder probands support these findings (Leonard et al., 1992; Pauls et al., 1995). The rates of Tourette's syndrome and CT were significantly elevated among the obsessive-compulsive disorder probands and their relatives. Although the data were consistent with the hypothesis that a form of obsessive-compulsive disorder is related to Tourette's syndrome, the family patterns suggest that not all forms of the disorder are related to Tourette's syndrome (Pauls et al., 1995). If all forms of obsessive-compulsive disorder were related to Tourette's syndrome, the rate of Tourette's syndrome and CT should be the same among relatives of obsessive-compulsive disorder probands with and without tics. It was not; the rate of tics was higher among relatives of obsessive-compulsive disorder probands with tics.

Additional evidence that there is a subtype of obsessive-compulsive disorder more likely to be etiologically related to Tourette's syndrome comes from some treatment studies conducted by McDougle and colleagues (1994). Haloperidol addition to serotonin-reuptake inhibitor treatment of obsessive-compulsive disorder patients significantly improved outcome in those individuals who also had a concurrent tic disorder. Furthermore, those obsessive-compulsive disorder individuals without a concurrent tic disorder who responded positively had a positive family history of tics and/or Tourette's syndrome. Although treatment studies are at least a step removed from the underlying etiology, these results are consistent with the hypothesis of a shared etiology.

At the present time, it is not known what proportion of obsessive-compulsive disorder cases are etiologically related to Tourette's syndrome. It is clear that not all obsessive-compulsive disorder families have members with a diagnosis of Tourette's syndrome or CT. Furthermore, it is not clear whether the nature of the obsessions and compulsions that occur among relatives of Tourette's syndrome patients is the same as those experienced by patients with obsessive-compulsive disorder. Recent work suggests that there are differences in symptomatology between obsessive-compulsive disorder individuals with a personal and/or family history of Tourette's syndrome or tics and that exhibited by obsessive-compulsive disorder subjects without such a history (Baer, 1994; Eapen, Robertson, Alsobrook, & Pauls, 1997; Holzer et al., 1994; Leckman, Grice, et al., 1995; Leckman, Grice, et al., 1997; A. Zohar et al., 1997). More work is needed to determine if those differences reflect genetic differences between obsessive-compulsive disorder that appears to be related to Tourette's syndrome and that which apparently is not.

FAMILY GENETIC RELATIONSHIP BETWEEN TOURETTE'S SYNDROME AND OTHER DISORDERS

Although the diagnosis of Tourette's syndrome is quite straightforward, the degree to which other behaviors may be associated with the syndrome has been the subject of some debate. From the beginning, CT was assumed to be a variant expression of the syndrome in relatives of Tourette's syndrome patients. In addition, Jagger et al. (1982) reported that inattention and hyperactivity were among the first symptoms observed in a large percentage of clinic patients. These findings and the observation that many Tourette's syndrome patients seen in clinics had a number of comorbid conditions urged Comings and Comings (1987a, 1987b, 1987c, 1987d, 1987e, 1987f) to propose that a large number of other behavioral disorders were also variant expressions of the Tourette's syndrome gene. These investigators claimed that, in addition to CT and obsessive-compulsive disorder, the following were all variant expressions of Tourette's syndrome: attention deficit disorder, learning disabilities (including specific reading disability), speech and language disorders (including stuttering), conduct disorder, panic disorder, generalized anxiety disorder, phobic disorders, schizoid behaviors, major depressive disorder, bipolar affective disorder, sleep disorders, and disorders of sexual inhibition. Findings from our work (Pauls et al., 1993, 1994; Pauls, Hurst, et al., 1986) did not support these hypotheses. Our work was based on the premise that, if any disorder is genetically related to Tourette's syndrome, the patterns within families should be similar to those observed for obsessive-compulsive disorder. That is, the rate of an etiologically related disorder alone (i.e., not in the presence of Tourette's syndrome) should be elevated among the relatives of Tourette's syndrome probands independent of the comorbid diagnosis of the proband.

Tourette's Syndrome and ADHD

In a family study of Tourette's syndrome in which all available family members were personally interviewed, the data were not consistent with the hypothesis that ADHD is a variant expression of the genetic factors important for the expression of Tourette's syndrome (Pauls et al., 1993). Overall, the rate of ADHD among relatives of Tourette's syndrome probands was not significantly increased when compared to a control sample. ADHD occurred most often among the relatives of Tourette's syndrome probands who themselves had a diagnosis of ADHD, suggesting that there might be a separate type of Tourette's syndrome that included symptoms of inattention, impulsivity, and hyperactivity. Furthermore, there was a higher than expected occurrence of ADHD among relatives who had a diagnosis of Tourette's syndrome (25% versus 8.9% overall). But this occurred in relatives of both Tourette's syndrome with ADHD and Tourette's syndrome without ADHD probands. Taken together, these data suggested that individuals who had Tourette's syndrome were at greater risk for exhibiting symptoms of inattention and impulsivity. However, because ADHD without tics did not occur with a higher frequency among all relatives, the data did not support the hypothesis that ADHD alone was a variant manifestation of the Tourette's syndrome spectrum. It is possible that Tourette's syndrome and some forms of ADHD share some common pathways of expression. Alternatively, it is possible that having Tourette's syndrome interferes with an individual's ability to attend appropriately to stimuli in the surrounding environment. Arguing against this explanation is the fact that many Tourette's syndrome patients appear to have symptoms of inattention prior to onset of tics. It follows that not all of the attentional problems experienced by individuals with Tourette's syndrome are secondary to the expression of Tourette's syndrome.

Further analysis of these family data were completed to determine if there were differences among relatives who had both Tourette's syndrome and ADHD. First, relatives with both ADHD and Tourette's syndrome were compared to relatives who had ADHD alone. The age at onset of

ADHD for relatives with both disorders was compared to the age at onset of ADHD among relatives who had only ADHD. Although the sample size was too small to allow rigorous statistical examination of the patterns observed, the findings were suggestive of possible etiological differences. The average age at onset of ADHD was 6.3 for relatives with both Tourette's syndrome and ADHD, compared to 5.5 for relatives with ADHD alone. Furthermore, examining the actual ages at onset for all relatives with both diagnoses revealed that, for all but one individual, the onset for ADHD occurred either concomitantly with the onset of tics or after the onset of tics. This suggests that the ADHD experienced by relatives with Tourette's syndrome might be secondary to the presence of tics.

It could be hypothesized that earlier-onset ADHD is more likely to be etiologically independent of Tourette's syndrome. If that were true, then to the extent that ADHD is familial, the risk of ADHD alone among relatives of Tourette's syndrome probands with early-onset ADHD should be higher than the risk of ADHD alone among relatives of Tourette's syndrome probands who have later-onset ADHD. Examining the relatives in these two types of families revealed that the rate of ADHD alone among relatives of Tourette's syndrome probands with earlier-onset ADHD was 25%, compared to only 12.2% among the relatives of Tourette's syndrome probands with later-onset ADHD. These findings suggest that there might be at least two types of Tourette's syndrome probands with ADHD: those who have a form of ADHD independent of Tourette's syndrome (probands with onset of ADHD prior to onset of Tourette's syndrome) and those who have a form that is secondary to the expression of Tourette's syndrome (probands with concurrent or later-onset ADHD). These findings need to be interpreted with caution. Retrospective data about age at onset are not optimal. Thus, these findings regarding the sequence of onset of Tourette's syndrome and ADHD should be considered as hypothesis-generating. In future work designed to more fully understand the relationship between Tourette's syndrome and ADHD, it will be important to study younger individuals who are closer to their age at onset and their families and/or to prospectively follow very young children at risk for Tourette's syndrome to collect data about the early developmental and clinical course of these individuals. Thus, a more rigorous examination of this hypothesis will be possible.

Tourette's Syndrome and Other Psychopathology

A second set of analyses examined the proposed relationship between Tourette's syndrome and other psychopathology (Pauls et al., 1994). As a first step, the rates of the following disorders were estimated among the probands in this family study and compared to those obtained from a control sample: conduct disorder, alcohol abuse, drug abuse, antisocial personality disorder, depressive personality disorder, minor depression, major depressive disorder, chronic hypomanic disorder, bipolar disorder, schizophrenia, schizoaffective disorder–depressed type, schizoaffective disorder–manic type, generalized anxiety disorder, overanxious disorder, separation anxiety, simple phobia, social phobia, agoraphobia, panic disorder, speech disorder (nonstuttering), stuttering, specific developmental disorder, pervasive developmental disorder, and mental retardation. The rates of major depressive disorder, panic disorder, simple phobia, stuttering, other speech problems, and specific developmental disorders were significantly elevated among the probands. No other psychiatric diagnoses were elevated in probands.

Logistic regression analyses were undertaken to understand more completely the relationship of major depressive disorder, panic disorder, and phobias to Tourette's syndrome, CT, and obsessive-compulsive disorder among relatives of Tourette's syndrome probands. The most parsimonious model for major depressive disorder included age, sex, the relative's diagnosis of obsessive-compulsive disorder, and the proband's diagnosis of major depressive disorder. No interactions reached statistical significance. Major depressive disorder occurred most often in those individuals who had obsessive-compulsive disorder. However, major depressive disorder was also significantly elevated among relatives of probands who themselves had a diagnosis of depression. This was expected, as major depressive disorder is a familial disorder. Inspection of the age at onset for major depressive disorder and obsessive-compulsive disorder in relatives who had both revealed that the onset of major depressive disorder in these individuals most often followed the onset of the obsessive-compulsive disorder. This was particularly true for the relatives of Tourette's syndrome probands who did not have major depressive disorder. Thus, much of the depression in these families was chronologically secondary to obsessive-compulsive disorder.

The results of the logistic regression analyses for panic disorder and simple phobia were similar to those for major depressive disorder. The significant predictors for the presence of either panic disorder or simple phobias among the relatives were age, sex, and obsessive-compulsive disorder diagnosis of the relative. The significant increase of panic disorder and simple phobias among relatives of Tourette's syndrome probands appears to be due to the presence of obsessive-compulsive disorder. These findings are consistent with reports in the phobic and panic disorders literature (Rasmussen & Eisen, 1991).

In sum, the results of these analyses suggest that there may be some relationship between Tourette's syndrome and attentional difficulties. Furthermore, the data are consistent with reports that obsessive-compulsive disorder individuals are at greater risk for major depressive disorder and panic disorder. But these family data do not support the hypothesis that ADHD, major depressive disorder, or panic disorder alone are variant expressions of the same underlying genetic factors that are important for the expression of Tourette's syndrome.

GENETIC LINKAGE AND ASSOCIATION STUDIES

The available evidence suggests that genetic factors are important in the expression of both Tourette's syndrome and obsessive-compulsive disorder. It is also clear that some forms of CT and obsessive-compulsive disorder are most likely variant expressions of the genetic factors conferring susceptibility to Tourette's syndrome. A more complete understanding of that genetic basis and of the interactions between relevant genotypes and relevant environmental factors will be important for eventual clarification of the etiology and pathogenesis of these complex disorders. As noted above, results from several investigations suggest that the underlying genetic mechanisms for both Tourette's syndrome and obsessive-compulsive disorder involve genes of major effect. The next logical step in our goal of understanding the genetics of the Tourette's syndrome spectrum is to localize and characterize the genes that confer susceptibility.

One of the strongest forms of evidence for a genetic factor is the demonstration of genetic linkage. Genetic linkage is detectable if a known genetic marker locus is sufficiently close to a locus segregating for alleles affecting a disorder so that nonrandom segregation of alleles at the two loci results in an association of phenotypes within a family. Thus, if it is possible to demonstrate genetic linkage between a locus for Tourette's syndrome and/or obsessive-compulsive disorder and a known marker locus, that demonstration will provide convincing evidence that there are genes of major effect contributing to the expression of Tourette's syndrome and/or obsessive-compulsive disorder. Demonstration of linkage is as important as identifying an aberrant enzyme or structural protein as a marker for an abnormal gene. Once located, the genetic marker provides an extraordinarily powerful research tool for dissecting out the specific genetic defect, identifying the relevant environmental risk factors, and characterizing their interactions. If linkage can be demonstrated, it will be possible to localize the genes and provide the framework for a complete characterization of them. Any additional insight gained into the genetics of Tourette's syndrome and obsessive-compulsive disorder will increase our knowledge of genetic control of the central nervous system and provide another reference point for use in conceptualizing the ways genetic factors can influence complex human disorders.

Genetic linkage has long been recognized as one of the methods useful in clarifying the role of genetic and environmental factors in the expression of complex disorders like Tourette's syndrome. Historically, the method has had limited applicability because of the small number of sufficiently polymorphic genetic markers available for study in humans. This situation has changed dramatically. Advances in DNA technology have made it possible to detect many highly polymorphic genetic markers. Extensive linkage mapping of all human chromosomes has resulted in several human genomic maps (Buetow et al., 1994; Gyapay et al., 1994). It is clear that the application of these techniques will help to clarify the underlying genetic mechanism of Tourette's syndrome, obsessive-compulsive disorder, and related behaviors. Theoretical and empirical work suggests that linkage studies can identify the location and thereby verify the existence of genetic loci important in the expression of complex disorders (Kramer, Pauls, Price, & Kidd, 1989; Kruglyak & Lander, 1995; Price, Kramer, Pauls, & Kidd, 1989). However, multiple strategies need to be employed in the study of complex non-Medelian disorders.

As discussed in Pauls (1993), a possible shortcoming of most previous linkage studies of complex disorders has been the reliance on large, multigenerational families. There are distinct advantages to using large families, including increased statistical power, so that it is possible to establish linkage within one family (assuming that the diagnosis is unambiguous and that the disorder is genetically homogeneous), and increased probability of genetic homogeneity. However, there are also limitations of large pedigrees. D. Greenberg (1992) lists five caveats to keep in mind when considering the use of large, multigenerational pedigrees: (a) it is less likely that the findings from large pedigrees will generalize to the more common form of the disease in the larger population; (b) it is not clear that large pedigrees guarantee homogeneity; as more branches of the family are included, it becomes more likely that individuals who marry in carry a distinct susceptibility gene for the disorder; (c) results from large families are sensitive to changes in the phenotypes of critical individuals in the family; (d) large, multigenerational families are hard to find; and (e) large pedigrees are less useful for different kinds of studies (e.g., sib-pair studies, association studies, and segregation analysis studies). A large sample of small families provides distinct advantages over a small sample of large families; the former allows the examination of hypotheses about the transmission of possible subtypes of disorders and the application of a wider range of analytic methodologies.

One alternative strategy is the use of families with affected sib-pairs. Although it has recently been shown that smaller samples of discordant sib-pairs have greater power for detecting linkage for quantitative traits (Fulker et al., 1991; Risch & Zhang, 1995), there are no currently available assessments that allow us to measure either Tourette's syndrome or obsessive-compulsive disorder as quantitative phenotypes. Thus, for the time being, the affected sib-pair paradigm is the method of choice.

The sib-pair approach has been available for some time, but only recently has it become evident that its application is increasingly important in the genetic study of disorders where there may be genetic heterogeneity and where the mode of inheritance is complex. The most important advantage in the use of sib-pairs is that no prior assumption regarding specific genetic model parameters is required. That is, the sib-pair method is a model-free procedure. The analytic approach relies on the comparison of the number of alleles at a given locus being shared by two affected sibs. If the number of affected individuals sharing alleles is significantly higher than expected by chance, it suggests that a gene of etiological importance for the trait in question is close to the marker being examined. Sib-pair analyses are statistically less powerful than family pedigree analyses and do not allow the estimation of the recombination fraction and the strength of the linkage. However, the sib-pair approach can provide important preliminary evidence for linkage that can form the basis for more powerful techniques.

Another strategy that has been employed recently is the use of association studies to examine the role of specific genes in the manifestation of a disorder. Genetic association studies are an efficient way to identify genotype-phenotype relationships, but in application, they are perilous. The susceptibility of association studies to false positive results is becoming well-known. False positive results are most likely when marker polymorphisms, rather than coding region polymorphisms affecting structure, are used, and when selection of affected and unaffected groups does not control for ethnicity (Gelernter et al., 1993).

It is possible to reduce or eliminate these problems. First, by preferentially studying polymorphisms in or near the coding region of a gene, the first cause of false positive results is minimized. Ideally, the polymorphism should affect protein structure. An example of such a polymorphism is the variable number of tandem repeats (VNTR) located in the region of the gene corresponding to the third cytoplasmic loop of the D4 dopamine receptor (van Tol et al., 1992). Second, by making allele frequency comparisons only between individuals in the same racial groups (unless it has been demonstrated that racial groups do not differ in allele frequency for a particular marker), it is possible to essentially eliminate the problem of ethnic differences in gene frequencies. One way of perfectly matching for ethnicity is by applying the haplotype relative risk (HRR) method (Falk & Rubinstein, 1987; Terwilliger & Ott, 1992). This method controls for variation in allele frequency due to ethnicity by constructing a control group of nontransmitted parental alleles. The HRR method requires collection of DNA from affected individuals and both biological parents (a family trio) and controls for population stratification. After genotyping each trio, transmitted and nontrasmitted alleles can be identified. The nontransmitted parental alleles are used as a perfectly matched comparison group of alleles. The proband's two alleles are considered to be in the ill group. The nontransmitted parental alleles (determined by subtracting the set of the offspring's two alleles from the set of parents' four alleles) are considered to be in the control group. Because the two parents each donate one allele to the ill group and one allele to the comparison group, it is clear that both groups are perfectly matched for ethnicity, as contributions to the two sets of alleles are completely balanced. Thus, the strength of the HRR method lies in the parental alleles that are not transmitted to the proband; these alleles form an independent control sample, thereby avoiding problems related to ascertaining control individuals appropriately matched for ethnicity.

Finally, Spielman, McGinnis, and Ewens (1993) described a test for association-linkage disequilibrium between a genetic marker and disease susceptibility. This transmission disequilibrium test (TDT) examines the transmission of alleles from parents heterozygous for the marker in question to affected offspring. Using data from families with at least one affected child, the test examines whether the marker allele has been transmitted to affected offspring more often than would be expected by chance. Ewens and Spielman (1995) showed that the TDT is a valid test for linkage and association, even when the association is caused by population subdivision and admixture. However, linkage is detected by this test only if true association is also present. Figure 11.1 provides a schematic for understanding the HRR and TDT designs.

Genetic Linkage Studies of Tourette's Syndrome

Considerable work has been done to localize and characterize genes important for the expression of Tourette's syndrome and associated behaviors.

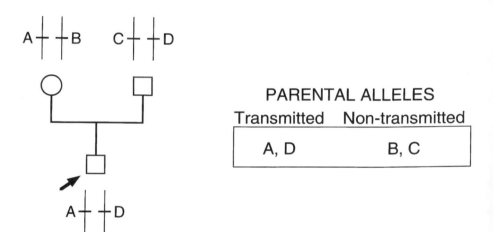

Figure 11.1 Schematic depicting the design of haplotype relative risk (HRR) and transmission disequilibrium test (TDT) studies. The parents are depicted by a circle (mother) and a square (father) connected by a solid line. The affected offspring is depicted as a son (a square) at the lower level. The maternal and paternal alleles at a hypothetical disease vulnerability locus are A and B for the mother and C and D for the father. The alleles transmitted to the affected son are A and D, and the nontransmitted alleles are B and C. In this example, the index case had a 50-50 chance of receiving allele A (the putative vulnerability allele) from his mother. In both the HRR and TDT designs, if the candidate allele was transmitted to the affected offspring at a rate much higher than the chance expectancy across multiple families (typically > 100 triplets [parents plus ill offspring] are genotyped), this constitutes evidence for association. The TDT is a special case of the HRR and requires that at least one parent is heterozygous for the allele of interest, as depicted in the schematic. A positive TDT constitutes evidence for association and linkage. See text and Falk and Rubinstein (1987), Spielman, McGinnis, and Ewens (1993), and Terwilliger and Ott (1992) for additional details.

Clinical and genetic studies have been carried out in approximately 25 families (Barr et al., 1994; Heutink, 1993; Pakstis et al., 1991; Pauls et al., 1990). Altogether, more than 800 genetic market loci have been screened for linkage to a hypothetical gene for Tourette's syndrome and related disorders.

In addition to this genomic screen, several candidate gene loci (focusing generally on the dopamine system) have been examined to determine whether they might be genetically linked to Tourette's syndrome. Linkage has been excluded between Tourette's syndrome and the D_2 dopamine receptor gene (DRD2; Gelernter et al., 1990) and between Tourette's syndrome and the D_1 dopamine receptor gene (Gelernter et al., 1993). More recently, close linkage between Tourette's syndrome and the serotonin 7 receptor gene (HTR7; Gelernter, Pakstis, & Kidd, 1995) and between Tourette's syndrome and the dopamine transporter protein gene was also excluded (Gelernter et al., 1995). Other candidate loci that have been excluded include pro-dynorphin (PDYN), proopiomelanocortin (POMC), and the gastrin-releasing peptide (GRP).

Overall, no strong positive evidence for linkage with Tourette's syndrome has been obtained. If it is assumed that (a) Tourette's syndrome is a homogeneous disorder, (b) the genetic model parameters obtained from segregation analyses are correct, and (c) all chronic tics are related to Tourette's syndrome, then approximately 85% of the genome has been excluded by the pooled results from all of the laboratories.

The possibility of heterogeneity needs to be considered. Genetic heterogeneity could mask a positive result given that LOD scores are summed over all families. Each family is always analyzed separately to examine whether there may be evidence for heterogeneity. One of the advantages of studying large families is that each is large enough to yield statistical significance by itself. However, to date, no compelling evidence has been obtained to suggest that Tourette's syndrome is linked to a marker in any of these families.

Genetic Association Studies of Tourette's Syndrome

Given the lack of success to localize a gene using these traditional linkage approaches, several investigators have begun to employ association strategies in the hopes of identifying loci that increase the risk of Tourette's syndrome. Comings et al. (1991) reported an association between Tourette's syndrome and alleles at the D_2 dopamine receptor. In particular, these investigators proposed that severity of Tourette's syndrome was associated with the number of specific alleles present at this locus. Gelernter, Pauls, and colleagues (1994) were unable to confirm this finding. The study design employed by Gelernter and colleagues differed from that employed by Comings; in the former, only within-family severity comparisons were used. This approach circumvents the problem with population stratification that, as discussed above, could lead to false positive results with association studies.

In a second study, the HRR method of Falk and Rubinstein (1987) and the TDT of Spielman et al. (1993) were employed to examine the possible association between alleles of the DRD4 locus and Tourette's syndrome (Grice et al., 1996). The DRD4 locus contains a polymorphism in the putative third cytoplasmic loop of the protein. The 7 allele of DRD4 (DRD4.7R, so designated because it has 7 repeats) has different pharmacological properties from the other major alleles (van Tol et al., 1992). The frequency of DRD4 alleles in 93 Tourette's syndrome family trios (24 unrelated trios and 69 trios from four large kindreds) was examined. HRR and TDT analyses of transmitted and nontransmitted alleles were completed. The DRD4.7R allele was found more frequently in the transmitted group of alleles than in the nontransmitted group. That is, it was transmitted more frequently to Tourette's syndrome patients than the other alleles at this locus. However, the increased transmission of the DRD4.7R allele was found to be concentrated in only two sections of two larger multigenerational families. Attempts to replicate these results in independent samples have been unsuccessful (Barr, Wigg, Zovko, Sandor, & Tsui, 1996; van de Wetering, personal communication).

Genetic Linkage and Association Studies of Obsessive-Compulsive Disorder

Linkage and association studies have also been initiated in obsessive-compulsive disorder families. As noted above, genes important in the serotonin neurotransmitter system are candidate genes for the expression of obsessive-compulsive disorder. Thus, a study was undertaken to examine the role of the serotonin transporter (SLC6A4) in the manifestation of obsessive-compulsive disorder (Alsobrook, 1996). Serotonin transporter protein is the site of presynaptic retrieval of serotonin and is the target of the specific serotonin-reuptake inhibitors that are the most efficacious for the treatment of obsessive-compulsive disorder. A polymorphism has been identified at this gene (Gelernter & Freimer, 1994) and was used to evaluate SLC6A4 as a candidate gene for obsessive-compulsive disorder. Initial typings were completed in one large obsessive-compulsive disorder kindred. A LOD score slightly less than 1 was obtained with SLC6A4. To follow up this finding, additional markers in the region (D17S33, D17S1293, D17S798, D17S250, and D17S975) were typed. Typings were completed on the obsessive-compulsive disorder family as well as two large Tourette's syndrome kindreds. Pairwise linkage analyses suggested that all of these loci could be excluded for Tourette's syndrome. However, D17S33 yielded a moderately positive LOD score in the large obsessive-compulsive disorder kindred. A linkage map of markers D17S33, D17S1293, D7S250, D17S975, and two additional markers, D17S58 and D17S73, was developed. Multipoint analyses were undertaken with SLC6A4 and D17S33. All LOD scores were significantly negative. Nonparametric linkage analyses were consistent with exclusion of this region.

Thus, it is unlikely that SLC6A4 is a gene of major effect in the manifestation of obsessive-compulsive disorder.

FAMILY GENETIC COUNSELING AND THE RISK OF TOURETTE'S SYNDROME AND RELATED CONDITIONS WITHIN FAMILIES

It is clear from the work summarized in this chapter that genetic and familial factors are important in the expression of Tourette's syndrome and obsessive-compulsive disorder. Although the specific genetic mechanisms are not yet clearly understood, it is possible to provide some estimates for recurrence risks within families. Data from several family studies (Eapen et al., 1993; Hebebrand et al., 1997; Pauls, Raymond, et al., 1991) are quite consistent in demonstrating that the risk for Tourette's syndrome among family members of an individual with Tourette's syndrome is about 10%–11%, and the risk for chronic tics is approximately 15%. In addition, it appears that the risk for obsessive-compulsive disorder without tics among first-degree relatives of Tourette's syndrome individuals is approximately 11%–12%. Thus, there is a significant risk (approximately 35%) for a first-degree relative of an individual with Tourette's syndrome to have either Tourette's syndrome, CT, or obsessive-compulsive disorder. Male relatives appear to be about three times more likely than female relatives to show tics, whereas mothers, sisters, and daughters appear to be about twice as likely to have obsessive-compulsive disorder without tics as fathers, brothers, and sons.

Unfortunately, it is not yet possible to predict the severity of the disorder among relatives. Nor is it possible to detect an affected individual prenatally. On the positive side, most longitudinal and follow-up studies of individuals with Tourette's syndrome suggest that the disorder often becomes less severe as the individual gets older and very often will be essentially unnoticeable when the individual reaches adulthood. Thus, although the risk for recurrence is quite large, the prognosis for affected individuals is quite good.

THE PROMISE OF GENETIC STUDIES

Despite the slow progress in defining the genes associated with Tourette's syndrome and related phenotypes, there is compelling evidence that such factors do exist. The identification and characterization of these genes will likely prove to be a major step forward in our understanding of the pathogenesis of this disorder. Even with an imprecise specification of a particular chromosomal region from genetic linkage studies, it should be possible in many families to gain some insight into who is at risk for developing Tourette's. It is also possible that by grouping patients according to their genotypes, patterns may emerge concerning symptom profiles, neuropsychological findings, course, and treatment response that will have predictive value for clinicians.

On the one hand, the identification of a linked marker will permit the design of much more incisive studies to illuminate the physiological and biochemical etiology of Tourette's syndrome and obsessive-compulsive disorder by examination of the gene product and its impact on the development of the disorders. With the eventual isolation and sequencing of specific Tourette's syndrome genes, we can expect a fundamental advance. We should be able to chart the normal expression pattern of each vulnerability gene. Specification of when during the course of development and in which brain regions the normal copies of these genes are expressed should clarify some aspects of function. Sequence studies should reveal conserved regions of the genes and some clues as to function of the protein(s) that they code for. We imagine that they collectively code for key portions of a multicomponent system involved in the acquisition and control of behavioral action plans that may have emotional and cognitive features as well as motoric ones. Examination of the regulatory regions of these genes may indicate which environmental factors at the level of the cell influence gene expression.

Twin studies have provided evidence that genetic factors are important for the expression of Tourette's syndrome and related conditions. Those twin studies have also demonstrated that nongenetic factors too play an important role. The localization and characterization of susceptibility genes will also allow the potential identification of nongenetic factors associated with the manifestation or the amelioration of the symptoms of the disorders. By controlling for genetic factors, through the genetic case–control research paradigm, it will be possible to document more carefully the environmental and nongenetic factors important for the expression of Tourette's syndrome, obsessive-compulsive disorder, and other disorders. Currently, a prospective longitudinal study is underway that is collecting data about the importance of nongenetic factors in the expression of Tourette's syndrome and obsessive-compulsive disorder. Studying genetic marker data together with data characterizing phenotypic expression in the context of specific environments should allow a more complete examination of the comorbid contribution of genetic and nongenetic factors.

The development of animal models of Tourette's should also be possible, by recreating in laboratory rodents crucial aspects of the genetic makeup of individuals with Tourette's syndrome. Such animal models may prove to be invaluable in rigorously defining the role of various nongenetic factors as well as in the development of new pharmacological treatments.

Despite these advances, knowledge of the vulnerability genes will neither easily nor immediately transform the clinical landscape. Although such advances will doubtless catalyze research, they will probably not readily answer some of the most pressing clinical questions: how best to cope with specific symptoms, how best to prevent or minimize the long-term emotional sequelae of having tics and obsessive-compulsive symptoms and how best to prevent adult exacerbations.

In addition, we should point out that the identification of specific genetic risk factors is not always an unmixed blessing. Ethical questions are likely to arise: Who should be told and when about their increased risk? Would it make sense to do prenatal testing? These questions emphasize the need for collaborative relationships among patients, their families, and the scientists involved.

SUMMARY OF CHAPTER 11

Family studies demonstrate that the risk of Tourette's syndrome, chronic tic disorders, and obsessive-compulsive disorder are significantly elevated among relatives of Tourette's syndrome probands. Twin studies demonstrate that genetic factors play a significant role in the manifestation of Tourette's syndrome and related conditions. Genetic linkage studies and association studies are currently underway to localize and characterize genes that may be important for the manifestation of these conditions. The localization and characterization of genes important in the expression of Tourette's syndrome, obsessive-compulsive disorder, and related disorders will be a major step forward in our understanding of the genetic-biological risk factors important for the expression of these disorders.

PREVIEW OF CHAPTER 12

The slow, steady progress on the genetic front is strongly complemented by notable gains concerning the role of a variety of epigenetic factors. Particular attention has been focused on the likely role of perinatal factors active early in brain development. Another emerging story concerns the role of postinfectious immune factors. The full story of Tourette's pathogenesis will undoubtedly involve multiple gene-environment interactions that occur over the course of brain development. Some aspects of this story can now be told in outline.

CHAPTER 12

Environmental Risk and Protective Factors

BRADLEY S. PETERSON, JAMES F. LECKMAN, PAUL LOMBROSO,
HEPING ZHANG, KIMBERLY LYNCH, ALICE S. CARTER, DAVID L. PAULS,
and DONALD J. COHEN

> Neurosis will always produce its greatest effects when constitution and ex-
> perience work together in the same direction. Where the constitution is a
> marked one it will perhaps not require the support of actual experiences;
> while a great shock in real life will perhaps bring about a neurosis even in
> an average constitution. (Incidentally, this view of the relative aetiological
> importance of what is innate and what is accidentally experienced applies
> equally to other fields.)
>
> —*Sigmund Freud, 1905*

The etiology of Tourette's syndrome is not yet known. Nevertheless, twin
and family studies have consistently implicated genetic factors in its pathophysiology (see Chapter 11), and they have suggested the importance of
nongenetic factors in determining aspects of the clinical phenotype, such as
the severity of tic symptoms and the presence of psychiatric comorbidities.
Nearly 90% of 30 monozygotic (MZ) twin pairs, for instance, were reported to be concordant for the expression of the full complement of symptoms of Tourette's syndrome (Walkup et al., 1988); the majority of these
twin pairs, however, had worst-ever and current tic symptom severities that
differed substantially (Hyde et al., 1992; Leckman et al., 1987). These differences in symptom severities cannot be due to genetic influences, because
MZ twin pairs are by definition genetically identical. Hence, the inciting
events that determine symptom severity differences between these comorbid twins must be nongenetic in nature. As will be seen, these nongenetic
determinants appear to include both pre- and postnatal experiences. Certain
environmental factors, moreover, appear to be important in determining
whether the putative gene is expressed as chronic tics, Tourette's syndrome,

obsessive-compulsive disorder, attention deficit/hyperactivity disorder (ADHD), or some combination of these. Nongenetic factors also seem to be important in determining whether the severity of symptoms of each clinical syndrome will be mild or severe.

In these studies, the constraints imposed by the genetic determinants facilitate the study of the impact of environment on disease development and progression—much like holding constant the important variables in a laboratory experiment can facilitate the study of other variables. Conversely, identification of environmental risk and protective factors may facilitate the study of the genetic determinants of the disorder by suggesting which regions of the genome should receive special scrutiny as candidate genes in linkage analyses. The environmental variable of interest, for example, may exert some of its pathophysiological effects through modification of the transcription rates of genes having either minor or major effects on the clinical phenotype, and knowing where on the genome that environmental variable interacts will prompt us to explore that region of the genome more carefully in our linkage studies. The strong genetic determinants of Tourette's syndrome therefore provide the opportunity to understand the importance of both epigenetic disease determinants and critical gene-environment interactions. For these reasons, Tourette's syndrome has become an increasingly important model for the study of disease mechanisms in other neuropsychiatric disorders. The kinds of risk and protective factors that putatively affect current symptom severity and the long-term outcome of Tourette's-related disorders include perinatal complications, sex-specific factors, stress, infectious and autoimmune processes, stimulant exposure, prior symptom severity and psychological resilience, the presence of comorbid neuropsychiatric disorders, and maturational and developmental factors. Each of these will be discussed in turn.

PERINATAL FACTORS

Evidence in Tourette's Syndrome

Birth Weights in MZ Twins

Preliminary MZ twin studies indicate that certain characteristics of the perinatal period of neural development may predispose individuals who have Tourette's syndrome to developing more severe disease later in life. Among six MZ twin pairs who were found to be discordant for the presence of Tourette's syndrome, for instance, the more severely affected co-twin invariably had the lower birth weight (Leckman et al., 1987). We have confirmed this finding in a larger series of 15 adult MZ twin pairs, in which seven twins differed in worst-ever severity ratings by 10% or more from their co-twins' ratings. In six of the seven twin pairs, the more severely affected twin had at least a 5% lower birth weight than did the comorbid twin (B. Peterson & Leckman, unpublished data). Similar findings were seen in yet another 16 MZ twin pairs: 13 of the pairs had differing birth weights, and in 12 of the pairs, the lower birth-weight twin had a higher tic score (Hyde et al., 1992).

Singletons

An early study reported that 51 children who had clinically identified tic disorders had sustained significantly more complications in pregnancy than did an equal number of matched control subjects. The number of subjects unfortunately did not permit an analysis of the risk associated with specific obstetrical events (Pasamanick & Kawi, 1956). A subsequent study of 31 Tourette's syndrome singleton children reported even higher rates of obstetrical complications: preeclampsia (10.3%), hypertension (10.3%), gestational diabetes (24.1%), use of medication during pregnancy (58.6%), use of forceps (41.4%), cord problems (13.8%), and nonvertex presentation (17.2%) (Leckman, Dolnansky, et al., 1990). Although no controls were included in this study, the rates are greater than those reported in the general population (Kochenow, 1990).

In this same study, the severity of maternal life stress during pregnancy and the presence of severe nausea and/or vomiting during the first trimester were found to be significantly associated with current tic severity, accounting for nearly 50% of the variance in tic symptom severity (Leckman, Dolnansky, et al., 1990). In addition, the severity of maternal emotional stress during the pregnancy (as measured by a 5-point ordinal scale with anchored descriptors) was positively associated with tic severity and the quality of psychosocial functioning.

Family Studies

The significance of prenatal and obstetrical risk factors for Tourette's syndrome-related diseases was assessed as a component of the largest extant Tourette's syndrome family genetic study (Santangelo et al., 1994). In the 60 Tourette's syndrome child probands, boys were 9 times more likely to have experienced some type of delivery complication; this excessive rate of obstetrical complications was primarily accounted for by an increased rate of forceps deliveries in boys (44% of the boys compared with 14% of the girls). Furthermore, the Tourette's syndrome boys delivered by forceps were 8 times more likely to have comorbid obsessive-compulsive disorder than those not delivered by forceps ($p < 0.05$). These findings together imply that perhaps this obstetrical maneuver specifically predisposes boys to a relatively increased risk of Tourette's syndrome (potentially explaining the higher frequency of Tourette's syndrome in boys) and to the obsessive-compulsive disorder seen in TS families (explaining to some degree who develops obsessive-compulsive disorder in genetically predisposed individuals). An additional five-fold elevated risk of obsessive-compulsive disorder comorbidity was associated in this study with the mother's daily use of coffee (more than two cups per day), cigarettes (more than 10 per day), and alcohol (more than two drinks each day; $p < 0.05$).

Evidence in Obsessive-Compulsive Disorder

Only two other studies have, to our knowledge, investigated the potential association of early developmental risk factors with the development of obsessive-compulsive disorder. One studied 103 adult patients diagnosed with "obsessional neuroses" and an age- and sex-matched control group diagnosed with nonobsessional neuroses (Grimshaw, 1964). Nearly 20% of the obsessional group and 8% of the control subjects had a history of neurological illness, such as encephalitis lethargica, Sydenham's chorea (the description of which sounds much like misdiagnosed Tourette's syndrome), poliomyelitis, meningitis, and neonatal seizures. A later study retrospectively assessed the birth histories of 33 adult patients diagnosed with obsessional neuroses and 33 age-, sex-, and date-of-referral-matched patients who had nonobsessional illnesses, such as depression, schizophrenia, schizoaffective illness, manic-depression, and anorexia (Capstick & Seldrup, 1977). Eleven patients in the obsessional group and two of the control subjects reported histories of abnormal birth that were not further characterized (matched odds ratio analysis $p < 0.01$). Within the obsessional group, those subjects reporting an abnormal birth tended to show "bizarre" rituals compared to those who had normal births ($p = 0.06$).

Evidence in ADHD

An increased rate of obstetrical complications has been reported in non-familial ADHD (Sprich-Buckminster et al., 1993). In this retrospective study, all ADHD probands together ($n = 73$) had an increased rate of delivery complications (odds ratio > 4.0) compared with normal control ($n = 26$) subjects; this was accounted for primarily by elevated rates of complication in subjects with nonfamilial ADHD ($n = 52$) compared with familial ADHD ($n = 21$). Delivery complications, in fact, were 22 times more likely in nonfamilial than in familial forms of the disorder. Delivery complication rates did not significantly differ, however, between the ADHD group and a heterogeneous psychiatric control population, suggesting that the risk posed by delivery complications to developing psychopathology is nonspecific. The nonfamilial variety of ADHD that these obstetrical complications produce therefore seems to be a phenocopy of the ADHD produced by a putative ADHD vulnerability gene.

Prenatal risk factors for ADHD have been assessed in more detail in two large studies. The first, a prospective longitudinal study of the prenatal determinants of "minimal brain dysfunction" (which, prior to *DSM* nosology, subsumed what is now ADHD) in more than 10,000 pregnancies, found a small to moderate risk (relative risk = 1.25) of hyperactivity/impulsivity in the offspring of mothers who smoked cigarettes compared with the offspring of mothers who had never smoked (Nichols & Chen, 1981a). This relative risk increased to 1.41 when heavy smokers alone were considered in the analyses (Nichols & Chen, 1981b). The elevated risk for the entire sample seemed to derive primarily from an elevated risk for Caucasian male offspring. Other risk factors associated with the development of hyperactivity/impulsivity included very low birth weight (less than 2500 grams, relative risk = 1.75) and breech delivery (relative risk = 1.31). These findings should be considered preliminary in light of the number of statistical comparisons performed (with the likelihood that positive findings may be attributed to chance), and the possibility that other potential confounds may be responsible for the observed association between the putative risk factor and symptoms of hyperactivity and impulsivity. Genetic and other familial factors that may manifest as hyperactivity and impulsivity, for instance, also may predispose to cigarette smoking and other forms of substance abuse, as well as to delivery complications.

One retrospective study of 140 ADHD children confirmed the association between heavy maternal smoking (at least one pack per day for three months of the pregnancy) and the subsequent development of ADHD (Milberger et al., 1996). The strength of the association of prenatal exposure to maternal smoking with ADHD was stronger than seen in the prospective study (odds ratio = 2.7; 95% confidence interval: 1.1–7.0) despite greater statistical control in the latter study for potentially confounding variables, such as the presence of ADHD in the parents, parental IQ, and socioeconomic status. Because of the smaller sample size in this study (140 in each diagnostic group), the level of statistical significance was less than it was in the larger prospective study ($p = 0.04$). If this significance level were corrected for the number of statistical tests performed (including tests of significance for maternal drug or alcohol abuse and maternal age), the association would not have attained the level of statistical significance ($p < 0.05$).

Evidence in Other Neuropsychiatric Disorders

The kinds of prenatal risk factors identified in the pathophysiologies of other neuropsychiatric disorders are similar to those implicated in disorders related to Tourette's syndrome. These include reports of more frequent family discord, maternal stress, and obstetrical complications in autistic children (Nelson, 1991; A. Ward, 1990), and prenatal exposure to influenza virus, maternal malnutrition, and obstetrical complications in genetically vulnerable children associated with the development of schizophrenia (Cannon et al., 1993, 1994; Marcus, Hans, Auerbach, & Auerbach, 1993; Mednick, Machon, Huttunen, & Bonett, 1988; Sham et al., 1992; Susser & Lin, 1992; Takei et al., 1994). The similarities of these risk factors to those implicated thus far in Tourette's syndrome pathophysiology raise the question of their specificity in producing any given neurodevelopmental disorder. Recall that at least in the case of ADHD, obstetrical complications appear to predispose equally to ADHD and to general neuropsychiatric illness, and that the nonfamilial ADHD that they produce may represent phenocopies of a putative ADHD gene (Sprich-Buckminster et al., 1993). Thus, it is possible that pre- and perinatal insults may either produce sporadic phenocopies of genetic disorders, or may otherwise non-specifically induce more severe symptomatology within genetically pre-disposed individuals.

Possible Mechanisms of Perinatal Complications

Many of the perinatal complications implicated in Tourette's syndrome—preeclampsia, hypertension, gestational diabetes, low birth weight, oligo-hydramnios, and placental insufficiency—are associated with impaired fetal blood flow to watershed areas of perfusion in the CNS, such as the basal ganglia and the periventricular brain parenchyma (Vannucci, 1989). We and others have speculated on the possible role of the basal ganglia in the pathophysiology of Tourette's syndrome (see Chapter 13). It is possible that perinatal complications produce hypoxic injury to the basal ganglia and related neurotransmitter system in utero (Arregui, Hollingsworth, Penney, & Young, 1994; Gross, Lun, & Berndt, 1993), which then predisposes the genetically vulnerable fetus to more severe tic symptoms. Similar mechanisms have been postulated in other movement disorders (Choi, Lee, & Choi, 1993; Hawker & Lang, 1990; Scott & Jankovic, 1996). It must be noted, however, that the genetic vulnerability to Tourette's syndrome could conceivably predispose the fetus to developing perinatal complications, and this then could produce the reported association between perinatal complication and the symptom severity of Tourette's syndrome. The available experimental data do not yet permit the assignment of a direction of causality to the observed associations.

Neuroimaging studies nevertheless provide supportive evidence for the hypothesis that adverse perinatal events injure the basal ganglia in Tourette's syndrome. MRI studies have demonstrated that basal ganglia volumes in Tourette's syndrome are smaller than are those of normal control subjects (B. Peterson, Riddle, Cohen, Katz, Smith, Hardin, et al., 1993; Singer et al., 1993). In addition to volume reductions, the basal ganglia of Tourette's syndrome subjects lack an asymmetry seen in the normal controls. The observation of these brain changes in children who have Tourette's syndrome (Singer et al.) places the temporal origin of the structural changes well into early childhood, suggesting that the structural changes are not likely to be a consequence of having the disorder. Other neuroimaging studies have provided additional evidence for aberrant cerebral lateralization in Tourette's syndrome, and include a reduced cross-sectional area of the corpus callosum on midline sagittal images (B. Peterson, Leckman, Duncan, et al., 1994) and abnormal lateralization of T2 relaxation times in the basal ganglia, frontal white matter, and amygdala (B. Peterson, Gore, Riddle, Cohen, & Leckman, 1994). In addition, functional tests of CNS lateralization (including line bisection and rotational bias) indicate that the cerebral lateralization seen in normal right-handed individuals (e.g., leftward shift in line bisection and leftward turning bias) may be reduced in adult subjects who have Tourette's syndrome (Yazgan, Peterson, Wexler, & Leckman,

1995), providing some degree of functional corroboration for what is seen structurally.

If abnormal lateralization of the CNS in Tourette's syndrome is confirmed in future imaging studies, the asymmetry abnormalities could be interpreted as arising either from a direct manifestation of the vulnerability gene(s) for Tourette's syndrome or from nongenetic factors that are somehow associated with the disorder. Preclinical studies of the determinants of CNS lateralization thus far suggest that the failure to develop normal brain asymmetries is due to nongenetic mechanisms active during the prenatal period of CNS development. Animal studies have shown, for instance, that loss of normal fetal brain asymmetries can be effected by exposing pregnant mothers to a variety of stresses (Fleming, Anderson, Rhees, Kinghorn, & Bakaitis, 1986). These neuroanatomical changes are thought to be induced by alterations in the magnitude and timing of normally occurring fetal hormonal surges that produce normal CNS hemispheric lateralization (M. Diamond 1991; Peterson et al., 1992). In addition, animal studies have shown that exposing pregnant mothers to a variety of stresses can induce in the fetus both a heightened neurobiologic responsivity to stress that endures into adulthood (Henry, Kabbaj, Simon, Le Moal, & Maccari, 1994; Takahashi, Turner, & Kalin, 1992) and an altered neurochemical and neuroendocrine CNS milieu (Fride & Weinstock, 1988, 1989; Henry et al., 1995; Insel, Kinsley, Mann, & Bridges, 1990; Peters 1982, 1990). Taken together, these considerations suggest that perhaps in visualizing the loss of normal hemispheric asymmetries we have imaged in Tourette's syndrome patients the residua of one or more adverse perinatal events.

SEX-SPECIFIC FACTORS

Evidence

Clinical evidence that sex-specific neuronal or hormonal systems affect symptom severity in Tourette's syndrome include case reports of the use of anabolic steroids, androgens, antiandrogens, and antiestrogens in Tourette's syndrome patients, as well as reports of tic exacerbation in women prior to and during their menses (Leckman & Scahill, 1990; B. Peterson, Zhang, Leckman, Scahill, et al., 1994; Sandyk, 1988; Schwabe & Konkol, 1992; M. Weiss, Baerg, Wisebord, & Temple, 1995). Only one controlled study has so far examined the role of sex steroid hormones in Tourette's syndrome. Flutamide, an antagonist of the androgen receptor, produced a modest though statistically significant reduction in motor but not phonic tic symptom severity in 13 adult subjects (B. Peterson, Zhang, et al., in press). Changes in hormone levels during flutamide administration provided evidence for the existence of physiological mechanisms that compensate for blocking of the androgen receptor, possibly explaining the seemingly short-lived effects of the medication. Because of the complicated compensatory response to this medication that has very specific direct effects, it currentl·

is not possible to say conclusively what specific effects the many sex hormones have on tic symptoms.

Possible Mechanisms

Certain brain regions are believed to be responsible for many of the range of normal affective, cognitive, and behavioral differences between the sexes. These regions are said to be sexually dimorphic; by definition they differ between the sexes in either anatomic structure or neurophysiologic function. Numerous human brain regions have been reported to be sexually dimorphic, including the preoptic and medial preoptic areas, the suprachiasmatic and arcuate nuclei in the brain stem, and the anterior commissure, corpus callosum, thalamic massa intermedia, medial amygdala, and bed nucleus of the stria terminalis in the forebrain. Several of these regions contain neurotransmitters such as oxytocin and arginine vasopressin that are important in learning, attachment, and sexual and aggressive behaviors (Leckman et al., 1994b; B. Peterson et al., 1992).

The sexual dimorphism of these brain structures seems to be established in utero by steroid hormone surges that occur during critical periods of CNS development. Changes in the magnitude and timing of these hormone surges in animals appear to alter the morphologies and neurochemical specifications of the dimorphic regions (deVries, Best, & Sluiter, 1983; deVries, Buijs, van Leeuwen, Caffe, & Swaab, 1985; Henry et al., 1995; Simerly, Swanson, & Gorski, 1985). These neurochemical and morphological changes are thought to induce in turn the dramatic alterations in some of the behaviors evidenced by these animals (I. Ward, 1984; Ward & Weisz, 1984). Although no direct evidence yet exists for the involvement of sexually dimorphic brain regions in the pathophysiology of Tourette's syndrome, it seems likely that one or more of these brain regions comprise at least a portion of the neurobiologic substrate of Tourette's syndrome. In addition, these regions probably mediate the sex-specific prevalence differences in phenotypic expression of the disorder, and they may modulate the severity of Tourette's syndrome symptom expression as well. These possibilities appear plausible because most of the known sexually dimorphic brain regions are thought to be regulators of other brain regions (such as the basal ganglia, CSTC circuits, and frontal cortex) that are probably crucially involved in the pathogenesis of Tourette's syndrome.

STRESS AND HEIGHTENED EMOTIONALITY

e

gical and psychosocial stress have long been thought to produce m symptom exacerbation in Tourette's syndrome. Life transitions of any kind, whether they are painful or enjoyable, can be considered a potential source of psychological stress in children and a possible risk factor for exacerbation of tic symptoms over the short term. Thus, family discord, school examinations, exciting holidays, and the beginning of a new school term are times when symptom exacerbation commonly prompts clinical reevaluation (Silva et al., 1995). Similarly, physical illness of all kinds can produce acute exacerbation of symptoms, which usually returns to baseline with time. Death and divorce in family members have also been linked to the onset of obsessive-compulsive disorder symptoms in one study of 20 obsessive-compulsive disorder children (Thomsen, 1995). One particularly stressful medical procedure (a lumbar puncture) has been shown to produce greater elevations in plasma ACTH in Tourette's syndrome than in control subjects, and an increase in urinary excretion of catecholamines in direct proportion to the severity of tic symptoms. These changes suggest the presence of an exaggerated stress reactivity that worsens tic symptom severity in Tourette's syndrome (Chappell, Riddle, et al., 1994). It should be emphasized that although acute stress seems to produce an exacerbation of symptoms over the short term, it is unknown whether acute or chronic stress alters the natural history of tic symptoms or comorbid illnesses. The long-term effects of stress warrant closer study in Tourette's syndrome-related conditions.

Possible Mechanisms

The human physiological stress response is multifaceted and complex, involving the entire hypothalamo-pituitary-adrenal axis and its effects on the brain, cardiovascular, and musculoskeletal systems (Herman & Cullinan, 1997). It is therefore undoubtedly an oversimplification to attribute tic symptom exacerbation to a single aspect of this stress response. Nevertheless, the correlation of the severity of tic symptoms with levels of stress is generally attributed to the effects of norepinephrine in the CNS, primarily because of the efficacy of clonidine (a presynaptic adrenergic agonist that decreases postsynaptic adrenergic system tonus) in reducing the severity of tic symptoms (Leckman et al., 1991). The increase in CNS norepinephrine during stress may either enhance dopaminergic tone or impair the function of other (primarily frontal) systems that tend to attenuate or inhibit tic symptoms (Chappell et al., 1990; Peterson & Cohen, 1998).

INFECTIOUS AND AUTOIMMUNE PROCESSES

Infectious processes have recently been suggested as one possible environmental factor associated with Tourette's syndrome and obsessive-compulsive disorder (Kiessling et al., 1993a; Swedo et al., 1994). The hypothesis is that some cases are caused by an autoimmune process in response to either a viral or a streptococcal infection (A. Allen et al., 1995).

Evidence

In the past several years, elevated levels of antineuronal antibodies have been reported in patients who have either tic or obsessive-compulsive disorders (Kiessling et al., 1993a, 1993b; Swedo, Kilpatrick, Schapiro, Mannheim, & Leonard, 1991; Swedo, Rapoport, Leonard, et al., 1989). In one study, children with movement disorders were found to be almost twice as likely to have antineuronal antibodies in their sera as children without movement disorders (Kiessling et al., 1993a). In addition, these same children were more likely than the control group to have had a previous streptococcal infection as indicated by at least one elevated antistreptococcal titer. The authors concluded from these findings that a subset of tic disorders is caused by a previous streptococcal infection (Swedo et al., 1998). Although these preliminary findings are intriguing, they must be viewed with caution, as the sera of many normal individuals contain antibodies that are immunoreactive against brain tissue, and it is not clear whether an ascertainment bias contributed to the findings (i.e., it is possible that the subjects were selected because their clinical histories suggested a recent streptococcal infection).

Possible Mechanisms

Several hypotheses have been advanced to explain how an immunological response could produce these disorders. The *molecular mimicry hypothesis* suggests that host proteins share immunological epitopes with proteins in the organism. The host responds to the infection by producing antibodies directed against proteins from the infecting organism; these antibodies, the theory postulates, are then able to cross-react with, and presumably damage, host tissues.

The *superantigen hypothesis* postulates that certain peptides and toxins from infectious organisms act as superantigens, which produce a tremendously broad range of host immune responses. Superantigens inappropriately bind to and activate a significant subset of the population of T cells, some of which are autoreactive. The expansion of these T cells results in the release of large amounts of inflammatory cytokines and the activation of antibody-producing B cells. The molecular mimicry and superantigen hypotheses are not mutually exclusive theories, and it is likely that different combinations of these immune responses are at work in different autoimmune disorders. These are testable etiologic hypotheses, and future research will aim to determine which model, if either, is operative in tic-related disorders.

Related Conditions

The current immunological explanations have grown out of earlier studies of another movement disorder, Sydenham's chorea. Sydenham's chorea is thought to be a late sequela of rheumatic fever. The evidence for an autoimmune response to an antecedent streptococcal infection is considerably stronger for this disorder than for Tourette's syndrome. A protein on the surface of streptococcal bacteria, termed the M protein, has been implicated as the antigen responsible for the autoimmune response in Sydenham's, although other components of the bacterial wall may be involved as well (Zabriskie, 1986). The M protein, located on the outer surface of the streptococcus bacterium, is a highly polymorphic protein used to subtype group A β-streptococci. Certain strains are rheumatogenic, as they are associated with rheumatic fever, carditis, and chorea. Others are nephritogenic and are associated with glomerulonephritis.

A marked structural similarity was noticed between the M protein molecule and a number of structural proteins found in muscle (Manjula & Fichetti, 1980). Antibodies raised against purified M protein have been shown to cross-react with heart tissue, thus proving that a shared epitope exists between M protein and heart muscle (Bronze & Dale, 1993; Dale & Beachey, 1985; Kisher & Cunningham, 1985).

Antibodies directed against brain tissue have been detected in the sera of patients with Sydenham's chorea. Sera from some of these patients are immunoreactive against neurons from caudate, thalamus, and subthalamic nuclei (Husby et al., 1976); the immunoreactive response against other brain regions, such as cerebral cortex, is less dramatic. The presence of antineuronal antibodies has been found to be considerably higher in Sydenham's chorea patients than in the control group of rheumatic fever patients who have carditis but no chorea and in patients with no antecedent streptococcal infection. In addition, Sydenham's chorea is associated with higher than expected rates of obsessive-compulsive disorder (Swedo et al., 1993) and is associated with abnormalities (7%–10% increases) of basal ganglia volume (Giedd et al., 1995), suggesting that its immunological mechanism may be relevant to that in Tourette's syndrome.

The mechanism by which these antibodies gain access to the CNS remains unclear, as the blood-brain barrier had previously been considered inpenetrable to these macromolecules. It is possible that the action of other factors, such as cytokines or complement, or the infectious process itself, increases the permeability of the blood-brain barrier and allows the antibodies entry. In either case, one would expect to find elevated titers of antistreptococcal and antineuronal antibodies in the CSF of patients with tic-related disorders, or infiltrating T cells in the affected tissue. CSF antibodies are present in other autoimmune disorders that affect the CNS, such as multiple sclerosis, Lupus erythymatosis, Stiff Man's syndrome, and the paraneoplastic cancers. Antineuronal antibodies have been reported in the CSF of patients with acute rheumatic chorea (Zabriskie, 1986), although these findings have not yet been replicated. If it is to be proved that some forms of tic and obsessive-compulsive disorders truly are autoimmune sequelae of streptococcal infection, similar antineuronal antibodies with activity directed specifically at particular neuronal tissues such as the basal ganglia will need to be demonstrated.

STIMULANT EXPOSURE

Evidence

Clinical anecdotes have long suggested that stimulant medications can either produce or worsen tic symptoms. Retrospective studies have indicated a worsening of tics in 30%–50% of children who have ADHD and tics and who take stimulants, and the de novo development of tics in 10% of ADHD children who did not have tics previously (Erenberg, Cruse, & Rothner, 1985; Golden, 1974; Lipkin, Goldstein, & Adesman, 1994; Price et al., 1986). One prospective crossover study administered low- to mid-range dosages of methylphenidate for two weeks to children who had ADHD and tics. A dose-related increase in motor and vocal tic severity was seen, although teachers rated vocal tic severity as being improved on medication (Gadow, Sverd, Sprafkin, Nolan, & Ezor, 1995). This apparent contradiction between clinician and teacher ratings of the severity of vocal tics might be explained by the improvement in behavioral disruption that stimulants can produce, which the teachers could then have interpreted as an improvement in tic symptoms. The long-term effects of stimulant use on the natural history of tics is unknown.

Cocaine use has also been implicated as a risk factor for developing obsessive-compulsive disorder (Crum & Anthony, 1993). In the Epidemiologic Catchment Area survey of 1980–1984, the Diagnostic Interview Schedule (DIS) was administered to 13,306 adult participants at baseline, and again during a one-year follow-up. New-onset obsessive-compulsive disorder, as diagnosed in 105 participants by the DIS at follow-up, was significantly associated with cocaine abuse in the preceding year (8 new cases among 414 active cocaine users, and 97 cases among the 12,892 nonusers), with a relative risk of 2.6 ($p = 0.02$). Female sex also was associated with a three-fold increased risk of developing obsessive-compulsive disorder ($p < 0.01$). Conditional and unconditional multiple logistic regression analyses that controlled for important potential confounding demographic variables (including sex of the subject) confirmed the elevated risk of developing obsessive-compulsive disorder associated with active cocaine use (relative risks 4.1–7.2) but not with other drugs of abuse. These findings should be interpreted with caution, since they likely were post hoc, and not driven by an a priori hypothesis.

Possible Mechanisms

The commonly accepted mechanism for the exacerbation of tics by stimulant medications is that the direct dopaminergic effects of the stimulant medications increase an already overactive dopamine tonus at the level of the striatum. Cocaine increases dopaminergic activity at nerve synapses in the striatum by blocking reuptake of synaptic dopamine by the presynaptic dopamine transporter. Tics and obsessive-compulsive disorder symptoms may be similarly aggravated by stimulation of dopaminergic pathways in these brain regions, which are thought to be involved in the pathophysiologies of both disorders.

SYMPTOM SEVERITY AND PSYCHOLOGICAL RESILIENCE

Preliminary follow-up studies suggest that the relative severity of tic symptoms in childhood is a weak but positive predictor of symptom severity in adulthood, so that relatively mild or severe tic symptoms in childhood tend to predict mild or severe symptoms, respectively, in adulthood (Bruun, 1988a). Childhood tic symptom severity, however, is probably a poor predictor of the long-term occupational, social, and emotional adjustment of Tourette's syndrome children. Tic symptom severity in childhood, in other words, explains only a fraction of the overall variance in long-term outcome, if outcome is interpreted broadly as academic and occupational success and the ability to love and to be loved.

As reviewed in Chapter 6, objective tic symptom severity (the number, frequency, and intensity of tic symptoms) at any given time also seems to be a poor predictor of a child's current level of adaptive functioning. Children with severe tic symptoms, for example, can be in every discernible respect happy, confident, well related, popular, academically successful, and comfortable with their families; other children with relatively mild tic symptoms, on the other hand, can be disproportionately sad and have a paucity of friendships, an impoverished self-esteem and lack of confidence, and poor academic achievement. This does not mean that objective tic symptom severity has no role in determining adaptive functioning. More severe tic symptoms are more likely to interfere with intended motor or speech acts, and children with more severe tic symptoms are in a probabilistic sense more likely to be teased and to suffer in self esteem; but these sources of interference are not assured in any particular child.

Intelligence and quality of socialization have been shown repeatedly to be the best long-term predictors of outcome, regardless of diagnosis (Masten & Coatsworth, 1995). Bright, academically successful children who have close and enduring friendships are likely to continue to be successful interpersonally and professionally throughout their lives, regardless of their future severity of tic symptoms. The child's responses to past hardship and challenges to self-esteem, and to the presence of tics currently, are important predictors of the child's future resilience to the effects of life stress, of which the presence of tics is only one. These coping abilities can often be assessed early in the course of clinical evaluation. Tic symptoms that seem to be impairing self-esteem need to be taken seriously by clinicians when planning treatment strategies, because the relatively ineffective coping strategies that are responsible for this breakdown in the resiliency of self-image are likely to remain relatively stable during the chronic course of tic symptom evolution through childhood, adolescence, and adulthood (see Chapters 1, 8, and 15).

NEUROPSYCHIATRIC COMORBIDITY

Common comorbidities seen in Tourette's syndrome, including obsessive-compulsive disorder, ADHD, affective disorders, and anxiety, are most often chronic or recurring (Harrington, Fudge, Rutter, Pickles, & Hill, 1990; Leonard et al., 1992; Mannuzza et al., 1993) and can profoundly affect social, occupational, and emotional functioning. The presence or absence of these comorbidities will therefore often have a much greater importance for prognosticating long-term outcome than will the presence of tics. ADHD, for instance, affects nearly 50% of children in clinic populations of Tourette's syndrome. Inattention and distractibility often impair academic performance, and impulsivity can disrupt relationships with family and friends. The risk that continuing ADHD poses in general for the future development of conduct disorder, substance abuse, anxiety, and affective disorder is well documented (Biederman et al., 1991a; Mannuzza et al., 1993) and warrants close clinical attention and diligent attempts at intervention. Similarly, the presence of comorbid obsessive-compulsive disorder confers a greater likelihood for a longer period of functional impairment, usually at least into later adolescence, when tic symptoms are generally on the wane. Unlike tics, the presence of tic-related obsessive-compulsive disorder also carries a higher risk for additional comorbid illnesses that include depression, anxiety disorders, and simple phobias (Pauls et al., 1994; Thomsen, 1994a, 1994b, 1994c). Children with tics should not be considered safe from the risk for new-onset obsessive-compulsive disorder until they reach later adolescence (Leonard, Goldberger, Rapoport, Cheslow, & Swedo, 1990; Swedo, Rapoport, Leonard, et al., 1989).

MATURATIONAL AND DEVELOPMENTAL FACTORS

Tics at their onset (usually in early grade school) are most often infrequent and mild. They eventually increase in frequency, forcefulness, or number until they are brought to clinical attention. Families usually have noted by then a distinct tendency for tics to fluctuate in severity, worsening predictably during times of stress. This waxing and waning can be expected to continue in the future. Such symptom fluctuation is likely to be superimposed on a trajectory of tic symptom severity that gradually increases up to and during puberty, and that then gradually decreases through adolescence until it reaches a relatively stable level by early adulthood. This typical trajectory of tic symptom severity is only a probabilistic one; predicting whether this will be the course an individual child follows, or whether his or her tics will unexpectedly either worsen or improve, is currently an impossibility. No blood test and no character-istic of the clinical phenotype of a given individual is known to predict clinical course.

Despite the limitations in prognosticating for individuals, the general long-term prognosis for tic symptoms is relatively optimistic. By early adulthood, nearly one-third of Tourette's syndrome patients will no longer have tic symptoms (Leckman, Zhang, et al., 1998). Another third will have milder tic symptoms than they had in childhood, and the remaining third will continue to have relatively severe tic symptoms and functional impair-ment (B. Peterson et al., 1995). Severely debilitating Tourette's syndrome in adulthood is a rarity, and represents the furthest extent on a very broad spectrum of symptom severity.

The causes of this overall trajectory of tic symptom severity are un-known. Nevertheless, the characteristic ages of onset, exacerbation, and attenuation strongly suggest the importance of maturational and develop-mental factors in shaping this trajectory. Among the multitude of possible maturational factors that have been proposed to influence this trajectory in-clude myelination of the CNS, neurotransmitter system imbalances in early childhood, and increasing gonadal steroid levels and synaptic pruning in adolescence (B. Peterson et al., 1992, 1995; B. Peterson, Leckman, Dun-can, et al., 1994).

Another important developmental consideration is the relatively unusual exacerbation of tic symptoms in mid- to late adulthood. The rapid or sus-tained severe exacerbation of tic symptoms in adulthood warrants a com-plete medical, neurological, and psychiatric evaluation. In our clinical experience, thyroid abnormalities, new-onset anxiety or affective distur-bances, substance abuse, early dementing illnesses, and menopause in women seem to be the most common underlying causes of late-life symp-tom exacerbation.

CONCLUSIONS

Despite the obvious importance of genetic factors in the pathophysiology of Tourette's syndrome, they can account for only a portion of the vari-ability in certain crucial aspects of the clinical phenotype. It appears from theoretical and empirical considerations that environmental risk factors may be important codeterminants of the syndrome. The multigenerational transmission of Tourette's syndrome therefore might be most appropri-ately regarded as the transmission of a background of genetic vulnerabil-ity to acquiring a constellation of potential symptoms; upon this genetic background are superimposed environmental events that account for the remainder of the overall phenotypic variability. Whereas genetic determi-nants confer a *vulnerability* to developing Tourette's syndrome, the pres-ence or absence of specific nongenetic risk factors might be considered to contribute to the *specificity* of phenotypic outcomes (B. Peterson et al.,

1995). Moreover, specific environmental events are likely to have very different effects depending on the specific genetic endowments of the individual, so that gene-environment interactions are likely to play a role of paramount importance in the determination of clinical phenotype.

The risk conferred by the interaction of genes and environment in producing a given disorder within a particular child is further contextualized by maturational and developmental timetables, concurrent illnesses, and by the child's adaptive capacities and psychological resilience. In many instances, this psychosocial context may prove to have a much greater impact on long-term outcome in terms of what is most tangible and salient for the child: academic and later occupational success, intimacy and love, and general well-being. As an important determinant of disease and long-term outcome, this psychosocial context must therefore be accounted for and studied.

SUMMARY OF CHAPTER 12

Although genetic factors in many families may set the stage for a vulnerability to develop Tourette's syndrome or a related disorder, the unique developmental history of the individual may determine the actual range of phenotypic expression: which comorbid conditions are present and how severe the syndrome is at different points in time.

PREVIEW OF CHAPTER 13

This chapter reviews the neural circuitry of Tourette's syndrome, obsessive-compulsive disorder, and ADHD. Beginning with clues from animal studies, early neurosurgical procedures, and experiments of nature (accidents, infections), the basal ganglia and related structures in the thalamus and cortex have become the prime focus in this research domain. Initial hypotheses are being tested using a variety of neuroimaging techniques that permit an in vivo examination of brain structure and function, with remarkable spatial and temporal resolution. The work thus far provides us with tantalizing hints of what may be possible in the future: monitoring in real time the complex patterns of neural activations associated with tics and obsessive-compulsive symptoms.

CHAPTER 13

Neuroanatomical Circuitry

BRADLEY S. PETERSON, JAMES F. LECKMAN, AMY ARNSTEN,
GEORGE M. ANDERSON, LAWRENCE H. STAIB, JOHN C. GORE,
RICHARD A. BRONEN, ROBERT MALISON, LAWRENCE SCAHILL,
and DONALD J. COHEN

> J'ai embrassé l'aube d'été . . . à la cime argentée je reconnus la déesse.
> Alors je levai un à un les voiles. Dans l'allée, en agitant les bras.
> Par la plaine, où je l'ai dénoncée au coq.
> A la grand'ville, elle fuyait parmi les clochers et les dômes, et,
> courant comme un mendiant sur les quais de marbre, je la chassais.
>
> [I embraced the dawn of summer . . . at the silvered summit I recognized the
>   goddess.
> I raised then one by one her veils. In the alley while waving my arms.
> On the plain, where I denounced her to the coq.
> In the city, she escaped among the belltowers and domes, and,
> running like a beggar on the marble quay, I chased her.]
>
> —*Arthur Rimbaud, "Aube" (Dawn)*

Human diseases, and brain disorders in particular, are inherently difficult to study. Informative experiments in living human beings—maneuvers either of scientists, clinicians, nature, or environment that definitively influence the symptoms of a disease—have profound and inherent limitations in the knowledge they provide of pathophysiology. The most that such maneuvers can definitively provide is circumstantial evidence about which proximal or distal brain systems influence disease symptoms, or which symptoms are capable of producing a phenocopy of the syndrome. Almost all of modern biological psychiatry involves this kind of experimentation. Although it has led to the elaboration of hypotheses about the brain circuitry involved in various neuropsychiatric disorders, experimental neuroscience has almost never in itself identified the cause of any particular disorder, and Tourette's syndrome is no exception.

Just as the causes of Tourette's syndrome are unknown, so are the regions of the brain that generate and regulate its symptoms. If knowledge of disease mechanisms is to improve, we must first understand and fully acknowledge not only what limits the current state of knowledge of substrate and pathophysiology of Tourette's, but also what is likely to limit what we can hope realistically to learn in the near future. Many investigators, for instance, place hope and emphasis for the improved understanding and treatment of the disorder on the identification of an animal model or on the identification of the putative Tourette's vulnerability gene. Although an animal model of Tourette's syndrome would no doubt be a boon to the research effort, it is unlikely that the experimental lesion producing tic symptoms artificially in an animal would be similar in kind or would involve the same brain regions as those that produce tic symptoms naturally in humans. An animal model could tell us much about the brain systems that produce symptoms similar to those of Tourette's syndrome, and perhaps even about which brain systems may be involved in modulating tic symptoms. But it would not give us a definitive answer as to precisely where in the brain things are going wrong to cause the disorder.

The most salient exception to this generalization of research impediments in human clinical research is in the genetic research of highly specific developmental disorders. The truly dramatic future advances of neurobiological research in Tourette's syndrome no doubt similarly await the identification of the putative vulnerability genes for the disorder. It should be stated clearly, however, that although the identification of these genes will advance and catalyze research efforts, knowledge of the genes will neither immediately nor easily address some of the clinically most relevant and pressing questions of patients suffering from Tourette's syndrome. Those questions include asking what is responsible for symptom exacerbations and remissions, how varying coping strategies affect the response to specific symptoms, what emotional effects the illness has on different individuals, and what determines the natural history and long-term outcome for any given child. Knowledge of the neurobiological substrate affected by the genes for Tourette's syndrome, and of how these neural systems interact with other systems that influence these most important clinical determinants, will still be necessary once the vulnerability genes are identified. Thus, although researchers, clinicians, and patients alike currently tend to regard the future identification of vulnerability genes as a Rosetta stone that will immediately provide the key to deciphering all of the central mysteries of the disorder, this hope for the discovery, however understandable it may be, is overly optimistic. A deeper understanding of the function and interaction of these various neural systems will still be necessary for broad advances in the understanding and treatment of these complex human conditions.

Despite the profound limitations that neurobiological studies of human beings have in identifying the brain-based substrate of either normal or pathological mental processes, a considerable body of circumstantial evidence has contributed to an increasingly sophisticated and specific hypothesis of the circuitry involved in subserving and modulating symptoms of Tourette's syndrome. Like beggars on a marble quay chasing after enlightenment, we must at once inflame and content ourselves with whatever brief and distant views of her are at hand. The clearest and most consistent views of Tourette's syndrome pathophysiology thus far are those pertaining to the importance of genetic factors in the disorder, and to the impressively high rates of obsessive-compulsive disorder and attention-deficit/hyperactivity disorder (ADHD) comorbidity that appear to be related to the genetic vulnerability for Tourette's syndrome; it may be most prudent, therefore, to begin our search for the Tourette's syndrome substrate here, in whatever can be gleaned from knowledge of the relatedness of this triad of disorders. The genetic relatedness of these conditions and their co-occurrence in the same individuals suggests that the intermediary between the gene and its clinical phenotype—brain organization and functioning—is also likely to be related for these same conditions.

Relationship to Obsessive-Compulsive Disorder

As noted in Chapters 2 and 3, complex tics can be extremely difficult to distinguish from compulsions. It is perhaps not surprising, then, that 30%–60% of Tourette's syndrome patients also are diagnosed as having comorbid obsessive-compulsive disorder. The obsessive-compulsive disorder that occurs comorbidly with Tourette's syndrome, however, is not simply misdiagnosed complex tics. Tourette's syndrome patients who have obsessive-compulsive disorder are plagued by the recurrent, intrusive thoughts, mental images, and urges to action of classically defined obsessive-compulsive disorder. Nevertheless, true obsessions and compulsions in Tourette's syndrome-related obsessive-compulsive disorder bear enough of a resemblance to complex tics to suggest that they might lie on a spectrum of compulsory behaviors. Those having a prominent ideational component belong to obsessive-compulsive disorder on one end; those with little or no ideational component (simple tics) lie on the other; and complex tics lie somewhere between these two extremes.

Family genetic and twin studies have provided compelling evidence that Tourette's syndrome is a genetic disorder (Pauls & Leckman, 1986; Pauls, Raymond, et al., 1991; Price et al., 1985). Family studies have also demonstrated that the obsessive-compulsive disorder that occurs in Tourette's syndrome patients is found in families of Tourette's syndrome patients much more often than it is found in families of normal control subjects (Pauls, Raymond, et al., 1991; Pauls, Towbin, et al., 1986), regardless of whether or not the Tourette's syndrome probands have obsessive-compulsive disorder themselves. This finding suggests that at least one form of obsessive-compulsive disorder is a manifestation of the genes that confer a vulnerability to developing Tourette's syndrome.

It is remarkable that disorders whose clinical phenotypes differ, at least superficially, so dramatically (one consisting of motor and vocal tics, the other of obsessions and compulsions) are produced from the same gene or genes. This suggests that their neurobiological substrate—the region or regions of the CNS whose disordered functioning produces the symptoms of Tourette's syndrome and obsessive-compulsive disorder—may be closely related because the Tourette's gene product is expressed in those regions. The substrates of Tourette's syndrome and obsessive-compulsive disorder cannot be identical, however, because the disorders are phenomenologically distinct, and these distinctions ultimately must be brain-based. The phenomenological similarities and the genetic relatedness of Tourette's syndrome and obsessive-compulsive disorder may nevertheless provide important clues in the search for their neurobiological determinants.

Relationship to ADHD

Approximately 50% of all clinically identified Tourette's syndrome patients also have ADHD. The genetic relationship between Tourette's and ADHD is not as clear, however, as the one between Tourette's syndrome and obsessive-compulsive disorder. An initial family study suggested that ADHD is not a manifestation of the Tourette's syndrome vulnerability gene (Pauls, Towbin, et al., 1986). However, a later analysis of the same data that included more families suggested that at least some of the ADHD in Tourette's syndrome families may in fact be caused by the Tourette's syndrome gene, particularly when it occurs together with Tourette's syndrome (Pauls, Hurst, et al., 1986). Despite the possible genetic relatedness between Tourette's syndrome and at least some cases of ADHD, however, it seems clear that at least a portion of the high rate of ADHD in clinically identified cases of Tourette's syndrome can be attributed to an ascertainment bias: children who have both Tourette's syndrome and ADHD are more likely to present to clinic for evaluation and treatment than are children who have either disorder alone. This ascertainment bias will be even stronger, and the proportion of ADHD in Tourette's syndrome clinic populations will be even greater, if ADHD and Tourette's syndrome share portions of the same neurobiological substrate. Disordered functioning of neural systems due to the presence of ADHD, for instance, is likely to worsen tic symptoms if the latter are dependent on the functioning of neural systems closely related to those of ADHD.

As was true for the symptoms of obsessive-compulsive disorder, it is possible that the symptoms of ADHD also bear a phenomenological resemblance to the tics of Tourette's syndrome. Tics can be thought of as a hyperkinesia, and motoric hyperactivity is one hallmark of ADHD. Tourette's syndrome patients can inhibit their tics only for brief periods of time, and an impaired inhibition of impulses is another hallmark of ADHD. Thus, both ADHD and Tourette's syndrome children appear to have excessive motor activity and difficulty inhibiting specific behaviors.

Regardless of the causal relationship between Tourette's and ADHD—whether it is due to variable expression of the Tourette's syndrome gene, to shared neurobiological substrate, or to both—this relatedness should, like that between Tourette's and obsessive-compulsive disorder, provide important clues to aid in identifying the substrate for these disorders.

THE SEARCH FOR A SUBSTRATE

Modern neuropsychiatry has never fully shed the tethers of the methods of brain function localization made popular in preclinical and clinical lesion studies in the earlier part of this century (Ferrier, 1890; R. Young, 1990). Despite the recognized importance of the distributed, nonlocalized nature of neural processing, it is still common to think of normal and disordered brain functioning as localized to small, discrete brain regions. Like Descartes, we would have the seat of the soul localized to the pineal gland. Although function is at least in part regionally specific within the CNS, regional function also depends critically on brain function at spatially remote sites. Thus, in searching for the substrate for Tourette's syndrome, we must remember that the Tourette's syndrome gene product, instead of producing a discrete, localized lesion in the brain, may instead produce disordered functioning of a more distributed network and circuitry.

With this caveat in mind, it may be worthwhile beginning the search for a substrate by considering the many common clinical features of Tourette's syndrome, obsessive-compulsive disorder, and ADHD. The hyperkinesia of Tourette's syndrome indicates that the substrate must involve, at least in part, motor regions of the brain. This would also be supported by the hyperactivity seen in ADHD and by the compulsive behaviors and stereotypies in obsessive-compulsive disorder. The premonitory urges of Tourette's syndrome and the obsessions of obsessive-compulsive disorder suggest that another portion of the substrate includes brain regions that support higher cognitive or ideational processes. Finally, the difficulty with inhibition of inappropriate behaviors in Tourette's syndrome, ADHD, and, to a lesser extent, obsessive-compulsive disorder suggests involvement of inhibitory brain regions. Motor, association, and inhibitory neural systems therefore are likely to subserve the symptoms of these disorders. One of the leading candidate neural systems that subserves these diverse processes is the circuitry that loops between cortical and subcortical brain regions, the name of which derives from the successive components of the loops: the cortico-striato-thalamo-cortical (CSTC) circuits.

NORMAL CSTC CIRCUITRY

CSTC circuits are composed of multiple, partially overlapping but largely parallel circuits that direct information from the cerebral cortex to the subcortex, and then back again to specific regions of the cortex, thereby forming multiple cortical-subcortical loops (Figure 13.1). Although multiple anatomically and functionally related cortical regions provide input into a particular circuit, each circuit in turn refocuses its projections back onto only a subset of the cortical regions initially contributing to that circuit's input. Within the basal ganglia and thalamus, each of the circuits appears to be microscopically segregated from others that course through the same macroscopic structure—hence the conceptualization of these pathways as parallel.

Although the number of anatomically and functionally discrete pathways is still the subject of some controversy (Alexander, Crutcher, & DeLong, 1990; Goldman-Rakic & Selemon, 1990; Parent & Hazrati, 1995a), the current consensus holds that CSTC circuitry has at least three components: those initiating from and projecting back to sensorimotor (SM), orbitofrontal (OF), or association (AS) cortices. Other functional

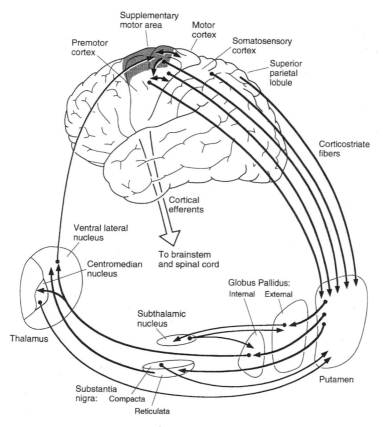

Figure 13.1 CSTC circuits. Cortical regions send projections to the striatum (either the caudate or putamen), which in turn project to the external globus pallidus, then either to the internal segment of the globus pallidus or to the substantia nigra, then to the thalamus, and back up to the cerebral cortex. This drawing has the subcortical sites located outside of the cerebrum, when actually they are located deep within the brain.

components of CSTC circuitry likely exist, and probably include those traditionally associated with the limbic system (Table 13.1).

Cortical projections to the caudate and putamen, which together compose the striatum, appear to be oriented in parasagittally elongated, somatotopically organized domains. From here, information leaves the basal ganglia principally through the internal segment of the globus pallidus (GPi) and its brainstem counterpart, the substantia nigra pars reticulata (SNr), before ascending to the thalamus and cortex. Striatal projections to the external segment of the globus pallidus (GPe), in contrast, give rise to projections directed primarily to the reticular thalamic nucleus, subthalamic nucleus, and GPi. Because the reticular thalamic nucleus in turn exerts on other thalamic nuclei powerful inhibitory influences mediated by gamma-aminobutyric acid (GABA), the GPe/reticular

TABLE 13.1   CSTC Circuitry Implicated in Tourette's Syndrome-Related Disorders

CSTC Component	Sensorimotor (SM) —TS—	Orbitalfrontal (OF) —OCD—	Association (AS) —ADHD—	Limbic (L) —OCD—
Cortical afferents	Somatosensory, Primary motor, Supplementary motor	Orbitalfrontal, Superior temporal gyrus, Inferior temporal gyrus, Anterior cingulate	Dorsolateral prefrontal, Posterior parietal, Arcuate premotor	Anterior cingulate, Hippocampal cortex, Entorhinal cortex, Superior temporal gyrus, Inferior temporal gyrus
Striatum	Dorsolateral putamen, Dorsolateral caudate, (Dorsolateral subthalamic nucleus)	Ventral caudate, Ventral putamen	Dorsolateral caudate	Ventral caudate, Ventral putamen nucleus, Accumbens, Olfactory tubercle
Pallidum/SNr	Ventrolateral GPI Caudolateral SNr	Dorsomedial GPi Rostromedial SNr	Dorsomedial GPi, Rostrolateral SNr	Rostrolateral GPi, Ventral pallidum, Rostrodorsal SNr
Thalamus	Ventrolateral nucleus, Centromedian & intralaminar nuclei	Medial dorsal nucleus (parvocellular)	Ventral anterior nucleus (parvocellular)	Medial dorsal nucleus (posteromedial)
Cortical projections	Supplementary motor	Orbitalfrontal	Dorsolateral prefrontal	Anterior cingulate

thalamic nucleus projection is viewed as one that can intrinsically modulate activity in CSTC pathways involving GPi (Parent & Hazrati, 1995a). The GPe projection to GPi may similarly modulate CSTC activity coursing through the GPi.

Pallidal projections to the thalamus, whether of GPi or GPe origin, are tonically active and primarily GABAergic. Projections from striatum to pallidum are also GABAergic. Thus, increased striatal activity (associated with movement, for instance) will phasically silence the tonically active GPi and SNr neurons. Silencing these neurons, in turn, reduces GABAergic transmission to the thalamus, thereby activating thalamic target neurons. Activation of thalamic nuclei is essential for the initiation of movement. Thus, increased striatal activity can be regarded as disinhibiting thalamic nuclei and cortical regions to produce movement, because the striatal activity activates the two GABAergic connections leading into and out of the GPi/SNr. This, however, is not the whole story—it becomes more complicated. Increased striatal activity in projections to GPe will similarly disinhibit reticular thalamic nuclei. Because these reticular nuclei in turn inhibit other thalamic nuclei, increased striatal activation of GPe will ultimately inhibit those same thalamic nuclei. GPe inhibition of the GPi will produce functionally similar thalamic inhibition. Therefore, increased striatal activity can either inhibit or disinhibit the same thalamic nuclei and cortical regions (and therefore either initiate or inhibit movement), depending on whether the GPe or GPi, respectively, is the target of striatal activity (Figures 13.1 and 13.2).

The subthalamic nucleus (STN) is also an important element of CSTC circuitry. Although STN projects to all basal ganglia elements, excitatory projections to both pallidal segments and SNr are particularly massive. Individual subthalamic axons, which project to both GPi and GPe, arborize extensively throughout their rostrocaudal extent and appear to influence uniformly large subpopulations of neurons in both pallidal segments (Parent & Hazrati, 1995b). Intracellular recordings suggest that STN may modulate the potential of pallidal neurons, thereby modifying pallidal response and sensitivity to incoming striatal signals (Figure 13.2; Kita & Kitai, 1991).

Interhemispheric Connectivity

Interhemispheric coordination appears to be important for CSTC functioning. Single GPi and GPe axons project both ipsilaterally and, through the thalamic massa intermedia, contralaterally to thalamic nuclei. Pallidal axons are thought thereby to influence CSTC functioning bilaterally (Hazrati & Parent, 1991; Parent & Hazrati 1995a). Cortical projections from the projective fields of the CSTC—from AS, supplementary motor area (SMA), and anterior cingulate—cross through the callosum to the contralateral striatum; in the SMA, at least, the strength of contralateral

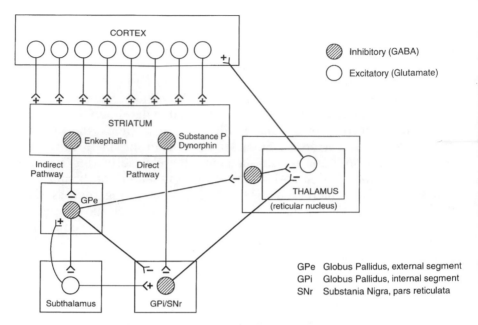

Figure 13.2   Schematic of normal CSTC connectivity. The striatum comprises the caudate nucleus and putamen. GPe is the external segment of the globus pallidus, GPi is the internal segment of the globus pallidus, and SNr is the substantia nigra pars reticulata. Adapted from Leckman, Peterson, et al., 1997.

projections are comparable to those of the ipsilateral projections. Contralateral projections to the putamen appear to be stronger than those to the caudate. These crossed projections from the cortex to the striatum appear to have important functional consequences: intracellular recordings have demonstrated that stimulation of ipsi- or contralateral frontal cortex can produce monosynaptic excitatory postsynaptic potentials in the same striatal cells (C. Wilson, 1986). Taken together, these data suggest that interhemispheric coordination is important for normal CSTC functioning (McGuire, Bates, & Goldman-Rakic, 1991), a hypothesis further supported by demonstrations that corpus callosum lesions disrupt the behavioral manifestations of unilateral basal ganglia and substantia nigra lesions in animals (Sullivan, Parker, & Szechtman, 1993).

EVIDENCE FOR CSTC INVOLVEMENT

Basal Ganglia

Basal Ganglia in Tourette's Syndrome

Single-cell recordings of normal basal ganglia neurons have shown that cell firing in the putamen is related to highly specific aspects of limb movement, including velocity and direction. Thus, motor portions of CSTC circuitry appear to be involved in the control of movement direction and in the scaling of movement force and speed. Because tics typically are parts of normal behavioral repertoires that are executed more frequently, rapidly, and forcefully than their normal behavioral counterparts, it is possible that focally disinhibited CSTC functioning could produce tic-like behaviors.

Other neurobiological studies of normal basal ganglia functioning implicate these structures in Tourette's syndrome. The application of stimulants directly to ventral basal ganglia nuclei, for instance, often produces tic-like stereotypies in animals (Kelley, Lang, & Gauthier, 1988). Similarly, chemical or electrical stimulation of inputs into the putamen in both primates and humans can produce motor and phonic sterotypies similar to the tics seen in persons who have Tourette's syndrome (Alexander & DeLong, 1985; Baldwin, Frost, & Wood, 1954; MacLean & Delgado, 1953). Conversely, chemical interference of the functioning of nigrostriatal afferents with neuroleptic agents is the mechanism whereby these medications are thought to attenuate tic symptoms. Dopamine-depleting agents, such as a-methyl-para-tyrosine and tetrabenazine, can suppress tic symptoms (Jankovic, Glaze, & Frost, 1984; Sweet, Bruun, Shapiro, & Shapiro, 1976), whereas L-dopa and stimulants, dopaminergic agonists, can with varying reliability exacerbate tic symptoms (Gadow, Sverd, et al., 1995; Golden, 1974; Lowe, Cohen, Detlor, Kremenitzer, & Shaywitz, 1982).

Other human studies support the importance of basal ganglia in Tourette's syndrome pathophysiology. One postmortem study reported that Tourette's syndrome basal ganglia were hypoplastic. Histological characterization of the hypoplasia revealed an increased number of small neurons and an increased neuron-packing density in the putamen and caudate nuclei, similar to the basal ganglia of young infants (Balthazar, 1956; Richardson, 1982). As discussed in Chapter 14, another postmortem study found markedly increased numbers of presynaptic dopamine-uptake sites in the caudate and putamen of four Tourette's syndrome adults (Singer et al., 1991). Levels of dopamine and its metabolites in these same subjects were not significantly different from control levels (G. Anderson et al., 1992a, 1992b; Singer et al., 1991). Postmortem studies in these four Tourette's syndrome subjects also demonstrated reduced glutamate levels in the projection areas of the STN (GPi, GPe, SNr; Anderson et al., 1992a, 1992b), as well as absent or markedly reduced dynorphin A (1–17) immunoreactivity in striatal projection neurons to dorsal GPe and ventral pallidum (Haber, Kowall, Vonsattel, Bird, & Richardson, 1986; Haber & Wolfer, 1992).

The first in vivo structural imaging study to examine basal ganglia morphology in Tourette's syndrome examined 14 unmedicated, neuroleptic-naïve, strongly right-handed patients and 14 matched normal control subjects. Based on the one detailed postmortem report of basal ganglia hypoplasia in Tourette's syndrome, the volume of the lenticular nucleus (i.e., the putamen and globus pallidus combined) was hypothesized to be smaller in the Tourette's group. This hypothesis was confirmed for the left- but not the right-sided structures: mean reduction in left lenticular nucleus volume was 10.7% compared to the controls ($p < 0.025$), and that on the right was 3.8% ($p =$ NS). Globus pallidus and putamen contributions to the lenticular nucleus volume reductions were proportionately similar (B. Peterson, Riddle, Cohen, Katz, Smith, Hardin, et al., 1993). The unilateral findings raised the possibility that lateralized neural systems might be uniquely affected in Tourette's syndrome, although this was a post hoc hypothesis.

Basal ganglia volumes are larger on the left in normal right-handed subjects (Castellanos et al., 1994; B. Peterson, Riddle, Cohen, Katz, Smith, & Leckman, 1993; Singer et al., 1993). The Tourette's syndrome subjects in this imaging study appeared to have a reduced asymmetry in the globus pallidus ($p < 0.005$), lenticular nucleus ($p = 0.03$), and total basal ganglia ($p < 0.05$). The magnitude of group differences was greatest in the globus pallidus, where asymmetries were either absent or reversed in direction in Tourette's syndrome subjects compared with controls (B. Peterson, Riddle, Cohen, Katz, Smith, Hardin, et al., 1993).

The initial findings of left-sided lenticular nucleus volume reductions and reduced basal ganglia asymmetry in Tourette's syndrome adults were largely replicated by an independent laboratory in a sample of Tourette's syndrome children (Singer et al., 1993). Studying a sample of 37 Tourette's syndrome children (29 boys, 8 girls, ages 7–16, mean age 11.5 years, mixed handedness) and 18 normal control children (14 boys, 4 girls, ages 6–15, mean age 9.8 years), analyses including only the boys of both groups revealed a trend toward reduced left putamen volumes ($p < 0.08$) that would have been significant if one-tailed significance tests had been used (this approach would have been justified given the prior findings of lenticular nucleus volume reduction). An absent or reversed (right larger than left) asymmetry of the lenticular nucleus was confirmed in the entire Tourette's syndrome group and in the male-only Tourette's syndrome subgroup.

Other investigators compared basal ganglia volumes between members of 10 monozygotic (MZ) twin pairs (ages 9–31, mean age 16.3 years) who were discordant for the severity of tic symptoms (Hyde et al., 1995). Because these twins were by definition genetically identical, any differences between co-twins in symptom severity and basal ganglia volumes must have been due to nongenetic factors. Although lenticular nucleus volumes and asymmetry coefficients did not differ significantly between co-twins, the more severely affected twins were found to have caudate nucleus volumes that were on average 6% smaller than the less severely affected co-twin ($p < 0.01$). A shortcoming of this study was the failure to characterize sufficiently the obsessive-compulsive disorder and ADHD status of the twin pairs. It may be that differences between co-twins in the presence or severity of these comorbid conditions were responsible for the differences either in tic symptom severity or in volumes of the caudate nucleus. This is particularly salient given the likely participation of the caudate nucleus in attentional processes and the reports of reduced caudate nucleus volumes in obsessive-compulsive disorder (Robinson et al., 1995). The Tourette's syndrome MZ twin findings, if confirmed, nevertheless suggest that right caudate nucleus volume reductions could be attributable to nonshared environmental determinants, and not to the effects of the Tourette's syndrome gene. An additional limitation of the study that is relevant to this interpretation, however, was the failure to examine a normal MZ comparison group to help ascertain whether *both* members of the Tourette's syndrome MZ twin pairs could have lenticular nucleus volume abnormalities, which if present would reflect both genetic and environmental contributions to the abnormal morphology.

Additional evidence for abnormalities in structural lateralization of basal ganglia was seen in particular measures of MRI signal change with time (termed relaxation times). When appropriate covariates were employed in group comparisons, abnormalities in relaxation time were seen in the putamen and caudate nuclei of the group of 14 Tourette's syndrome subjects whose basal ganglia volume reductions have already been described (Peterson, Gore, Riddle, Cohen, & Leckman, 1994). Although the physical determinants of these asymmetry abnormalities are presently unknown, they indicate that not only are basal ganglia volumes abnormal in Tourette's syndrome, but that actual tissue characteristics in those structures are abnormal as well.

In vivo PET and SPECT studies suggest that the basal ganglia volume reduction seen in structural studies is accompanied by decreased basal ganglia metabolism and blood flow. In both the structural and functional studies, basal ganglia abnormalities appear to be most prominent in the left cerebral hemisphere. One preliminary [^{18}F]-FDG PET study of 12 Tourette's syndrome adults reported a 15% decrement in nonnormalized glucose utilization in the inferior striatum, with a significant inverse correlation seen between tic symptom severity and striatal metabolism ($p < 0.01$; Chase, Geoffrey, Gillespie, & Burrows, 1986). A second FDG PET study of 16 medication-free Tourette's syndrome adults also found reduced metabolism in the ventral striatum (nucleus accumbens, ventromedial caudate, and left anterior putamen) compared with 16 normal control subjects; decreased metabolism was most prominent in the left hemisphere (Braun et al., 1993; Stoetter et al., 1992). A preliminary HMPAO SPECT study of 9 Tourette's syndrome and 9 individually matched control subjects also found a statistically significant 4% reduction in blood flow to the left putamen–globus pallidus complex (Riddle, Rasmusson, Woods, & Hoffer, 1992). However, a subsequent HMPAO SPECT blood flow study of 20 Tourette's syndrome subjects (mean age 28 ±12 years, 10 with comorbid obsessive-compulsive disorder) and 5 normal control subjects (mean age 34.7 ±12.5 years) failed to find differences in basal ganglia blood flow (George et al., 1992). In this latter study, the small number of control subjects and limitations in scanner resolution diminish the force of its negative findings. A larger HMPAO SPECT blood flow study of 50 Tourette's syndrome patients (ages 7–65 years) and 20 normal controls (mean age 23 years, range not listed), after correction for multiple comparisons, found reduced blood flow to the left basal ganglia (Moriarty et al., 1995). This study suffers from numerous serious methodological limitations, including poor subject matching (neither on age, sex, nor handedness), current neuroleptic use in nearly one-third of the patient group, and the use of two different SPECT scanners having resolutions that did not allow differentiation of basal ganglia subregions. Despite these limitations, the study's findings are consistent with findings of left-sided basal ganglia hypoperfusion in Tourette's syndrome.

Although the findings of predominantly left-sided blood flow and metabolism are reasonably consistent among studies, the pathophysiological significance of the findings is unclear. They could represent either a decreased activity per unit volume of striatal tissue, or they could represent only relative decreases that would not reach statistical significance if the metabolism and blood flow rates were normalized by the volumes of the structures being measured. These considerations emphasize the need for structural and functional measures in the same individuals.

Other preliminary functional studies of Tourette's syndrome have focused on quantifying dopaminergic transmitter systems in the striatum. An ^{18}F-dopa PET study of 10 Tourette's syndrome adults, for example, indicated normal functioning of presynaptic dopaminergic terminals, and a ^{11}C-raclopride PET study in another 5 Tourette's syndrome subjects suggested that D_2 receptor density was similar to control values (Turjanski et al., 1994). Similarly, D_2 and D_3 receptor availability, as assessed with the SPECT ligands ^{123}IBZM and ^{11}C-NMSP, have not been found to differ from control levels in Tourette's syndrome adults (George, Robertson, et al., 1994; Singer et al., 1992).

In contrast, a pilot study of striatal $[^{123}I]\beta$-CIT uptake, a measure of presynaptic dopamine transporter levels, in five medication-free Tourette's syndrome and five individually matched healthy control adults (two men, three women, ages 27 ±8 years) showed a nearly 50% mean elevation (range 6–79% increase) in striatal dopamine transporters in the Tourette's syndrome subjects (10.4 ±2.3 versus 7.7 ±1.4; mean ± SD ratio of specific to nonspecific uptake; Malison et al., 1995). This SPECT study is thus consistent with the postmortem findings of elevated transporter levels but normal dopamine metabolite levels in Tourette's syndrome basal ganglia (Anderson et al., 1992; Singer et al., 1991). In contrast to postmortem findings, however, where transporter abnormalities were more prominent in the putamen (Singer et al.), the in vivo SPECT results suggest relatively greater elevations of $[^{123}I]\beta$-CIT binding in caudate (30%) compared with putamen (17%). An IBZM SPECT study of MZ twins with Tourette's syndrome has recently demonstrated an increased dopamine receptor availability in the caudate nuclei of the more severely affected cotwins (Wolf et al., 1996).

The findings of increased striatal presynaptic dopamine transporter sites and increased postsynaptic dopamine receptor availability, if confirmed, would suggest a hyperinnervation of the striatum by dopaminergic neurons and a subsequent increase in striato-pallidal inhibitory activity, a decrease in pallido-thalamic inhibition, and therefore an overall disinhibition of thalamo-cortical activity, consistent with theories of hyperkinetic disorders. As discussed in Chapter 14, dopaminergic hyperinnervation of the striatum could also produce inhibition of the subthalamic nucleus and reduced glutamate levels in its projection areas (the GPe, GPi, and SNr), thereby further compounding an overall disinhibited excitation in thalamo-cortical projections (Figure 13.3).

More recently, the basal ganglia have been implicated in a functional MRI study of tic suppression in 22 adult Tourette's syndrome conducted at

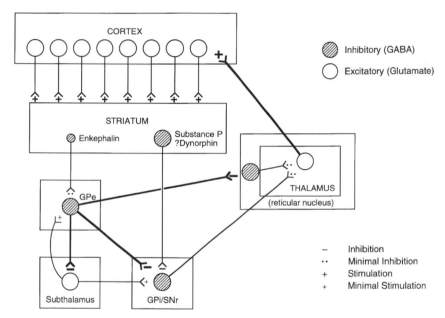

Figure 13.3 Hypothesized dysfunction of CSTC circuitry in Tourette's syndrome. The neurobiological and neuroimaging studies of Tourette's syndrome suggest that CSTC circuitry is dysfunctional in Tourette's syndrome. We propose that activity in the normal inhibitory (GABAergic) projections from striatum to GPe is reduced in Tourette's syndrome, either as an intrinsic, pathogenetic "lesion," or as a distal consequence of some more proximal cause. Reduced inhibition (or a net increased activity) of GPe inhibitory projection neurons to the subthalamic nucleus and GPi/SNr would in turn decrease activity in thalamo-cortical excitatory neurons. Decreased activity in the thalamo-cortical neurons then initiates movement, which in Tourette's syndrome manifests as a tic (figure adapted from Leckman, Peterson, et al., 1997). As discussed in Chapter 14, hyper-dopaminergic innervation of the striatum, seen in some imaging and neurobiological studies of Tourette's syndrome, would produce even greater impairment in the inhibition of GPe (see Figures 14.1a and 14.1b).

the Yale Child Study Center (Peterson, Skudlarski, et al., 1998). Significant changes in signal intensity in the basal ganglia were observed comparing periods of voluntary tic suppression to periods when the patients were instructed not to inhibit their tics. Remarkably, the magnitude of the regional signal change in most areas of the basal ganglia was found to be reduced during tic suppression and inversely related to the patient's current tic severity. This suggests that patients who are able to reduce the metabolic activity in the putamen and globus pallidus are more likely to experience fewer and less severe tic symptoms. Other notable findings from this study were that the signal intensity in the right caudate nucleus increased during periods of tic suppression, and the magnitude of this increase was positively associated with current tic severity ($r = 0.46$, $p < .02$). These observations combined with the increases in signal intensity seen in several frontal cortical regions suggests that the head of the caudate may be an important way station in efforts to voluntarily suppress unwanted tics.

Basal Ganglia in Obsessive-Compulsive Disorder

Numerous disorders of presumed basal ganglia origin, in addition to Tourette's syndrome, have been associated with an increased frequency of comorbid obsessive-compulsive disorder. Postencephalitic Parkinson's disease is characterized by an array of abnormal movements and vocalizations, as well as compulsive actions (Von Economo, 1931). Sydenham's chorea, a sequela of streptococcal-induced rheumatic fever that is associated with specific antibodies directed against caudate and putamen neurons (Husby et al., 1976), degeneration of striatal neurons, and perivascular infiltrates (Greenfield & Wolfsohn, 1922), is also associated with elevated rates of obsessive-compulsive disorder. Various basal ganglia ischemic lesions have been associated with complex stereotypies and obsessive-compulsive disorder symptoms (Bhatia & Marsden, 1994; Laplane et al., 1989). In addition, ablative lesions of the ventromedial caudate nucleus are known to produce perseverative interference in behavioral set (Butters & Rosvold, 1968; Divac, Rosvold, & Szwarcbart, 1967). Finally, serotonergic agents have proven remarkably successful in treating the symptoms of obsessive-compulsive disorder. A possible substrate upon which these agents may act to produce their therapeutic effects is the ventromedial striatum, an area that includes the head of the caudate nucleus and accumbens; the ventral striatum has strong serotonergic innervation directly from the raphe nucleus, and it receives many projections from orbitofrontal and anterior cingulate cortices (Parent, 1990), regions that also have heavy serotonergic inputs.

Neuroimaging studies also support the hypothesis that basal ganglia portions of CSTC circuitry are important in the pathophysiology of obsessive-compulsive disorder. Reduced caudate nucleus volumes were first reported in a computerized tomography study of 10 adult obsessive-compulsive disorder men (Luxenberg et al., 1988). Two poorly controlled, low-resolution MRI studies, however, failed to confirm caudate nucleus volume reduction (Kellner et al., 1991; Scarone et al., 1992). Another study of 24 adult-onset obsessive-compulsive disorder and 21 normal controls that was better controlled, but that had equally low resolution and that did not permit resampling of the data in orthogonal imaging planes, also showed no group differences (Aylward et al., 1996). A methodologically more rigorous MRI study of 26 adult obsessive-compulsive disorder subjects and 26 controls reported a significant 11% bilateral volume reduction in the caudate nuclei of the obsessive-compulsive disorder subjects (Robinson et al., 1995).

Two FDG PET studies of obsessive-compulsive disorder adults reported caudate nucleus hypermetabolism at rest (Baxter, Phelps, Mazziotta, Guze, & Schwartz, 1987; Baxter et al., 1988). A subsequent ^{15}O CO_2 PET study demonstrated increased blood flow to the right caudate nucleus in eight obsessive-compulsive disorder subjects during symptom provocation (Rauch et al., 1994). An fMRI study of 10 adult obsessive-compulsive disorder patients and 5 normal controls using a similar symptom provocation paradigm yielded similar findings of right caudate nucleus activation, as well as bilateral lenticular nucleus activation (Breiter et al., 1996). Caudate nucleus hypermetabolism appears to normalize in response to successful antiobsessional treatment (Baxter et al., 1992; Schwartz, Stoessel, Baxter, Martin, & Phelps, 1996).

Basal Ganglia in ADHD

Abnormalities in striatal functioning, and in the functioning of related association cortex circuitry, have been hypothesized to contribute to ADHD pathophysiology. Preclinical and clinical evidence supporting this theory includes reports of hemispatial neglect in ADHD subjects and in animals with nigrostriatal lesions (Damasio, Damasio, & Chui, 1980; Heilman, Voeller, & Nadeau, 1991; Kertesz, Ferro, & Black, 1986). Striatal and thalamic relays are also important for the performance of saccades made during shifts in visual attention, and ADHD children consistently show deficits both in saccade pursuit and in maintaining steady fixation on a target. In addition, stimulant medications, the most effective known treatment for ADHD symptoms, increase dopaminergic transmission in the striatum and in frontal cortices.

In vivo imaging data also support the hypothesized involvement of striatum in ADHD pathophysiology. A recent MRI study of 50 ADHD and 48 normal children demonstrated an absence of normal right-greater-than-left caudate nucleus asymmetry in the ADHD subjects that appeared to be due to smaller right-sided structures (Castellanos et al., 1994, 1996). In addition, a ^{18}Xe PET study of 13 children with ADHD, the majority of whom had significant comorbid neurologic deficits, reported significantly reduced metabolic rates in the striatum (Lou et al., 1989). An MRI study of Tourette's syndrome children demonstrated abnormalities in globus pallidus asymmetry that were even more accentuated in those children who had comorbid ADHD, suggesting that this important comorbidity is associated with CSTC structural abnormalities that are greater than those found in Tourette's syndrome alone (Singer et al., 1993). This suggestion of globus pallidus involvement in ADHD pathophysiology has been supported by a more recent study of 57 ADHD and 55 normal control boys, 5–18 years of age, in which a significantly ($p < 0.006$) smaller right globus pallidus nucleus was seen (Castellanos et al., 1996).

Thalamus

Thalamus in Tourette's Syndrome

Evidence for thalamic involvement in Tourette's syndrome derives primarily from the effects of either space-occupying or neurosurgically induced thalamic lesions (Leckman, deLotbiniere, et al., 1993; B. Peterson, Bronen, & Duncan, 1996). Surgical lesions to ventral, medial, and intralaminar thalamic nuclei appear to attenuate tic symptoms in some patients (I. Cooper, 1969; de Divitiis, D'Errico, & Cerillo, 1977; Hassler & Dieckmann, 1970; Korzen, Pushkov, Kharitonov, & Shustin, 1991; Rauch, Baer, Cosgrove, & Jenike, 1995). Irritative space-occupying lesions in ventral thalamic nuclei, on the other hand, may exacerbate symptoms (B. Peterson et al., 1996). In addition, intraoperative microelectrode stimulation of the ventral intermediate and other ventral thalamic nuclei has produced sensations of the urge to move, or feelings of tightness, pulling, or compression in contralateral body regions that are similar to the premonitory urges associated with tics (Tasker & Dostrovsky, 1993).

The thalamus has been implicated in a recent functional MRI study of tic suppression (Peterson, Skudlarski, et al., 1998). Significant changes in signal intensity in the thalamus were observed comparing periods of voluntary tic suppression with periods when the patients were instructed not to inhibit their tics. The magnitude of the regional signal change in the thalamus was found to be reduced during tic suppression and inversely related to the patient's current tic severity. This suggests that patients who are able to reduce the metabolic activity in the thalamus are more likely to experience fewer and less severe tic symptoms, a finding consistent with our general supposition that tics occur, in part, as the net result of a disinhibition of thalamocortical projections.

Thalamus in Obsessive-Compulsive Disorder

The thalamus has not been extensively implicated in the pathophysiology of obsessive-compulsive disorder. Increased resting right hemithalamus metabolism has been reported in adults with childhood-onset obsessive-compulsive disorder (Swedo, Schapiro, et al., 1989). Trends toward increased left hemithalamus activity in response to symptom provocation have been seen (Rauch et al., 1994), and left hemithalamus metabolic activity has been shown to decrease in response either to successful medication therapy or behavioral therapy (Baxter et al., 1992; Schwartz, Stoessel, Baxter, Martin, & Phelps, 1996). However, several structural imaging studies, albeit with suboptimal measures of this vaguely defined structure, have reported normal thalamic volumes (Jenike et al., 1996).

Thalamus in ADHD

The thalamus repeatedly has been implicated as important in normal attentional processing. Numerous PET studies have shown thalamic activation during attentionally demanding tasks (George, Ketter, et al., 1994; Kinomura, Larsson, Gulyas, & Roland, 1996; B. Peterson et al., 1996). The only human imaging studies implicating the thalamus in ADHD is an FDG PET study of 10 medication-free ADHD and 10 normal control adolescents that reported a 12% reduction in left hemithalamus metabolism in the ADHD sample.

Premotor and Supplementary Motor Cortices

SMA in Tourette's Syndrome

Electrical stimulation of the SMA produces complex movements, vocalizations, and speech arrest, in addition to sensations that in some patients are described as an urge to move the somatotopically stimulated contralateral body region (Fried et al., 1991; Lim et al., 1994). These urges to move are reminiscent of the premonitory urges that Tourette's syndrome adolescents and adults describe prior to the performance of their tics (Leckman, Walker, et al., 1993). Increased metabolism was seen in the premotor and SMA cortices and in primary sensorimotor regions in one FDG PET study (Braun et al., 1993).

SMA in Obsessive-Compulsive Disorder

Cortical premotor and supplementary cortices have not been the focus of extensive study in obsessive-compulsive disorder. One FDG PET study reported increased right lateral prefrontal metabolism (Baxter, Schwartz, Guze, Bergman, & Szuba, 1990), and another found bilaterally increased prefrontal and increased left premotor metabolism (Swedo, Schapiro, et al., 1989). Blood flow studies have suggested increased blood flow to left posterior frontal regions (probably lower SMA and premotor regions; R. Rubin, Villanueva-Meyer, Ananth, Trajmar, & Mena, 1992) that normalized in response to successful antiobsessional therapy (R. Rubin, Ananth, Villanueva-Meyer, Trajmar, & Mena, 1995).

SMA in ADHD

Reduced metabolic rates have been reported in the left sensorimotor area in ADHD children (Lou et al., 1989) and in the premotor and somatosensory cortices of ADHD adults (Zametkin et al., 1990). An FDG PET study of 10 adolescents with ADHD and nonaffected controls found reduced metabolic rates in, among other regions, the left anterior frontal area that correlated negatively with numerous symptom severity measures (Zametkin et al.,

1993). These findings support the hypothesis that portions of CSTC circuitry, particularly association cortex and possibly its premotor connections, are involved in ADHD pathophysiology. Reduced activity in the left frontal regions, and possibly in related sensorimotor systems, may reflect underactivity in cortical systems subserving attentional mechanisms and motor hyperactivity. This hypothesis is supported by numerous studies demonstrating reductions in the size of regions of the corpus callosum—the genu and the isthmus (Hynd et al., 1991), the rostrum and rostral body (Giedd et al., 1994), and the splenium (Semrud-Clikeman et al., 1994)—that contain interhemispheric axons connecting association, SMA, and parietal cortices, regions thought to mediate symptoms of motor hyperactivity and inattention.

Orbitofrontal Cortex

The orbitofrontal (OFC) cortex is intimately connected with the anterior cingulum (ACA) and other limbic structures. OFC may subserve the capacity to perform successive discrimination, Go/No-Go, and response-reversal tasks (Diamond & Goldman-Rakic, 1989; Drewe, 1975; Rosvold & Mishkin, 1961). Lesions of this region result in perseverative interference with an animal's capacity to make appropriate changes in behavioral set (Divac et al., 1967; Iverson & Mishkin, 1970; Mishkin & Manning, 1978) and produces affective dysregulation and impulsive, socially inappropriate behaviors (Luria, 1980). OFC lesions are thought to interfere with the ability to generate internal cues that guide goal-directed behaviors (Goldman-Rakic, 1987). Neurosurgical lesions of the OFC or ACA can produce marked improvement in treatment-resistant obsessive-compulsive disorder (Baer et al., 1995), suggesting that such lesions may disrupt an overly active (disinhibited) orbitofrontal-striatal circuit. Obsessive-compulsive symptoms frequently have sexual or aggressive content, which may derive from functional contributions to this circuitry from closely associated limbic and paralimbic regions, such as the amygdala and hypothalamus.

The hypothalamus is the site of production of the neurotransmitter hormone oxytocin and, consistent with the hypothesized contribution of paralimbic regions to obsessive-compulsive disorder pathophysiology, elevated oxytocin levels appear to be elevated in obsessive-compulsive disorder subjects whose illness is not tic-related (Leckman, Goodman, et al., 1994a). The content of most obsessions and compulsions—checking for threat and harm, concern for cleanliness and grooming, avoidance of germs and contagion, sex, and aggression—like tics, are part of normal cognitive and behavioral repertoires. In moderation, these concerns and behaviors are generally adaptive. Dysregulation of inhibitory neural mechanisms for the orbitofrontal-limbic circuitry, however, could produce the impulsive, compulsive, and perseverative cognitive and behavioral patterns seen in Tourette's syndrome, obsessive-compulsive disorder, and ADHD.

OFC in Tourette's Syndrome

One Tourette's syndrome FDG PET study reported a significant decrement in metabolism of the medial and lateral OFC (Braun et al., 1993). Deficient frontal inhibition to basal ganglia portions of CSTC circuitry may contribute either to the generation of tic symptoms or to their impaired suppression.

OFC in Obsessive-Compulsive Disorder

Only one structural study thus far has measured prefrontal cortex volumes, with no differences seen between obsessive-compulsive disorder subjects and controls (Robinson et al., 1995). The prefrontal volume measurement, however, consisted of the entire frontal cortex anterior to the genu of the corpus callosum, and so did not assess specifically OFC volumes. Functional imaging studies have much more consistently implicated the OFC in obsessive-compulsive disorder pathophysiology. Obsessive-compulsive disorder symptom severity, for instance, has been reported to correlate with prefrontal and OFC metabolism (Swedo, Pietrini, et al., 1992; Swedo, Schapiro, et al., 1989). In addition, several investigators have found that regional hypermetabolism and elevated blood flow not only normalize in response to successful antiobsessional therapies, but the improvement in symptoms correlates with the decrement in metabolic activity (Benkelfat et al., 1990; R. Rubin et al., 1995; Swedo, Pietrini, et al., 1992). One group of investigators, however, has failed to replicate this correlation between change in symptom severity and change in OFC metabolism (Baxter et al., 1992; Schwartz et al., 1996). A SPECT blood flow study found increased rCBF to the medial-frontal cortex of 10 obsessive-compulsive disorder patients compared with controls (Machlin et al., 1991) that attenuated during fluoxetine treatment (Hoehn-Saric, Pearlson, Harris, Machlin, & Camargo, 1991). Symptom provocation, moreover, appears to increase blood flow in the OFC bilaterally (Breiter et al., 1996; Rauch et al., 1994).

These imaging studies provide compelling evidence for the involvement of the OFC portion of CSTC circuitry in the pathophysiology of obsessive-compulsive disorder. Several methodologic limitations interfere with interpretation of the findings, however: (a) small numbers of subjects, especially in the functional studies; (b) the total absence of studies of children, which would elucidate early developmental aspects of the disorder; and (c) the difficulty in ascribing directions of causality to the association between overactivity of OFC circuitry and increasing obsessive-compulsive symptoms. The OFC hypermetabolism, for instance, could represent OFC activity directed at inhibiting compulsive urges or suppressing obsessive thoughts. In neuropsychological terms, OFC activation may represent the generation of the internal cues necessary for goal-directed behavior (Goldman-Rakic, 1987), which in this instance is the inhibition of compulsive behaviors (Insel, 1992b). As treatment attenuates symptoms, the effort required to suppress symptoms would decrease, which could account for the normalized frontal metabolism seen during successful antiobsessional therapies.

OFC in ADHD

Children with ADHD typically perform poorly on tests of frontal lobe functioning, such as continuous performance tasks and Go/No-Go, Stroop Word Color Interference, and Wisconsin Card Sort tests (Barkley et al., 1992). Moreover, frontal lobe lesions in humans and animals that involve association, OF, and ACA cortices often produce the ADHD-like symptoms of inattentiveness, distractibility, and impairment in response inhibition.

LIMBIC SYSTEM CIRCUITRY

The limbic system consists of the amygdala and hippocampus in the temporal lobe; the cingulum, the caudate nucleus, and other basal ganglia structures in the subcortex; the hypothalamus and periaqueductal gray matter in the brainstem; and connections with the associated frontal cortex (Figures 13.4a and 13.4b). The functions of the limbic system are classically regarded as regulating (a) physiological homeostasis, particularly through neuroendocrine modulation; (b) feeding and foraging behaviors; (c) defense and attack; and (d) sexual and reproductive behaviors. This list underscores the interconnectedness of the limbic system with many of the regions that have been implicated in Tourette's syndrome-related conditions. The components of the limbic system have also been postulated to constitute a disinhibited, reverberating neural circuit that gives rise to obsessive-compulsive disorder symptoms (Insel, 1992b) and other repetitive behaviors.

Temporal Lobe

Remarkably few neurobiological investigations of temporal lobe regions have been undertaken in Tourette's syndrome–related illnesses, despite the hypothesized involvement of these regions in Tourette's syndrome pathophysiology by several investigators (Jadresic, 1992; B. Peterson et al., 1992). The sexual and aggressive content of many complex motor and vocal tics, and many obsessions and compulsions, is probably the most compelling aspect of the clinical phenotype that suggests involvement of the amygdala and related circuitry. The human amygdala and related portions of the limbic circuitry are densely populated by steroid hormone receptors that may mediate the sex-specific differences in prevalence of tic symptoms in the general population, as well as the sexual and aggressive content of tics within specific individuals. Indirect evidence in support of this hypothesis is provided by reports that antiandrogens can improve, though perhaps only transiently, the symptoms of Tourette's syndrome and obsessive-compulsive disorder (Casas et al., 1986; B. Peterson, Leckman, Scahill, et al., 1994; B. Peterson, Zhang, et al., in press; Sandyk, 1988; Swedo & Rapoport, 1990).

In preclinical studies, unilateral electrical or chemical stimulation of the amygdala has been reported to produce tic-like stereotypies and vocalizations in animals and humans (Baldwin et al., 1954; MacLean &

(a)

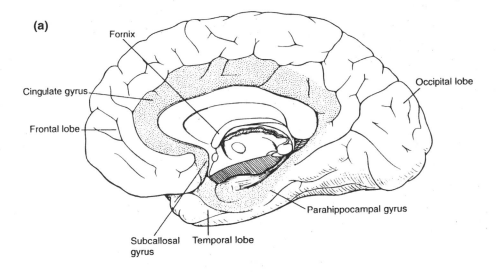

(b)

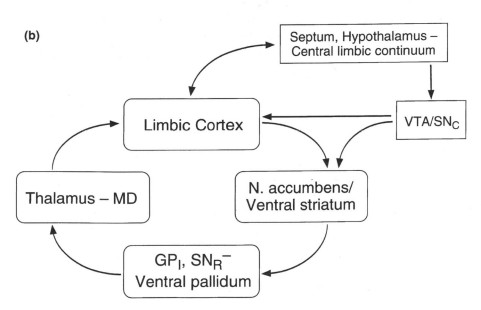

Figures 13.4a and 13.4b   Limbic system components. (a) The limbic system is a collection of broadly distributed anatomical regions that include the cingulate gyrus, the amygdala, hippocampus, and parahippocampus in the temporal lobe (pictured here); the associated portions of frontal cortex; and brainstem regions that include the hypothalamus, periaqueductal gray matter, the fornix, and mamillary bodies (not shown here). Represented in this figure is the midsagittal view of the brain, with the cingulate gyrus, frontal lobe, and temporal lobe portions of the system. (b) Some of the circuitry of the limbic system is depicted in this schematic diagram.

Delgado, 1953). One human neuroimaging study of T_2 relaxation times found evidence of abnormal tissue characteristics in the left ($p < 0.05$) and right ($p < 0.002$) amygdala of 14 Tourette's syndrome adults compared with an equal number of normal controls (B. Peterson, Gore, et al., 1994). Volumetric measures of temporal lobe regions have not yet been reported in Tourette's syndrome. Only one functional imaging study thus far has looked closely at temporal lobe activity. In 16 adult medication-free Tourette's syndrome subjects and an equal number of normal controls, decreased regional metabolism was seen in the parahippocampal (entorhinal) cortex bilaterally and the left inferior insular region ($p < 0.0005$), as well as in the left anterior superior temporal cortex ($p < 0.01$; Braun et al., 1993).

Cingulate Cortex

Cingulate in Tourette's Syndrome

The cingulate has been portrayed as a component of the neurobiological substrate of Tourette's syndrome (Bonnet, 1982; Devinsky, Morrell, & Vogt, 1995). Anterior cingulate regions receive input from thalamus, amygdala, and motor cortex, and send projections primarily to motor cortex, striatum, periaqueductal gray, and brainstem motor nuclei (Bates & Goldman-Rakic, 1993; Vogt, Finch, & Olson, 1992). Electrical stimulation of the anterior cingulate in humans can produce semi-involuntary movements that resemble complex motor tics (Talairach et al., 1973). Anterior cingulotomies have been reported, in uncontrolled studies, to alleviate tic symptoms in some patients (Kurlan, Kersun, Ballantine, & Caine, 1990; Robertson, Doran, Trimble, & Lees, 1990). An [18F]-FDG PET study of 12 Tourette's syndrome adults demonstrated a 15% decrement in cingulate metabolism (Chase et al., 1986), although cingulate metabolism appeared normal in a technically superior FDG PET study of 16 Tourette's syndrome adults (Braun et al., 1993). Finally, preliminary data suggest the presence of changes in opioid receptor binding in the cingulate cortices of Tourette's patients (Weeks, Turjanski, & Brooks, 1996).

The right cingulate cortex has been implicated in a recent functional MRI study of tic suppression (Peterson, Skudlarski, et al., 1998). Significant changes in signal intensity in the right cingulate were observed comparing periods of voluntary tic suppression with periods when the patients were instructed not to inhibit their tics. The magnitude of the regional signal change in the right singulate was found to be increased during periods of voluntary suppression. Taken with the finding of similar increases in signal intensity in the right caudate, this suggests that patients who are able to increase the metabolic activity of regions of the cingulate cortex and related areas of the striatum are more effective in suppressing tics.

Cingulate in Obsessive-Compulsive Disorder

Ablation of the cingulate cortex in rats interferes with, among other behaviors, nest building and maternal care, both of which have been postulated to relate to phylogenetically conserved cognitive, affiliative, and sexual behaviors that in the extreme present as obsessive-compulsive disorder symptoms (Leckman, Goodman, et al., 1994a). Numerous studies have found increased metabolism or blood flow to anterior cingulate regions in adults with obsessive-compulsive disorder (Breiter et al., 1996; Rauch et al., 1994; Swedo, Schapiro, et al., 1989). Decreases in the severity of obsessive-compulsive disorder symptoms correlated with decrements in right anterior cingulate metabolic activity during successful medication therapy (Baxter et al., 1992). Surgical lesions to the cingulate or regions related to it have been reported to reduce symptoms in the treatment of refractory obsessive-compulsive disorder (Baer et al., 1995).

Cingulate in ADHD

Experimental evidence supports the hypothesis that the anterior cingulate subserves executive functioning, or the controlling and organizing of visceromotor, endocrine, and skeletomotor behaviors (Vogt et al., 1992). Lesions confined to the anterior cingulate can produce indifference, inattention, and disinhibition (Angelini, Mazzucchi, Picciotto, Nardocci, & Broggi, 1980). The anterior cingulate has been identified in several human imaging studies, sometimes in a highly localized fashion (Gevins, Smith, Leong, McEvoy, Whitfield, Du, & Rush, 1998), as being important in attentional processes (George, Ketter, et al., 1994; Pardo, Pardo, Janer, & Raichle, 1990).

Hypothalamus

The cingulate gyrus and hypothalamus are integrally interconnected, and both have been implicated in obsessive-compulsive disorder and compulsive behaviors. The hypothalamus, for instance, is the site of oxytocin production, and oxytocin levels have been shown to be elevated in obsessive-compulsive disorder that is not genetically related to Tourette's syndrome (Leckman, Goodman, et al., 1994a). Oxytocin is one of the mediators of numerous behaviors that are subserved by hypothalamic functioning and that could be considered phylogenetically conserved precursors to the content of common obsessions and compulsions. Oxytocin mediates behavioral aspects of grooming, maternal care and affiliation, and sexual and aggressive behaviors, all of which are components of common obsessive-compulsive symptoms (Leckman, Goodman, et al., 1994b).

Periaqueductal Gray

The periaqueductal gray (PAG) matter is a vaguely defined cell mass that is continuous rostrally with the ventromedial and lateral hypothalamus and caudally with the dorsal raphe nucleus. Stimulation of the PAG can produce a wide array of behavioral responses, including sexual behaviors, vocalization of emotion, aggressive and defensive posturing, and activation of the sympathetic nervous system (Nieuwenhuys & Voogd, 1988), similar to many of the tic-related behaviors seen in Tourette's syndrome. Disturbances in the PAG have been hypothesized to produce motor and vocal tics associated with encephalitis lethargica (Devinsky, 1983). In addition, noradrenergic fibers ascend from the locus ceruleus to pass through the PAG, and lesions in this midbrain region could worsen tic symptoms by disrupting the function of these fibers of passage, in addition to disturbing the function of PAG and midbrain cell bodies (Nieuwenhuys, 1985). This was the mechanism postulated to produce symptom exacerbation in an adult male Tourette's syndrome patient whose PAG was calcified in association with a pineal tumor (Lakke & Wilmink, 1985).

OTHER CORTICAL REGIONS

Given the apparent abnormalities in structural lateralization of basal ganglia portions of CSTC circuitry in disorders related to Tourette's syndrome, it is possible that aberrancies might also be seen in other structurally lateralized neural systems in Tourette's syndrome. The brain structure that participates most directly in both the segregation and integration of lateralized neural systems is the corpus callosum (CC), the massive cerebral commissure through which funnels the majority of interhemispheric axons. Measurement of CC size consequently has the potential to be a sensitive index of abnormalities in interhemispheric cortical lateralization and connectivity.

The first report to carefully examine CC size in Tourette's syndrome studied the same 14 Tourette's syndrome and 14 normal control subjects as those included in the first report of Tourette's syndrome basal ganglia volume abnormalities. Thus, the studies cannot be considered an independent investigation of structural lateralization in Tourette's syndrome, because the determinants of lateralization, whatever they may be, might have affected both basal ganglia and CC morphology in this particular subject sample. With this caveat in mind, an overall decrease in CC cross-sectional area of 18% in the Tourette's syndrome group ($p < 0.006$) supported the hypothesis of abnormal brain lateralization and interhemispheric connectivity in Tourette's syndrome (B. Peterson, Leckman, Duncan, et al., 1994). Subregional areas were all reduced to a similar degree. A technical limitation of the study was the use of imaging data that could not be resampled (resliced) to a more accurate sagittal midline, making the data dependent on correct head positioning of the subjects. Any inaccuracies in head positioning would increase measurement variance and render the data vulnerable to spuriously and erroneously suggest the existence of group differences (Type I error).

The second study to examine CC morphology in Tourette's syndrome compared 16 Tourette's syndrome children with 21 children who had both Tourette's syndrome and ADHD, 13 children with ADHD alone, and 21 control children (Baumgardner et al., 1996). Their ages ranged from 6 to 16, and they were predominantly boys. In contrast to the study of

Tourette's syndrome adults, this investigation reported larger CCs in Tourette's syndrome children, with relative CC size reductions evident in children who had ADHD, whether or not they had Tourette's syndrome. Thus, pure Tourette's syndrome children had the largest CCs, Tourette's syndrome plus ADHD children had CC sizes intermediate between pure Tourette's syndrome and normal controls, and ADHD children had the smallest CCs. After covarying appropriately for age and intracranial volume, size increases that otherwise appeared to be generalized throughout the CC were significant only in the rostral body of the CC, approximately 17% larger than controls in that region. The authors interpret this finding as evidence for the involvement of premotor and supplementary motor regions (which send interhemispheric axons through the rostral body of the CC) in the pathophysiology of Tourette's syndrome. The same technical limitations apply to this study of children as those noted in the adult study, and Type I error may account for the two studies' contrary findings. In addition, obsessive-compulsive disorder comorbidity was not taken into account in this study of children, and this may have confounded CC size analyses. Finally, the differences in the findings of the two studies may reflect real differences in CC morphology in Tourette's syndrome children compared with those in adults. We hypothesize that smaller CCs in symptomatic adults may explain in part symptom persistence in these subjects, whereas in most Tourette's syndrome subjects, symptoms subside by adulthood. The Tourette's syndrome adults of the first study had larger ventricles than the adult controls, which may reflect loss of white matter surrounding the ventricles. Decreased white matter volume would likely reduce CC size as well. Adult white matter loss (and smaller CC area in Tourette's syndrome) may therefore reflect the presence of some process or morphological marker that is associated with symptom persistence.

OTHER BRAINSTEM REGIONS

The brainstem has been implicated already as a possible component of the substrate of Tourette's syndrome-related disorders. The hypothalamus and periaqueductal gray as components of limbic system circuitry, and the substantia nigra pars reticulata as a component of CSTC circuitry, in general are likely candidates for the substrate of Tourette's syndrome. Other candidates include the numerous brainstem centers that produce catacholamine and indoleamine neurotransmitters (which probably play important neuromodulatory roles in the disorder), motor nuclei of the cranial nerves, and the more recently described brainstem pathways of simple motor learning.

Neuromodulators

Catecholamine and indoleamine systems that project to the basal ganglia are thought to exert a modulatory effect on tic symptoms. Dopaminergic afferent systems that ascend to the basal ganglia from the midbrain substantia nigra are believed to modulate tic symptoms. Noradrenergic systems from the locus ceruleus are also thought to exert indirect effects on basal ganglia function through modulatory effects on midbrain dopamine systems and on frontal inhibitory centers that may help to suppress tic-related behaviors. Noradrenergic systems also may mediate the exquisite stress responsivity seen in the disorder (Chappell, Riddle, et al., 1994). In addition to these neurotransmitter systems, limbic regions are also hypothesized to be important in modulating tic symptoms, particularly symptoms that are of predominantly sexual or aggressive content. Limbic regions exert these effects presumably through direct afferent projections to the ventral striatum, and indirectly through projections to midbrain dopaminergic neurons (Jadresic, 1992; B. Peterson et al., 1992).

Brainstem Motor Nuclei

Abnormalities in the regulation of motor discharge of brainstem motor nuclei, perhaps through dysfunction of descending cortical or subcortical afferents, could produce motor and vocal tics having the characteristic somatotopy of Tourette's syndrome. The brainstem motor nuclei innervating muscles of the face (motor nucleus of cranial nerve VII in the midpons), neck and shoulders (spinal accessory cranial nerve XI in the medulla), larynx and pharynx (nucleus ambiguus, a portion of the vagus cranial nerve X in the medulla), tongue (hypoglossal nucleus of cranial nerve XII in the medulla), and diaphragm (descending brainstem control of high cervical spinal cord) are all situated close to one another, and this musculature is most commonly affected by tics. In contrast, the musculature of the extremities is much less commonly affected by tics. Their neural control is from descending corticospinal motor neurons of the pyramidal tract, whose cell bodies reside in motor cortex rather than in the brainstem. Perhaps dysregulation of these motor nuclei produces tic symptoms, a hypothesis supported in part by the finding of increased R2 amplitude of the blink reflex in 26 adult Tourette's syndrome subjects compared with 10 normal controls. This finding has been interpreted as indicating the presence of increased excitability of regulatory interneurons in the Tourette's syndrome brainstem (Smith & Lees, 1989). The activity of these brainstem interneurons and motor nuclei is in turn regulated by descending projections from motor cortex and basal ganglia nuclei.

In addition to dysregulation of brainstem motor nuclei, disruption of the brainstem sensory pathways for this musculature could also contribute to tic symptoms. The mesencephalic nucleus of the fifth cranial nerve in the pons, for instance, relays unconscious proprioceptive information from the face. Disturbing this relay could affect the reflex reactivity of facial muscle spindles, thereby possibly producing the clonus-like activity of muscle groups affected by tics. The basal ganglia and descending dopaminergic systems from the midbrain are also known to influence the activity of these brainstem motor nuclei (Larumbe, Vaamonde, Artieda, Zubieta, & Obeso, 1993; Lawrence & Redmond, 1985).

Brainstem Pathways of Reflexive Motor Learning

Additional motor pathways that could subserve some aspect of the tic symptomatology are those involved in learning the semireflexive or semiautomatic behaviors that are similar in appearance to stereotypies and tics. The paradigm developed to study these kinds of behaviors has been classical eyeblink conditioning. This elementary learning involves circuitry of the cerebellar cortex, the deep cerebellar interpositus nucleus, the pontine and red nuclei in the brainstem, and then the lower motor neurons of effector brainstem motor nuclei (B. Anderson & Steinmetz, 1994; Gruart & Delgado-Garcia, 1994; Raymond, Lisberger, & Mauk, 1996).

Clinical anecdote suggests that learning or habit may be involved in the development or maintenance of specific tic behaviors. Often, for instance, Tourette's syndrome patients who speak of specific tics that they had in the past but that are no longer present will then immediately develop those tics again. It is as if recalling the tics somehow reactivated previously overlearned motor programs. Parents often report that their child's vocal tic symptoms began with sniffing or throat clearing due to an obvious cold, and then continued long after other cold symptoms abated. Moreover, many motor tics, such as eyeblinking, forehead wrinkling, neck turning, and shoulder shrugging, are components of normal behavioral repertoire and are only distinguished from that repertoire by the intensity and frequency of the movements. Often these normal behaviors serve to relieve muscular tension, particularly after prolonged periods of inactivity. These subtle tic-like movements abound in people sitting in meetings and lectures, for instance, and can be seen readily by an observing eye. Perhaps these motor acts are overlearned in Tourette's syndrome subjects, either due to heightened stress reactivity and awareness of muscular tension (producing the premonitory urge of Tourette's syndrome), or to an intrinsic abnormality in the neural basis of learning these normal, stereotyped fragments of motor behavior. If the pathways involved in learning these normal motor subroutines are similar to those involved in learning other rapid, semispontaneous or involuntary behaviors such as reflexive eyeblink conditioning, then cerebellar and related brainstem subregions warrant investigation as part of that circuitry.

The recent interest in cerebellar-related circuitry as a portion of the substrate for attentional and other higher cognitive processes (Courchesne et al., 1993; Gao et al., 1996; Petersen et al., 1996) could be relevant to understanding ADHD comorbidity in Tourette's syndrome, if the cerebellum were to prove important in Tourette's syndrome pathophysiology. Although the cerebellum and lower brainstem centers have not been implicated in the pathophysiology of obsessive-compulsive disorder, many of the phylogenetically primitive, stereotyped compulsions of obsessive-compulsive disorder—such as grooming, cleaning, checking, and sexual behaviors—could be considered overlearned behaviors that are the product of the disordered functioning of broadly distributed learning pathways that probably include cortical, subcortical, limbic, and brainstem regions. Similar habit learning systems, in fact, have been postulated in the neostriatum as well (Knowlton, Mangels, & Squire, 1996).

CONCLUSIONS

Despite the formidable obstacles that clinical investigation presents for a deep understanding of the substrate that produces and modulates the symptoms of complex neuropsychiatric disorders, a remarkable confluence of mostly circumstantial data has yielded a theory of the neural circuitry in Tourette's syndrome that has surprising explanatory power and detail. The model is one in which CSTC circuitry plays a prominent though not exclusive role in subserving and modulating the symptoms not just of Tourette's syndrome, but of obsessive-compulsive disorder and ADHD as well. Cortical, subcortical, and brainstem regions are all likely important in Tourette's syndrome-related pathophysiology. This model is integrated parsimoniously with current theories of genetic and environmental determinants of these disorders. The neurobiological substrate is in part unique to and in part shared among each of these disorders, explaining in large measure how a given genetic vulnerability to Tourette's syndrome can manifest as one or more of these symptom complexes. It also explains how a child with more than one of these disorders (e.g., Tourette's syndrome and ADHD) is more likely to require clinical attention because of the multiple sources of disturbance to regions of shared neural substrate.

Future advances in the delineation of the relevance of this circuitry to the pathophysiologies of Tourette's syndrome-related disorders will no doubt come from identification of the Tourette's syndrome vulnerability genes and examination of the regional expression of those genes in transfected laboratory animals. Postmortem and in vivo neuroimaging studies can then focus more precisely on the structural, functional, neurochemical, and neurotransmitter characteristics of those regions, perhaps aiding in predicting longitudinal course, suggesting new pharmacological interventions, and following or predicting medication responsiveness. This, however, will provide only a part of the story.

Broadly ranging advances in the understanding of genetically programmed and environmentally modified pre- and postnatal vulnerability, neuronal and neurochemical maturation, organizational plasticity and adaptation, and, perhaps above all, the integration of neural activity across a wide range of behaviors and spatially distant brain regions and circuitries, will be of greatest importance in understanding the clinically most salient issues for children who actually have these disorders: how to intervene in the circuitry now to improve both symptoms and adaptive functioning; how to know what the circuitry holds in terms of future core and comorbid symptom severities; how to prevent dysfunction in these systems from producing dysfunction in other systems; and how to avoid long-term harm to these systems from present interventions.

SUMMARY OF CHAPTER 13

*The complexities of the design and circuitry of the human brain are begin-
ning to be more fully understood. Of particular relevance to studies of
Tourette's syndrome, obsessive-compulsive disorder, and ADHD are cortico-
striato-thalamo-cortical circuits involved in the learning, selection, and monitoring of behavioral programs. Our brains contain a vast repertoire of such
programs, most of which need to be inhibited most of the time. Our current
hypotheses concerning Tourette's syndrome and obsessive-compulsive disorder focus on the disinhibition and inappropriate expression of fragments of
these programs in the form of tics or harm-avoidant compulsions. Functional
in vivo neuroimaging studies are leading the way in these research endeavors.*

PREVIEW OF CHAPTER 14

*Recent studies have continued to implicate dopaminergic projections to the
striatum in the pathobiology of Tourette's and related disorders. Dopaminergic pathways—and possibly other ascending monaminergic and cholinergic pathways—appear to have a key role in linking behavioral programs to
salient perceptual cues coming from the inner world of the body or the external environment. However, definitive studies remain to be done. It is
likely that Tourette's symptoms can appear as the result of more than one
set of neurochemical alterations.*

CHAPTER 14

Neurochemical and Neuropeptide Systems

GEORGE M. ANDERSON, JAMES F. LECKMAN, and DONALD J. COHEN

> It is impossible to meet a whale-ship on the ocean without being struck by her near appearance. The vessel under short sail, with look-outs at the mastheads, eagerly scanning the wide expanse around them, has a totally different air from those engaged in regular voyage.
>
> —*From the "Extracts" in the preface to* Moby-Dick,
> *by Herman Melville, 1851*

Tourette's syndrome is a neuropsychiatric disorder characterized by multiple motor and vocal tics, with symptoms typically occurring in bouts of seconds and minutes. As discussed in Chapter 2, although Tourette's syndrome is a chronic condition with onset in childhood, the severity and pattern of tics typically change over time. Long-term fluctuations in symptom expression tend to occur over months and years. Along with this waxing and waning, there appears to be a general pattern of exacerbation between 8 and 12 years of age, followed by a gradual diminution of severity in adulthood (Leckman, Zhang, et al., 1998; Shapiro et al., 1988). Although the diagnosis of Tourette's can often be made with relative certainty, the situation is complicated by associated comorbidity. About half of children seen with Tourette's also meet criteria for attention-deficit hyperactivity disorder (ADHD). In addition, a majority of Tourette's patients display obsessive-compulsive behaviors and will, at least at times, meet criteria for obsessive-compulsive disorder. The relationship of the obsessive-compulsive and ADHD-related symptoms to the symptoms and pathophysiology of Tourette's awaits clarification. Difficulties in trying to distinguish Tourette's patients from those with tics and associated behaviors arising from alternative etiologies further complicates this area (Comings, 1995a; Kurlan, 1989; Leckman et al., 1992;

Palumbo, Maughan, & Kurlan, 1997; Pauls et al., 1993; Robertson, 1989).

Investigations into the etiology and pathophysiology of Tourette's and related forms of obsessive-compulsive disorder have included research in the areas of psychopharmacology (Chappell, Scahill, & Leckman, 1997; B. Peterson, Zhang, et al., 1997; Scahill, 1996), brain imaging (B. Peterson & Klein, 1997), neuropsychology (R. Schultz et al., 1998), genetics (Leckman, 1997; Sadovnick & Kurlan, 1997), and neurochemistry (Leckman, Peterson, et al., 1997; Singer, 1997). There has been increasing overlap among these approaches as they have focused on central processes and systems that might be altered in patients with Tourette's. For practical purposes, the neurochemical research can be defined as those studies involving chemical analyses of postmortem brain tissue, cerebrospinal fluid (CSF), plasma, platelets, and urine, as well as ligand-based neuroimaging studies. As previously reviewed (G. Anderson & Cohen, 1996; Chappell et al., 1990; Chokka, Baker, Bornstein, & de Groot, 1995; Leckman et al., 1992; Leckman, Peterson, et al., 1997; Rogeness, Javors, & Pliszka, 1992), the neurochemical research has been undertaken in an attempt to assess the functioning of specific central neurotransmitter systems in Tourette's. It was hoped this endeavor would lead to the identification of alterations in Tourette's patients that would be useful in diagnosis and subgrouping. Additional impetus for the neurochemical research comes from the promise that through a better understanding of etiology, improved treatment and even cure might be possible. Researchers have taken heart from the advances that have resulted from neurochemical studies of Huntington's, Parkinson's, and Alzheimer's disorders.

Most of the neurochemical research has been concerned with the assessment of monoaminergic neurotransmitters and a limited number of neuropeptide and neuroendocrine systems. Much of the rationale for examining the monoamines, including dopamine, norepinephrine, and serotonin, comes from a consideration of the possible neuroanatomical/neurophysiological correlates of the behavioral and neurological aspects of the disorder. Hypotheses regarding the monoamines have also arisen from observations of the effects of various pharmacological agents on symptom expression. The apparent influence of a range of actions and events, including perinatal complications, day-to-day stress, and central infections and lesions, has also contributed to theories implicating one or another of the monoaminergic neurotransmitters (Leckman, Peterson, et al., 1997).

The attempt to identify neurochemical alterations in Tourette's is characterized by its complexity. Along with the issue of comorbid behaviors, one must try to sort out early epigenetic environmental influences that can modulate the disease process, while attempting to clarify whether the system under study has a fundamental or more distal role in the pathophysiology of the disorder. The extensive interconnections of the monoamine systems with one another and with other central neurotransmitter systems further complicate the attempt to isolate specific alterations. In addition, most of the available neurochemical measures have fundamental limitations in terms of just how much can be inferred concerning the functional significance and regional location of differences that are seen (G. Anderson & Cohen, 1996; Rogeness et al., 1992). However, recent advances in understanding basal ganglia function have, in some respects, simplified the task. As reviewed in Chapters 8 and 12, increased knowledge of basal ganglia pathways, especially elucidation of their role in the modulation of cortico-striato-thalamo-cortical (CSTC) circuits, has led to a number of testable hypotheses concerning the pathophysiology of Tourette's syndrome.

DOPAMINE

To a large extent, Tourette's can be considered a movement disorder. The predominance of motoric features in Tourette's, as well as the associated behaviors in the realms of inattention and hyperactivity, has led to a considerable focus on the basal ganglia as a possible site of altered brain function in Tourette's. The continuing advances in basal ganglia research have confirmed a critical role for dopamine (DA) in controlling basal ganglia output (Albin, Young, & Penney, 1989, 1995; Graybiel, 1996; Parent & Hazrati, 1995a, 1995b; A. Young & Penney, 1984). As seen in Figures 14.1a and 14.1b, dopaminergic nigral efferents project to striatal areas where they influence the activity of GABAergic and peptidergic neurons of the direct and indirect pathways. These pathways are, in turn, crucial in the modulation of the major basal ganglia output nuclei, the medial globus pallidus and the reticulata. Not shown are important dopaminergic nigral projections to pallidal and cortical areas, as well as projections from the ventral tegmentum to limbic areas, including the accumbens (ventral striatum) and limbic cortex.

Although theoretical considerations of the role of midbrain DA systems in adaptive motor control have been taken to implicate DA in Tourette's (see Devinsky, 1983; Graybiel, Aosaki, Flaherty, & Kimura, 1994; Singer, Butler, Tune, Seifert, & Coyle, 1982), the most compelling evidence for DA involvement in Tourette's probably comes from observations of the effects of pharmacological agents influencing the DA system. The pharmacological observations are consistent with a hyperfunctional DA system: Agents and actions that increase DA functioning, such as L-dopa administration, stimulant medication (Golden, 1974; Price et al., 1986), and neuroleptic withdrawal (Klawans, Falk, Nausieda, & Weiner, 1978; Riddle, Hardin, Towbin, Leckman, & Cohen, 1987; Singer, 1981), have been reported to exacerbate Tourette's. Drugs that lower or block the action of DA, including typical (Sallee, Nesbitt, Jackson, Sine, & Sethuraman, 1997; Seignot, 1961; E. Shapiro et al., 1989) and atypical neuroleptics (Lombroso,

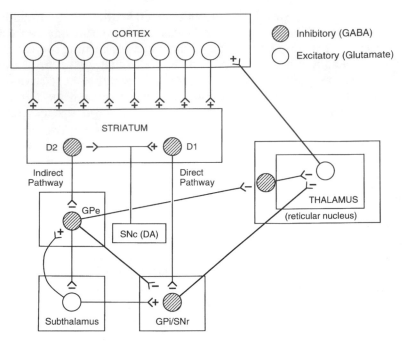

Figure 14.1a   The role of dopamine in the modulation of CSTC circuitry. The role of nigrostriatal dopamine projections in mediating the output of the basal ganglia appears to depend on the balance of D1 versus D2 dopamine receptor stimulation in the striatum. Indeed, the stimulation of D1 and D2 receptors produces opposing effects in both rodents and primates. Adapted from Leckman, Peterson, et al., 1997.

Scahill, King, et al., 1995), tetrabenazine (Jankovic, Glaze, & Frost, 1984), and α-methylpara-tyrosine (Sweet et al., 1974), tend to improve tic symptoms in Tourette's.

Neurochemical Assessment of Dopamine Function in Tourette's

The neuroanatomical considerations and pharmacological observations have served to spur a wide range of neurochemical investigation on DA. Much of the early work involved the measurement of CSF levels of the principal DA metabolite, homovanillic acid (HVA). Studies using probenecid to block the egress of the acid metabolite from CSF found, somewhat surprisingly, reduced accumulation of HVA in Tourette's patients (Butler, Koslow, Seifert, Caprioli, & Singer, 1979; D. Cohen, Shaywitz, Caparulo, Young, & Bowers, 1978; D. Cohen, Shaywitz, et al., 1979; Singer, Tune, Butler, Zaczek, & Coyle, 1982). Researchers were led to suggest that the apparent reduction in presynaptic synthesis and release of DA was in compensation for a presumed postsynaptic hypersensitivity. Although a compensatory mechanism was plausible, the data could not be taken to strongly support the idea of hyperfunctional central DA in Tourette's. Other studies of baseline CSF HVA

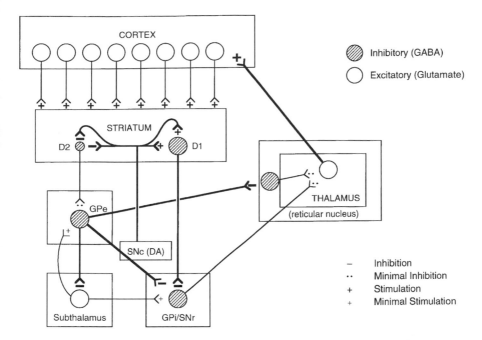

Figure 14.1b   The hypothesized role of dopamine in Tourette's syndrome and tic-related obsessive-compulsive disorder. If Tourette's syndrome is associated with a dopaminergic hyperinnervation of the striatum, this hyperinnervation would result in a further inhibition of the indirect pathway and stimulation of the direct pathway, both resulting in increased thalamo-cortical stimulation. Adapted from Leckman, Peterson, et al., 1997.

levels have been discrepant, with reports of reduced (Butler et al., 1979), unchanged (Leckman et al., 1988), and elevated (Takano & Ishiguro, 1993) levels in Tourette's. Recently, a large study of CSF HVA in Tourette's syndrome has provided more definitive data (Leckman, Goodman, et al., 1995). Not only were substantially larger groups of subjects examined, but complications arising from the use of probenecid were avoided and patients were carefully characterized with respect to comorbid behavior—especially with respect to obsessive-compulsive symptoms. In this latest study, no mean differences in CSF HVA levels were seen across groups of Tourette's patients, Tourette's patients with obsessive-compulsive disorder, and normal controls (Leckman, Goodman, et al., 1995).

On the whole, the CSF research would suggest that there is no marked and global alteration in central DA turnover. Other attempts at addressing this issue have been made through the measurement of plasma HVA levels and urine excretion rates of HVA. Whereas plasma HVA was reported to be lower in more severely affected Tourette's patients (Riddle et al., 1989), studies of urine HVA have found higher rates of excretion in Tourette's (Bornstein & Baker, 1988; Messiha, Knopp, Vanecko, O'Brien, & Corson, 1971).

The most direct tests of possible alterations in central DA synthesis have been accomplished through postmortem brain studies. In these studies, levels of DA and of HVA, as well as the rate-limiting synthetic enzyme, tyrosine hydroxylase (TH), were measured in cortical and subcortical regions of postmortem brain tissue from Tourette's patients. The postmortem studies have been consistent in finding similar group mean levels of the neurotransmitter and its major metabolite in Tourette's and control subjects (G. Anderson et al., 1992a, 1992b; Singer, Hahn, Krowiak, Nelson, & Moran, 1990; Singer et al., 1991). In addition, TH activities were not found to be altered in Tourette's syndrome (Anderson et al., 1992a, 1992b). The conclusion that central DA synthesis and metabolism are largely unaltered in adult Tourette's patients is thus strongly supported by the postmortem studies.

As discussed briefly in Chapter 12, a number of PET and SPECT imaging studies have examined postsynaptic dopamine receptor densities in Tourette's. The studies have concentrated on assessing the density of D_2 receptors in the basal ganglia: two have found similar receptor densities in the Tourette's and control groups (George, Robertson, et al., 1994; Turjanski et al., 1994), and a third study reported an elevation in Tourette's patients (Singer et al., 1992). The PET study of Turjanski and colleagues also found normal rates of ^{18}F-DA accumulation in Tourette's patients after administration of ^{18}F-labeled amino acid precursor dihydroxyphenylalanine (^{18}F-dopa), indicating the presence of normal rates of DA synthesis in Tourette's. At this point, the bulk of the neurochemical and neuroimaging data paint a picture of normal presynaptic metabolism and unaltered D_2 receptor functioning in Tourette's.

However, two recent studies present consistent and intriguing data suggesting that Tourette's patients have an increased density of the presynaptic DA uptake site. The transporter protein is found on the cell membrane; its critical role in the regulation of DA neurotransmission can be appreciated by considering the marked effects of agents like cocaine that block DA transport and by the striking hyperactive behavior shown by rats lacking the transporter protein (Jones, Jaber, Giros, Wightman, & Caron, 1996). In the postmortem study of Singer and colleagues (1991), increased binding of the transporter ligand ^{3}H-mazindol was observed in homogenates of caudate and putamen tissue obtained from Tourette's patients, compared to controls. In the SPECT neuroimaging study of Malison and coworkers (1995), increased binding of a DA transporter ligand was observed in the striatum of Tourette's patients. Although the studies were both limited by small subject number, their agreement is impressive.

It is unclear how the DA transporter results, if replicated in larger groups, should be interpreted. Typically, monoaminergic transporter densities have been considered to be presynaptic markers that can be used as an index of innervation. However, in this case, all the other markers of presynaptic dopamine neurons, including DA levels, HVA levels, and TH activity, have been reported as normal in Tourette's.

Another possible explanation for the elevation in transporter density involves an up-regulation of transporters occurring in response to excessive DA release or activity. As reviewed in Chapter 11, acute hypoxic insults in the perinatal period and maternal stress during pregnancy can prompt such an outpouring of DA and the up-regulation of the striatal DA transporters (Arregui et al., 1994; Gross et al., 1993; Henry et al., 1995). However, the relevance and time course of these changes has yet to be established in Tourette's.

More extensive postmortem and imaging research is warranted to replicate the basic findings and to explore implications of possible increased striatal DA transporters in Tourette's. Parenthetically, although decreased rates of platelet DA uptake have been reported for Tourette's patients (Rabey, Oberman, Graff, & Korczyn, 1995), it should be pointed out that a distinctively different transporter, the vesicular amine transporter (VAT), was assessed in that study.

Neurochemical Assessment of Dopamine in Obsessive-Compulsive Disorder and ADHD

Dopamine has been suggested to be altered in obsessive-compulsive disorder and in ADHD based on the symptomatology of the syndromes and their response to dopaminergic agents. There is only limited neurochemical data of relevance to dopamine's possible involvement in patients with obsessive-compulsive disorder and Tourette's-related obsessive-compulsive symptoms. As mentioned, studies of CSF HVA have not found differences among the patient groups or with controls (Leckman, Goodman, et al., 1995); however, a study of baseline plasma prolactin, a hormone under strong inhibitory dopaminergic control, found increased levels in a Tourette's plus obsessive-compulsive disorder group compared to a pure obsessive-compulsive disorder group (Hanna, McCracken, & Cantwell, 1991). The situation regarding DA in ADHD is complicated. Although there have been a large number of studies assessing neurochemical indices of DA functioning in ADHD (Rogeness et al., 1992; Zametkin & Rapoport, 1987a, 1987b), there are no robust, well-replicated alterations. There is a sense that comorbid ADHD symptoms in Tourette's patients are closely associated with tic symptoms; however, neurochemical studies comparing Tourette's patients with and without associated ADHD are lacking. It is worth noting that stimulants can ameliorate symptoms of ADHD while exacerbating or precipitating tic symptoms. This striking pharmacological dissociation between the symptom domains suggests that DA alterations in Tourette's and, particularly, in Tourette's with comorbid ADHD may be complex.

Future Directions on the Role of Central Dopamine Pathways

Future neurochemical research on the DA system in Tourette's will probably focus on postmortem and in vivo neuroimaging studies. The DA transporter will be of particular interest; however, the full range of DA receptor subtypes is worthy of study. The D_4 receptor is of special interest given genetic studies suggesting linkage between Tourette's and the seven repeat allele of the exon 3 VNTR at the D_4 locus (Grice et al., 1996). The D_2 receptor remains of interest given the recent report of a relationship between D_2 receptor density and severity in monozygotic twins (Wolf et al., 1996), and given the efficacy of D_2 agents in treating tics. Imaging studies will continue in parallel with the postmortem research; they will also permit functional aspects, such as the relative concentrations of synaptic or released DA, to be examined (see Szymanski et al., 1997).

Developmental changes in the relative abundance of D_1-type versus D_2-type receptors in the striatum have been hinted at in earlier postmortem studies (Seeman et al., 1987). If confirmed, the balance of D_1 to D_2 receptors could influence the onset and time course of tic symptoms. Similarly, the number of DA transporter sites in the striatum is known to decline with age (van Dyck et al., 1995). The time course of this decline roughly parallels the reduction in tic severity toward the end of the second decade of life (Leckman, Zhang, et al., 1998). Longitudinal studies of Tourette's subjects could test for an association between tic severity and striatal DA transporter density and tic symptoms (Leckman, Zhang, et al.).

Another promising lead concerns the interaction of dopaminergic pathways and androgenic steroids. In the CNS of rodents, there are high levels of androgen receptors (in the absence of estrogen receptors) in the dopaminergic cells within the substantia nigra and the ventral tegmental area (VTA) as well as many nuclei in the brainstem that mediate the muscular contractions associated with both motor and vocal tics (Simerly, Chang, Muramatsu, & Swanson, 1990). A full understanding of the developmental impact of early exposure to androgenic gonadal steroids on these midbrain and brainstem structures in the male fetus may contribute in an important fashion to our emerging models of pathogenesis (see Chapters 9 and 12 for further discussion of the role of gonadal steroids).

Finally, of heuristic interest is the suggestion that dopaminergic and other monoamine pathways are part of a *salience* system in the brain that detects perturbations in the environment that hold special significance for the organism (Edelman, 1987; Edelman & Tononi, 1995; W. Schultz et al., 1997). As discussed in Chapters 1, 2, and 8, Tourette's is a disorder of heightened sensitivity to environmental stimuli—internal somatosensory as well as external environmental cues. A similar case can be made for the brain's error-detection system being set too high in obsessive-compulsive disorder (see Chapter 3). These increases in sensitivity to environmental cues may relate in part to the genetically and developmentally induced changes in central DA pathways. However, caution is warranted. The available data directly implicating central DA pathways are preliminary. Whether alterations in the DA system exist in Tourette's remains an open question; whether possible alterations might be fundamentally etiologic, part of a pathophysiological cascade, or of modulating influence is also unclear.

NOREPINEPHRINE

The intensity and frequency of tics displayed by patients with Tourette's have long been observed to be affected by levels of emotional stress. Based on the indispensable role of central noradrenergic neurons and the peripheral sympathetic nervous system in eliciting and mediating the stress response, the noradrenergic system has been suggested to play a part in Tourette's. The noradrenergic neurons originating in the locus ceruleus, a compact cell group of about 25,000 neurons in the brainstem, project to all cortices and thalamic and hypothalamic nuclei. Projections to the hypothalamus promote the release of corticotropin-releasing hormone (CRH), as shown in Figure 14.2. Appreciation of the extensive noradrenergic projections to dopamine neurons in the basal ganglia, and to areas of the frontal cortex involved in attentional mechanisms and in the control of cortical-striatal circuits, has lent further weight to norepinephrine (NE) hypotheses. Of particular relevance to Tourette's and ADHD are projections to the

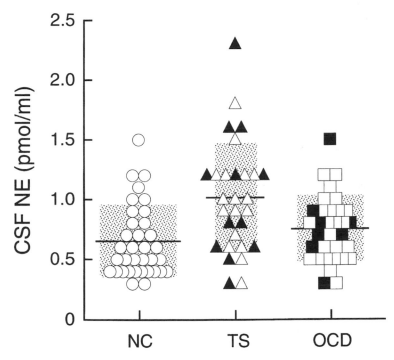

Figure 14.2 CSF norepinephrine (NE) levels are elevated in Tourette's syndrome (TS). Compared to normal controls (NC, circles) and patients with obsessive-compulsive disorder (OCD, squares), patients with TS (triangles) have elevated levels of CSF NE. No differences were observed comparing TS patients with OCD versus those without OCD (filled triangles versus empty triangles). Similarly, no differences were found comparing OCD patients with tics (filled squares) versus OCD patients without tics (empty squares). For additional details of this study, see Leckman, Goodman, et al. (1995).

frontal cortex that, upon activation, appear to inhibit spontaneous discharge and facilitate attentional processes (Arnsten, Steere, & Hunt, 1996).

As with DA, observations from drug trials have tended to support the idea that NE plays at least a modulating role in Tourette's. Studies of the α_2-noradrenergic agonist clonidine have usually shown it to reduce tic symptoms (Chappell, et al., 1997; Leckman et al., 1983, 1991); rapid clonidine withdrawal has been observed to cause acute exacerbation of Tourette's (Leckman, Ort, et al., 1986). The facilitating role of NE in the stress response and the beneficial effects of clonidine, an agent that tends to reduce NE functioning through its action at somatodendritic α_{2C} autoreceptors, led to a search for neurochemical evidence of a hypernoradrenergic state in Tourette's.

Neurochemical Assessment of Central Noradrenegeric Systems in Tourette's

Most early studies of NE-related measures found either lowered or unchanged levels in patients with Tourette's. Measurement of 3-methoxy-4-hydroxyphenylglycol (MHPG), the principal central metabolite of NE, found lower urinary excretion rates (Ang, Borison, Dysken, & Davis, 1982; Baker, Bornstein, Douglass, Carroll, & King, 1990; Sweeney, Pickar, Redmond, & Maas, 1978), while normal plasma (Riddle, Leckman, Anderson, Ort, et al., 1988) and CSF MHPG (Singer, Tune, et al., 1982) levels were reported. Unchanged levels of plasma dopamine-β-hydroxylase (DBH, an NE synthetic enzyme released along with NE from sympathetic neurons; Lake, Ziegler, Eldridge, & Murphy, 1977; A. Shapiro, Baron, Shapiro, & Levitt, 1984) and normal plasma NE concentrations (Eldridge, Sweet, Lake, Ziegler, & Shapiro, 1977; Lake et al., 1977) were reported for Tourette's patients. A contrasting study of salivary amylase did find elevated secretion of the enzyme in Tourette's patients, suggestive of increased β-adrenergic receptor functioning in the acinar cells of the parotid gland (Selinger, Cohen, Ort, Anderson, & Leckman, 1984).

In other studies, the neurochemical and neuroendocrine effects of acute (Muller et al., 1994; J. Young et al., 1981) and chronic (F. Silverstein, Smith, & Johnstone, 1985) clonidine treatment and of clonidine withdrawal (Leckman, Ort, et al., 1986) were examined and found to influence NE-related measures in the expected directions. Although the withdrawal study did provide neurochemical confirmation of hypernoradrenergic functioning during withdrawal-induced symptom exacerbation (Leckman, Ort, et al.), the challenge studies have not led to a useful method for predicting drug response.

Two more recent studies have examined indices of noradrenergic functioning in large groups of Tourette's and control subjects receiving lumbar punctures (Chappell, Riddle, et al., 1994; Leckman, Goodman, et al., 1995). The studies were unique in obtaining CSF levels of both MHPG and NE itself, and in their use of the lumbar puncture procedure as a robust and relatively reproducible stressor. Also examined were neuroendocrine measures relevant to the functioning of the hypothalamic-pituitary-adrenal (HPA) axis, the other major component of the stress response (Chappell et al., 1996; Chappell, Riddle, et al., 1994). Most striking was the large group mean elevation (+55%, $p < .001$) in CSF NE levels observed in the Tourette's group (Figure 14.2) and that CSF NE was correlated with motor tic severity. A trend toward slightly (approximately 10%) higher levels of MHPG was also reported (Leckman, Goodman, et al.). Significantly higher CSF levels of corticotropin-releasing factor (CRF) were observed (Chappell et al.), along with elevated plasma concentrations of adrenocorticotropin hormone (ACTH; Chappell, Riddle, et al.). Surprisingly, no difference between Tourette's and controls was seen for cortisol secretion over a six-hour period including the spinal tap (Figure 14.3). However, urinary excretion of NE was elevated in Tourette's subjects in the 21-hour period leading up to the tap (Chappell, Riddle, et al.). The results, when considered in the context of previous research in the general area of stress responsivity in Tourette's, suggest that Tourette's patients do tend to have an increased stress response. However, patients may not have a detectable increase in baseline functioning of the noradrenergic system or the HPA axis. Thus, the stress response systems appear more likely to be involved in influencing severity of symptoms, rather than being directly related to fundamental etiologic processes.

Neurochemical Assessment of Norepinephrine Function in Obsessive-Compulsive Disorder and ADHD

As is the case with DA, there is very limited data regarding NE function in obsessive-compulsive disorder, whereas a number of studies have examined NE-related measures in ADHD. In the obsessive-compulsive disorder domain, the most recent and useful data are the measures of CSF NE and MHPG in large groups of patients with obsessive-compulsive disorder, obsessive-compulsive disorder plus tics, and Tourette's plus obsessive-compulsive disorder (Leckman, Goodman, et al., 1995). No differences were seen in the two groups with primary obsessive-compulsive disorder; the group with Tourette's plus obsessive-compulsive disorder had an elevation in CSF NE similar to that observed in the Tourette's alone group. It was somewhat surprising that the obsessive-compulsive disorder patients, with a diagnosis in the anxiety disorders family, did not appear to show the increased stress response to the lumbar puncture seen in the Tourette's group (and the Tourette's plus obsessive-compulsive disorder group).

Although a good number of studies have examined NE-related measures in ADHD, there is little consensus regarding possible noradrenergic alterations in ADHD (Rogeness et al., 1992). In addition, there are no studies attempting to examine neurochemical correlates of this behavioral domain in patients with Tourette's. It is interesting that a recent report of noradrenergic function in ADHD proposes that children with ADHD have

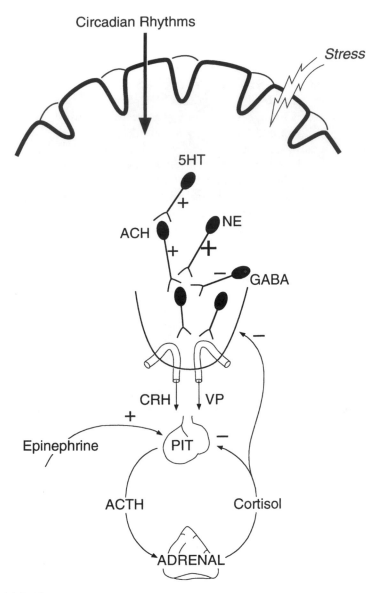

Figure 14.3 Schematic diagram of the hypothalamic-pituitary-adrenal axis. This figure depicts aspects of the hypothalamic-pituitary-adrenal (HPA) axis, highlighting the role of central serotonin (5HT), norepinephrine (NE), and cholinergic (ACH) pathways, as well as the negative feedback loop from the adrenal gland to the hypothalamus. Other abbreivations include: corticotrophin-releasing hormone (CRH), arginine vasopressin (VP), the pituitary gland (PIT), adrenocorticotrophin homone (ACTH), and gamma-aminobutyric acid (GABA). In one series of studies, Tourette's syndrome patients had elevated levels of CSF, NE, and CRH, as well as plasma ACTH (see Chappell, Leckman, et al., 1996; Chappell, Riddle, et al., 1994; Leckman, Goodman, et al., 1995).

slightly elevated basal noradrenergic activity, but are less able to mount a robust release of noradrenaline in a stressful situation. This is counter to the findings regarding the noradrenergic and sympathetic nervous systems in Tourette's patients and, again (as with the differences in DA-related pharmacology between tic and ADHD behaviors), speaks to the complexity of the relationship between Tourette's and ADHD.

Future Directions for Research on Noradrenergic Pathways

Future work in this area should be directed toward assessing, and trying to modulate, the mechanisms involved in the elicitation of the stress-response systems. Further neurochemical/neuroendocrine assessment could make use of probes of the NE and HPA systems. The use of more specific agents—such as the α_{2A}-receptor-specific agent guanfacine (Chappell, Riddle, et al., 1995)—acting at noradrenergic receptors and the availability of new agents affecting the HPA axis may be beneficial in this regard and in terms of developing new pharmacological interventions. The increasing availability of postmortem brain tissue is also promising, as postmortem studies should permit a much more complete assessment of the NE and HPA systems.

Other studies should explore the neural substrates associated with the profound tic reductions that occur during sleep. Alterations in noradrenergic activity during the sleep-wake cycle make it an important candidate for such studies (Aston-Jones & Bloom, 1981). Similarly, this system may be involved when severe tic symptoms persist into adulthood in a minority of adults.

SEROTONIN

Initial speculation regarding a role for serotonin (5-hydroxytryptamine, 5HT) in Tourette's centered on the neurotransmitter's generally inhibitory influence on behavior. Serotonergic neurons of the raphe nuclei project throughout the brain, with particularly rich innervation of the limbic areas and basal ganglia. This rich serotonergic innervation of paleocortical areas provides a route for influencing motor symptoms and affecting emotional content of tics and related compulsive behaviors. Apparent benefit from treatment with the 5HT precursor 5-hydroxytryptophan (van Woert, Rosenbaum, & Enna, 1982) and worsening after administration of the $5HT_2$ antagonist cyproheptadine (Crosley, 1979) were consistent with the idea that central 5HT functioning was reduced in Tourette's. On the other hand, it should be mentioned that treatment studies with serotonin-reuptake inhibitors have not found this class of drugs to be useful in reducing tics (Riddle, Leckman, Hardin, Anderson, & Cohen, 1988). Lately, the association of Tourette's with 5HT has been strengthened due to the increasingly appreciated clinical relationship between Tourette's and obsessive-compulsive disorder.

Neurochemical Assessment of Serotonin Function in Tourette's

The first neurochemical assessment of 5HT functioning in Tourette's consisted of measurements of the major 5HT metabolite 5-hydroxyindoleacetic acid (5HIAA) in CSF (Butler et al., 1979; D. Cohen, Shaywitz, et al., 1978, 1979). Postprobenecid and baseline levels of 5HIAA tended to be reduced in Tourette's patients compared to controls. In contrast, more recent studies of CSF 5HIAA have not found group differences (Leckman, Goodman, et al., 1995; Leckman et al., 1988); the later studies have studied larger, better-characterized groups and have used improved analytical methods.

Additional neurochemical studies have examined a variety of peripheral 5HT-related measures, including urine indoles (Bornstein & Baker, 1992), plasma tryptophan and kynurenine (Chappell, Anderson, et al., 1995; Comings, 1990; Dursun, Farrar, et al., 1994; Leckman et al., 1984; Rickards et al. 1996), platelet 5HT (Leckman et al.), and platelet 5HT transporter binding (Weizman et al., 1992). Reports of lowered platelet 5HT (Comings) and of greatly increased plasma kynurenine (Dursun, Farrar, et al., 1994; Rickards et al., 1996) have not been substantiated by other studies (Chappell, Anderson, et al., 1995; Leckman et al., 1984). An uncontradicted finding is that of lowered plasma tryptophan in Tourette's patients (Comings, 1990; Leckman et al., 1984). As has been pointed out (Chappell, Anderson, et al., 1995; Rickards et al., 1996), this slight but significant decrease in plasma tryptophan could be a result of increased stress reactivity in the Tourette's group leading to activation of tryptophan pyrrolase (the major catabolic enzyme for tryptophan). In a preliminary study of tryptophan depletion in Tourette's patients, some effects on relevant behaviors were observed (Rasmusson et al., 1997).

The finding of lower plasma tryptophan is also made more interesting by the report of reduced tryptophan in a range of subcortical and cortical brain regions from Tourette's patients (Akbari et al., 1993; G. Anderson et al., 1992a, 1992b). The postmortem studies also found reduced levels of 5HT and 5HIAA in nearly all of the brain areas examined. The decreases in the precursor, neurotransmitter, and metabolite occurred in spite of apparently normal levels of the 5HT transporter. The situation seems to be the converse of that seen with striatal DA, where increased levels of transporter were seen despite normal levels of precursor, neurotransmitter, metabolite, and synthetic enzyme.

Relevant Serotonergic Studies in Obsessive-Compulsive Disorder and ADHD

The effectiveness of serotonergic agents in treating obsessive-compulsive disorder (Lydiard, Brawman-Mintzer, & Ballenger, 1996; McDougle, Goodman, Leckman, & Price, 1993), as well as some limited neurobiological evidence for serotonergic alterations in obsessive-compulsive disorder (Jenike, Rauch, Cummings, Savage, & Goodman, 1996), have made 5HT of substantial interest in research and treatment of the obsessive-compulsive disorder. The increasing awareness of the prevalence of obsessive-compulsive disorder–related behavior in Tourette's and of the apparent genetic relationship between some forms of obsessive-compulsive disorder and Tourette's have also served to increase interest in 5HT in Tourette's. The recent studies of CSF 5HIAA probably provide the best neurochemical data concerning possible serotonergic alterations in Tourette's-related obsessive-compulsive disorder and obsessive-compulsive disorder itself. The absence of differences across control and patient groups indicates that global alterations in innervation or metabolism are probably not present in either form of obsessive-compulsive disorder. The research on possible 5HT mechanisms in ADHD and the disruptive behavior disorders have been prompted less by pharmacological evidence and more from a consideration of the role of 5HT in impulsivity, aggression, activity, learning, and memory (G. Anderson, 1993; Zubieta & Alessi, 1993). Although there are some suggestive CSF 5HIAA findings in the areas of aggression and impulsivity, there are little or no useful or replicated data regarding the 5HT system in ADHD patients (see Zubieta & Alessi).

Future Directions

At present, it is difficult to reconcile the more recent CSF findings of normal 5HIAA and tryptophan levels with the observations of reduced indoles in brain tissue. Certainly, additional genetic, in vivo imaging, and postmortem research is needed to resolve these questions and to provide a more comprehensive assessment of the serotonergic system in Tourette's syndrome and related disorders.

AMINO ACID NEUROTRANSMITTERS

Glutamate and γ-aminobutyric acid (GABA) are, respectively, the major excitatory and inhibitory neurotransmitters in the mammalian central nervous system. This preeminence alone forces a consideration of their possible role in Tourette's. Interest in GABA has been further stimulated by the critical role of striatal GABAergic projections in modulating movement. Both the direct and indirect pathways from the striatum to the pallidum and related structures utilize GABA as their principal neurotransmitter (see Figures 14.1a and 14.1b). It is especially relevant that the loss of these striatal GABAergic neurons has been established to be a major neuropathological lesion in Huntington's disease (Albin et al., 1989, 1992). In addition to this association with hyperkinesis, there is some suggestion that agents that increase GABA functioning, such as the benzodiazepine clozapam and the agonist progabide, can be beneficial in Tourette's (Mondrup, Dupont, & Braengaard, 1985). Glutamatergic neurons (shown as open circles in Figures 14.1a and 14.1b) are intimately involved in the functioning of the CSTC circuits. A potential role for glutamate in Tourette's syndrome has been suggested based on glutamate's critical involvement in basal ganglia circuitry, specifically in corticostriatal and subthalamopallidal projections (Albin et al., 1989, 1995; Parent & Hazrati, 1995a, 1995b; Young & Penney, 1984). Possible glutamate-induced excitotoxicity in Huntington's disease has also drawn attention to glutamate in Tourette's (Comings, Goetz, Holden, & Holtz, 1981).

Neurochemical Assessment of Amino Acid Neurotransmitters in Tourette's

The limited neurochemical research on GABA has consistently found little or no difference between Tourette's patients and control subjects: normal levels of whole blood and CSF GABA have been reported for Tourette's patients (van Woert et al., 1982). More important, analyses in postmortem brain regions found activities of the major GABA synthetic enzyme glutamic acid decarboxylase (GAD) and GABA levels to be unaltered in Tourette's patients (G. Anderson et al., 1992a, 1992b; Singer et al., 1990).

Only two glutamate-related neurochemical studies have been carried out in Tourette's. In the first (Comings et al., 1981), normal rates of fibroblast glutamate uptake were observed in Tourette's patients. In a more recent study (G. Anderson et al., 1992a, 1992b), glutamate was measured in subcortical and cortical regions of postmortem brain tissue from Tourette's and control subjects. In general, glutamate levels, as well as the levels of a number of other amino acids, were similar in the Tourette's and control tissue. However, significantly reduced levels of glutamate were observed in the medial globus pallidus of the four Tourette's brains examined. A group mean reduction of 30% was seen whether glutamate concentration was expressed as $\mu g/g$ or $\mu g/mg$ protein, and nonoverlapping distributions were seen for the Tourette's and control groups. Trends to lower levels of glutamate also were seen in the lateral globus pallidus and the substantia nigra reticulata. It was noteworthy that the reductions in glutamate occurred in the three major projection areas of the subthalamic nucleus (STN), suggesting that excitatory output from the STN was reduced (Figure 14.1b).

The glutamate finding is congruent with emerging concepts of basal ganglia function that hold the STN to play a critical role in regulating the activity of the major inhibitory output nuclei of the basal ganglia (the medial globus and substantia nigra reticulata). Underactivation or disregulation of these nuclei has been suggested to play a role in the hyperkinetic symptomatology seen in hemiballismus and Huntington's disease (Albin et al., 1989, 1992).

Future Directions for Research on Amino Acid Neurotransmitters

Given the neuroanatomical specificity of the glutamate finding, follow-up studies probably will need to examine glutamate and related neurochemical measures in postmortem tissue. A complete investigation of excitatory amino acid (EAA) receptors in the areas of interest, as well as analysis of other potential presynaptic markers, including specific membrane and vesicular EAA transporters, is called for. Given the relatively high concentrations of these neurotransmitters in the brain, the application of magnetic resonance spectroscopic techniques may prove to be a valuable adjunct to planned, ongoing large-scale postmortem studies.

ACETYLCHOLINE

Based on the importance of cholinergic interneurons in the striatum, a case can be made for the involvement of acetylcholine in Tourette's. The cholinergic interneurons exert an influence on CSTC circuits through their inputs to striatal neurons in an analogous, if opposing, fashion to that exerted by dopaminergic afferents. Interestingly, the interneurons are themselves apparently regulated by dopaminergic input and likely participate in the brain's putative salience system. The emerging importance of the cholinergic tonically active neurons (TANs) in modulating movement and sensorimotor learning has stimulated interest in their role in movement disorders (Graybiel et al., 1994). Previous consideration of the critical and opposing relationship between dopamine and acetylcholine in the striatum led to the concept of Tourette's as an acetylcholine-deficiency syndrome (Stahl & Berger, 1982). The pharmacological data, however, are inconsistent, with the cholinesterase inhibitor physiostigmine reported to both improve (Stahl & Berger, 1981) and worsen tics (Tanner, Goetz, & Klawans, 1982). A muscarinic antagonist was seen to be of benefit (Tanner et al., 1982), but precursor administration has not been observed to be useful (G. Rosenberg & Davis, 1982). Finally, studies using nicotine, either alone or as an augmentation to neuroleptics, have found some beneficial effects on tics (Dursun, Hewitt, King, & Reveley, 1996; McConville et al., 1991; Silver & Sanberg, 1993); however, the clinical utility of nicotine remains to be established.

Neurochemical Assessment of Cholinergic Function in Tourette's

The neurochemical research on cholinergic functioning is limited. Two studies from Hanin and colleagues have reported elevated red blood cell choline in Tourette's (Hanin, Merikangas, Merikangas, & Kopp, 1979; Sallee, Kopp, & Hanin, 1992). Normal activities of the catabolic enzymes acetyl- and butyrylcholinesterase were seen in the CSF of Tourette's patients (Singer, Oshida, & Coyle, 1984). Activities of the synthetic enzyme choline acetyltransferase have been observed to be unaltered in cortical (Singer et al., 1990) and subcortical (G. M. Anderson, unpublished data) regions of postmortem brain tissue of Tourette's patients. Binding site densities of the muscarinic cholinergic receptor, as assessed by binding of the ligand ^{3}H-quinuclidinyl benzilate (^{3}H-QNB), were reported to be decreased in lymphocytes (Rabey, Lewis, Graff & Korczyn, 1992). In contrast, ^{3}H-QNB binding appeared to be normal in postmortem cortical tissue obtained from Tourette's patients (Singer et al., 1990).

Future Directions

Given the sparseness of the data, it is clear that the hypocholinergic hypothesis has not been meaningfully tested. Intensive research on cholinergic mechanisms in Alzheimer's should contribute to the development of new agents and approaches for assessing possible alterations in acetylcholine in Tourette's syndrome. For instance, newer, more specific cholinergic agents may be usefully employed in neuroendocrine protocols and in ligand-based neuroimaging studies. In addition, continued advances in defining and characterizing cholingergic receptors will permit more complete examination of acetylcholine-related systems using genetic, neuroimaging and postmortem approaches.

NEUROPEPTIDES

Neuropeptides of the dynorphin and met-enkephalin opioid peptide families occur in high concentration in the basal ganglia (Nieuwenhuys, 1985). There, the opioids are involved in the regulation of striatal dopaminergic activity and are found in important striato-pallidal projections (Haber, 1986; Parent & Hazrati, 1995a, 1995b). The striato-pallidal neurons are of special interest in hyperkinetic disorders, and it is clear that enkephalin is colocalized in GABAergic neurons of the indirect pathway (see Figure 14.1); less clear is the distribution of dynorphin in the striato-pallidal system. The opioid peptides are also involved in modulating HPA axis and noradrenergic functioning among many other brain systems (Christie, Williams, Osborne, & Bellchambers, 1997; A. Grossman, Moult, Cunnah, & Besser, 1986). These links to systems thought to be involved in Tourette's symptom mediation have led to the use of opioid agents both as neuroimaging probes (Weeks et al., 1996) and experimental pharmacological treatments (Chappell et al., 1992, 1993; Kurlan et al., 1991; Sandyk, 1985a, 1985b). The pharmacological data are not entirely consistent; there have been indications of some limited benefit from both opioid agonists and antagonists (McConville et al., 1994; Meuldijk & Colon, 1992; Sandyk, 1985a, 1985b). As has been pointed out (Chappell, 1994), the complexity of the relevant opioid receptor systems and the relative nonspecificity of the agents employed make interpretation difficult.

The two neuropeptides oxytocin and arginine-vasopressin (AVP) form another peptide family of potential importance in Tourette's and obsessive-compulsive disorder. These two very similar nonapeptides are synthesized in neurons of the supraoptic and paraventricular nuclei of the hypothalamus (AVP, but not oxytocin, is also synthesized and released from other hypothalamic and limbic centers). Well-studied projections of oxytocin- and AVP-containing neurons to the posterior pituitary release the hormones into the bloodstream, while other oxytocin- and AVP-containing neurons project to limbic, brainstem, and spinal cord areas; release can also occur directly into the CSF. The behavioral effects of oxytocin and AVP and their synthetic analogues, especially the role of oxytocin and AVP in repetitive grooming behaviors and the involvement of oxytocin in affiliative and maternal behavior, have prompted their study in obsessive-compulsive disorder (Insel, 1992a, 1997; Leckman, Goodman, et al., 1994b).

Neurochemical Assessment of Neuropeptides in Tourette's and Obsessive-Compulsive Disorder

Neurochemical research on the opioids in Tourette's has been restricted to two postmortem studies of dynorphin-A (1–17) and a study of CSF levels of dynorphin-A (1–8). The postmortem studies reported lower dynorphin levels in basal ganglia areas, with an especially marked decline in the globus pallidus of Tourette's patients (Haber et al., 1986; Haber & Wolfer, 1992). The findings could reflect a deficit in peptidergic striato-pallidal projections; such a loss would be expected to have a major effect on the regulation of basal ganglia output and, hence, of motor behavior. In contrast to the observations from postmortem brain research, CSF levels of dynorphin-A (1–8) were found to be elevated in Tourette's patients (Leckman et al., 1988). Initial neuroendocrine challenge studies revealed apparent abnormal endocrine responses to the nonspecific antagonist naloxone (Sandyk, 1989). However, more recent research has found normal ACTH, cortisol, and lutenizing hormone release after naloxone challenge (Chappell et al., 1992). Use of spiradoline, a specific κ agonist, did, however, reveal increased growth hormone release in Tourette's patients compared to controls (Chappell et al., 1993).

Assessment of AVP functioning in obsessive-compulsive disorder and Tourette's is limited to two studies of CSF levels. In the initial study (Altemus et al., 1992), increased AVP concentrations were observed in patients with obsessive-compulsive disorder. However, in a more recent study, normal levels were seen in obsessive-compulsive disorder, Tourette's, and tic-related obsessive-compulsive disorder patients (Leckman, Goodman, et al., 1994a). In the same study, levels of oxytocin were found to be elevated in obsessive-compulsive disorder patients when compared to normal controls, patients with tic-related obsessive-compulsive disorder, or Tourette's patients. The CSF level of oxytocin was correlated with the severity of compulsive and obsessive-compulsive behavior, with the correlation being most apparent in the non-tic-related obsessive-compulsive disorder group. Although these relationships were not seen in an earlier study of children and adolescents with obsessive-compulsive disorder, an inverse relationship between the AVP-oxytocin ratio and measures of obsessive-compulsive disorder symptomatology had been reported (Swedo, Leonard, et al., 1992).

Future Directions

Altered prohormone (prodynorphin) processing has been suggested as a possible explanation for the apparent discrepancy between the brain and CSF dynorphin data, but expanded CSF and brain studies are needed before definitive statements can be made concerning the dynorphin family of peptides in Tourette's. The virtual lack of neurochemical and neuro-endocrine research in Tourette's concerning met-enkephalin and β-endorphin indicates a pressing need for studies on these other two important opioid neuropeptides. Further studies examining CSF oxytocin levels in obsessive-compulsive disorder and tic-related obsessive-compulsive disorder are necessary to replicate the basic finding of an elevation in obsessive-compulsive disorder. More specifically, an examination of the diurnal rhythm for oxytocin in patients and controls would be of interest given the possibility of phase shifting. Other approaches to the oxytocin and AVP systems such as genetic, neuroimaging, postmortem studies as well as pharmacological and neuroendocrine challenge studies may also provide useful data.

CONCLUSIONS

There are several potentially important findings derived from preliminary postmortem, in vivo neuroimaging, CSF, and peripheral neurochemical studies. Although most of these leads need to be confirmed and better characterized, it seems likely that central monoaminergic systems may play an important role in the pathobiology of Tourette's and related disorders. Future neurochemical research might most fruitfully concentrate on examination of postmortem brain tissue and in vivo neuroimaging studies using ligand-based and magnetic resonance spectroscopy techniques. Continuous sampling of CSF over the course of a day may also clarify some of the earlier results. Preliminary postmortem and imaging findings, as well as the CSF results, can serve to guide these studies.

Basic advances in systems in neuroscience and neuropharmacology will enhance the ability of the neurochemical and neuroendocrine approaches to assess central transmitter function in Tourette's. For example, clarification of the normal functional role of the ascending monoaminergic systems should illuminate aspects of the natural history of Tourette's. An increasing recognition of the complexity of the clinical phenomena and the importance of careful subject characterization will improve the power of future studies. These factors, particularly when coupled with the genotyping of relevant alleles, should lead to significant advances in our understanding of the etiology and pathophysiology of Tourette's syndrome.

SUMMARY OF CHAPTER 14

Investigations into the etiology and pathophysiology of Tourette's and related forms of obsessive-compulsive disorder have included research in the areas of psychopharmacology, neuropsychology, genetics, and neurochemistry. There has been increasing overlap among these approaches as they have focused on central processes and systems that might be altered in patients with Tourette's. Undertaken in an attempt to assess the functioning of specific central neurotransmitter systems in Tourette's, the neurochemical research can be defined as those studies involving chemical analyses of postmortem brain tissue, ligand- and spectroscopy-based neuroimaging studies, as well as studies utilizing cerebrospinal fluid, plasma, platelets, and urine. As reviewed in Chapters 9 and 13, increased knowledge of basal ganglia pathways, especially elucidation of their role in the modulation of cortico-striato-thalamo-cortical circuits, has led to a number of testable hypotheses concerning possible neurotransmitter abnormalities in Tourette's syndrome.

PREVIEW OF CHAPTER 15

Having completed a review of the various elements that likely contribute to the pathogenesis of Tourette's and related disorders in Section Two, we move on to consider approaches to treatment and prevention. This first chapter of Section Three describes the approach to care taken by the clinical teams at the Tic and Obsessive-Compulsive Disorder Specialty Clinics at the Yale Child Study Center. The underlying principles of care that have evolved over the past two decades are highlighted, and specific guidelines for assessment and treatment are provided.

SECTION THREE

Partnerships for Making the Best of Tourette's

In practice this [evaluation and treatment] requires an understanding of and an appreciation for the biological and psychological developmental transformations and reorganizations that occur over time . . . an analysis and appropriate weighting of the risk and protective factors and mechanisms operating in the individual and his or her environment throughout the life course.

—Dante Cicchetti and Donald J. Cohen, 1995

CHAPTER 15

Yale Approach to Assessment and Treatment

JAMES F. LECKMAN, ROBERT A. KING, LAWRENCE SCAHILL,
DIANE FINDLEY, SHARON I. ORT, and DONALD J. COHEN

> Assessment refers to gathering data with which to identify the distinguishing features of individual cases.
>
> —*Thomas Achenbach, 1995*

> Tourette's syndrome illuminates the need to see the child as a growing, differentiating whole person, a psychosomatic entity, living in the complex environment of home and family, not just the bearer of symptoms in need of elimination. In the treatment of Tourette's syndrome, our primary focus must be on the individual child's navigation through the normal tasks of development.
>
> —*Donald J. Cohen, Jill Detlor, Bennett Shaywitz,*
> *and James F. Leckman, 1982*

The challenge of a thorough clinical assessment and long-term case management is the coordination of a multidisciplinary team that is informed by the latest scientific knowledge, yet sensitive to the needs and priorities of the patient and family. In this chapter, we discuss the principles that have guided our assessments and treatment recommendations over the past two decades. Figure 15.1 depicts the key elements of this approach.

A HOLISTIC PERSPECTIVE

Tics, obsessive-compulsive symptoms, and other concerns that threaten a sense of well-being are only a part of a larger story. The larger context includes the family's and patient's strengths and vulnerabilities, their

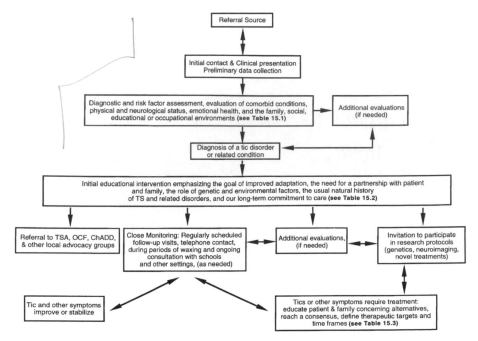

Figure 15.1   Yale approach to care. This flowchart provides a summary of the Yale approach to the evaluation and care of patients with Tourette's syndrome, obsessive-compulsive disorder, and related conditions.

personal histories and life circumstances. Typically, we begin our evaluation sessions by acknowledging this larger context and discussing in a positive tone the interests and accomplishments of the identified patient. This inquiry is informed by materials prepared and sent in by the family prior to the evaluation (see Appendices 1 and 2). Depending on the age of the individual, this exchange will frequently touch on hobbies, sports, special talents, and other areas of expertise and enthusiasm. We are looking for strengths and signs of resilience: What aspects of the patient's life are "on course" and seen in a positive light? Our objective is to start the consultation on a positive note and to establish the perspective that, whatever the realities are about the tics and other vulnerabilities, there are circumstances and potentialities in the patient's life that have a positive valence. Whether these aspects are formally viewed as protective factors or simply as areas where a person's life is proceeding normally, they point toward a shared goal of discovering and sustaining pathways to competence.

PARTNERSHIPS TOWARD A COMMON GOAL

In our experience, it is important that the family comes to feel positive regard from the treating professionals. Tics and other symptoms that frequently accompany Tourette's syndrome are almost always a threat to self-esteem that can jeopardize the daily interaction with parents and peers or challenge the order and decorum of the classroom. In the midst of this distress, it is easy for patients and families to blame themselves or at least to harbor doubts about their attitudes or conduct. It is best to be respectful of the patient's and family's attempts to deal with the unwanted tics—to acknowledge their anger and confusion and offer them reassuring, but true, stories of other patients and families whose lives and development were not permanently damaged by these disorders. The task is not to blame anyone or to examine too closely the mistakes of the past, but to idealize the patient, the family's struggle, and their future. A large measure of respect is conferred as the family realizes that the clinicians involved are willing to make a long-term commitment to their care and that their feelings and values matter. This is easier with some families than others.

Another aspect of this partnership is the expectation on the part of the clinicians that the patient and families learn as much as they would like or are able about these conditions so that when they participate in decision making, they are well-informed. Practically at the outset of the consultation, we invite patients and families to frame the question or questions that they would like to have answered. This request might be posed as follows: "We have a few hours today. Are there particular questions that you would like us to focus on during our time together?" The outcome of this exercise is never quite the same. Fears emerge, stated or unstated. Despite our prior written or telephone contacts, the family's anxiety level is usually high. Family roles and tensions are revealed as someone takes the lead. After hearing from one or more family members, we ask each person present the same question. In a brief period, we often gain an understanding of what the family collectively knows about these conditions and how the symptoms are regarded in the family. We also learn directly, by the explicit questions asked, how they perceive we can be helpful to them. We take these initial questions seriously and endeavor to return to them before the session concludes. This initial approach is an invitation to collaborate from a position of mutual respect as we begin to investigate the family's and the individual's functioning in the context of developmental expectations and environmental influences.

KEY ELEMENTS IN THE EVALUATION

Table 15.1 presents an outline of clinically relevant areas that should be assessed in patients presenting with a tic disorder or a potentially related form of illness. One goal of the initial assessment consultation is to determine the individual's overall level of adaptive functioning and to identify areas of impairment and distress. Relevant dimensions include the natural history of tic and obsessive-compulsive symptoms; comorbid mental, behavioral, developmental, or physical disorders; history of important life

TABLE 15.1   Clinical Evaluation of Tic Disorders and Closely Related Conditions

Tics: Anatomic location and symmetry, number, frequency, intensity, complexity, degree of interference (family and clinician ratings of current and worst-ever severity).

    Onset: Age, characteristics (sudden, gradual, associated with stressful life events, infections [particularly recurrent streptococcal infections]).

    Course: Boutlike occurrence, waxing or waning course, and changing repertoire (most occurring in the eyes, face, head, and shoulders); tic complexity likely to increase with increasing age; momentary suppressibility, reduction during fine motor or vocal tasks that require mental effort, marked diminution during sleep, and usual improvement during the second half of the second decade of life; intramorbid factors associated with worsening or improvement (stress, fatigue, recent infections); current treatment regimen; history of response to medications (efficacy, side effects, adequacy of trials); history of other interventions.

    Associated Perceptual Phenomena and Disinhibited Behavior: Premonitory sensory urges, mental tics, site sensitization, trigger stimuli; socially inappropriate urges or behaviors (calling out in libraries or other quiet public places, urges to do prohibited actions).

    Comorbidity: Obsessive-compulsive symptoms; attention-deficit/hyperactivity disorder; mood and anxiety disorders.

    Impairment: Impact on self-esteem, family function, social acceptance, educational or job performance; risk of physical injury to self or others.

Obsessive-Compulsive Symptoms and Behaviors: Range of obsessive worries and thoughts with aggressive, sexual or religious content; need for symmetry or exactness; a need for things to look, feel, or sound "just right"; contamination fears; thoughts about saving or hoarding; simple compulsive rituals ("evening-up," ordering behaviors); full-fledged obsessive-compulsive disorder (time-consuming ego-dystonic obsessive thoughts and compulsive rituals that are "resisted" and interfere with normal cognitive function); pathological doubting; family and clinician ratings of current and worst-ever severity and assessment of obsessive-compulsive symptom dimensions.

    Onset: Age, characteristics (associated with recurrent streptococcal infections, associated with the onset of puberty, recent moves, separations or losses).

    Course: Time spent and types of obsessions and compulsions; level of autonomic arousal and anxiety; level of control and resistance; perceived distress if prevented from performing compulsions; role of environmental cues and avoidance behaviors; progression from ego-neutral to ego-dystonic compulsions; changing repertoire of obsessions and compulsions; intramorbid factors associated with worsening or improvement (stress, fatigue, recent infections); current treatment regimen; history of response to cognitive behavioral interventions, medications (efficacy, side effects, adequacy of trials); history of other interventions.

    Comorbidity: Depression and other mood and anxiety disorders; obsessive-compulsive personality; schizophrenia; developmental disorders (autism, Asperger's syndrome, Prader-Willi syndrome).

    Impairment: Impact on self-esteem; subjective distress; pervasive slowness and getting stuck in routine behaviors; impact on family function (level of involvement of the family in the performance of compulsions); effect on social adaptation, educational or job performance; risk of physical injury to self or others.

Attention-Deficit/Hyperactivity Disorder: Distractibility and impulsive behavior; poor sustained attention, motoric hyperactivity and fidgetiness; associated disruptive behaviors; need for multiple sources of information, especially teachers and other school personnel.

    Onset: Age, timing (before or after onset of tic syndrome).

TABLE 15.1   (*Continued*)

> **Course:** Context dependence: settings where these difficulties are less apparent versus settings of greatest difficulty; history of tutoring and other special educational services; current treatment regimen; history of response to stimulants (efficacy, side effects, adequacy of trials); history of other nonsomatic interventions.
>
> **Comorbidity:** Oppositional defiant disorder, conduct disorder, and substance abuse disorders; specific learning disabilities; depression and other mood and anxiety disorders; developmental disorders (Fragile X syndrome and other mental retardation syndromes).
>
> **Impairment:** Impact on self-esteem; impact on family function, especially difficulties with siblings; effect on peer relationships; school underachievement; job performance.

Prenatal and Birth History: Prenatal events (severe nausea and vomiting, maternal emotional stress during pregnancy, history of smoking and alcohol use, other drug and hormonal exposures); birth history (hypoxic episodes, prolonged labor, use of forceps).

Developmental, Neurologic, and Pediatric Histories: Developmental delays; exposure to toxins (lead); medication exposures; infectious diseases (streptococcal pharyngitis and other infections such as varicella, rheumatic fever, rheumatic carditis, and Sydenham's chorea); head injuries; seizures; asthma; allergies; migraine; disorders of arousal (night terrors, sleep walking).

Comorbid Developmental, Behavioral, Emotional, Personality, or Substance Abuse Problems: Presence of pervasive developmental disorders (autism, Asperger's syndrome, and PDD not otherwise specified), specific developmental disorders, mood liability and increased irritability, major depression, bipolar disorder, anxiety disorders (panic disorder, phobias including social and agoraphobia, generalized anxiety disorders), perfectionism and other obsessive-compulsive personality traits, other personality disorders, any history of substance abuse.

Family and Social Environment, Stress, and Adaptive Function: Premorbid history; family environment—stability of family life, coping skills, and social supports; relationship of life events (major losses or moves, changes in family circumstances) to onset and exacerbations of symptoms; current adjustment (patient's general knowledge and attitude toward tics, obsessive-compulsive symptoms, and problems with impulsivity and attention, willingness to teach others about symptoms, and the level of understanding and acceptance of the symptoms by close family members); existence of close and lasting friendships; marital status.

School Status: Cognitive level, special talents or gifts, specific learning problems, adequacy of placement, level of understanding and acceptance of the symptoms by school personnel and classmates.

Employment Status: Current occupation, job difficulties associated with tic behaviors or related phenomena, adequacy of placement given patient's native abilities, level of understanding and acceptance of the symptoms by employer and coworkers.

Family History of Developmental, Autoimmune, Behavioral, and Emotional Disorders: Review of family pedigree with regard to tics, Sydenham's chorea, other movement disorders; rheumatic fever; attentional problems and hyperactivity; learning problems; developmental disorders; obsessive-compulsive behaviors; personality disorders; major depression and other mood and anxiety disorders; schizophrenia; alcoholism and other substance abuse disorders.

Neuropsychological Assessment: Estimate of cognitive ability, visual-motor integration.

Continued

TABLE 15.1   *(Continued)*

Physical and Neurological Evaluations: Health history; evidence of recent physical examinations throat culture and titers for antistreptolysin O and antiDNase B (if requested); presence of soft, nonlocalizing neurological signs; consider more extensive workup (EEG and structural MRI scan) in atypical cases (negative family history, positive seizure history, history of severe hypoxia, head trauma, marked symptom severity, atypical pattern of response to medication).

Awareness of and Relationship to Advocacy Organizations: How aware is the patient and family of the existence of national and local advocacy organizations such as the Tourette Syndrome Association (TSA), Obsessive Compulsive Foundation (OCF), and the Children and Adults with Attention Deficit Disorder (ChADD).

Source: Adapted from Leckman et al. (1988).

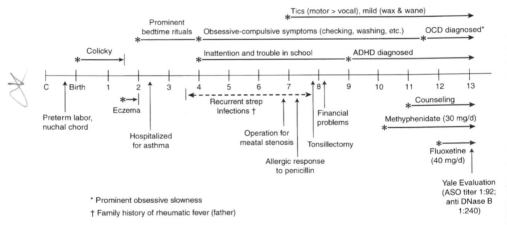

Figure 15.2a   This figure (case #4001) depicts the natural history of a 13-year-old boy diagnosed with attention-deficit/hyperactivity disorder at 9 years of age and obsessive-compulsive disorder at 11 years of age. His most troublesome symptom at present is marked obsessional slowness. This slowness and his difficulty in making transitions are having their most devastating effects in school. His strengths include a positive attitude, an above-average IQ, a strong support system (parents, peers, and teachers), a talent in art, and good athletic skills. A worrisome feature in the natural history of his tic and obsessive-compulsive symptoms is the recurrent streptococcal pharyngitis from 3 to 8 years of age. Taken with the family's clear history of rheumatic fever and chronic tic disorders (see Figure 15.3a), some autoimmune process may be at work in this case. Despite the tonsillectomy, his recent serum titers suggest that exposure to streptococcal antigens is continuing. Management of this case will be complicated by his allergy to penicillin. At present, the workup continues, with a volumetric MRI scheduled and work in the laboratory to determine if there are specific antibodies in his sera that are immunoreactive to proteins in the basal ganglia regions.

events; family history of psychiatric and/or neurological disease; relationships with family and peers; school and/or occupational performance; physical and neurological examination; and awareness of and relationship to potentially useful advocacy organizations.

In this section, we review each of these domains in turn. We also refer specifically to clinician rating instruments in use in the Yale Clinic. In addition, we have found that creating a time line can be enormously helpful in the course of the initial evaluation. This time line is used to mark major medical and life events as well as prior assessments and treatment trials (Figures 15.2a and 15.2b).

Tics

As noted in Chapter 2, it is important to document the current and worst-ever tic severity. We have developed a set of psychometrically sound clinician- and family-rated scales of tic severity that focus on the nature of the tics as well as their anatomic location, number, frequency, intensity, complexity, and degree of interference (D. Cohen, Leckman, & Shaywitz, 1984; Leckman et al., 1989). As discussed in Chapter 16, the Yale Global Tic Severity Scale (YGTSS) and the Tourette Syndrome Symptom List–Revised (TSSR) are currently the instruments in use at the Center.

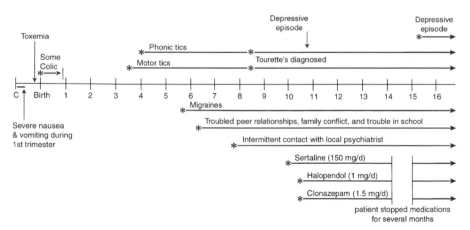

Figure 15.2b   This figure (case #4005) depicts the natural history of a 16-year-old adolescent boy diagnosed with Tourette's syndrome at 8 years of age. His tic symptoms began at 3.5 years of age. His tics remain quite noticeable. In many respects, his story is a classic one, with a positive family history of Tourette's syndrome (his father, see Figure 15.3b) and clear prenatal risk factors (severe nausea and vomiting in the first trimester of gestation and toxemia prior to delivery). His strengths include a supportive and knowledgeable family (his father is a physician) and an IQ in the superior range. This young man remained with his parents throughout the evaluation, wanting to know as much as they did about pathogenesis and prognosis. A good deal of time was focused on the school setting and the need to develop an alternative placement and what might be done to best prepare for college.

These ratings have proven useful in monitoring the waxing and waning course of the disease and are invaluable during open and double-blind clinical trials. A family-rated version of the YGTSS is included in Appendix 1 as part of our Tourette's Syndrome–Obsessive-Compulsive (TS-OC) questionnaire. Documenting the ages and circumstances of motor and phonic tic onset on the time line mentioned above may point to the involvement of specific risk factors. For example, the precipitous onset of severe tics in the wake of a streptococcal pharyngitis may suggest that postinfectious autoimmune mechanisms are involved.

We have found it helpful to inquire about the bout-like occurrence of tics, the changeable nature of an individual's tic repertoire, and its waxing and waning course. It usually takes patients and families some time to appreciate fully these near-universal features of tics, yet being aware of these characteristics can help families sustain their hopefulness in the dreadful hours when bouts-of-bouts of tics are virtually nonstop. It is also important to note the usual fluctuations in tic severity over the course of a day. For example, children frequently report that their tics are much worse at home compared to in the classroom. Although families are usually well aware of the marked reduction of tics during sleep, they may be less aware of the reductions that typically accompany fine motor and vocal tasks that simultaneously require mental effort. The unconscious or conscious suppressibility of tics is often a source of confusion for families and teachers that can lead to conflict and recrimination. Thus, the issues of tic suppression and control are well worth a brief discussion. Similarly, many patients and families report that tics worsen usually during periods of increased stress, emotional excitement, and fatigue. These observations should be confirmed; if no spontaneous comment is made, a direct inquiry may be required. Indeed, many of these features are so characteristic of tics that their absence would cast doubt on the validity of the diagnosis and prompt a more extensive evaluation.

It is important to document any ongoing or prior treatments. A patient's history of response to the usual therapeutic agents, such as haloperidol, pimozide, risperidone, and clonidine, should be noted along with the adequacy of the trials in terms of dosage and duration. We typically collect this information as part of our initial TS-OC questionnaire and include it on the patient's time line.

Associated Perceptual Phenomena and Disinhibited Behaviors

This area is reviewed in Chapter 2. It is rare for these symptoms to be spontaneously reported. The premonitory urges are hypothesized to reflect a heightened sensitivity to internal somatosensory cues (Bliss, 1980; A. Cohen & Leckman, 1992; Leckman, Walker, et al., 1993). They are described as insistent and nearly irresistible urges that are only relieved with the performance of a particular tic or set of tics. On many occasions, patients have expressed surprise on being asked about these internal signals, as they have never before spoken of or tried to describe these feelings. We have found a full exploration of these phenomena is often helpful to the patient and family, as it provides a compelling explanation concerning why a particular tic is performed in a particular fashion at a particular moment. It is also important to recall that children younger than 10, unless they are unusually precocious, are unlikely to be aware of these urges. Given the elusive nature of these urges and the difficulties associated with putting the experience into words, a focused inquiry about these symptoms has the added benefit of enhancing the credibility of the clinician in the eyes of the patient and family. Practically, this information is included in the TS-OC questionnaire. We review this information prior to the family's first visit and make further inquiries during the formal clinical consultation.

The clinical interview surveys other perceptually mediated phenomena, such as site sensitization, trigger phenomena, and disinhibition. Each of these refers to a heightened sensitivity to external sensory stimuli. In the case of site sensitization, patients report the need to remove tags and labels from clothing and to avoid restrictive articles of clothing such as neckties, tight belts, and socks because of the discomfort and heightened sensitivity they produce. Some older patients report that certain sounds will trigger a bout of tics; hearing a certain word or a particularly irritating sound may unaccountably prompt an outburst of tics. Disinhibition usually occurs in the context of specific prohibitions. Signs such as "Quiet Please" or "Danger, Do Not Touch, High Voltage" are common cues that prompt patients to do the proscribed behavior. Other common examples include the urge to touch hot or sharp objects or to shout out racial slurs or other socially inappropriate remarks about someone's appearance or ethnic background.

On occasion, some patients are able to trace the origin of particular complex tics to particular movements, sounds, or events that they had witnessed and were instantly urged to reproduce: a strange laugh, an odd pointing gesture, or a peculiar grimace. All of this directs our attention to the fundamental importance of sensorimotor learning in Tourette's syndrome and the hope that efforts to understand the way in which perceptual phenomena normally sculpt the acquisition of adaptive behavioral routines will lead to a deeper understanding of this disorder.

Impairment

Another key area of assessment is determining the level of impairment across the dimensions of self-esteem, family functioning, social adaptation, and educational and job performance. This forms a routine part of the severity ratings included in the YGTSS (Appendix 1). For some patients, the insistent premonitory urges are more impairing than the tics. Many other historical and context-dependent variables need to be considered in judging impairment. For example, the level of understanding and acceptance that the patient currently encounters, and has encountered during his or her lifetime, in the various social, educational, and community settings is often a crucial factor. Indeed, although the nature, frequency, and forcefulness of the tics are important, the patient's and family's emotional responses to the tics are crucial determinants of the patient's level of impairment.

Obsessive-Compulsive Symptoms and Behaviors

Documenting the current and past history of obsessive-compulsive symptoms is a routine part of the clinical interview. Once it is clear that true obsessions and compulsions form part of the clinical presentation, the types, frequency, and intensity of current and past symptoms are noted. We and others have developed a set of psychometrically sound clinician- and family-rated scales of obsessive-compulsive symptom severity that focus on the nature of the symptoms as well as other indices of severity, including the time occupied by these symptoms, the degree of interference and distress associated with them, how actively the patient resists, and the degree of control the patient has over the symptoms (Berg, Whitaker, Davies, Flament, & Rapoport, 1988; J. Cooper, 1970; Goodman, Price, Rasmussen, Mazure, et al., 1989; Goodman, Price, Rasmussen, Mazure, Delgado, et al., 1989; Scahill et al., 1997). A family-rated version of the Yale-Brown Obsessive-Compulsive Scale (Y-BOCS), developed by Wayne Goodman and his colleagues here at Yale and Steven Rasmussen at Brown University and used in our clinic, is included in Appendix 1. This version of the Y-BOCS is based in part on modifications made by ourselves and Rosenfeld and his colleagues (1992).

In addition to composite ratings of severity, several specific areas of symptomatology warrant careful exploration (Baer et al., 1994; Leckman, Grice, et al., 1997), including the presence and severity of aggressive, sexual, somatic, and religious obsessions and related checking compulsions. This set of symptoms usually involves some element of harm avoidance and is a frequent concomitant of obsessive-compulsive symptoms seen in conjunction with chronic tics. A second dimension includes compulsions of ordering, arranging, doing, and redoing, and counting and related obsessional worries concerning symmetry, exactness, and the need for things to look, feel, or sound just right. This category is also commonly associated with Tourette's syndrome. A third dimension is restricted to contamination fears and washing and cleaning compulsions, and a fourth category includes obsessions and compulsions related to hoarding. At a practical level, we invite the patient and family to document any of these symptoms on a 58-item checklist that forms a part of our TS-OC questionnaire.

In some cases, certain compulsive behaviors can appear quite tic-like. For example, complex touching rituals may be performed in a tic-like fashion or repeated a certain number of times to prevent some feared event. In some of these instances, it may be more important simply to note these symptoms rather than to struggle over their proper classification, as the boundary between complex tics and compulsions can be indistinct. Another particularly troublesome obsessive-compulsive symptom concerns the emergence of a pervasive slowness in which the patient has difficulty starting or finishing tasks; in extreme cases, patients can become stuck for hours in the midst of a routine task such as bathing, dressing, eating, and speaking. Finally, children with co-occurring pervasive developmental disorders may exhibit repetitive behaviors and time-consuming preoccupations; however, these symptoms are generally not distressing to the patient.

In contrast to the ratings of overt tic symptoms, the assessment of obsessive-compulsive symptoms has several problematic aspects, not the least of which is their subjective nature and their distressing and often embarrassing content. Indeed, for many patients, it is only after their symptoms begin to improve that they are able to reveal the full extent of their obsessive-compulsive preoccupations. This means, in part, that initial ratings of severity must be seen as provisional and in need of reexamination as the clinicians gain the trust and confidence of the patient (Scahill et al., 1997). Despite this limitation, periodic severity ratings are useful in monitoring the course of obsessive-compulsive symptoms and are invaluable during open and double-blind clinical trials.

Documenting on a time line the ages and circumstances of the onset of obsessions and compulsions can be revealing (Figures 15.2a and 15.2b). Intriguingly, many children will report the presence of compulsions well before the onset of obsessional worries. The inquiry should include possible precipitants of obsessive-compulsive symptoms such as separations, geographical moves, or the illness or loss of a close family member, as well as any relationship to the occurrence of infections or hormonal changes, such as the onset of puberty.

Another essential feature of obsessive-compulsive symptomatology is the setting in which the obsessions and compulsions occur. Commonly, this condition is most noticeable in the home environment. Issues touching on the safety and security of the home and close family members are often explicit features of the symptoms and offer a clinically useful evolutionary perspective of the disorder (Leckman & Mayes, in press). This feature may also relate to the heightened sense of responsibility that Rachman (1993) has emphasized.

It may also be of interest to elicit a history concerning the normal period of heightened obsessive-compulsive-like symptoms that typically begin at 2 years of age or earlier (Evans et al., 1997). This is when children develop certain strongly held, but usually transient, preferences for certain foods and articles of apparel, for example, a certain cap that needs to be worn in a certain way every day. This is also the time when bedtime rituals become elaborated, as a joint enterprise of parents and children. Although such histories are commonplace among younger children, empirical studies have yet to clarify whether there are any features of these normal behaviors that carry prognostic significance for the later development of obsessive-compulsive disorder.

Perceptual Cues and Avoidance Behaviors

This area is reviewed in Chapter 3. It is not uncommon for obsessive-compulsive symptoms to be prompted by some perceptual cues, which roughly fall into two categories: known stimuli that regularly prompt obsessive worries or compulsive behaviors (Scahill, Vitulano, Brenner, Lynch, & King, 1996; Woods et al., 1996) and unexpected cues of something in the environment not being just right (Leckman, Grice, et al., 1995; Leckman, Walker, et al., 1994). Perceptual cues of the first sort frequently are associated with deliberate avoidance behaviors, for example, avoiding contact with certain substances, animals, or people or avoiding certain rooms or locations that have become conditioned stimuli for specific obsessive-compulsive symptoms. Actual, or even possible, contact may lead to specific washing or decontamination rituals. Such behaviors can be a source of bewilderment and frustration when other family members fail to comprehend or assist the patient in the avoidance maneuvers. Parental participation in avoidance behaviors or decontamination procedures appears to be common in childhood-onset obsessive-compulsive disorder and serves as a marker of severity (Riddle et al., 1990; Scahill et al., 1996).

Perceptual cues of the unexpected sort, for example, noticing that something does not look right in its position or alignment, can prompt time-consuming bouts of adjusting and readjusting, suffused with doubt and anxiety, as if something dreadful will occur if such remedial actions are not undertaken. As with premonitory urges, we have found a full exploration of this phenomenon is often helpful to the patient and family, as it provides a credible explanation concerning certain otherwise inexplicable behaviors. Practically, some of this information is included in our TS-OC questionnaire.

Impairment

As with tic disorders, another key area of assessment involves determining the level of impairment across the dimensions of self-esteem, family functioning, social adaptation, and educational and job performance. The nature, frequency, and distress caused by the obsessions and compulsions are important determinants of impairment, as is the level of understanding and acceptance that the patient has encountered. Although not all patients with a chronic tic disorder have obsessive-compulsive disorder, most patients exhibit some degree of vulnerability in this area. Many may have clear obsessions or compulsions but fall short of the prevailing impairment or severity criteria.

Attention-Deficit/Hyperactivity Disorder

As reviewed in Chapter 4, another common feature of the clinical presentation in our clinic is comorbid ADHD. Often, the most prominent symptoms are distractibility and impulsive behavior. These symptoms can blend readily with tic symptoms, making it difficult to disentangle what is due to a tic disorder from the hyperactivity per se. The situation is further complicated by the possible presence of premonitory urges and obsessional worries, either of which could compound any preexisting distractibility.

As the behaviors associated with ADHD are usually context-dependent, it is essential that information is gathered from multiple sources, especially teachers and other school personnel. It is usually informative to contrast current severity with the worst-ever period of symptom severity. As discussed in Chapters 4, 5, and 17, a number of useful and well-established parent and teacher ratings are available (Conners, 1969; DuPaul & Barkley, 1990; DuPaul, Barkley, & McMurray, 1994). Laboratory-based measures of sustained attention can also be a valuable adjunct. We typically collect information relevant to ADHD using semistructured interviews as well as parent and teacher reports. In ideal circumstances, all of these data have been reviewed prior to sitting down with the family.

Onset and Course

Parents will frequently report that their children with ADHD have always been hyper and difficult to manage. Clinically, inattention often leads to daydreaming and difficulties completing tasks that require a sustained effort. As their attention wanders, they often give parents and teachers the impression that they are not listening. The impulsivity and fidgetiness can lead to disruptions in the classroom, confrontations on the playground, accidents and injury. Combined, these symptoms frequently result in underachievement at school, impaired interpersonal relationships, chronic frustration, and lowered self-esteem. In adolescence, symptoms of hyperactivity and impulsivity may diminish in a minority of cases, but the majority of these adolescents remain at high risk for lower self-esteem; poor relationships with parents, siblings, and peers; conflict with teachers and others in positions of authority; delinquency; and smoking and substance abuse.

Noting on the patient's time line when the parents first became aware of these problems is useful (Figures 15.2a and 15.2b). It is important to document any history of tutoring and other special educational services as well as any ongoing or prior treatments. Treatment history including medication trials are important to document; of particular interest is the patient's response to stimulant medications if such trials have been undertaken in the past.

Oppositional defiant disorder, conduct disorder, substance abuse disorders, dyslexia and other specific learning disabilities, and depression and other mood and anxiety disorders frequently co-occur with ADHD (Biederman et al., 1992). As noted in Chapter 4, this comorbidity has been documented in both unselected population-based samples as well as referred study populations.

Impairment

Symptoms of ADHD and their effect on school performance and peer acceptance can have a major adverse impact on self-esteem and can restrict academic and occupational options. Marital discord, family dysfunction, and parental depression can be compounded by these symptoms as well as foster their development (Barkley, 1990; Biederman, Faraone, et al., 1995).

Prenatal and Birth History

Although the mechanisms are not well understood, evidence suggests that some prenatal events may have a profound influence on the later course of tic disorders and related conditions. These data are reviewed in detail in Chapter 12. Specific features that have been implicated include nutritional status, severe nausea and vomiting during the first trimester, severe maternal emotional stress during pregnancy, alcohol and drug use, including cigarettes, as well as hormonal exposures (Leckman & Peterson, 1993; Leckman, Peterson, et al., 1997). Birth complications including hypoxic episodes, evidence of fetal distress, prolonged labor, and the use of forceps have also been implicated. This information is typically collected by parental report or by direct interview in the context of a more complete history of gestation and parturition. A copy of our modified Risk and Protective Factors in Early Development (RPED) instrument appears in Appendix 2. We also ask permission to receive copies of relevant medical records from the obstetrician and the birth hospital. In most instances, the maternal report has proven to be quite accurate.

Developmental, Neurologic, and Pediatric Histories

The RPED instrument also includes sections on the child's developmental history through the first five years of life. A normal developmental course and a benign pediatric history are usual and considered to be a good prognostic indicator. Evidence of developmental delay, mental retardation, severe head trauma, seizures, coma, or other neurological insults complicates the picture and may adversely affect prognosis. In such cases, we often will conduct a more elaborate evaluation that includes a structural MRI, EEG, and formal neurological consultation.

Thanks to the work of Susan Swedo and her colleagues at the National Institutes of Mental Health, we are more aware of the potential role of postinfectious immune processes in the pathogenesis of Tourette's syndrome (Swedo, 1994; Swedo et al., 1998). We record the timing of prior streptococcal infections, their treatment, and the occurrence of any complications. Rheumatic fever, rheumatic carditis, and Sydenham's chorea should be documented and included on the patient's time line. As noted below, if the history is suggestive, we collect serum to titer streptococcal-related antibodies at the time of our initial evaluation. The timing of other major infections, such as varicella (chicken pox), should also be noted.

We pay special attention to our patients' allergic and asthmatic history. Although compelling evidence has not emerged concerning the prognostic significance of these conditions, the attendant stress and chronic use of sympathomimetics and antihistamines may contribute in vulnerable patients to a worsening of tic, obsessive-compulsive, and ADHD problems or interact with pharmacotherapy routines.

Comorbid Developmental, Behavioral, Emotional, Personality, or Substance Abuse Problems

Another important set of prognostic indicators that must be assessed is comorbid developmental, behavioral, emotional, personality, or substance abuse problems. As discussed in Chapter 16, we collect this information using semistructured interviews. For children and adolescents, we are currently using the Schedule for Affective Disorders and Schizophrenia (K-SADS) (J. Kaufman et al., 1997). In the case of adult patients, we use the Structured Clinical Interview for *DSM-IV* (SCID). We are particularly concerned about the presence of a pervasive developmental disorder (autism, Asperger's syndrome, and PDD not otherwise specified), specific developmental disorders, mood lability and increased irritability, major depression, bipolar disorder, anxiety disorders (panic disorder, phobias including social and agoraphobia, and generalized anxiety disorder), perfectionism and other obsessive-compulsive personality traits, other personality disorders, as well as any history of substance abuse. As noted by David Comings and others, it is commonplace to encounter prominent symptoms of depression and anxiety in this population (Comings & Comings, 1987a, 1987b, 1987c, 1987d, 1987e, 1987f, 1987g). In our experience, bipolar disorder can be a particularly troublesome comorbidity and may be associated with a poor prognosis unless adequately treated. Again, we have found it helpful to have some preliminary knowledge of the presence of these disorders, as well as their course and treatment prior to the actual clinical consultation.

Stress and Adaptive Functioning

Levels of stress, emotionality, and individual and family adaptive functioning exert an exacerbating or protective influence on symptom expression and severity. Reciprocally, symptom severity can be an important source of stress and can undermine adaptive functioning. The purpose of measuring life events and individual and family functioning is to evaluate the relationship between these variables and symptom severity.

As reviewed in Chapter 16, this information is collected using a series of self- and family reports supplemented by direct interviews. We currently interview parents to rate the socialization domain of the Vineland Adaptive Behavior Scales (Sparrow et al., 1984). The parental or self-reports include the Family Inventory of Life Events and Changes (McCubbin & Patterson, 1991), the Child Behavior Checklist (Achenbach & Edelbrock, 1978), and Family Environment Scale (Moos & Moos, 1976a, 1976b). It is crucially important to assess the impact of the tic disorder, obsessive-compulsive disorder, or ADHD on these dimensions of adaptive function. We frequently inquire about how things were different prior to onset. It is important to understand the patient's general knowledge and attitude toward tics and obsessive-compulsive symptoms, willingness to teach others about symptoms, and the level of understanding and acceptance of the symptoms by close family members. As in most disorders, an accepting, supportive, and noncritical family and social environment is a positive prognostic sign; the same can be said for the presence of close friendships.

School Status

In addition to collecting the teacher ratings noted above, we make an effort to collect school records prior to the initial clinical consultation. If the circumstances warrant and the family gives permission, we make direct contact with school personnel prior to or during the family's first visit. Points to document include the teachers' perceptions of the patient's cognitive level, special talents or gifts, specific learning problems, adequacy of placement, level of understanding, and acceptance of the symptoms by school personnel and classmates. These issues are discussed in greater detail in Chapters 17 and 19.

Employment Status

In the case of adolescent and adult subjects, we routinely inquire about current occupation, job difficulties associated with tics or related phenomena, adequacy of placement given the patient's native abilities, and the level of understanding and acceptance of the symptoms by the employer and coworkers.

Family History of Developmental, Autoimmune, Behavioral, and Emotional Disorders

Another critically important part of the assessment includes a review of the family pedigree with regard to tics, Sydenham's chorea, other movement disorders, rheumatic fever, attentional problems, hyperactivity, learning problems, obsessive-compulsive behaviors, personality disorders, major depression, alcoholism, and anxiety disorders. The acquisition of family genetic data is an important determinant in the classification of subjects and may inform clinical management. For example, in cases where there is an absence of any positive family history of tics or obsessive-compulsive symptoms, we may initiate a more comprehensive neurological evaluation to rule out other causes or occult injuries. Similarly, a positive family history of rheumatic fever or rheumatic carditis may prompt closer monitoring with regard to streptococcal infections.

Practically, we make inquiries concerning a family history of tics, obsessive-compulsive symptoms, and ADHD as part of the TS-OC questionnaire. We also construct a family pedigree. Examples of such family trees are presented in Figures 15.3a and 15.3b.

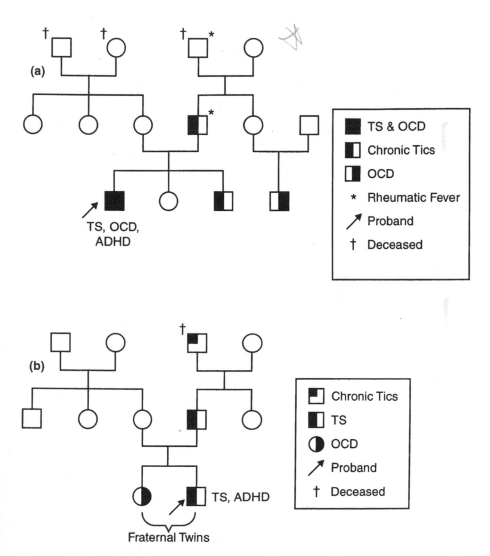

Figures 15.3a and 15.3b Family pedigrees. The two pedigrees presented (a and b) correspond to the two cases briefly presented in Figures 15.2a and 15.2b.

Neuropsychological Assessment

There has been a recent increase in the investigation of neurocognitive functioning among individuals with Tourette's syndrome and obsessive-compulsive disorder (see Chapters 5 and 17). Based on findings that have emerged from these studies, we have selected an experimental battery of tests to provide a detailed characterization of the neuropsychological phenotype. For the most part, we have not included these measures in our routine clinical assessments. The one exception to this is our inclusion of the Beery-Buktenica test of Visual Motor Integration (1989), as a review of the neuropsychological literature suggests that the most consistently observed deficits occur on tasks requiring the accurate copying of geometric designs, that is, visual-motor integration or visual-graphic ability (R. Schultz et al., 1998). We also routinely administer the Kaufman Brief Test of Intelligence (A. Kaufman & Kaufman, 1990) to obtain an estimate of the patient's cognitive abilities.

Physical and Neurological Examinations

In addition to routine physical and neurological examinations, we note the anatomic location of motor tics, as well as any tremors and myoclonic, choreiform, athetotic, dystonic, or dyskinetic movements. As part of the YGTSS, we record the number, frequency, intensity, complexity, and interference of motor and phonic tics. Symptoms of restlessness, incoordination, and difficulty with sustained contractions can accompany postinfectious Sydenham-like presentations, as can apathy, mental confusion, and delusions, in severe cases. Any compulsive rituals, pervasive slowness, or disturbances of inertia are also noted. As part of the physical examination, we also document the patient's Tanner stage.

At present, we do not routinely screen patients using laboratory-based measures. If there is some evidence of a postinfectious process, we will collect a throat culture and titers for streptococcal-related antibodies: anti-streptolysin O (ASO or ASLO) and antiDNase B. These specimens may be collected even if there is no history of pharyngitis or a recent febrile episode, as we have encountered cases where the history and physical examination are negative (Tucker et al., 1996). Elevated ASO titers usually reflect a fairly recent streptococcal infection, whereas the antiDNase B titers can remain elevated for months after the initial infection. In some instances, it has proven valuable to perform a drug screen. We typically do not screen our patients for Wilson's disease unless there is a positive family history of hepatic and neurologic disease.

We do not routinely perform other diagnostic procedures. A decade ago, we ordered EEG on all patients, but the low yield led us to discontinue this practice in most cases. However, any hint of a history of recent seizures or postictal states should prompt an EEG and a neurological consultation. Similarly, we do not recommend in vivo imaging studies for clinical reasons unless the presentation is atypical or the symptoms unusually severe or un-responsive. Other laboratory tests may be ordered in preparation for a clinical trial or long-term monitoring for unwanted physical effects of psychopharmacological agents.

For research purposes, as described in the earlier chapters, we routinely invite families to participate in our genetic studies (by donating DNA by either a blood draw or a brushing the inside of the cheek) and our brain imaging studies.

PRINCIPLES OF CARE

There are certain principles of care that guide our therapeutic endeavors. First is a nearly universal effort to inform the patient and family and other concerned professionals (pediatricians, internists, teachers) about Tourette's syndrome and any related disorders. Given the chronic nature of these disorders, a second principle involves assisting the family to find a long-term treatment setting where continuity of care is possible. A third principle involves making clear to everyone that the goal of treatment is keeping the patient's life on track—not necessarily to be entirely tic- or symptom-free. In selecting a specific form of treatment, a fourth principle consists of reaching a consensus in all interested parties about which symptoms to treat and how. The remaining principles of care include a commitment to involve advocacy organizations and to invite participation in ongoing research projects, when appropriate. Each of these principles is discussed below and highlighted in Tables 15.1 and 15.2.

Education

Tic and obsessive-compulsive symptoms are often frightening and can con-jure dreadful images of the future. Regrettably, families' initial attempts to educate themselves may only serve to reenforce these stereotypes: If he is this bad now, just imagine how awful things will be when he is an adult. In our experience, the more the family knows, the better. Fortunately, much of this knowledge is reassuring: that many children with Tourette's syn-drome do grow up and succeed in life, that the tics usually do get better by early adulthood, and that just because the tics are horrible today does not mean that they will not markedly diminish over the succeeding weeks. What is true for tics is also true for obsessive-compulsive disorder and ADHD. Parents are often the most effective advocates for their children, and it is frequently the case that more can be done in the school setting and at home to ease the burdens associated with these disorders if the families know what to advocate for.

The commitment to provide educational support is not limited to the ini-tial phases of treatment but is a continuing obligation, especially because

TABLE 15.2   Treatment Modalities

Intervention	Circumstances	Focus	For Additional Information
Education concerning the symptoms, natural history, and treatment of Tourette's syndrome, obsessive-compulsive disorder, and ADHD.	Always.	Patient, family, and school personnel, if the patient is a child.	Entire volume, particularly Chapters 2, 3, 4, 9, 12, 15, 17–21.
Supportive psychotherapeutic interventions with regularly scheduled appointments, access by telephone or e-mail, and a commitment to long-term care.	Always, provided that the family is in the same geographic region.	Patient, family, and school personnel, if the patient is a child.	Chapter 18.
Close monitoring without specific treatment.	Symptoms of Tourette's, obsessive-compulsive disorder, and ADHD are not severe enough to warrant cognitive behavioral or pharmacological interventions, or the treatment team is waiting to see what beneficial effects may follow from the initial round of supportive and educational interventions.	Patient, family, and school personnel, if the patient is a child.	Chapters 2, 3, 4, 18.
Specific psychotherapeutic, cognitive-behavioral, or pharmacological treatment.	If tic, obsessive-compulsive, or ADHD symptoms are moderate or severe, or if some other comorbid disorder is present and is of sufficient severity, such as major depression or panic disorder.	Patient, family, and school personnel, if the patient is a child.	See Table 15.3, Chapters 17–20.

the shock that accompanies a diagnosis may make it difficult for some individuals to grasp the available information.

Continuity of Care

During the course of discussing specific treatment recommendations, it is necessary to determine who will be providing the care. It is not unusual for us to offer to follow the patient long term and to provide case management services in an open-ended fashion. This means, among other things, that the family should feel free to contact the clinic at any point to seek consultation and to provide information concerning any changes in the course of the illness. We have followed hundreds of families for more than a decade and highly value such continuity. We are also pleased to serve as consultants to other clinicians engaged in the care of patients and their families.

Optimizing Adaptation and Keeping Development on Track

As emphasized in Chapters 1 and 8, this is our most important principle of clinical care. Although it applies regardless of the patient's age and clinical status, it can be easily lost from view in the crisis of the moment. If families or clinicians get too caught up in the process of counting tics or keeping track of how much time patients lose to their obsessive-compulsive symptoms, this attention to pathology can have adverse effects. Such preoccupations can amplify the traumatic effects of Tourette's syndrome or obsessive-compulsive disorder. The affected family member may begin to consider him- or herself as a Tourette's case rather than a young person with many strengths who is being challenged by unwanted symptoms that are easily misunderstood. We usually encourage families *not* to make decisions based on how bad the tics are at present. Although these disorders are, to some degree, stress-sensitive, it rarely makes things better to remove the children from school or discourage them from pursuing sports or activities that they and their friends enjoy. Indeed, the task is to emphasize the positive. As clinicians, we need to get to know children and families and do what we can, in partnership with them, over the course of years, to foster their normal development despite the challenges posed by Tourette's syndrome. This goodness-of-fit approach means learning about the strengths and weaknesses of the individuals and about the environments in which they live and work. How can we build on their strengths? How can we help them envision their struggle with Tourette's syndrome as an endeavor that will lead them to be stronger and more compassionate adults?

The Role of Comorbid Diagnoses

Our threshold for suggesting specific treatments, including psychopharmacological interventions, is straightforward. If the comorbid ADHD, obsessive-compulsive disorder, or depression are severe, we will frequently encourage treatment of these symptoms first, either with cognitive-behavioral approaches or psychopharmacological agents. If the tics, even at their best, are severe and if the comorbid diagnoses have been adequately addressed, we will focus our interventions on the tics themselves. Having reached this point, we usually make an effort to educate the patient and family concerning the alternatives, including cognitive-behavioral approaches. Unfortunately, we have not had much success with habit reversal or other cognitive-behavioral approaches to Tourette's syndrome, so our interventions are usually psychopharmacological in character. In the beginning,

TABLE 15.3   A Guide to Choosing a Specific Treatment Modality

Intervention	Circumstances	Focus	For Additional Information
Supportive and educational approaches.	Always.	Patient, family, and school personnel, if the patient is a child.	Table 15.2.
Cognitive-behavioral treatments.	Exposure and response prevention: First choice in cases of obsessive-compulsive disorder with a significant anxious or avoidant component. This may be a useful adjunct in other obsessive-compulsive cases (e.g., concerns that things do not look just right), but compelling data are not yet available.	Patient and family.	Chapter 18.
	Habit reversal: Consider in cases of trichotillomania and simple compulsions without an avoidance component; in Tourette's syndrome, consider especially if single tic interferes with daly living; however, compelling efficacy data are not yet available.	Patient and parents.	Chapter 18.
	Parent training, daily report cards, regular teacher consultation, and paraprofessional classroom aide: First choice for moderate to severe ADHD with or without adjunctive medication.	Patient, family, and teachers.	Chapter 19.
Pharmacological treatments.	Symptoms of Tourette's, obsessive-compulsive disorder, and ADHD are severe enough to warrant treatment. Usually not the first choice of treatment for tics. Frequently an adjunctive treatment for obsessive-compulsive disorder or ADHD.	Patient, family, and school personnel if the patient is a child.	Chapter 20.
Patient support groups.	Encourage participation. Warn families that some of the individuals in the support group may have severe tic or obsessive-compulsive symptoms, which may be frightening for some individuals or families.	Patient, siblings, and parents.	Chapters 18 and 21.

TABLE 15.3   (*Continued*)

Intervention	Circumstances	Focus	For Additional Information
Traditional individual or family psychotherapy.	If the family's or the individual's long-term adjustment to the disorders is problematic, consider a trial of psychotherapy. More generally, referrals are made if other individual or family problems are stress producing.	Patient and/or family.	Chapter 18.
Alternative treatments.	Not encouraged, as compelling data are not available to support their use. If family is determined to give one or more treatments a try, encourage them to share the results of the trial with the treatment team.	Patient and family.	Other sources: Word of mouth, Internet chat rooms, and local practitioners.

families are typically grateful for this instruction, but usually expect the clinician, in the end, to make specific recommendations; it is only with time that patients and families become full participants in the decision-making process of determining treatment. As with any treatment trial, being clear about the target symptoms, the time frame, possible side effects, and the need for everyone to be satisfied with the treatment are the usual ingredients for success.

In many clinics, it is still often the case that if a family presents when the tics are severe, the patient stands a good chance of leaving the consulting room with a prescription for a powerful psychotropic medication. This is usually followed by a diminution of symptoms and a positive appraisal of the initial interaction. Unfortunately, this improvement may only be short-lived, or sufficiently problematic unwanted side effects may appear that further complicate the clinical picture. In contrast, in cases where the tics remain suppressed, the patient may remain on these medications for years—often despite serious side effects affecting physical appearance, mental acuity, and subtle shifts in personality and demeanor. Each of these outcomes is troublesome and should be avoided, if at all possible. The greatest difficulty with these medications is how difficult it is to withdraw them, as withdrawal-emergent dyskinesias and tic exacerbations are commonplace.

Although it is a more difficult initial course, patience, education, and reassurance are often the best medicine. The occasional case will continue to be severe, requiring medication, but in many cases, a watch-and-wait strategy works best. It is also the case that giving families something to do in response to the symptoms is helpful. Often, this takes the form of learning more about Tourette's and other comorbid conditions and sharing this knowledge with teachers and other school personnel. Table 15.3 offers some guidance concerning our usual approach to deciding which treatment to recommend. It also notes where additional information can be found in this book concerning each of these treatments.

Advocacy Organizations

Another important aspect of our assessment is to determine the patient's and family's awareness of the existence of national and local advocacy organizations such as the Tourette Syndrome Association (TSA), Obsessive Compulsive Foundation (OCF), and the Children and Adults with Attention Deficit Disorder (ChADD). As described in Chapter 21, these organizations have made an important and positive contribution to the lives of many patients and their families by providing support and information to them. They can also be a valuable outlet for families intent on making a difference, for example, to advance research and raise the general level of awareness among health care professionals, educators, and the public at large.

Integrating Research and Clinical Care

The goal of the research enterprise is to advance knowledge and to improve care. As such, we have found it worthwhile to describe our efforts and to invite most families to join us in this joint endeavor. Learning of the range of studies, families come to feel a part of an important and larger process. The presentation of the results of research studies in the clinical context constitutes a form of direct dissemination of the latest findings. Appeals to families' altruism and their help, either now or in the future, place them in an honored position that may enhance their self-esteem. Of course, there is a need not to burden the families with such requests and to make it clear that the quality of care does not depend on their willingness to assist us in these efforts.

Actual treatments rarely satisfy the hopes of patients or clinicians. The chronicity of Tourette's, obsessive-compulsive disorder, and ADHD means that some accommodation to the presence of unwanted symptoms is a painful necessity. Here the clinician becomes the trusted advisor, modeling for the patient and the family an attitude toward disease that is optimistic, deliberate, and uncowed. We are grateful that in so many instances, the long-term outcomes of our patients allow their initial distress and impairment to recede into the recesses of memory.

SUMMARY OF CHAPTER 15

Tics and obsessive-compulsive symptoms appear in the unfolding of latent strengths and vulnerabilities during the first decades of life. The meaning and impact of these symptoms are conditioned by multiple neurobiological, psychological, social, and environmental factors. This chapter points to some of the dimensions and the distinguishing features of individual cases that need to be considered. The chapter closes with an examination of the principles that have guided our therapeutic interventions. Tables 15.2 and 15.3 briefly summarize the various treatment options that are presently available and indicate where the reader can find additional information concerning these choices.

PREVIEW OF CHAPTER 16

Diagnostic interviews and rating instruments are becoming commonplace in the practice of psychiatry and neurology. These assessment tools are useful in the clinical care of patients with Tourette's syndrome and related disorders and are essential in research studies. This chapter reviews commonly used assessment instruments and offers guidance for selecting rating scales and diagnostic interviews.

CHAPTER 16

Selection and Use of Diagnostic and Clinical Rating Instruments

LAWRENCE SCAHILL, ROBERT A. KING, ROBERT T. SCHULTZ, and
JAMES F. LECKMAN

> Empiricism means the habit of explaining wholes by parts, and rationalism
> means the habit of explaining parts by wholes.
>
> —*William James, 1909*

The importance of valid measuring instruments in psychiatry and neurology is underscored by the considerable increase in the number of interview schedules and rating scales that have been developed over the past 30 to 40 years. Diagnostic and rating instruments are now routinely used in clinical assessment to ensure comprehensive and systematic data collection. In the case of children and adolescents, comprehensive and systematic data collection means gathering data from multiple informants. Rating measures may be used to identify comorbid conditions, quantify the severity of primary symptoms, and organize clinical data for statistical analyses (Costello & Angold, 1988; Jensen, Salzberg, Richters, & Watanabe, 1993; Kazdin, 1989; Rutter, Tuma, & Lann, 1989; Scahill & Ort, 1995). By enhancing the efficiency of data collection, clinical measurement tools can sharpen the focus of the clinical consultation and ensure broad coverage of behavioral problems not specified in the chief complaint. Quantification of symptom severity can also promote clarification of target symptoms that can be monitored over time to evaluate treatment response. Health services research aiming to understand changes in referral patterns and treatment conventions will also be aided by more systematic data collection methods in clinical practice.

The value of reliable and valid quantitative ratings in research is perhaps more firmly established than in clinical practice. For example, demonstrating the effectiveness of a new pharmacologic agent in a clinical trial relies on the measurement of change from baseline. Indeed, most of the early developmental work on diagnostic interviews and rating scales was prompted by the demand for more reliable diagnostic determination and outcome measurement (Conners, 1969; Feighner, Robins, & Guze, 1972; Hamilton, 1959; Rutter, Tizard, & Whitmore, 1970). Structured diagnostic interviews have become standard in epidemiological studies, family genetic studies, and large treatment trials. Despite advances over the past two decades, the need for additional work in this area (especially in pediatric populations) has been emphasized by prestigious commissions (Institute of Medicine, 1989).

There are several types of clinical assessment measures, including diagnostic interviews, semistructured severity ratings, parent and teacher checklists, patient self-reports, family questionnaires, and direct observational tools. The purpose of this chapter is to describe currently available rating instruments for tics, obsessive-compulsive symptoms, and attention-deficit/hyperactivity disorder (ADHD) to guide the selection and use of clinical assessment measures. The last section of the chapter reviews diagnostic interview schedules, general behavior scales, and adaptive functioning.

MEASURES USED IN TIC AND RELATED DISORDERS

There are three methods of estimating tic severity: self-reports (parent reports, in the case of children), clinician-administered ratings, and direct observational methods such as tic counts. Each of these methods has advantages and disadvantages. For example, the validity of self-reports may be threatened by inaccurate information about the nature of tics on the part of the child or parent leading to over- or underendorsement of symptoms. On the other hand, self-reports are efficient and potentially cost-effective. Clinician ratings offer some protection against the problem of over- or underendorsement, but they require time and effort from an experienced clinician to complete. Direct observational methods such as tic counting would appear to be an objective measure of tic severity; however, it has been observed by many clinicians that individuals with Tourette's syndrome may suppress their tics during clinical visits.

Self-Reports of Tic Severity

The Tic Symptom Self-Report (TSSR) is a self-report measure that consists of a checklist of simple and complex motor and phonic tics over the prior week (D. Cohen et al., 1984). The original instrument, called the Tourette's Syndrome Symptom List, asked the patient or a parent to rate a discrete list of simple and complex motor and phonic tics as well as a brief set of behavioral characteristics on a 0 to 5 scale. These items could be rated either daily for seven days or retrospectively over the past week. In a clinical trial with clonidine, the scale showed sensitivity to change, but it was apparently not as sensitive as the clinician-rated measure that was also used in that study (Leckman et al., 1991). The TSSR has also been used to describe the severity of tic symptoms in a clinical series of patients (de Groot, Janus, et al., 1995). Nonetheless, the reliability and validity of the TSSR have not been well studied. Questions about the psychometric properties arise from the somewhat restricted pool of items, the unbalanced set of motor and phonic symptoms, and the inclusion of behavioral symptoms that might be more reliably measured by existing instruments designed for that purpose. These limitations prompted our recent efforts to revise the instrument.

In the recently revised version, the instrument includes a brief definition of tics and asks the subject or parent to rate tic symptoms on a 4-point scale, with 0 being absent and 3 being both frequent and forceful. In most applications, the time reference is the previous week, but in some situations, the form can be completed daily. Preliminary analyses of 50 children with Tourette's syndrome rated by their parents with the TSSR indicate excellent consistency (Cronbach alpha coefficient = 0.88) and respectable correlation with a semistructured clinician measure of tic severity (Pearson $r = 0.60$ for the total score). Also, in our ongoing neuroimaging study, parents of normal control subjects have rarely endorsed tic behaviors in their children, suggesting that the revised TSSR does not result in false positive scores (Scahill, unpublished data).

Clinician-Rated Instruments

The Yale Global Tic Severity Scale (YGTSS) is a clinician-rated, semistructured interview developed by members of the Tic Disorders Clinic at Yale (Leckman et al., 1989). The interview begins with a systematic inquiry of tic symptoms that the clinician rates as present or absent over the past week. Current motor and phonic tics are then rated separately according to number, frequency, intensity, complexity, and interference on a 6-point ordinal scale (0 = absent; 1–5 for severity) yielding three scores: Total Motor, Total Phonic, and Total Tic score. The YGTSS has shown excellent interrater agreement with intraclass correlation coefficients of 0.78, 0.91, and 0.84 for Total Motor, Total Phonic, and Total Tic scores, respectively (Leckman et al.). The structure of the interview ensures an orderly review of motor and phonic tic severity and allows the clinician to observe tics that may not be endorsed by the patient or parent. Because the YGTSS permits the clinician to incorporate direct observation with historical information, it requires both training with the instrument and clinical experience with tic disorders. At present, most investigators consider the YGTSS to be the best available clinician rating of tic severity.

Other clinician-rated scales include the Tourette Syndrome Severity Scale (TSSS; A. Shapiro et al., 1988), Tourette Syndrome Global Scale (TSGS; Harcherik, Leckman, Detlor, & Cohen, 1984), and the Hopkins Motor and Vocal Tic Scale (Hopkins scale; Walkup et al., 1992). Although both the TSSS and TSGS have been used in numerous published reports, both scales have unconventional scoring procedures and unstable psychometric properties. For example, the TSSS combines items with different ranges; the TSGS multiplies tic frequency by degree of disruption that may exaggerate small differences in severity. Indeed, the YGTSS was developed at Yale as a second-generation instrument to redress some of the shortcomings of the TSGS.

The Hopkins scale is a more recently developed instrument that combines self-report data with clinician assessment, resulting in a composite rating. This scale consists of a series of analog scales that are tallied to yield a 1–5 score for motor, phonic, and total. This scale has shown promise as a global measure of tic severity in a preliminary study of 20 children, but has not entered into common use. When compared to other measures of tic severity, the Hopkins scale showed the strongest correlation with the YGTSS (Walkup et al., 1992).

A study group convened by the Tourette Syndrome Association (TSA) has developed and tested a scale called the Unified Tic Rating Scale (UTRS; Kurlan & McDermott, 1993). Like the Hopkins scale, the UTRS includes a historical component and an examiner-rated component that is completed by the clinician. The first version of the scale proved to be cumbersome and did not produce encouraging results with respect to reliability and validity. The revised version has recently been tested and results are pending.

Another approach to blending parent and self-reported information with clinician validation has been adopted by the TSA in the collaborative Affected Sib-Pair Study. In this study, parents are given detailed questionnaires concerning tics, obsessive-compulsive symptoms, and symptoms of ADHD about themselves, the identified patient, and the patient's siblings. The self-report portion of the questionnaire for tic symptoms is based on the YGTSS. These responses are then verified in a follow-up semistructured interview by an experienced clinician. Preliminary analyses of 20 cases in our clinic revealed a high correlation ($r = 0.86$, $p = 0.0001$) between the family self-report and independently measured YGTSS derived by clinical interview. If this correlation were to hold up with larger numbers of Tourette's patients, this self-report with clinician validation may be an effective and efficient way of gathering data on tic symptoms and severity. Additional experience is also needed to determine whether this method is valid in nonclinically ascertained samples and whether it is acceptable to families. A version of this family- (or self-) rated version of the YGTSS is included in Appendix 1.

Direct Observational Methods for Tic Severity

Observational methods include videotaped tic counting procedures (Chappell, McSwiggan-Hardin, et al., 1994; Goetz, Tanner, Wilson, & Shannon, 1987) and in vivo evaluation of tic symptoms (Nolan, Gadow, & Sverd, 1994). The challenge confronting any direct observation method is the tremendous variability of tic symptoms. In addition, the well-known capacity of individuals with Tourette's syndrome to suppress their symptoms for brief periods of time may limit the value of direct observation unless the duration of observation is long, Yet, if the duration of observation is too long, it could present a threat to reliability. Videotaped tic counting methods have demonstrated high levels of interrater reliability and at least moderate correlation with clinician ratings in some studies (Goetz et al., 1987), but in other studies this correlation varied depending on the clinician measure used (Chappell, McSwiggan-Hardin, et al., 1994). Tic counting procedures appear to be most useful for pharmacological challenge studies (Chappell et al., 1993; Riddle et al., 1995); periods of five minutes or more appear to provide a valid and reliable index of tic severity in most cases (Chappell, McSwiggan-Hardin, et al., 1994).

In vivo methods are appealing because the investigator can evaluate the number, frequency, and intensity of tics in natural settings. However, the findings to date are not convincing. The recent report by Nolan and colleagues (1994), in which trained observers assessed tic symptoms in classroom settings, found only modest correlations with the YGTSS subtotal scores (0.33 and 0.31 for motor and phonic tics, respectively). Correlations were slightly better for a subgroup of children with more severe tics. Compared to the classroom, other school settings, such as the lunchroom and the playground, showed ever lower correlations with the YGTSS subscale scores, suggesting that these settings may not be suitable for naturalistic observation. Given the expense of direct classroom observation for tics and the limited return for the effort, classroom observation of tic severity does not appear to be a cost-effective strategy.

MEASURES USED IN OBSESSIVE-COMPULSIVE DISORDER

Self-Reports

Most available self-report measures of obsessive-compulsive disorder are for adults; thus, because of the reading level required and because not all questions can be answered by a parent, they may not be practical for children. In addition, many current measures suffer from undocumented reliability, incomplete coverage of symptom types, or inadequate inclusion of impairment data, making diagnostic determination difficult (Steketee, 1993).

The 20-item Leyton Survey was derived from successive revisions of the original Leyton Obsessional Inventory (Berg et al., 1988; Berg, Rapoport, & Flament, 1986; J. Cooper, 1970). This version of the Leyton consists of 20 yes-no questions which are then rated for level of interference on a 0 to 3 scale. A yes score ≥ 15 or an interference score ≥ 25 were highly predictive of an obsessive-compulsive disorder diagnosis in an epidemiological study of adolescents (Flament et al., 1988). In a recent clinical series of 65 children and adolescents with obsessive-compulsive disorder, the yes score and the interference score were highly intercorrelated, suggesting that the two scores could be combined into a single total. The total score showed a correlation of 0.62 with a clinician measure of obsessive-compulsive severity (Scahill et al., 1997). As one of the few available instruments for which data are available from both community (Flament et al., 1988) and clinical samples (Berg et al., 1988; Riddle, Scahill, et al., 1992; Scahill et al., 1997) in the pediatric age group, the Leyton appears to be a useful self-report measure of obsessive-compulsive symptoms in children and adolescents. It may also be useful for adults as a screening measure, but this has not yet been carefully evaluated. Children below the age of 9 will probably need to have the questions read to them for yes or no response and then will need to be asked about the degree of interference. The chief disadvantage with the Leyton Survey is the restricted range of items; also, the wording of some of the items may be unfamiliar to children.

Clinician-Rated Instruments

The Yale-Brown Obsessive Compulsive Scale (Y-BOCS) is a clinician-rated, semistructured interview for rating the severity of obsessive-compulsive disorder. Each of the 10 items is scored on a 5-point scale from 0 (not present) to 4 (most symptomatic). The CY-BOCS is a slightly modified version of the original instrument that was developed to rate severity of obsessive-compulsive disorder in children and adolescents. The primary difference between the two versions is the symptom checklist, reflecting the slight differences in obsessive-compulsive disorder symptomatology in children and adults. There are no differences with respect to scoring. Thus, both versions yield a total obsession score (0–20), a total compulsion score (0–20), and combined total (0–40).

Considerable data support the reliability and validity of the adult version (Goodman, Price, Rasmussen, Mazure, et al., 1989; Goodman, Price, Rasmussen, Mazure, Delgado, et al., 1989; Kim, Dysken, & Kuskowski, 1990). In the study of Goodman, Price, Rasmussen, Mazure, et al. (1989), the interrater reliability (intraclass correlation coefficient) was 0.97 for obsession subtotal, 0.96 for compulsion subtotal, and 0.98 for the total score. Most investigators consider the Y-BOCS to be the best available instrument for rating obsessive-compulsive symptomatology.

Recent data for the CY-BOCS show respectable intraclass correlation as well: 0.91 for obsession subtotal, 0.66 for compulsion subtotal, and 0.84 for the total score (Scahill et al., 1997). Findings from this investigation strongly suggest that valid assessment of obsessive-compulsive symptom severity in children requires input from parents as well as the child. In addition, clinicians must carefully weigh information provided by parent and child to determine the frequency, interference, and distress caused by compulsive behavior and, to a lesser extent, obsessive thoughts.

Recently, self-report versions of the Y-BOCS have been introduced (Leckman, Grice, et al., 1995; Rosenfeld et al., 1992). Both versions follow the format and scoring of the Y-BOCS. The study by Rosenfeld et al.

collected data with a computerized questionnaire from 31 adults with obsessive-compulsive disorder, 16 adults with other anxiety disorders, and 23 controls. The self-administered Y-BOCS was highly correlated with the clinician-rated Y-BOCS done on the same day (r values were 0.88, 0.87, and 0.86 for the total, obsessions, and compulsions, respectively). Control subjects got equally low scores on both versions of the Y-BOCS. This self- or family-rated version of the Y-BOCS is included in Appendix 1.

Leckman, Grice, and colleagues (1995) evaluated responses on a self-report version of the Y-BOCS provided by 177 obsessive-compulsive disorder patients between the ages of 16 and 72 years. Of these 177 patients, 56 had a chronic tic disorder. The self-report instrument was able to detect a wide range of symptom severity (0–40) with no difference in mean scores between those with and without tic disorders. The group with comorbid tic disorders, however, reported a greater number of obsessive-compulsive symptoms. They were also more likely to report obsessions involving aggressive, sexual, and religious themes as opposed to contamination themes. Those without a history of tics were more likely to endorse cleaning and washing habits. By contrast, those with tic disorders reported more checking, counting, ordering and arranging, and touching than the group without tic symptoms. Similar findings were reported in a previous study of 70 adults with obsessive-compulsive disorder using the clinician-rated version of the Y-BOCS (Holzer et al., 1994). Additional study is needed to see if these trends are also present in children and adolescents with obsessive-compulsive disorder.

The Y-BOCS has also become the foundation for the obsessive-compulsive symptom section of the TSA-sponsored Sib-Pair Study. As with the tic symptom section, the obsessive-compulsive disorder section consists of a self/parent-report instrument that is verified by subsequent clinical interview. Based on the data from Rosenfeld et al. (1992) and Leckman, Grice, et al. (1995), this self-report version of the Y-BOCS ought to perform well for older adolescents and adults who can complete the questionnaire themselves. Younger age groups, however, will probably rely on parent report. Given the private nature of some obsessive-compulsive symptoms, it is uncertain whether parent report alone will provide a satisfactory picture of the child's obsessions and compulsions. Hence, verification of the parent report with the child present by an experienced clinician is an important step in the validation of this self/parent-report instrument in pediatric populations.

Another area of recent interest in evaluating the severity of obsessive-compulsive disorder concerns the organization of the symptoms. The Y-BOCS retains obsessions and compulsions as the conceptual framework, but behavioral therapists have suggested that patients can be classified by symptom cluster—for example, checkers and washers (Foa & Emmelkamp, 1983). Recent factor analyses support the view that obsessive-compulsive symptoms do cluster on certain themes (Baer, 1994; Leckman, Grice, et al., 1997). Both studies used the Y-BOCS checklist. Baer derived a three-factor solution that accounted for 50% of the variance (factor 1: ordering, arranging, counting, hoarding; factor 2: contamination, cleaning, checking; factor 3: sexual and aggressive obsessions). Leckman, Grice, et al. found similar groupings (factor 1: checking; factor 2: need for symmetry, ordering and arranging; factor 3: cleanliness and washing; factor 4: hoarding). These four factors accounted for over 60% of the variance.

Direct Observational Measures

Several versions of behavioral avoidance tests (BAT) have been introduced over the past two decades with some success (Steketee, Chambless, Tran, Worden, & Gills, 1996). These ratings include observable behavior with self-reported anxiety during the performance of assigned tasks. Although these methods have not been employed to any wide extent in pediatric populations, they appear to be a valuable addition to clinical trials in adult subjects. The major drawback of these direct observational measures in OCD is that they are complicated to conduct and score.

MEASURES USED IN ADHD

ADHD is a relatively common disorder affecting an estimated 2–11% of school-age children (Costello, Angold, Burns, Stangl, Tweed, Erkanli, & Worthman, 1996; Jensen et al., 1995; Szatmari et al., 1989). The cause is unknown and available evidence indicates that no single etiology is likely to explain all cases of ADHD (see Chapter 4). Although there is continued controversy concerning whether ADHD is etiologically related to Tourette's syndrome, it is well established that ADHD is a common comorbid condition in clinical samples of Tourette's syndrome (Walkup et al., 1995). In many of these cases, the ADHD may be of greater clinical importance than the tic symptoms. Thus, comprehensive evaluation of children with Tourette's syndrome for either clinical or research purposes should include a review of ADHD symptoms.

Accurate diagnosis and estimation of the severity of ADHD in children and adolescents depend on data from multiple informants, especially parents and teachers. Because the impressions of both parents and teachers are essential in the assessment of ADHD, rating scales are often used to collect data about the child's behavior across settings (Barkley, 1990; Hinshaw, 1994). Parent and teacher checklists may consider a range of behavioral problems or may be focused more narrowly on ADHD. In general, these questionnaires have the advantage of brevity and provide a simple method of obtaining information about the child's behavior in school and home. A number of available rating scales have also shown sensitivity to change and are therefore valuable for assessing response to a medication trial.

Potential problems with these rating scales are that some parents may misunderstand particular items either because of parents' reading level or cultural background. Thus, clinicians may have to verify parental responses on the questionnaire and confirm whether the available norms are relevant to the individual patient or patient group being evaluated. Another source of bias, especially for teachers, is the presence of conduct problems, which may cloud perceptions about inattention and hyperactivity. Thus, although highly useful in the clinical evaluation of ADHD in children and adolescents, these rating scales alone cannot be relied upon for establishing the diagnosis of ADHD. In response to these concerns, some researchers recommend the use of direct observational methods either in a simulated or actual classroom setting (Abikoff, Gittelman, & Klein, 1980; Atkins, Pelham, & Licht, 1989; Barkley, 1990; Nolan et al., 1994). Although these observational methods offer a measure of objectivity, those that rely on actual classroom observation are expensive to conduct. Simulated classroom methods may have problems with validity in that the child is alone in the room without the usual distractors of the typical classroom.

Specific ADHD Scales

The two most commonly used ADHD rating scales are the Parent and Teacher Questionnaires developed by Conners (1969). There is an ongoing controversy concerning the use of the Conners rating scales. Although generally regarded as reliable, some argue that the Conners scales do not discriminate between ADHD and conduct disorder (Loney & Milich, 1982). In addition, the items on the Conners scales do not correspond with current diagnostic criteria. On the other hand, the Conners scales have been used for almost three decades, providing powerful testimony to their practical utility (Barkley, 1990).

The Conners Parent Questionnaire (CPQ) is completed by a parent and concerns the child's conduct, activity level, attention, impulsiveness, and somatic complaints for children age 3 to 17 years. Commonly used versions of the CPQ are the 48-item questionnaire and the abbreviated 10-item questionnaire. The items are rated from 0 to 3 corresponding to *not at all, just a little, pretty much,* or *very much.* In the 48-item version, items have been organized by factor analysis into five mutually exclusive dimensions and a hyperactivity index that uses items from the other five subscales. The abbreviated 10-item version contains the items that compose the hyperactivity index.

The Conners Teacher Questionnaire (CTQ) is a 28-item questionnaire for teachers of school-age children. It is also available in a shortened 10-item version. The 28-item questionnaire is divided into three statistically derived factors and the hyperactivity index. As with the CPQ, items are rated from 0 to 3. Several studies have shown that the 28-item scale (and the 10-item hyperactivity index) correlate with a clinical diagnosis of

ADHD and are capable of detecting change in treatment trials (Barkley, 1990; Conners, 1969; Conners & Barkley, 1985).

The CPQ and the CTQ can be usefully applied in both clinical and research settings. Both ratings have recently revised norms for school-age children, which allow raw scores to be transformed into standard scores by age and gender (Conners, 1989). However, concern that the CPQ and CTQ overemphasize conduct problems and do not reflect contemporary conceptualizations of ADHD suggests that they may be more useful as a measure of change in treatment trials rather than as a diagnostic measure. These concerns have prompted several investigators to introduce new parent and teacher rating scales (Barkley, 1990; Pelham, Gnagy, Greenslade, & Milich, 1992; Ullmann, Sleator, & Sprague, 1985a).

The ADD-H Comprehensive Teacher Rating Scale (ACTeRs) was developed by Ullman, Sleator, and Sprague (1985b) to collect diagnostic and severity data on school-age children from their teachers. It contains 24 items that reside in one of four factors: attention, hyperactivity, social skills, and oppositional. The items are scored from 1 to 5 with norms for boys and girls age 5 to 11 years for each of the four factors. Pelham and colleagues (1992) developed the Disruptive Behavior Disorders Rating Scale (DBD) to be completed by teachers and parents. The DBD is based on *DSM-III-R* criteria and contains 14 items for ADHD, 9 items for oppositional defiant disorder, and 13 items for conduct disorder. Items are rated on a 0 to 3 scale with a score of 3 indicating a clinically meaningful symptom. In a nationwide sample of 931 boys between the ages of 5 and 14 years, the authors found 61 boys (6.5%) with eight or more symptoms of ADHD. There was substantial overlap between oppositional defiant disorder and ADHD symptoms. A high percentage of conduct disorder items was listed as unknown by teachers, suggesting that it may be more appropriate for parents to complete this portion of the rating. To date, the DBD has not been widely used.

The ADHD Rating Scale was introduced by DuPaul and Barkley (reviewed in Barkley, 1990). It has recently been revised to reflect *DSM-IV* criteria. Each item is rated from 0 to 3 with responses of 2 or 3 accepted as a positive symptom response. Because it consists of *DSM-IV* criteria, some researchers believe that it might be a more useful aid to the diagnosis of ADHD with less overlap with conduct problems. However, empirical support for this scale is not yet available. The ADHD Rating Scale has been used in a pharmacological trial as a primary outcome measure (Kurlan et al., 1997).

Adult ADHD

In recent years there has been increased interest in adult ADHD. Data from longitudinal studies suggest that ADHD does indeed persist into adulthood in 30–40% of those clinically diagnosed in childhood (Mannuzza,

Gittelman-Klein, Horowitz-Konig, & Giampino, 1989). The diagnosis of ADHD in adulthood entails establishment of current symptoms as well as evidence of childhood onset. Diagnostic data can be elicited by using the ADHD modules from interview schedules such as the K-SADS or the DISC.

MEASURES USED IN THE DIAGNOSIS OF PSYCHIATRIC DISORDERS

Diagnostic Interviews

Diagnostic interviews survey a wide range of emotional and behavioral symptom clusters to establish the presence or absence of psychiatric disorders. These interviews may be highly structured, in which case they may be conducted by a specifically trained interviewer who is not a clinician; semistructured instruments, by contrast, require clinical skill to elicit valid answers and interpret responses. Hence, these instruments are typically administered by a clinician or an extensively trained lay interviewer. The choice of a structured or semistructured interview depends on time, cost, and available personnel. Because they require clinical judgment to discern the presence or absence of a symptom, semistructured diagnostic interviews are more expensive to administer.

There are several diagnostic interviews currently in use for the assessment of psychiatric disorders in children (Hodges, 1993; Robins, 1995). The informant (adult patient, parent, child, or teacher) is asked a set of screening questions for each disorder. If the screening questions elicit a negative response, the interviewer proceeds to the next section of the interview. When the responses to the screening probes are positive, the interviewer follows with more detailed questions within that diagnostic category. One exception to this format is the Child Assessment Schedule, which is organized by domains of daily living such as friends, family, and school (Hodges, McKnew, Burbach, & Roebuck, 1987; Hodges, McKnew, Cytryn, Stern, & Kline, 1982).

Commonly used structured diagnostic instruments for children and adolescents include the Diagnostic Interview Schedule for Children (DISC) and the Diagnostic Interview for Children and Adolescents (DICA). These instruments have undergone substantial revision and have been studied in both clinical and community samples (Boyle et al., 1993; Piacentini et al., 1993; Shaffer et al., 1996; Welner, Reich, Herjanic, Jung, & Amado, 1987).

The most commonly used semistructured diagnostic interview in pediatric populations is the Schedule for Affective Disorders and Schizophrenia for School-Age Children (K-SADS). Earlier versions showed acceptable test-retest reliability (kappa coefficients were 0.54 for depression, 0.63 for conduct disorder, and 0.53 for separation anxiety); mean intraclass correlation for symptom counts was 0.60 (Chambers et al., 1985). The K-SADS has been revised for *DSM-IV* and appears to retain adequate reliability and validity (J. Kaufman et al., 1997).

A semistructured diagnostic interview that has been recently introduced is the Child and Adolescent Psychiatric Assessment (CAPA; Angold et al., 1995), designed to be administered by clinicians or extensively trained lay interviewers. A strength of this instrument is that it allows the interviewer to follow up leads in the interview in a fashion that mimics clinical practice. Another advantage is that it establishes the presence or absence of psychiatric symptoms as well as the level of impairment caused by the symptoms. The CAPA was used in an epidemiological study and exhibited good to excellent test-retest reliability for parents on child interviews (Costello, Angold, Burns, Stangl, Tweed, Erkanli, & Worthman, 1996). Surprisingly, the reported prevalence for ADHD was 1.9%, which is considerably lower than most other surveys. This difference may reflect differences in the CAPA or the diagnostic algorithm used by the investigators.

Informants

In clinical practice with children, most practitioners collect and weigh information from multiple informants, such as the child, parent, and teacher. Unfortunately, the unstructured techniques, such as play interviews, used by clinicians to gather data from children cannot be easily translated into a structured interview format with younger children. Studies with the DISC and the DICA-R found poor test-retest agreement among children age 6 to 12 years, suggesting that direct questions about psychiatric symptoms may not be an effective method of data collection (Boyle et al., 1993; Schwab-Stone, Fallon, Briggs, & Crowther, 1994). In their analysis of the DISC test-retest data, Schwab-Stone and colleagues concluded that the primary threats to reliability were male gender, age less than 8 years, open-ended questions about time, and requests requiring self-reflection (Fallon & Schwab-Stone, 1994). In both studies, children endorsed fewer symptoms in the second interview. By contrast, mothers showed good agreement over both brief (Schwab-Stone et al., 1994) and more extended periods of time (Faraone, Biederman, & Milberger, 1995). The poor test-retest reliability in younger children is presumably due to their incomplete understanding of the presence, intensity, and duration of psychiatric symptoms. Older children (ages 12 to 18 years) appear to be more reliable in their responses.

In addition to differences in test-retest reliability, parents and children often give discrepant responses to queries about psychiatric symptoms. Disagreement varies according to symptom category. Nor surprisingly, agreement is typically better for behavioral symptoms than for symptoms of depression; anxiety symptoms appear to elicit intermediate agreement (Boyle et al., 1993; Chambers et al., 1985; Jansen et al., 1995; Schwab-Stone et al., 1994; M. Weissman & Klerman, 1978). Exceptions to this general trend have been reported with clinical samples in which agreement between parents and children is better (Welner et al., 1987).

Diagnostic Interviews for Adults

The Structured Clinical Interview for *DSM-III-R* (SCID–nonpatient version) developed by Spitzer, Williams, Gibbon, and First (1992) was designed to gather data concerning both current and lifetime psychiatric diagnoses in adults. The multisite study conducted by Williams et al. (1992) revealed respectable test-retest reliability (kappa coefficients were 0.54–0.84 for current and lifetime). The overall weighted kappa coefficient (accounts for percentages of cases within each diagnosis) for interrater reliability was in the fair range of 0.61 (range 0.40–0.86). The SCID is based on *DSM-III-R;* as such, the diagnostic criteria are embedded in the interview. Like the K-SADS, it has been designed to be administered by clinicians or trained interviewers. Also like the K-SADS, it allows the interviewer some flexibility in the conduct of the interview.

Diagnostic Judgments

Psychiatric diagnoses may be determined by a careful subject-by-subject review of all available information by one or two expert diagnosticians (Leckman, Sholomskas, Thompson, Belanger, & Weissman, 1982). Alternatively, for the highly structured interviews, responses from the parent and/or the child can be entered into a computer database that permits the use of computerized algorithms to determine diagnosis (P. Cohen, Velez, Kohn, Schwab-Stone, & Johnson, 1987; Costello, Angold, Burns, Stangl, Tweed, Erkanli, & Worthman, 1996; Piacentini et al., 1993). These computer-based diagnostic algorithms may be especially advantageous for large research data sets, but less relevant for clinical practice and smaller clinical research projects.

The use of expert diagnosticians to integrate data from multiple sources is appealing because it resembles clinical practice. Although computerized algorithms offer efficiency, reproducibility, and flexibility in the diagnostic threshold, expert clinicians may weigh diagnostic data from multiple sources in subtle ways that may not easily transfer to a computerized decision tree. However, the reliability and validity of the best-estimate method are limited by the quality of data on which diagnostic decisions are made.

Selection of a Diagnostic Interview

The primary application of diagnostic interviews is in research. Structured diagnostic interviews have become standard in epidemiological research because, although costly, they are the least expensive method of establishing diagnostic status in large community-based samples. Family genetic studies are another common application of both semistructured and structured instruments (Pauls, Raymond, et al., 1991; Weissman et al., 1986). The chief advantage of structured interviews is that the researcher can feel confident that a wide range of psychiatric symptoms has been systematically examined. However, reliability and validity have not been demonstrated for all structured interviews currently in use (Hodges, 1993). In addition to cost, training, and demonstrated reliability, the time demand on families to complete the interview is also an important criterion for selecting a diagnostic interview.

Semistructured interviews, such as the SCID and the K-SADS, are often used in clinical research settings for establishing primary and comorbid diagnoses at the baseline of a treatment trial. Semistructured interviews are purported to mimic clinical practice in that they permit the clinician examiner to follow up clues in the interview. In practice, however, there is a trend toward the use of nonclinicians to administer semistructured interviews (Biederman, Faraone, et al., 1993). Hence, the contention that semistructured interviews have greater validity than the highly structured interviews seems weakened by the use of nonclinicians. On the other hand, the use of nonclinicians may substantially reduce the cost of the interviews. The use of diagnostic interview schedules in clinical practice is not yet routine. However, the potential reduction in clinician time to gather this wide range of diagnostic data is attractive.

CONCLUSIONS

We anticipate that clinical rating instruments will continue to evolve. As dimensions of obsessive-compulsive disorder and ADHD emerge more clearly into view, it may be possible to develop more refined instruments that monitor clinical change within each dimension. In the case of tic disorders, new technologies may emerge that will permit the long-term monitoring of tics using electromyography. This may set the stage for a new class of assessments that estimate key features of the dynamic properties of tics—reflecting how they cluster in bursts and how the bursts themselves cluster together in bouts (described in Chapter 2). Longitudinal tracking of symptom severity may also become more commonplace, particularly if investigators are able to demonstrate that specific features in the initial phase of Tourette's syndrome are predictive of disorder subtypes or long-term outcomes.

SUMMARY OF CHAPTER 16

Diagnostic interview schedules and rating instruments have become indispensable tools in clinical research and clinical practice in psychiatry and neurology. They can be used to ensure systematic clinical assessment and to evaluate progress over the course of treatment. However, diagnostic interviews and standardized ratings are not a substitute for careful clinical evaluation. Beyond issues of reliability and validity, selection of the diagnostic interview or rating instrument for a particular application depends on the purpose, availability of personnel, acceptability to patients and their families, and cost. Primary research applications include quantitative comparisons across study groups and correlation with neurobiological or neuroanatomical measures. Familiarity with common rating instruments is likely to be useful to clinicians and essential for researchers in child psychiatry and neurology.

PREVIEW OF CHAPTER 17

As presented in Chapter 15, a comprehensive evaluation of individuals with Tourette's and related disorders includes more than establishing a categorical diagnosis and an assessment of current levels of symptom severity. Other crucially important domains focus on cognitive strengths and weaknesses, academic achievement and classroom adjustment (in the case of children), and peer and family relationships.

CHAPTER 17

Comprehensive Psychological and Educational Assessments

ALICE S. CARTER, NANCY J. FREDINE, ROBERT T. SCHULTZ, LAWRENCE SCAHILL, DIANE FINDLEY, and SARA S. SPARROW

> Promoting the patient's development by supporting warm family and peer relationships, aiding socialization, facilitating school achievement or rewarding employment, and cultivating self-esteem carries greater developmental benefit than dedication to suppression of tics at any cost.
>
> —*Donald J. Cohen, Kenneth Towbin, and James F. Leckman, 1992*

This chapter describes a developmentally sensitive, comprehensive approach to conducting psychological and educational evaluations with individuals who are affected with Tourette's syndrome and associated conditions. This comprehensive assessment approach (Sparrow et al., 1995) can be applied to all individuals. In this chapter, we offer guidelines, based on current empirical knowledge, for adapting this approach for use with children and adolescents who have been diagnosed with Tourette's syndrome or closely related conditions (see Chapters 15 and 16 for details concerning diagnostic assessments). Empirical studies suggest that there are specific profiles of strengths and deficiencies that are more commonly observed in individuals with Tourette's syndrome. Based on these profiles, we propose domains that should be assessed and describe specific recommendations for intervention that are likely to optimize the performance of children and adolescents with Tourette's syndrome and related disorders in both home and school settings.

As described in Chapter 15, a comprehensive assessment approach facilitates capturing patterns of the strengths and weaknesses that are most relevant to developing an appropriate formulation of the whole child and that inform recommendations for effective interventions. A careful assessment also involves an evaluation of the environmental demands and challenges

viduals with Tourette's syndrome may encounter, as recommenda-
y include modifications of the child's behavior and/or environmental demands. For example, the requirement that a child inhibit all tics to
stay in a classroom is an inappropriate environmental demand; the more
appropriate recommendation would involve increasing the family's, peers',
and teacher's understanding of the nature of Tourette's syndrome and related conditions.

Consistent with our effort to assess functioning across situations, we advocate including in the evaluation all of the professionals who are involved
with the affected individual. With children and adolescents, this will involve, at a minimum, one or more teachers and the pediatrician. In more
complex cases, a physician with a specialized interest in childhood-onset
neuropsychiatric disorders (psychiatrist, child psychiatrist, neurologist, or
pediatrician, depending on the age of the patient and the expertise of the
physician) as well as a variety of other special education, health, and mental health professionals must be integrated into both the information-
gathering and recommendation phases of the evaluation. When all relevant
professionals share a genuine understanding of the manner in which
Tourette's syndrome and related conditions are *or are not* interfering with
a particular individual's developmental progress, more effective interventions are possible. Of course, contacting professionals involved in the life
of the affected individual requires written consent.

THE COMPREHENSIVE DEVELOPMENTAL
ASSESSMENT MODEL

In this model, *comprehensive* refers to an evaluation of multiple aspects of
an individual's functioning while paying careful attention to developmental and environmental influences. The goal of the comprehensive psychological assessment is to create a developmentally sensitive picture of
strengths and weaknesses across multiple domains of functioning to inform the understanding of the whole individual and lead to optimal functioning at school, work, and home.

To complete a comprehensive assessment, the evaluator must select a
number of domains that are deemed most relevant to capture an individual's
current functioning and potential. When evaluating children and adults
with Tourette's syndrome and associated conditions, relevant domains are
selected on the basis of the specific referral questions or complaints that
are presented as well as recent findings in the empirical literature regarding
general patterns of strengths and weaknesses among individuals with
Tourette's syndrome. No individual can be understood adequately on the
basis of a single score in one domain or subtest or a global summary score
that averages performance across subtests or domains. This is especially
important in a disorder such as Tourette's syndrome, where we expect a significant percentage of individuals to evidence specific deficits in some but

not all domains of functioning (Bornstein, 1990; Bornstein et al., 1983; Bornstein, Carroll, & King, 1985; Bornstein & Yang, 1991; Carter et al., 1994; Dykens et al., 1990; Ferrari et al., 1984; Incagnoli & Kane, 1983; R. Schultz et al., 1998; see Chapter 5).

Core Symptoms

A comprehensive list of all possible relevant domains is presented in Chapter 15 (Table 15.1). The current chapter focuses on those domains relevant to the psychological and educational evaluation of children, adolescents, and adults with Tourette's syndrome and closely related disorders. The psychologist must be mindful that tics are typically not the problem most likely to interfere with day-to-day functioning (Cohen, 1990). Moreover, many individuals with Tourette's syndrome do not have any difficulties in functioning beyond the vocal and motor tics that characterize the disorder; these individuals rarely require any school or work modifications. It is not unusual for the associated attentional, affective, behavioral, and learning difficulties to become the focus of intervention when an individual with Tourette's syndrome is not meeting developmental expectations in school, at work, or in the family.

Several methods of study, including genetic and epidemiological approaches (see Chapters 8 through 10), indicate that individuals with Tourette's syndrome are at increased risk for behaviors associated with attention-deficit/hyperactivity disorder (ADHD; Chapter 4) and obsessive-compulsive disorder (Chapter 3). In addition, many individuals show weaknesses in fine motor and visual-motor integration (Chapter 5). It is not yet clear whether the attentional and obsessive symptoms that emerge within the context of Tourette's syndrome are comparable to those that appear in its absence (Walkup et al., 1995).

With respect to ADHD, it is not surprising that children and adults with Tourette's syndrome, a disorder characterized by motor disinhibition, would also have difficulty inhibiting attentional shifts and motor movements that are not pure tics. Clinical observations suggest that 40–50% of individuals referred with Tourette's syndrome show signs of ADHD before the onset of Tourette's syndrome symptoms (D. Cohen, Friedhoff, et al., 1992; Comings & Comings, 1987a). Common manifestations of ADHD include difficulty concentrating, distractibility, calling out in class, talking excessively, and having trouble sitting still and staying seated. When assessing ADHD in children with Tourette's syndrome, the fidgety, restless, "on the go" behaviors that characterize ADHD must be distinguished from the typically abrupt, often explosive, staccatolike movements of tic behaviors (Scahill, Lynch, et al., 1995; Walter & Carter, 1997). ADHD symptoms often lead to a high rate of school underachievement (Barkley, Fisher, et al., 1990); in addition, difficulties in peer relations (e.g., Pelham & Bender, 1982) and conduct (Biederman et al., 1991a; Loney & Milich, 1982) are observed in many children with ADHD. Children with Tourette's syndrome and ADHD are more likely to exhibit maladaptive behaviors such as impulsivity and stubbornness and lower levels of adaptive behaviors than children with Tourette's syndrome alone (Dykens et al., 1990; Walkup et al., 1995).

Many children, adolescents, and adults with Tourette's syndrome have obsessive-compulsive disorder or experience significant obsessive-compulsive symptoms (Pauls, Raymond, et al., 1991; B. Peterson et al., 1995; Robertson et al., 1988b). Obsessive-compulsive disorder symptoms commonly emerge as children enter adolescence (Jagger et al., 1982), though in some cases they precede the onset of tics (Leonard et al., 1992). Obsessions are persistent thoughts, images, or impulses that are experienced as intrusive and senseless. The thoughts and images may be frightening or upsetting (e.g., family members being injured). The individual typically tries to suppress these thoughts or to neutralize them with another thought, image, or behavior. Compulsions are repetitive behaviors that are performed according to specific rules or in a stereotyped manner or in an effort to neutralize obsessions. For example, an individual may engage in a counting ritual (e.g., counting to 700 by 7s) to neutralize a silly, scary, or random thought. When an individual attempts to resist engaging in a compulsion, he or she typically experiences increasing tension, anxiety, or fear that is diminished after performing the compulsive behavior. For some individuals, the tension or anxiety is only diminished if the compulsion is performed properly, resulting in many repetitions of the compulsion until it is performed just right (Leckman, Walker, et al., 1994).

Thus, a child or adolescent with obsessive-compulsive disorder might feel the need to redo schoolwork many times because of a perceived imperfection, or because it does not look right or the doing did not feel right. Some get stuck rereading or rewriting a word over and over again. It may seem as if the child or adolescent is just a very slow worker or cannot or will not finish assignments (Walter & Carter, 1997). Individuals with Tourette's syndrome and obsessive-compulsive disorder or individuals with obsessive-compulsive disorder and a family history of Tourette's appear to experience more tension or anxiety concerning "just right" perceptions or things not feeling right than individuals with obsessive-compulsive disorder alone (Leckman, Grice, Barr, et al., 1995). At times, it may be difficult to distinguish a complex tic that involves several movements from a compulsion. Obsessive-compulsive symptoms may emerge early and often result in a sudden and unexpected decrease in academic performance. In contrast to tics and ADHD behaviors, obsessive-compulsive disorder symptoms are not always easily observed and children are often quite secretive about them. Some children and adolescents are so embarrassed and confused about the obsessions and compulsions that they prefer to be viewed as oppositional rather than reveal the real nature of their difficulties (Walter & Carter, 1997).

Other Domains

Many individuals with Tourette's syndrome who present for psychological evaluations may also exhibit other difficulties, including problems in executive functioning (i.e., mental flexibility and planning), specific learning disabilities, social-emotional problems, and various other secondary emotional disorders (e.g., anxiety, depression; cf. B. Peterson et al., 1995; Walter & Carter, 1997). When conducting an evaluation with an individual who presents with Tourette's syndrome and these other difficulties, it is very important to recognize that these difficulties may not be related to Tourette's syndrome and may have very different etiologic and maintaining factors. Although the etiology may not be shared, learning difficulties may influence the course of Tourette's due to general stress or overall adaptation (D. Cohen, Bruun, & Leckman, 1988). It should be noted, however, that despite the reported association of Tourette's with a wide range of problems, most of these studies have recruited subjects from clinical settings (e.g., child psychiatry or neurology clinics) rather than community samples. As children with multiple problems are more likely to be referred to clinics, the co-occurrence of these problems with Tourette's syndrome must be interpreted with great caution (Caine et al., 1988; Como, 1993; Walkup et al., 1995). Indeed, Caine et al. demonstrated that children with Tourette's syndrome and ADHD were much more likely to be seen by a clinician than those affected with Tourette's syndrome alone. Another methodologic problem is that many studies combine children, adolescents, and adults within a given sample. This approach minimizes the influence of development in the emergence of psychopathology and assumes that symptoms are the same throughout development (Carter et al., 1994).

As presented in Chapter 6, many children and adults affected with Tourette's syndrome have significant difficulties with peer relations (Cohen, 1990; D. Cohen, Friedhoff, et al., 1992; Dykens et al., 1990; Stokes et al., 1991), including both withdrawal and increased aggression (Stokes et al.). Deficits in parent-reported adaptive socialization skills have also been found among children with Tourette's syndrome (Carter, Lidsky, Scahill, Schultz, & Pauls, 1997; Dykens et al., 1990). Of importance for the evaluator, there does not appear to be a consistent association between social-emotional problems and tic severity (de Groot, Janus, et al., 1995; Edell & Motta, 1989; Frank et al., 1991; L. Rosenberg, Harris, & Singer, 1984; Stokes et al., 1991; R. Wilson, Garron, Tanner, & Klawans, 1982). Furthermore, no association has been reported between obsessive-compulsive disorder symptom severity and tic severity (Singer & Rosenberg, 1989) or family functioning and illness severity (Carter et al., 1994; Edell & Motta, 1989; Stokes et al., 1991). Thus, it is important to screen for social and emotional difficulties even if the symptoms of Tourette's syndrome and obsessive-compulsive disorder appear to be relatively mild. When clinic-referred children have ADHD in addition to Tourette's syndrome, they appear to have much more significant social-emotional difficulties than children with Tourette's syndrome alone (Carter et al., 1997).

It is not yet clear whether the peer and emotional symptoms that are observed are etiologically related to the disorder or are sequelae of living with uncontrollable physical symptoms and associated symptoms (Scahill et al., 1993a). It is quite likely that a component of the peer, emotional, and behavioral difficulties develops in response to being teased and misunderstood. Almost every child who has Tourette's syndrome can tell painful stories about being teased by peers. Family members may also contribute to social, emotional, and behavioral difficulties before they understand the nature of the disorder. Parents often report that in their efforts to develop an appropriate parenting strategy they felt confused and/or helpless and responded inconsistently or harshly to the symptoms of the disorder and to associated difficulties (e.g., ADHD). Identifying the factors that predict or lead to the emergence of associated behavior problems and comorbid disorders may improve prevention and intervention strategies (Carter et al., 1994). This research is especially critical because maladaptive behaviors that are not symptoms of Tourette's syndrome may cause more adaptive impairment than the Tourette's syndrome itself (D. Cohen, Riddle, & Leckman, 1992).

MULTIPLE SETTINGS AND INFORMANTS

Individuals with Tourette's syndrome, obsessive-compulsive disorder, and ADHD often show variable functioning across different settings (Nolan et al., 1994; Scahill, Lynch, et al., 1995; Walter & Carter, 1997). Thus, parents and teachers may have a very different view of a given individual (Scahill et al., 1993b). For example, it is not unusual for a child who has been suppressing tics very actively and evidencing excellent self-control skills throughout the schoolday to display intense bouts of tics and low frustration tolerance when he or she returns home from school. Rather than view one informant (e.g., teacher) as more reliable or valid than the other informant (e.g., parent), these apparent discrepancies may reveal important differences in the individual's functioning and in the environmental demands of home and school. Moreover, systematic patterns in these differences can inform the kinds of interventions that may be beneficial for an individual with Tourette's syndrome in any setting.

Also, it is important to assess not only informants' understanding of the individual's functioning, but their general understanding of these complex disorders. For example, when evaluating children and adolescents, it is critically important to learn what teachers and other relevant school personnel (e.g., the school psychologist) know about Tourette's and related conditions (Walter & Carter, 1997). For example, beliefs of intentionality and control regarding specific tic and other problem behaviors as well as convictions regarding the etiology of the disorder are often important targets for intervention. Because symptoms wax and wane and individual performance fluctuates from week-to-week and day-to-day, teachers often assume that children have greater control over their tics and attention than may be warranted (Scahill et al., 1993b). Moreover, some parents and teaches may not be aware that Tourette's syndrome is a neuropsychiatric disorder. It is imperative that the evaluator include an assessment of school professionals' knowledge regarding Tourette's syndrome, as beliefs and perceptions impact on the attributions that are made regarding a child or adolescent's behavior and the quality of interactions with the child or adolescent in the school setting. Further, teachers and other school professionals are critical players in educating peers about Tourette's syndrome. They can be extremely effective in helping other children understand and learn to cope with the unpredictable behaviors that the child with Tourette's syndrome may present in the classroom, minimizing fear and aggression.

Thus, information collected across many domains of functioning and across varied settings and informants provides the basis for generating a profile of strengths and weaknesses that informs our view of the whole individual and necessary recommendations for intervention.

DEVELOPMENTAL INFLUENCES

To appreciate the complexity of an individual's current functioning, a consideration of multiple developmental influences is required (e.g., the age of Tourette's syndrome onset, specific family stressors or losses, previous school experiences). One gains a richer understanding of the individual from longitudinal rather than from single cross-sectional or snapshot assessment. As children and adolescents with Tourette's, especially those with attentional difficulties, may be quite variable from day-to-day, including multiple testing sessions in the evaluation process is always preferable to a single long session. Thus, when conducting a psychological or psychoeducational evaluation within the framework of the comprehensive approach, every effort is made to understand the current sample behavior within the context of additional samples of observed and quantified behavior, informant reports about multiple settings, and knowledge of development across multiple domains of functioning.

DOMAINS OF ASSESSMENT AND TEST SELECTION

For each individual with Tourette's syndrome there is an interplay of immediate contextual factors as well as broader familial, social, and cultural influences. The immediate context refers to situational factors in the testing setting that can affect an individual's performance during the assessment. Examples of such factors that deserve consideration include the physical environment of the testing room, the gender and race of the examiner, the interpersonal style and comfort level of the examiner, the order and number of tasks presented, the individual's physical health, and the individual's understanding of the purpose of the testing. In addition to the central role of the family, broader contextual influences include the individual's culture, community, and institutional environments. Although formal assessments in each of these areas are not always feasible, it is important for the evaluator to be mindful of the contribution of proximal and distal contextual influences.

The selection of the most appropriate domains of assessment will be guided by the age of the individual and the nature of the individual referral questions (e.g., "Johnny doesn't remember what I ask him to do. Is it a memory problem?") as well as the empirical evidence regarding the kinds of difficulties that individuals with Tourette's syndrome typically exhibit. Thus, although not all individuals with Tourette's will evidence attention and visual-motor integration deficits, the competent evaluator will include these domains when administering a psychological evaluation to an individual who is affected with Tourette's syndrome. A best-practice guideline for answering the referral question regarding a memory deficit is to evaluate the domains of memory and attention. Determining that an individual has an attention deficit that could account for the observed difficulties in memory does not rule out the possibility that this individual also has a relative weakness in memory that is independent of the attentional difficulties.

Cognitive Abilities, Perception, and Motor Skills

As an individual's general problem-solving abilities provide a framework for a developmental understanding of all other domains of functioning, measurement of global cognitive functioning (i.e., IQ) is essential in any comprehensive evaluation. With children and adolescents, an assessment of academic achievement is also indicated to rule out the presence of learning difficulties. For mental level and academic achievement, no special modifications in test selection are indicated. However, it may be useful to include a test of academic achievement that includes a writing sample; because many children with Tourette's evidence fine-motor and visual-motor coordination difficulties, speed and neatness of written work may be affected.

It is critical to document such difficulties and specific deficits in fine-motor coordination, for example, by employing a peg task such as the Purdue Pegboard (Tiffen, 1968), and in visual-motor coordination, for example, with the Beery Developmental Test of Visual-Motor Integration (Beery & Buktenica, 1989), Bender Gestalt (Bender, 1938; Hutt, 1977), or Rey Osterreith Complex Figure Drawing (Rey, 1941). Some children with Tourette's syndrome will perform competently on the Beery but will have difficulty on the Rey, which requires a higher level of visual organization and planning. Although academic achievement may be consistent with the level predicted from the child's or adolescent's cognitive functioning, it is also important to address the child's academic functioning, or how he or she is managing day-to-day in the classroom. For children and adolescents, it is essential to obtain information from teachers as part of the assessment of academic functioning and also to determine whether attention and behavior problems occur across settings.

Thus, the psychological evaluation of individuals with Tourette's syndrome should begin with an assessment of global cognitive level, academic achievement and functioning, and fine- and visual-motor coordination. When difficulties in fine- and/or visual-motor coordination are observed, it is important to document whether the difficulties are limited to tasks that require motor coordination or whether visual-preceptual difficulties extend to motor-free tasks (e.g., Judgment of Line Orientation; Benton, Hannay, & Varney, 1975; Benton, Varney, & Hamsher, 1978). Observations of the individual during this portion of the assessment should greatly inform whether a more careful assessment of attention regulation and/or social-emotional functioning is indicated.

Although many individuals with Tourette's syndrome will have received a thorough psychiatric evaluation that describes the symptoms of Tourette's syndrome and associated conditions (i.e., obsessive-compulsive disorder and ADHD), this will not always be the case. The psychologist conducting the comprehensive assessment may need to include an assessment of psychiatric status as part of the evaluation (see Chapters 15 and 16 for information concerning diagnostic issues). At a minimum, screening for ADHD and obsessive-compulsive disorder is indicated, as the presence of these comorbid conditions tends to increase the likelihood of impairment in day-to-day adaptation.

When ADHD is a concern, a number of additional rating scales should be considered (see Chapters 4 and 16). In addition, although computerized performance tests do not yield information that is directly relevant to the diagnosis of ADHD, they are extremely beneficial for developing a broader understanding of the nature of the individual's attention regulation. In combination with information from interviews that address developmental aspects of attentional difficulties, rating forms that address current functioning, continuous performance tests, and other assessment data can inform a diagnosis of ADHD. If an evaluator believes that significant attentional problems are present, the domain of executive functioning should be examined. Specifically, tasks that are designed to address the individual's ability to develop and implement rules, maintain focus on a rule that is currently working, and planning, are subsumed within executive functioning (Chapter 5). Executive deficits are not assessed in a traditional clinical or school psychological evaluation. Yet, such difficulties in planning and organization can have a profound impact on day-to-day functioning. Studies of individuals with Tourette's syndrome that address coexisting conditions have shown that children with Tourette's syndrome at greatest risk for learning difficulties in the classroom appear to be those who are also experiencing attentional, obsessional, or depressive symptoms (e.g., Bornstein, 1991a, 1991b).

Even if attentional issues are not raised as a focus of concern, children and adolescents who are reported to be messy and disorganized, who forget books at school and fail to arrive at class in a timely manner may have an underlying neurocognitive deficit in executive functioning. As such behaviors are often attributed to laziness, documenting the presence of a specific pattern of neurocognitive, executive functioning deficits can have a significant impact on educational recommendations. Moreover, when school professionals understand that difficulties in organization and neatness are not volitional, they often develop increased empathy toward the individual affected with Tourette's and are more likely to implement suggested recommendations.

When obsessive-compulsive disorder appears to be part of the clinical picture, visual perception, including visual memory, should be assessed. One task that may be particularly informative is the Benton Judgment of Line Orientation (Benton, 1994). This test requires the child or adolescent to match two target lines—in the same position and pointing in the same direction—from an array of lines.

Dimensional Ratings of Behavior and Adaptive Functioning

Although individuals with Tourette's syndrome have friends, experience positive self-regard, and exhibit age-appropriate emotion and behavior regulation skills, the challenges that Tourette's syndrome presents (e.g., not being able to control one's movements, experiencing harsh teasing), places individuals with Tourette's syndrome at greater risk for difficulties in social and emotional functioning. At a minimum, it is useful to screen for social and emotional difficulties by asking parents, teachers, and child (when older than age 9 and able to make reliable judgments) about both difficulties and strengths.

Among the most commonly used parent and teacher questionnaires concerning general behavior problems and overall adaptive functioning are the Child Behavior Checklist (CBCL) and the Teacher Report Form (TRF; Achenbach, 1991a). Each contain over 100 items concerning the child's behavior and functional capacity. The first part of each questionnaire inquires about the child's interests, social skills, and academic performance. The second part contains a list of questions concerning a wide range of problem behaviors that the informant (parent or teacher) rates 0, 1, or 2, corresponding to *not true, somewhat true,* and *very true.* Items are grouped to form eight specific behavior problem scales and three competency scales. These scales also provide internalizing and externalizing scales which characterize broad domains of behavior. The established norms permit integration of the CBCL dimensions with the TRF into a single profile that is consistent across developmental stages and genders (Achenbach, 1991a).

In clinical practice, these questionnaires can be reviewed for obvious patterns of disruptive behavior, social isolation, and adaptive functioning. Furthermore, the availability of population norms for both the competency scales and the behavior problems scales make the CBCL and the TRF useful in research as well. For example, these instruments might be used to characterize a clinical sample of children with Tourette's syndrome (L. Rosenberg et al., 1994) or obsessive-compulsive disorder (Hanna, 1995). In a series of 65 children and adolescents with obsessive-compulsive disorder, we observed that those with greater obsessive-compulsive symptoms had lower social competence scores (Scahill et al., 1997).

The CBCL and TRF have been criticized for being too focused on behavior problems. Moreover, it has been argued that the competency scales contain too few items to be useful. Also, because the dimensions of the CBCL and the TRF have been derived by a statistical process, the clinical relevance of these dimensions is uncertain. Finally, there is evidence that parental psychopathology can bias parental response (Jensen, Traylor, Xenakis, & Davis, 1988). On the other hand, these instruments can be completed in approximately 15–20 minutes. They have been used in large community-based samples and in clinical populations, which provides a rich context for interpretation (Hanna, 1995; Jensen et al., 1988, 1993; King et al., 1995; L. Rosenberg et al., 1994; Scahill et al., 1997; Stanger, Achenbach, & Verhulst, 1994). Also, several studies have shown correspondence between the CBCL and categorical diagnosis (Biederman, Faraone, et al., 1993; Edelbrock & Costello, 1988). Of specific relevance to the assessment of ADHD, 10 items from the TRF have been shown to be highly predictive of the diagnosis of ADHD (Barkley, DuPaul, & McMurray, 1991; Edelbrock & Achenbach, 1984). Thus, the CBCL and the TRF have good statistical properties and appear to be useful measures of general psychopathology and adaptive functioning in children and adolescents. Achenbach and colleagues (Achenbach, 1991a) have also developed a companion self-report instrument for youngsters between 11 and 18 years.

The Vineland Adaptive Scales were developed at the Yale Child Study Center and consist of several domains reflecting adaptive functioning in children 6 to 19 years of age (Sparrow et al., 1984). The domains include socialization, communication, daily living skills, and motor skills. The Vineland is administered in a semistructured interview format and takes about 40 minutes to complete. It has shown excellent interrater reliability, and norms have been established for age and gender following assessment of a large national sample. The Vineland can readily discriminate between clinical and nonclinical populations and may be especially useful in the assessment of children with developmental delays. It may also be useful in delineating the functional implications of comorbidity. For example, Dykens and colleagues (1990) showed that children with Tourette's syndrome and ADHD scored lower on Vineland scales than those with Tourette's syndrome alone. A potential drawback of the Vineland is the cost, as interviewers require careful training and the interview itself takes time to complete.

The Social Adjustment Scale Self-Report (SAS-SR) is a written, self-administered version of the Social Adjustment Scale. The SAS is the most widely used adult social adjustment scale and extensive information is available on its psychometric properties and norms in community samples (Prien & Robinson, 1994). The SAS-SR, which takes 15–20 minutes to complete, is a 42-item questionnaire measuring performance in occupational, social, and leisure activities; family roles; and economic independence over the prior two weeks. The instrument has a high internal consistency (mean alpha, $r = 0.74$), test-retest stability ($r = 0.80$), and excellent agreement with the interview version of the SAS (M. Weissman, Sholomskas, & John, 1981).

Living with someone who has Tourette's can be extremely stressful for family members. Because Tourette's syndrome is a genetic disorder (Chapter 10), a parent or sibling in the family may also be affected. Parents may experience guilt about having passed the illness to a child (Scahill et al., 1993b). They may also be experiencing stress as a result of the unpredictability and chronicity of the disorder, which may include financial and time-management burdens as a result of negotiating appointments with the health care and school systems. Thus, a comprehensive assessment also includes inquiry about the impact of the illness on day-to-day family life and whether family members feel that they are able to find ways to enjoy family life. It is also important to inquire about the status of any unaffected siblings in the family. Although little research has focused on the siblings of children with Tourette's syndrome, research on siblings of children with other chronic illnesses (e.g., diabetes) suggests that siblings may become extremely responsible in reaction to the challenge of having an ill sibling or may develop social and emotional difficulties that reflect an inability to surmount the stress of the ill sibling (Gamble & McHale, 1989; Lavigne & Ryan, 1979; Sargent et al., 1995; S. Taylor, 1980; Tew & Laurence, 1973).

A number of assessment instruments are available to assess parenting stress: Parenting Stress Index (PSI; Abidin, 1983); family functioning: Family Environment Scale (FES; Moos & Moos, 1976a); marital functioning: Dyadic Adjustment Scale (DAS; Spanier, 1976); and family members' ability to cope with the ill child: Coping-Health Inventory for Parents (CHIP; McCubbin, McCubbin, Nevin, & Cauble, 1983). Many of these instruments have been normed or provide cutoff scores that indicate when a family may benefit from intervention or family-focused intervention. Despite the fact that no studies of family intervention with families affected by Tourette's syndrome and related conditions have been conducted, addressing ongoing sources of stress and conflict in the family is likely to benefit an affected child and his or her siblings (Hamlett, Pellegrini, & Katz, 1992; McKeever, 1983).

Finally, school personnel and other health professionals involved with a child or adolescent with Tourette's syndrome will vary greatly in their knowledge about the disorder. Part of a comprehensive evaluation should review the understanding of the adults in the affected individual's life. When information is limited or incorrect, a primary focus of the intervention becomes education, as discussed in Chapters 15 and 19.

SUMMARY OF CHAPTER 17

Tourette's syndrome and related conditions can have an impact on development in several areas, including educational progress, socialization, family relationships, and development of self-image. A comprehensive, developmentally sensitive psychological and psychoeducational evaluation of children and adolescents will facilitate appropriate recommendations for intervention. In addition to diagnostic assessments and ratings of symptom severity, the following domains are necessary to include in such an evaluation: global cognitive functioning, academic achievement, academic performance, fine-motor coordination, visual-motor integration and visual perception, attention regulation and executive functioning, social-emotional functioning, family stress, and parents' and school personnel's understanding of these conditions. An assessment of global cognitive level provides a developmental frame for understanding a child's or adolescent's functioning. As many children come to the attention of a psychologist because of questions about learning rather than because of tics per se, careful evaluation of the child's academic abilities as well as the implementation of these abilities in the classroom is essential. Findings from current research also suggest that attention, visual-motor integration, and fine-motor coordination are commonly deficient in Tourette's syndrome; hence, some form of screening should be included to determine the existence of these difficulties. Identifying parental and sibling stresses associated with coping with a chronic disorder should also be assessed.

PREVIEW OF CHAPTER 18

Supportive educational interventions are a crucial feature of the initial phase of treatment regardless of age. Cognitive-behavioral interventions, particularly the technique of exposure and response prevention, have a proven track record for the treatment of obsessive-compulsive disorder. Despite optimistic reports concerning the use of habit reversal and other behavioral approaches to the treatment of chronic tic disorders, they have not gained widespread acceptance. The chapter concludes with an exploration of the promise and limitations of dynamically oriented individual and family psychotherapies.

CHAPTER 18

Psychosocial and Behavioral Treatments

ROBERT A. KING, LAWRENCE SCAHILL, DIANE FINDLEY, and
DONALD J. COHEN

All perceivable Tourette's syndrome actions have the following three
phases: a beginning, the inception and emergence; a middle, their movement
and path; and an end, the consummation (incomplete). To recognize the beginning, to hold it briefly in abeyance, to survey it and study it, to banish it
if possible, are all terribly difficult; and, most important, the effort is only
intermittently successful. . . .

Often the effort to control these wild sensations seems to be more than
the human spirit can bear; there are really only two choices: let it all hang
out or keep fighting. . . .

Behavioral control may utilize (1) substitution of overt actions or (2) attempts at extinction of overt actions. Neither of these provides a satisfactory treatment, but they can offer realistic support through difficult
periods. . . . Extinction is based on the instant recognition and instant denial of emergent sensory signals. The signal is an extremely subtle sensation, a feel, and if it is detected and rejected quickly enough reflexively it
can be extinguished *without* a buildup of tension. . . . The accomplishment
of this state of instant recognition is not easy to achieve. It requires intensive and prolonged training. Motivation and persistence are indispensable
allies. When extinction of symptoms is achieved, the symptoms will con-
stantly recur and need to be confronted and extinguished endlessly. The result is a kind of half-life in which there is constant vigilance and divided
attention. . . .

No matter what the method of control . . . , the only true relief comes in
moments when no urge at all is perceived. To remember this fact at the
onset of an impulse is most trying because at that precise moment it does
not seem possible for the state to be relieved by anything other than the action in progress.

—*Joseph Bliss, 1980*

Although Tourette's syndrome and its frequently attendant obsessive-
compulsive, attentional, and cognitive difficulties have a primarily

neurobiological etiology, the model of pathogenesis we have proposed suggests that psychosocial factors can influence the developmental course, severity, and manifestations of the disorder. The diverse symptoms of the disorder—tics, obsessions, compulsions, and a propensity to emotional lability, anxiety, and learning difficulties—influence the child's development both directly and indirectly through coloring and shaping the child's interactions with the world of peers, family, and school. In turn, there is abundant evidence that nonspecific stressors, as well as individual and family psychological factors, can ameliorate or exacerbate symptoms and produce measurable neurobiological changes (Chappell, Leckman, et al., 1995, 1996; Silva et al., 1995; Surwillo et al., 1978). Furthermore, individual, family, and cultural factors shape the ways that patients, parents, peers, and teachers perceive, give meaning, and respond to the symptoms of Tourette's syndrome. Finally, psychosocial factors also influence patients' and families' engagement and compliance with various interventions, including medication. This broad biopsychosocial perspective on the disorder implies that psychosocial influences can be risk factors for increased impairment and comorbidity, as well as focal points for therapeutic and preventive interventions.

In this chapter, we discuss the range of psychological and behavioral interventions available for individuals with Tourette's syndrome. Some of these modalities, such as behavioral and cognitive-behavioral treatments for obsessive-compulsive disorder and tics, target specific symptoms; other approaches, such as more traditional interpersonal and psychodynamic therapies, address broader developmental issues and the fostering of new social, emotional, and adaptive competencies (D. Cohen, 1995).

The availability of effective pharmacological agents that can at least partially suppress tics or obsessive-compulsive symptoms and ameliorate attentional and affective difficulties should not obscure the fact that the goal of treatment is not merely symptom suppression. As discussed in Chapter 15, the clinician's broader goal is to help individuals move forward successfully with the developmental tasks of establishing sustaining attachments with family and peers, functioning competently in the world of work or school, and developing and maintaining a positive identity and sense of self-esteem (also see Chapters 1, 6, and 8; D. Cohen, 1980, 1995; R. King & Cohen, 1994).

EDUCATIONAL AND PSYCHOTHERAPEUTIC ASPECTS OF THE DIAGNOSTIC PROCESS

The process of the initial diagnostic assessment and evaluation has important therapeutic components in its own right. By the time they come to clinical attention, individuals with tic disorders and their families have often been distressed and puzzled by the various symptoms and frustrated in their attempts to find appropriate guidance. Having the opportunity to tell their story to a knowledgeable and empathic clinician familiar with the vicissitudes of the disorder and its developmental impact can provide a crucial element of support and an antidote to isolation or despair. In the course of the initial evaluation, it is often possible to reformulate previously puzzling and upsetting symptoms within the context of a disorder. For example, before diagnosis, patients may experience their tics, obsessions, or compulsive urges as shameful secrets or a form of private madness. Parents or teachers may regard facial and phonic tics and compulsions as voluntary, deliberately annoying acts of defiance or evidence of a woeful lack of self-control. The child with tics may have been frequently scolded or cajoled to suppress a tic or compulsion. Framing these symptoms as part of a disorder helps to decriminalize them and to begin a more informed discussion of what degree of control can be reasonably expected for different behaviors in various situations. Such a dialogue can de-escalate a vicious circle of recrimination leading to further tic exacerbation and help aggravated parents shift the focus from blame to problem solving.

It is often useful to begin by asking children if they know why their parents have brought them to see the clinician. If the child purports not to know, one can ask the parents what they have told the child. This will usually provide an entree into the child's symptoms, as well as the child's and family's vocabulary for discussing them. Often, a child will answer "My Tourette's syndrome" or "obsessive-compulsive disorder." Even when accurate, however, it is important to inquire what the child means by such a phrase. The clinician must remain alert as to whether such terms are invoked as a useful shorthand or as an unhelpful, obscuring intellectualization. Learning about the child's and family's shared language for talking about the child's symptoms and difficulties is an important part of exploring and clarifying their understanding of the disorder. Some children and parents may simply prefer to speak of habits, noises, or movements as convenient, nontechnical terms. On the other hand, for some families, certain terms may take on highly charged or dreaded personal meanings. For example, we usually ask parents on meeting them at the beginning of the evaluation if they would prefer us to start with both child and parents present or to begin with just the adults alone. Parents will sometimes take the opportunity of meeting alone to caution us not to use the word *tics* or *Tourette's* in front of the child. With exploration, it will often turn out that these terms carry frightening connotations for the parent, perhaps based on extreme cases they have seen on television talk shows or among family members.

Children may have developed their own theories and idiosyncratic ways of thinking about their symptoms (for a detailed example, see the case of Richard in Chapter 3). One 7-year-old girl developed the term "Sally Sourmind" to describe her intrusive obsessions and accompanying feelings of irritability and dysphoria. The Sally Sourmind feeling became a convenient shorthand for discussing the vicissitudes of her difficulties. Understanding the meanings the parents and child have given to the child's symptoms is also an important prerequisite to helping educate them concerning Tourette's. Education consists of more than a didactic presentation of facts about the disorder. It involves helping the family and child to bring their own experiences of the child's symptoms into relation with what is known about the condition. Such education must be geared to the child's developmental phase and degree of sophistication. Explanations about the neurobiology of the disorder and of the medications used to treat it may be important and useful. On the other hand, the clinician must take pains to identify and address the patient's and family's true concerns and to be alert to the possibility that overly didactic explanations may be used defensively, misunderstood, reified, or conflated with the child's idiosyncratic theories:

> **Case Example.** A 9-year-old boy with Tourette's syndrome spat frequently to relieve the urge to tic. Asked about this, he explained to his doctor the theory he had developed about how the "kaka" rising from his stomach collided with the "tics coming down from my brain" and ricocheted about his body, producing his various symptoms. His theory reflected his struggle to reconcile the neurological explanations he had heard with his own sense of uncontrollable "bad" impulses within.

BEHAVIORAL TREATMENT OF OBSESSIVE-COMPULSIVE DISORDER

As discussed in Chapter 20, the introduction of the serotonin-reuptake inhibitors (SRIs) constitutes a major advance in the treatment of obsessive-compulsive disorder. However, recent studies suggest that as many as 30–40% of patients with obsessive-compulsive disorder demonstrate little or no response after adequate trials of these agents (Greist, Jefferson, Kobak, Katzelnick, & Serlin, 1995; McDougle et al., 1993). Moreover, studies of both children (Leonard et al., 1989) and adults (Pato, Zohar-Kadouch, Zohar, & Murphy, 1988) find relapses of obsessive-compulsive disorder symptoms in up to nearly 90% of patients within a few weeks of withdrawal from clomipramine or specific SRIs such as fluoxetine (Pato, Murphy, & DeVabe, 1991). Finally, some patients or, in the case of children, some parents may be opposed to the use of medication for obsessive-compulsive symptoms because of real or potential side effects. Thus, clinicians who treat children and adolescents with obsessive-compulsive disorder may be called upon to provide nonpharmacological treatment either as an adjunct or as an alternative to medication.

Even prior to the widespread availability of the SRIs, a large body of studies established the utility of cognitive-behavioral therapy (CBT) using exposure and response prevention as a treatment for adults with obsessive-compulsive disorder (Foa, Steketee, Grayson, Turner, & Latimer, 1984; Marks, 1987; Rachman & Hodgson, 1980). Despite this persuasive body of evidence, systematic studies of CBT in children and adolescents have been considerably more limited. Numerous single-case reports of behavioral therapy techniques in the treatment of pediatric patients with obsessive-compulsive disorder have been published over the past two decades (see review by March, 1995); however, studies involving more than a single case are scarce (Apter, Bernhout, & Tyano, 1984; Bolton, Collins, & Steinberg, 1983; March, Mulle, & Herbel, 1994; Piacentini et al., 1994; Scahill et al., 1996). To date, only two studies have used a structured treatment protocol and rigorous methods for rating severity (March et al., 1994; Scahill et al., 1996). Twelve of 15 youngsters were responders (greater than 30% improvement) in the March study, and 5 of 7 patients showed a positive response in the series reported by Scahill et al. (In both of these studies, most children were also receiving medication.) Although neither of these studies was controlled, they support the feasibility of CBT in children and adolescents with obsessive-compulsive disorder.

Component analyses of CBT in adults find that the active ingredients in the successful treatment of obsessive-compulsive disorder are exposure and response prevention (Marks, 1987). *Exposure* consists of confronting a feared stimulus. For example, a person who is fearful of contamination may be instructed to touch a perceived "dirty" object. The therapeutic benefits of exposure stem from the fact that anxiety usually decreases with sustained contact with a feared stimulus. *Response prevention* refers to the instruction not to carry out the ritual (e.g., not to wash) or not to avoid the stimulus (i.e., continue the exposure). When these ingredients are paired, the patient usually experiences a rapid increase in anxiety after exposure, followed by a leveling off and gradual decline of anxiety during the response prevention. Anxiety typically decreases with successive repeated exposure to a given stimulus. With guidance and encouragement from the behavioral therapist, the patient gradually moves through a hierarchical list of feared stimuli (from less anxiety-producing to most) until they no longer provoke anxiety and the urge to ritualize. With children and adolescents, an important key to success is the patient's active collaboration in choosing the sequence of situations to which exposure is to be attempted.

Cognitive-behavioral treatment of obsessive-compulsive disorder in children and adolescents begins with a careful assessment of the obsessive-compulsive symptoms (see Chapters 3 and 15). This is likely to require two or three sessions involving the child and parents in separate and conjoint interviews. Following this step, the child is asked to record the obsessive-compulsive symptoms on a self-monitoring log sheet. The purpose of self-monitoring is to identify the events and situations that provoke the urge to ritualize. Self-monitoring allows therapist and child to refine their common vocabulary about the obsessive-compulsive symptoms. This discussion also provides an opportunity to educate the child that obsessive-compulsive symptoms may be triggered by environmental stimuli and that these triggering stimuli vary in their provocative power. These triggering stimuli are then ranked according to their severity and used in the exposure and reponse prevention exercises. Exposure consists of graded, but deliberate, confrontation with the triggering stimulus. In response prevention, the child agrees to delay the performance of the ritual for increasing periods of time. These exercises are first done in the therapy session and then at home. The exercises may be enhanced by encouraging the child to graph the rise and fall of anxiety during the response prevention period.

Although a variety of other techniques—including relaxation training, cognitive reevaluation of fears, cultivating psychological distance from symptoms (Schwartz, 1996), and systematic positive or negative reinforcement—do not appear to be beneficial when used in isolation, they may be helpful adjuncts as part of an overall treatment plan. These techniques may also help to maintain the child's compliance and to improve anxiety tolerance (March et al., 1994; Scahill et al., 1996). For example, rewards for bravery in the form of praise from the clinician and parents as well as small prizes for engaging in the homework exercises can be very helpful to maintain motivation.

The high rate of success in the case series reported by March et al. (1994) and Scahill et al. (1996) raises questions about which children are most likely to respond to behavioral therapy. In general, predictors of success include motivation, anxiety and avoidance, sufficient ability to report symptoms, and the presence of overt rituals and compulsions (Baer, 1992; Foa & Emmelkamp, 1983). Studies in adults suggest that comorbid depression or delusional beliefs about the obsessional worries predict poor response to CBT. In children, the presence of extensive comorbidity, family conflict interfering with compliance, or developmental factors, such as young age or comorbid pervasive developmental disorder, are associated with poor response.

Few of the treatment studies of exposure and response prevention in patients with obsessive-compulsive disorder provide information regarding the presence or absence of comorbid tic disorder. It remains an important unanswered question whether exposure/response prevention, either alone or in combination with medication, is equally effective for the various apparent subtypes of obsessive-compulsive disorder, such as tic-related, non-tic-related, putatively infection-triggered, and non-infection-triggered forms (King, Leonard, & March, 1998). Also remaining to be systematically studied is the relative utility of exposure/response prevention versus habit reversal techniques, such as those described in the next section, for tic-related compulsions.

As discussed in Chapter 3, tic-related and non-tic-related obsessive-compulsive disorder appear to have important phenomenological differences. For example, non-tic-related obsessive-compulsive disorder is often characterized by fears of harm to self or family members. Thus, washing rituals are performed to prevent the perceived harm of contamination; complex touching rituals are performed to prevent some feared outcome, such as the death of a parent. In contrast, individuals with tic-related forms of obsessive-compulsive disorder describe the urge to repeat an activity until it feels "just right" or until it yields an "even" or symmetrical arrangement. These compulsive urges are typically not preceded by fears of harm, but may be preceded by a feeling that something is not right or is incomplete. In trying to describe this feeling, one 17-year-old patient with

Tourette's syndrome observed that it was an intense variation of the familiar "I feel like I'm forgetting something" experience as one is about to walk out the door. Still other common tic-related obsessive-compulsive disorder symptoms include intrusive sexual and aggressive thoughts and urges. These thoughts may or may not be accompanied by compulsive actions.

Although anxiety may not be the initial felt motivation for compulsive repetition, the child with tic-related obsessive-compulsive disorder may experience mounting frustration and agitation in the effort to "get it right." For example, as 15-year-old Victor put it during his initial evaluation, "Even though I know intellectually I've done it enough, it somehow doesn't register." He then became bogged down in repetitive attempts to explain this feeling over and over again, resulting not in greater clarity but increasing agitation that he hadn't explained it well enough. He then became upset when, after several minutes of repetition, his parents, who tried to reassure Victor that he had described it well enough, wanted to go on to another topic. Victor also described having to wake up and get out of bed in a precise manner each morning. If, after several, time-consuming attempts, he was unable to get it right, Victor would become upset that the whole day would continue to be "messed up," quite literally feeling he had gotten up on the wrong side of the bed.

Even in such cases where clear-cut obsessional worries are not part of the sequence leading to rituals, graded exposure and response procedure may enable the patient to resist repetitions and may reduce and render more tolerable the feelings of incompleteness:

Case Example. At the age of 12 years, George came to the clinic describing multiple simple tics and complex touching habits. The tics, which consisted of facial movements, head jerks, shrugging, and throat noises, had started at the age of 8 years. Although his tics occurred on a daily basis and were noticed by others, they had not posed a major problem and, thus far, had not been the target of treatment. At about the age of 10 years, however, George began to repeat routine activities such as flipping light switches or setting down a glass four or five times. Gradually, he found that more and more activities had to be repeated, and the habits extended beyond ordinary activities to complex routines, such as touching the table corners four times or in multiples of four. This ritual evolved into touching a selected spot near the corner, tracing his finger around the corner, and then stopping at an equidistant point on the other side. If he was successful in landing on the equidistant point, he could move on with his day; if not successful, he would have to retrace the corner four times to get it right. In most instances, four repetitions were sufficient. Increasingly, however, driven by the feeling that it was not quite right, George found himself getting caught in a growing number of multiple repetitions. When caught in these multiple repetitions, he would feel a rising sense of urgency and a vague impression that something bad might happen if he did not get it right. George felt quite certain that the vague worry about harm only occurred when his initial efforts to get it right failed.

Cognitive-behavioral intervention with George included a reassessment of the anxiety that accompanied his failed attempts to get it right. This reassessment challenged his idea that the anxiety was produced by the possibility that something bad would happen and instead proposed reattributing this feeling to the frustrations associated with multiple repetitions to get it right. If true, then repetition would not be an effective strategy because the more he repeated, the more anxious he became. As an alternative strategy, George was instructed to wait and watch the contour of his anxiety without repeating. For example, he was encouraged to practice by tracing the corner once and only once while observing the change in his anxiety. Although these practice sessions were less anxiety producing than the occurrence of similar habits in everyday life, the rise and fall of anxiety served as a useful model for anxiety management outside of the office and homework sessions.

More systematic research is needed concerning the efficacy of behavioral techniques in the treatment of tic-related obsessive-compulsive disorder. Because the distinction between compulsions and complex tics is often not clear, such studies will need to include careful phenomenological description of the target symptoms, including the apparent internal and external triggers for the repetitive behaviors and urges. The relative efficacy of exposure/response prevention versus habit reversal paradigms for various tic-related obsessive-compulsive disorder symptoms also needs to be studied further. As noted below, habit reversal techniques may include implicit elements of exposure and response prevention; thus, careful component analyses of both techniques are desirable. Such studies are especially important in light of the evidence that the improvement produced by behavioral treatment of obsessive-compulsive disorder may have greater durability than that associated with antiobsessional medication, where relapse following discontinuation is common. Indeed, recent studies have shown that behavior therapy and medication can work well together (March & Mulle, 1995; Piacentini et al., 1993; Scahill et al., 1996; Wever, 1994) and can in many cases produce a greater and more sustained therapeutic response than medication alone (Cottraux, Mollard, Bouvard, & Marks, 1993; March et al., 1994). For example, March et al. found that addition of CBT to a stable medication regimen produced a substantial further improvement, and that two-thirds of CBT responders were able to successfully discontinue medication during a two-year follow-up.

BEHAVIORAL TREATMENTS FOR TICS

Over the past three decades, various behavioral treatments have been applied to tics with mixed success. This large literature consists of many case reports and single-subject experimental designs for habit disorders, including tics. Indeed, one of the difficulties in evaluating the efficacy of these behavioral treatments for tic disorders is that many of these studies have included subjects with a range of poorly characterized clinical pictures and habits that may or may not meet diagnostic criteria for chronic tic disorder or Tourette's syndrome. A second difficulty is the variety of treatments that have been used together in treatment packages without evaluation of the efficacy of the individual components. Third, as with studies of all biological and psychological treatments directed at tics, the natural waxing and waning of tic symptoms makes it difficult to determine whether changes in the tics are due to treatment or to the natural course of the disorder. Although many of the single-case experimental studies give careful attention to assessment of symptom severity and treatment integrity, the absence of a comparison group in many studies makes it difficult to exclude nonspecific treatment effects or natural fluctuations, especially in lengthy multisession protocols. Fourth, it is difficult to merge the findings of these various studies because they employed different methods for measuring tic severity.

Massed Negative Practice

Until recently, massed negative practice was the most frequently used behavioral treatment for Tourette's syndrome (Azrin & Peterson, 1988a; A. Peterson, Campise, & Azrin, 1994; Turpin, 1983). This procedure consists of having the patient deliberately perform the tic movement for specified periods of time interspersed with brief periods of rest (e.g., four minutes of movement alternating with one minute of rest). Azrin and Peterson concluded from their review that massed negative practice was somewhat effective, with about half of the studies reporting at least some decrease in tic frequency. Long-term benefit, however, is less clear. Turpin reviewed 22 studies that used massed negative practice and noted that only three maintained successful outcomes after six months' follow-up. Many subjects reported no change in tics, and a substantial number of subjects experienced an actual increase in tics. Turpin concluded that massed negative practice had limited therapeutic usefulness and theoretical validity.

Contingency Management

Operant conditioning in the form of contingency management has been another behavioral treatment technique frequently used with tics (Azrin & Peterson, 1988a; Turpin, 1983). Contingency management is based on the theory that the consequences of a behavior influence the recurrence of that behavior. Simply stated, when a behavior is reinforced, it will be maintained or increased; likewise, when a behavior is punished, it will be suppressed or extinguished. According to theory, if the consequence that follows a tic is reinforcing, the tic will be maintained or even increase; on the other hand, if the consequence is punishing, the tic will be reduced or eliminated. In general, contingency management is implemented by someone other than the patient (e.g., a parent); thus, contingency management may be useful for patients who cannot or will not engage in other techniques. Several studies (Doleys & Kurtz, 1974; Miller, 1970; Schulman, 1974; Tophoff, 1973; Varni, Boyd, & Cataldo, 1978) have employed contingency management with some degree of effectiveness. Unfortunately, most studies included this technique as part of multiple-component treatment packages and have not specifically evaluated contingency management, making it difficult to draw firm conclusions about the effectiveness of this technique in treating tics (A. Peterson, Campise, et al., 1994). Turpin (1983) concluded that outside of controlled settings such as schools and institutions, contingency management procedures may be limited in their utility for treating tics. Outside of such settings, situations and consequences are difficult to control and behaviors may be inadvertently maintained by unintended contingencies across time and settings. Such factors could account for the poor generalization of contingency management outside of the rigorously controlled treatment conditions that have been studied.

Despite these limitations, Azrin and Peterson (1988a) have suggested that positive reinforcement in the form of praise and encouragement from family members and others involved in the child's treatment and care may be useful. This approach entails acknowledging and praising the child's efforts when he or she is tic-free, and refraining from comment during bouts of tics. For example, Wagaman, Miltenberger, and Williams (1995) found that reinforcement for the absence of tic behavior was an effective treatment for a 9-year-old male with a vocal tic that was unresponsive to habit reversal procedures. Although this approach may be beneficial, it is important not to imply that periods of tic exacerbation represent some failure of self-control. Positive reinforcement should not be expected to reduce the frequency or intensity of tics, but it may be helpful in increasing the child's motivation to comply with other forms of treatment.

One potentially useful application of contingency management and related techniques would seem to be the management of disruptive behaviors associated with Tourette's syndrome. Although these techniques have been effectively employed with children with ADHD uncomplicated by Tourette's syndrome (Kazdin, 1993), their use in children with comorbid ADHD and tic disorders remains largely unstudied and underutilized.

Self-Monitoring

Self-monitoring consists of having the subject record tics by using a wrist counter or small notebook. Multiple baseline studies by Hutzell, Platzek, and Logue (1974) and Billings (1978) reported improvements using this method. An essential ingredient of self-monitoring is discrimination training, the ability of the individual to identify accurately when a tic occurs, as well as the situation in which it occurs. Immediate, rather than delayed, recording of tics appears to be essential. Thomas, Abrams, and Johnson (1971) demonstrated a reduction of tics using self-monitoring. However, self-monitoring was only one component of a treatment package, making it difficult to attribute these gains specifically to self-monitoring. In a study of two children, self-monitoring alone was effective for one and, in combination with competing response training, was effective for the other (Ollendick, 1981). Azrin and Peterson (1988b) speculated that self-monitoring may be successful in reducing some tics because it increases the individual's awareness of the tic behaviors. In a report of a multiple baseline design to treat head and eyebrow tics in a young man (Wright & Miltenberger, 1987), awareness training alone was successful in reducing the subject's tics, although his difficulty in consistently identifying occurrences of tics persisted throughout the treatment. These possible therapeutic effects of self-monitoring may pose problems when this technique is used as a method of assessing treatment effects.

Habit Reversal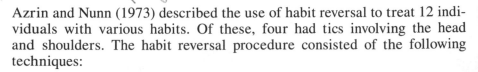

Azrin and Nunn (1973) described the use of habit reversal to treat 12 individuals with various habits. Of these, four had tics involving the head and shoulders. The habit reversal procedure consisted of the following techniques:

> *Recording.* Subjects estimated the frequency of the habit prior to treatment and kept a record of the habit after the initiation of treatment.
>
> *Awareness training.* This consisted of *response description* (while looking in a mirror, the subject describes each occurrence of the behavior in detail), *response detection* (the subject was told by the therapist each time the target behavior occurred until the subject was able to detect the occurrence unassisted), *early warning* (the subject practiced identifying early signs of the behavior), and *situation awareness training* (the subject described people, places, and situations in which the behavior occurred).
>
> *Competing response practice.* The subject was instructed to tense muscles that are incompatible with the habit movement. The authors described several characteristics presumed to be necessary for the competing response: it needs to be opposed to the tic or habit movement; and it must be sustainable for several minutes to produce an increasing awareness of the muscles involved in the movement, to be socially unobtrusive and easily compatible with ongoing behaviors, and to strengthen the muscles opposite the tic movement. Subjects were instructed to engage in the response either at the urge to tic or at the actual occurrence of the tic. Examples: for an eye blinking tic, "systematic, voluntary, soft blinking consciously maintained at a rate of one blink per 3–5 seconds and/or frequent downward shifting of gaze about every 5–10 seconds"; for arm movements, "push[ing] hand down on thigh or stomach and push[ing] elbow in towards hip"; for a phonic tic, "slow rhythmic deep breathing through the nose while keeping the mouth closed" taking care not to interrupt the flow of air (Carr, 1995, p. 455).

Habit control motivation. This component involved a habit inconvenience review as well as social support procedures, that is, having the subject describe how the habit or tic had caused problems and having the subject's friends and family provide praise and support for the nonoccurrence of the habit.

Generalization training. Symbolic rehearsal, practice, and instructions for controlling tics in everyday situations comprised this component. Symbolic rehearsal consisted of imaginal exposure in which the subject was instructed to imagine being in situations described in the awareness training phase. During the exposure, the subject is encouraged to imagine not performing the behavior and engaging in the competing response.

After only one treatment session, the reported mean reduction in habits and tics for all 12 subjects was 90%, with a 99% mean decrease at three-month follow-up. All data were self-report and did not involve direct observation.

Since this original description, numerous studies have evaluated this method for reducing habits, including trichotillomania (Vitulano, King, & Scahill, 1992) as well as tics. The focus of the following discussion is on those studies that have evaluated this method specifically for treating tic symptoms.

Finney, Rapoff, Hall, and Christophersen (1983) used the habit reversal procedure described by Azrin and Nunn (1973) to treat motor tics in two early adolescent boys, with the added component of a simple breathing and muscle relaxation exercise. Treatment was administered in three clinic visits ranging from one to one and one-half hours in duration. Because social embarrassment is often a reason for seeking treatment of tics, social validation was used as a measure of treatment success. This consisted of asking groups of judges (teachers and graduate students) who were not informed of the purpose of the study or the target behaviors to observe videotapes of the subjects at baseline and during treatment conditions. They were asked to answer whether they observed any distracting behaviors, to rate any distracting behaviors observed on a 7-point scale, and to answer whether they would seek treatment for similar behaviors. Observations were videotaped in the subjects' homes and segments were randomly selected and ordered. Results showed 50–98% reduction in tics; this was maintained at 5- and 12-month follow-ups. A strength of this study was its use of the social validation procedure and direct observation in a natural setting.

Miltenberger and his colleagues have focused much of their work on identifying the active components of the habit reversal procedure. Miltenberger, Fuqua, and McKinley (1985) compared treatments using the entire habit reversal procedure to a simplified procedure consisting of only self-awareness and competing response training. Nine subjects participated in the study, only three of whom appeared to have childhood-onset tics, two with eye blinking and one with shoulder and head jerking. The other six subjects had movements described as tics with onset in adulthood. All nine subjects were divided into two groups, with one receiving 4–10 sessions of the entire habit reversal procedure and the other receiving 4–10 sessions of the simplified procedure. All but one subject (an adult-onset subject in the habit reversal condition) showed significant decreases in the target behaviors as measured either by frequency count or by naïve raters' scores of six-second intervals of videotaped observations; these gains were maintained at 7- and 15-week follow-ups. There were no differences in treatment effects between subjects receiving the full habit reversal procedure and those receiving the simplified procedure. These results suggest that it is possible to obtain significant treatment gains using self-awareness and competing response training alone without the other components of the entire habit reversal procedure. Although these studies provide guidance for refining the competing response process, they should be viewed cautiously because of the small, heterogeneous samples employed and the brief observation periods used to assess efficacy.

Azrin and Nunn (1973) contend that the efficacy of the competing response component stems from its incompatibility with the habit (or tic) and the "heightened awareness [produced] by an isometric tensing of the muscles involved in the movement" (p. 623). In contrast, Miltenberger and Fuqua (1985) propose that the performance of the competing response contingent upon the occurrence of a tic is an effective treatment because it serves as a punishment.

Further component analyses of the competing response technique have been conducted to evaluate if the competing response must be similar to the tic or if a dissimilar competing response could be as effective. For example, for a head jerk, the dissimilar competing response was to tighten the left calf; the similar response was to tighten the neck by pressing the chin to the chest. The authors noted, "contingent practice of [a] similar competing response sometimes involves performance of a behavior that is either effortful . . . disruptive of on-going activities, or potentially embarrassing when performed in public" (Sharenow, Fuqua, & Miltenberger, 1989, p. 36). Using a multiple baseline design with three subjects, the authors found that a dissimilar competing response was successful in reducing tics and that the addition of a similar competing response did not lead to further reductions in tics. Social validation measures after intervention provided supportive evidence of the success of the treatment. These results suggest that incompatibility of the competing response with the tic movement is apparently not essential to efficacy (Miltenberger & Fuqua, 1985).

To perform a competing response, the individual must first be aware of the tic when it occurs. As previously described, self-monitoring can enhance self-awareness and has been shown to be effective for reducing tics in some people. Habit reversal components were analyzed in four children with tics to evaluate the effects of awareness training independent of competing response training (Woods, Miltenberger, & Lumley, 1996). The components were implemented in an additive sequential manner (from the least to the most effortful), to identify the treatment combination that was effective for each child. The rationale for this approach is based on the clinical observation that patients and their families will be more likely to comply with treatment procedures that require less effort. Results of this multiple baseline study were mixed. Although all four children experienced decreases or elimination of their tics, each one responded differently to the different combinations of treatment components. Thus, no clear indication as to which components are most likely to benefit a given child emerged from the study. As expected, a decrease in the level of compliance was noted as the demand characteristics of the procedures became more rigorous.

A. Peterson and Azrin (1992) suggest that self-monitoring be used as the initial approach because it will provide baseline data and may result in significant decreases in tics with minimal instruction. Carr and Bailey (1996) used an alternating treatments design to determine experimentally the optimal treatment rather than making an arbitrary selection. A 9-year-old boy with nasal tics (described as forced nasal exhalations, sniffling, snorting, and throat clearing) was assessed and treated in his home for a total of nine sessions (including baseline). After experimental sessions of self-monitoring, competing response practice, and dissimilar response practice were conducted, competing response practice was chosen as the treatment. After three treatment sessions, his tic frequency was reduced by 70% as measured by direct observation frequency counts; these gains endured at one-month follow-up.

In some cases, the benefits of habit reversal procedures for one tic are reported to have generalized to suppression of other tics not specifically treated with a competing response (Azrin & Peterson, 1988b; Woods et al., 1996). Although this can present a problem from an experimental design position, it is a positive bonus from a clinical standpoint, in that each tic may not need to be treated separately. Other studies did not observe this generalization of effect, but did find a decrease in the specific tics that were the focus of treatment (Finney et al., 1983).

Collectively, the preceding studies have reported success in treating individual tics using composite habit reversal procedures or simplified components. A major weakness of most studies is that they lacked diagnostic information about subjects and the severity of their tics. Hence, the generalizability of these findings to the often complex and persistent symptoms of chronic multiple tic disorders including Tourette's syndrome is unclear. Notable exceptions to this limitation are studies by Azrin and Peterson (1988, 1990). Azrin and Peterson (1988b) examined the efficacy of habit reversal in three adults diagnosed with Tourette's syndrome. Individual components of the procedure were not evaluated. Over a period of six to eight months, the frequency of tics decreased by 93–95% in the clinic and 64–99% at home, with concurrent decreases in severity. In a subsequent study (Azrin & Peterson, 1990), a waiting-list control group design was used to evaluate the habit reversal procedure for treating motor and vocal tics in subjects with Tourette's syndrome. Although treatment effects were less rapid than in previous studies targeting single tics, all subjects were reported to have improved substantially.

Turpin (1983) offers possible theoretical explanations for the success of habit reversal procedures. First, learning a response that competes directly with the tic behavior may provide motivational components that facilitate self-control. Second, the competing response practice, which is experienced as unpleasant by the subject, could be viewed as a self-administered punishment procedure paired with the tic, resulting in a reduction of the tic. A third possibility conceptualizes habit reversal as a form of response prevention. Given the sensory component of tics (Leckman, Walker, et al., 1993; Scahill, Leckman, et al., 1995), treatment procedures developed for obsessive-compulsive disorders, specifically response prevention, might also be useful for tic disorders. O'Brien and Brennan (1979) reported a multifaceted behavioral treatment for a woman with a severe chronic facial tic and vocal distortion. After several strategies were attempted, a physical restraint device was used to restrict excessive jaw movement, effectively serving a response prevention function. Results were reportedly dramatic, with greatly reduced movements within a few days that were maintained through a two-year follow-up.

Bullen and Helmsley's (1983) findings provided additional support for this interpretation. The subject was "instructed to 'ignore the itch' and it was suggested to her that the sensation would eventually disappear without her having to move" (p. 200). By following this instruction, improvement was noted within treatment sessions, but the subject was unable to continue this effort between therapy sessions. Bliss (1980) also reported being able to control his tics in this manner, emphasizing that it did not eliminate the urge but rather allowed some degree of control over the movements. In our clinical experience, some patients with Tourette's syndrome report that although they may be able to suppress a given tic transiently, for example in a potentially embarrassing situation, it is usually by dint of great effort and frequently followed by a more severe bout of tics.

Although competing response techniques may be useful in reducing the frequency of troublesome tics, the impairment associated with some tics may not be due to the actual tic movement so much as to the disruption of concentration on other activities, secondary to premonitory urges, the tic movement, and the effort to suppress it. Given the effort and concentration necessary to perform the competing response, it is unclear in any given case whether the competing response will be less burdensome than the tic symptom against which it is deployed. It is also unclear whether habit reversal techniques can be useful in reducing troublesome premonitory urges and sensory phenomena. Clearly, more systematic controlled treatment studies of the habit reversal and response prevention paradigms, using clinically appropriate measures, are needed in well-characterized patients with Tourette's syndrome.

At least in its naïve form, stimulus-response theory is sometimes taken to imply that all voluntary behaviors (as well as many autonomic ones) are potentially malleable, given the appropriate positive or negative contingent reinforcers. Behavioral researchers have recently begun to grapple theoretically with the likelihood that tics are maintained by multiple factors that include neurophysiological factors as well as environmental influences and contingent reinforcers (Carr, Taylor, Wallander, & Reiss, 1996). For example, one such approach suggests that, because performing the tic may relieve or reduce the sensory phenomena and premonitory urges that often precede tics, this reduction serves to reinforce further tics (Evers & van de Wetering, 1994). It is to be hoped that further theory building, based on increasingly sophisticated appreciation of the phenomenology of Tourette's syndrome, will facilitate the development of more effective methods of non-pharmacological intervention for tics.

TRADITIONAL PSYCHOTHERAPEUTIC CONSIDERATIONS

Indications for Formal Psychotherapy

In contrast to the specific behavioral therapy interventions discussed above, the core symptoms of tics, compulsions, and obsessions are usually not the immediate focus of psychodynamic psychotherapy for individuals with Tourette's syndrome. As discussed in Chapters 3, 4, and 5, a vulnerability to learning and attentional difficulties, anxiety, impulsivity, emotional lability, and affective difficulties is common in individuals with Tourette's syndrome. Not surprisingly, the commonest indications for formal psychothera-peutic interventions for such patients are low self-esteem, impairing anxiety or depression, and poor relationships with family, teachers (or employers), and peers. The goals of such dynamic and interpersonal psychotherapeutic interventions extend beyond the elimination of specific symptoms to facilitating progress in the crucial adaptive tasks of maintaining supportive relationships at home, developing friendships, acquiring a sense of mastery at school or work, and developing a coherent, positive identity (D. Cohen, 1995). Although the primary goal of such treatment is usually not the direct reduction of tics or compulsions, improving individual and family coping strategies may help ameliorate stress-related exacerbations of such symptoms and reduce the levels of medication needed for their control (Wolff, 1988). Unfortunately, there continues to be a lack of any empirical studies of traditional psychotherapy with individuals with Tourette's syndrome.

Technical and Developmental Issues

Psychodynamic and interpersonal interventions with individuals with Tourette's syndrome consist of many of the same psychotherapeutic components as with other patients. In addition, however, such work also often involves technical and dynamic issues specific to Tourette's syndrome and to the developmental phase of the patient.

Prepubertal Children

Although isolated transient tics are common in school-age children, especially boys, it is usually in the early school years that the multiplicity and chronicity of tics first become apparent in children who come to bear a diagnosis of Tourette's syndrome. In the primary grades, ADHD-associated difficulties, such as impulsiveness, poor social skills, and irritability, are usually more common indications for psychotherapeutic intervention than are tics per se. In fact, many young children are far less aware of their tics than are their parents. By third or fourth grade, however, children may have tics severe enough to cause them distress or embarrassment or to provoke adverse reactions from peers or teachers. In addition to the necessary direct interventions with school personnel, psychotherapeutic work can profitably explore how children represent their symptoms to themselves and others and how their attempts to deal with others' reactions may elicit support or counterproductively exacerbate interpersonal difficulties. For example, one common important therapeutic exercise is to help children work through how and with whom they will share the fact of having tics.

Adolescence

Like other adolescents, teenagers with Tourette's syndrome are concerned with issues of autonomy and acceptance by friends and members of the opposite sex. For the older adolescent, issues of identity, romantic and sexual intimacy, separation from parents, and vocational choices become more prominent developmental issues. As with other adolescents with chronic medical conditions, the wish to minimize difficulties in the service of not feeling weak, defective, or dependent renders many adolescents with Tourette's syndrome wary of psychotherapy or noncompliant with medication. Because such adolescents see involvement in treatment, whether psychological or medical, as a humiliating admission of weakness, it is often useful to emphasize the progressive aims of treatment, namely, helping the youngster to feel more in control of his or her feelings, actions, and important life choices.

Even when parents, peers, and school have been sympathetic and accommodating, adolescents with Tourette's syndrome may feel painfully different from peers. For some youngsters, the burden of constant vigilance against socially embarrassing or sexually or aggressively charged tics and compulsions may take its toll in the form of isolation, depression, or character constriction; other adolescents' personalities may become organized around their perceived lack of control. If compounded with perseverative stickiness, impulsiveness, and adolescent oppositionality, the outcome may be frequent, stormy, and stubborn confrontations with adults and peers.

Issues of Attribution and Locus of Control

A common and recurrent issue in work with children with Tourette's and their families concerns the extent to which the child, as opposed to the disorder, should be seen as responsible for various problematic behaviors. Closely related to these concerns is the task of determining what are reasonable expectations for the control of such behaviors. Although this question takes us to the heart of deep philosophical issues regarding volition and moral agency, the more pressing concern here is the practical clinical challenge posed.

Conferring a diagnosis of Tourette's syndrome is more than an exercise in clinical classification. In addition to helping make sense of a plethora of seemingly disparate symptoms (tics, compulsions, impulsiveness, perseveration, etc.) under a single explanatory rubric, this act of diagnosis also carries social meaning in implying that the individual is not to be held fully responsible for certain behaviors. As noted earlier, this reframing of behavior may have an important beneficial effect in reducing inappropriate parental recriminations or counterproductive demands for tic suppression, as well as ameliorating the child's own sense of guilt or shame over various tics. At the same time, however, it must be noted that the child with tics inevitably struggles with defining the shifting boundaries of his or her self-control (D. Cohen, 1980). To the extent that various impulses or acts are seen by the child or family as "not self, but Tourette's syndrome," culpability is reduced. The potential price of assuming this posture, however, is reduction of the scope of perceived efficacy and self-control.

On a practical level, the degree of control that can be exerted over different symptoms at tolerable cost varies across symptom class and individuals and can perhaps only be determined empirically in each individual case. For example, although many adult patients with Tourette's describe tics as straddling the boundary between voluntary and involuntary and may be able to transiently suppress or defer some tics, most patients find it ineffective and counterproductive to attempt to suppress all or most of their tics over sustained periods (Bliss, 1980; Kane, 1994; Leckman, Walker, et al., 1993). In contrast, although the impulsive behavior of many children with Tourette's syndrome most likely reflects a neurobiological vulnerability, environmental structure and firm, consistent parental expectations and limit setting are usually helpful to the child. Paradoxically, if the attribution of these behaviors to Tourette's is taken to imply that they are beyond the child's control, the failure to set appropriate limits may be detrimental to the child's overall development. Similarly, abrupt, unrehearsed, and unilateral parental fiats are usually not helpful to the child who is pathologically attempting to engage parents in the child's compulsive routines; however, consistent parental limit setting and resistance to colluding with the child's compulsive routines are important components of a systematic treatment plan (Knox, Albano, & Barlow, 1996; March & Mulle, 1995; March et al., 1994; Scahill et al., 1996). Although the malleability of each specific symptom area must be addressed individually, most children do best with an approach that helps to foster an internal locus of control through maintaining reasonable expectations and encouraging active problem solving.

Occasionally, one sees children and families whose overattribution of all problematic aspects of the child's behavior to Tourette's syndrome is a serious, partially iatrogenic problem:

Case Example. John, a 9-year-old boy, was seen for a second opinion concerning a putative diagnosis of Tourette's syndrome. Both on the symptom report form filled out prior to the interview and in the evaluation itself,

John described an extensive list of tics that ranged from simple facial and phonic tics through "energy tics, jumping up and down tics, head-standing tics, running around tics, angry tics, and mean tics." In the course of the two-hour evaluation, it became clear that John was an intelligent, active boy, who, despite a variety of mild to moderate simple tics, suffered greater impairment from his restless behavior, which sometimes took on an oppositional or provocative edge. His diligent and devoted parents, having been told that tics were involuntary and that demands for suppression were ill-advised, felt confused and stymied about how to deal with John's panoply of putative tics, which included cursing when he did not get his own way. An important part of the consultation involved helping the parents distinguish between John's true tics and his unrestrained provocative behavior. In the session itself, the clinicians were able to demonstrate that reasonable limit setting could be effective and tolerated by John (e.g., asking John, who was restlessly lying on the couch with his legs over his head, to sit up and take his feet off the wall).

Case Example. Naomi, a 14-year-old girl with Tourette's, was hospitalized for evaluation and adjustment of an ever-increasing number of medications on which she had been placed by her primary clinician. Naomi had been out of school for several weeks with a variety of physical and psychological symptoms, among which it was hard to disentangle medication side effects, depression, anxious somatization, angry outbursts in the midst of family conflicts, and normative adolescent issues, as well as several simple tics of moderate severity. Naomi came from a concerned and devout family with high moral standards, and she herself was a diligent student with perfectionistic expectations of herself and others. She and her parents spoke at distressed length about what they regarded as her alter "Tourettic" personality, whom they named Touretta, and whom they held responsible for many of Naomi's outbursts. Asked to describe one such episode in detail, Naomi provided what appeared to be a typical example of Touretta's troublemaking. After Naomi had been out of school for several weeks because of her symptoms, a close friend came over to visit but spent most of the time talking and playing with Naomi's older sister. Following this, Naomi, under what she described as Touretta's baleful influence, had yelled and thrown objects at her sister, conduct that Naomi assured us *she* never would have done herself. Here the issue was not some inexorable malignant neurological process, which the parents feared. Rather, it was the spurious attribution of the behavior to the disorder, in such a way as to give Naomi permission to act on (but disavow) impulses that should have been restrained. This view of the disorder provided a potential fault line for dissociation and repudiation of normal but poorly tolerated feelings. The therapeutic task was to help Naomi recognize her various difficult and conflictual feelings as legitimate aspects of herself and to develop more adaptive methods of coping with them, rather than to encourage her disavowal of them by medicalizing them as bizarre features of Tourette's.

Although these are extreme cases, they illustrate some of the hazards and misuses of diagnosis. Part of the clinician's task is to help maintain a focus on the patient's overall developmental trajectory. Although a small number of individuals are truly overwhelmed by the severity of their disorder, with few areas of functioning left unimpaired, for most individuals with Tourette's syndrome, their diagnosis is only one part of who they are. Together with the generally positive prognostic picture that it is now possible to convey to most children with Tourette's syndrome and their families (Leckman, Zhang, et al., 1998), parents need support in maintaining a balanced picture of the child, with all of his or her strengths and vulnerabilities, developmental challenges and accomplishments (R. King et al., 1995). To insist on the term "a child with Tourette's syndrome" rather than "a Tourette's syndrome child" is more than a nicety of diction or piece of political correctness; it reflects a clinical stance that places the child's symptoms and the interventions addressed to them in the context of the child's overall development and personality.

Family Issues

As with most chronic disorders, the impact of the symptoms of the child with Tourette's syndrome on overall family functioning, including effects on siblings and the parents' spousal relationship, must be carefully assessed. At the same time, serious family stresses or conflicts, especially those focused on the patient, may serve to exacerbate tic and obsessive-compulsive disorder symptoms as well as disrupt development in other ways. Because of the important genetic component to Tourette's syndrome, it is common for there to be another close family member affected with tics, obsessions, compulsions, anxiety, depression, or impulsiveness. In addition to the family burden of multiple affected siblings, parental symptoms may have a deleterious impact on the child. For example, a father who is himself reactive, irritable, or impulsive may have difficulty maintaining the structured environment and emotional modulation optimal for a child with the same problems. On the other hand, a parent who is overly anxious or obsessionally inflexible may be deleteriously intolerant of a child who is hyperactive with prominent tics. Goodness of fit among family members may be more important than the individual temperaments of family members and may need to be the explicit focus of family-oriented interventions.

When both a parent and a child share a symptom, this may be a useful source of mutual understanding. For example, a father with childhood or persistent tics is in a unique position to understand his young son's experience and to provide a model of successful perseverance in the face of similar difficulties. On the other hand, overidentification can be a problem when a parent sees his or her worst self-doubts (or worries about a spouse or sibling) reawakened by the appearance of similar symptoms in an offspring. This type of overidentification may also be a source of trouble when it elicits overprotection by a parent. Excessive guilt or blame over which parent's side of the family is to blame for the child's condition usually reflects deeper-lying marital tensions that need to be therapeutically addressed.

Duration and Dosing of Psychotherapy

The scope, duration, and frequency of psychotherapeutic intervention and the identified participants (child, sibling, and/or parents) will most often vary over time depending on the type and severity of symptoms, the child's level of overall adaptive functioning, family issues, and so on. At any one phase of development, interventions may range from single, one-shot interventions aimed at helping the child and family deal with an acute crisis, through long-term intensive psychotherapy and every shade of intensity and breadth in between (D. Cohen, 1991, 1995). What is most important is the continuity of care provided by a knowledgeable and flexible therapist who can remain available to the child and parents as a resource over the succesive phases of the child's development.

INTEGRATION OF
PSYCHOTHERAPEUTIC INTERVENTIONS

For many individuals, the optimal treatment of Tourette's syndrome requires a flexible coordination of different modalities over time. These modalities may include psychodynamic and interpersonal interventions, behavioral techniques, family education and guidance, and school consultation, as well as judicious use of medication (see Tables 15.2 and 15.3). Too often, however, a therapeutic tower of Babel exists, where the choices of therapies offered depend less on the patient's needs than on the guild preferences or theoretical predilections of the specialist consulted. Outside of tertiary care settings specializing in the multimodal treatment of Tourette's disorder, it may be difficult to find clinicians capable of individually providing this full range of treatment. Most commonly, patients and families are best served by the ongoing availability of a flexible, non-doctrinaire clinician who can coordinate a multidisciplinary team capable of providing different interventions as the child's symptoms change or different developmental challenges arise.

Although the various psychodynamic, behavioral, and cognitive approaches may appear quite divergent in theoretical terms, in actual practice there are often important commonalities among therapists of nominally different theoretical orientation (Arkowtiz & Messer, 1984; Wachtel, 1977) over and above the nonspecific elements of attention and support. Self-monitoring, identifying situational and affective triggers of problem behaviors, imaginal exposure, encouragement of graded exposure and response prevention, and reframing of expectations and beliefs are important shared elements of both psychodynamic and behavioral approaches.

SUMMARY OF CHAPTER 18

Supportive psychotherapeutic interventions with a strong educational component are hallmarks of the Yale approach to the long-term care of individuals with Tourette's syndrome and related disorders. Cognitive-behavioral treatments of obsessive-compulsive disorder are well established and should be considered early, particularly in cases where there is a strong element of anxiety or phobic avoidance. Despite a number of optimistic reports, behavioral approaches for the treatment of chronic tic disorders are not well established. The chapter closes with a review of traditional psychotherapeutic approaches and their relevance to the treatment of the emotional sequelae of Tourette's and related disorders.

PREVIEW OF CHAPTER 19

When individuals are having significant difficulties in the classroom, with peers, in the family, or emotionally, intervention is warranted. Although no educational methods specific to Tourette's or obsessive-compulsive disorder have been validated empirically, considerable information is available regarding strategies that have been reported to be helpful with tics and the related behaviors that often accompany Tourette's syndrome. Maintaining a focus on the affected individual's strengths and weaknesses is central to developing appropriate compensatory strategies within the child and in the environment. Teachers and other school professionals should consider not only interventions that involve the individual child or adolescent, but also more universal interventions that affect all of the children in the classroom. Educating teachers and classmates about the nature of Tourette's syndrome, obsessive-compulsive disorder, and ADHD can enhance empathy and understanding and facilitate a more positive learning environment for the child or adolescent, but also for all of the unaffected children in the classroom. Continued research is needed to validate current clinical recommendations for education both in and out of the classroom. Further, research integrating pharmacological treatment, behavioral modification, and different types of school and family interventions is needed.

CHAPTER 19

Recommendations for Teachers

ALICE S. CARTER, NANCY J. FREDINE, DIANE FINDLEY, LAWRENCE
SCAHILL, LYNNE ZIMMERMAN, and SARA S. SPARROW

> It is most helpful when teachers, like clinicians, view the child as a whole
> person, develop a broad view of a pupil's overall academic and social func-
> tioning, and avoid the temptation to fix upon target symptoms.
>
> —*Donald J. Cohen, Kenneth Towbin, and James F. Leckman, 1992*

Although not all children with Tourette's syndrome require special educational services, specific intervention is indicated when a child or adolescent is not making sufficient developmental gains in any domain of
functioning or is acquiring deviant behaviors that interfere with forward
progress. As discussed in Chapter 15, school-based interventions are recommended (a) when a child is falling behind academically; (b) when tics
are frequent, forceful, and directly interfere with the child's ability to
learn or participate in classroom activities; (c) when a child or adolescent
has no friends or has significant problems in peer acceptance; or (d) when
the child's self-esteem is in jeopardy (Cohen, 1990). The most beneficial
treatments are developmentally determined and tailored to the individual
affected with Tourette's syndrome and his or her family. Frequently, the
behavioral and learning problems that occur in association with Tourette's
pose the greatest obstacle to the child's ongoing developmental progress
and must be the first focus of treatment interventions (Chappell, Leckman,
et al., 1995). School psychologists are in an ideal position to collect information regarding a child's difficulties in the school setting as well as
changes in symptoms that may follow the introduction of specific interventions (Atkins & Pelham, 1991; Walter & Carter, 1997).

As discussed in Chapter 18, cognitive-behavioral approaches may be
particularly effective in obsessive-compulsive disorder and ADHD. Pharmacological interventions designed to reduce tic or obsessive-compulsive
symptoms should be carefully evaluated for their potential impact on the

overall development of the child; for example, a reduction in tics that is accompanied by drowsiness may well be counterproductive. Further, in our experience, only a minority of patients have tics of sufficient severity to warrant treatment with medications (Chappell, Leckman, et al., 1995; see also Chapter 20). In the case of a child with significant comorbid ADHD and obsessive-compulsive symptoms, the clinician may be faced with a real dilemma concerning which symptoms are the most problematic for the child's development at the time (Scahill, 1996).

STRATEGIES FOR PARENT-SCHOOL PARTNERSHIPS

Collaborative relationships between the families of children with Tourette's syndrome and related disorders and school personnel are essential to effective evaluation and treatment. Ongoing communication among parents, teachers, and other school and mental health professionals about changes in academic functioning or behavior is necessary to develop and maintain appropriate interventions, which are generally based on a shared understanding of the child's strengths and needs as well as changes in specific target symptoms. For many children with these conditions, no special modifications will be needed in school or at home, although it is generally beneficial to educate teachers and other school professionals about the nature of Tourette's syndrome, obsessive-compulsive disorder, and ADHD. For other children, specific modifications in expectations at school and at home will be necessary. A smaller number of these children may require special education services mandated by state and federal statutes. In addition, many children and families may benefit from adjunct psychotherapy that is focused on learning to cope with a chronic, erratic, and often stigmatizing illness (see Chapter 18).

Although there have been no formal studies evaluating the best approach to structuring the daily life of a child with Tourette's syndrome or related conditions (see Chapters 1 and 8), many approaches and guidelines are recommended by experienced clinicians and consumer advocacy groups such as the Tourette Syndrome Association (TSA; Scahill, Lynch, et al., 1995). The TSA, Obsessive Compulsive Foundation (OCF), and Children with Hyperactivity/Attention Deficit Disorder (CHADD) are national volunteer organizations that provide support, guidance, education, and comfort for affected individuals and their families. They can be valuable resources, offering a great deal of information specifically designed for educators, such as videos, books, educational pamphlets, and suggestions for speakers. Clearly, more empirical research that addresses the efficacy of school and parent interventions is needed. In the interim, however, parents may seek consultation from their school psychologist to assist in developing strategies to establish a baseline of performance, monitor the child's progress, and evaluate the child's response to any intervention that is introduced. By carefully evaluating interventions that are introduced in school and at home, parents and school professionals can have greater confidence that they are proceeding in a positive direction. The following sections outline and briefly describe approaches that we have found to be useful in structuring the child's home and school environment.

Strategies for Children with Tourette's Syndrome

Although there are some similarities across children with Tourette's syndrome, it is critical to acknowledge that each child with Tourette's is unique and presents with a singular educational and clinical profile. For example, children with Tourette's reflect the normal intelligence curve (Chapter 5; Hagin et al., 1982). Some will be excellent students, others artistically talented, and still others exceptional athletes. Children with Tourette's syndrome have the same needs and desires as other children— they differ in experiencing the effects of a neuropsychiatric disorder (Scahill, Lynch, et al., 1995; Walter & Carter, 1997). By understanding that there is no prototypic child with Tourette's syndrome, school professionals can be more creative and flexible in facilitating a particular child's academic adaptation (Walter & Carter).

The teacher's response and reaction to the child's tics can make a critical difference in the child's life. Teachers who are unfamiliar with Tourette's syndrome can benefit from support from the child's family and other school personnel, such as the school psychologist, the school nurse, and the principal, to understand that the tics are the result of a brain-based condition and are performed in response to insistent sensory urges—something like an itch (see Chapter 2 for a more detailed account of this phenomenon). Although tics can be annoying or disruptive in a classroom, expressing frustration, anger, or dismay is not an effective way to help the child stop the tics. Indeed, a negative emotional reaction by the teacher is likely to make a child or adolescent feel more anxious, isolated, or hostile. Further, as tics tend to be sensitive to stress, they may worsen if the child becomes more frustrated or fearful. A child or adolescent with Tourette's syndrome tends to perform optimally, as do most individuals, in a calm, supportive environment. It is remarkable what many teachers are able to achieve when they and their students are well informed and unfazed by even disruptive tics.

Teachers serve as role models for classmates and can actively educate students about Tourette's either alone or in the context of other chronic illnesses that children may experience. Classmates may be totally ignorant or misinformed about Tourette's syndrome and may harbor erroneous ideas such as believing that the tics are contagious. As classmates learn more about Tourette's syndrome, it becomes less frightening and mysterious, allowing them to be more supportive and less likely to tease the child about the tics (see Chapter 6; Hamilton, 1997). Because most children are frustrated and embarrassed by their tics, it may be possible to involve the child in developing strategies for coping with tics in the classroom and for educating his or her classmates. Level of involvement would depend, in part, on the child's age and comfort level. In devising strategies, a major dilemma for the teacher is how to balance the need for individualized approaches with the needs of the whole class, while minimizing stigmatization that can lead to difficulties with peer teasing. Strategies that minimize stigmatization include those that privately involve only the child with Tourette's syndrome or are directed in a universal manner to all children in the classroom or school. Teachers can learn about successful strategies from parents, who often have a fund of knowledge about their child's responses to a variety of approaches that is based on years of trial-and-error experiences. The school psychologist, who may have experience with behavioral methods, is another important resource for teachers. Teachers and school psychologists should also be encouraged to obtain materials from the TSA. As previously stated, the need for collaboration among all involved is essential.

Although collaboration can facilitate the development of appropriate strategies to cope with the disruption in learning that tics may cause in the classroom for both the child with Tourette's and his or her peers, the primary responsibility of implementation typically falls on the classroom teacher. In many cases, the most difficult aspect of Tourette's syndrome for teachers is determining where the boundaries are between the child's volitional states and the Tourette's syndrome: what is reasonable to tolerate, what should be accommodated, and how and when to set appropriate limits (Scahill et al., 1993b). Teachers often need support and encouragement to cope with feelings of frustration that could be transmitted to the child inadvertently. As the symptoms of Tourette's syndrome vary dramatically across children and within a particular child over brief periods of time, teachers are placed in the difficult position of needing to reevaluate and make appropriate modifications in their strategies quite frequently.

Often, accommodations can be implemented by the classroom teacher without the need for formal evaluations and intervention plans. Some of the strategies we and others (Burd, Kauffman, & Kerbeshian, 1992; Packer, 1997) have found useful include extending time limits on tests, allowing alternative ways to produce work (i.e., using a word processor, calculator, or books on tape), and allowing the child to choose where to sit. In regard to completing assignments, the focus should be on the work that has been done and programming for gradually increasing the quantity. The goal of providing modifications to the child's learning environment is to meet the child's individual needs by helping him or her to develop effective skills to compensate for specific areas of weakness (Burd, Kauffman, & Kerbeshian).

One of the most difficult situations for teachers arises when tics are disturbing the classroom learning environment. Tics occur in bouts and these bouts can occur at the most inopportune times. In our experience, the best strategy is to ignore the tics when they occur; this is possible only when teachers and classmates are well informed about Tourette's. Other options include asking children with Tourette's to request permission to leave the classroom briefly to release or let out tics that they have been suppressing.

Permission to take short breaks may diminish class disruption as well as the child's or adolescent's anxiety and increase his or her feelings of self-efficacy. When successful, the result of such a solution is that the child feels more able to focus on schoolwork rather than expending excessive energy on suppressing tics and worrying about upsetting peers. With less disruption in the classroom, there is a greater likelihood of peer acceptance.

Selected periods of separation may also be helpful. Specifically, it may be useful to allow a student with distracting or disruptive tics to take tests in a private room. This may optimize the performance of all of the students and minimize classmates' anger and frustration at the child or adolescent with Tourette's syndrome. Allowing the child to take breaks as needed should not be misconstrued to suggest that the child should be permanently removed from the regular education setting and placed in a self-contained special education classroom. Although some tics may be very disruptive, tics alone are not a sufficient or valid reason to remove a child from a regular classroom. In fact, according to the Individuals with Disabilities Education Act, or IDEA (PL 101-476), children must be maintained in the least restrictive educational setting (Office of Education, 1990).

The vast majority of children with Tourette's syndrome do not need special interventions, but others may need accommodations or modifications, some of which have been outlined above, that can be easily provided by the regular classroom teacher in collaboration with other school professionals and parents. Other children with Tourette's syndrome who also have problems in attention regulation, executive functioning, or academic and/or social-emotional functioning may need more specific programming and planning, which can be provided through the school's special education services and which are mandated by federal and state laws. Thus, it is incumbent on professionals who evaluate children and adolescents with Tourette's to be familiar with the rules and regulations for special education services in their state.

Educators generally do not receive training specific to these disorders, which may lead to misunderstanding and a lack of appropriate services. In our experience, it is not uncommon for children with Tourette's syndrome and associated disorders who are having difficulties in school not to meet the qualifying criteria for a learning disability as defined by special education laws. However, more thorough evaluations that extend beyond those typically performed by school systems often identify the more subtle neuropsychological difficulties having an impact on school performance (described in Chapter 5). Possibly because of the lack of training for school professionals in these disorders, children frequently are not identified as needing or eligible for special accommodations or special education services (Packer, 1997). If these difficulties interfere with the child's academic progress, school districts are obliged under the IDEA to provide educational assistance even if formal criteria for learning disabilities are not met. In some cases, a child advocate who is knowledgeable about educational law, regulations, and the school system itself can be very helpful to families who are unfamiliar with their rights under federal (PL 101-476) and state law.

However, both parents and educators are cautioned against creating an adversarial situation regarding services, as these conflicts can add stress to the child and may affect symptom severity.

Strategies for Children with Attention-Deficit/Hyperactivity Disorder

Children with Tourette's syndrome and ADHD appear to benefit from similar behavioral methods and interventions as children who have ADHD without Tourette's syndrome (Scahill et al., 1993b; Walter & Carter, 1997). Educational interventions for ADHD include specific behavioral strategies in the classroom that enhance attentional focus, diminish impulsive responding, and improve organizational skills (Packer, 1997). A significant degree of structure that includes well-defined expectations and consistency seems to be advantageous for children with attentional difficulties and impulsivity regardless of tic behavior. It should be remembered, however, that attempts to minimize attentional problems may not have a direct impact on the severity of tics (Nolan et al., 1994). Consistent with the approach for children with ADHD without Tourette's syndrome, the teacher's strategic deployment of attention—praising adaptive behaviors and ignoring tics or other disruptive behaviors—coupled with the use of tangible rewards and the prudent use of reprimands often yields improvement in the classroom (Pfiffner & Barkley, 1990). Training in self-management skills can provide strategies that children can use to structure their own environments (Brigham, 1989). Interventions directed at specific target behaviors (e.g., completing five math problems) appear to be more successful than those that are more general (e.g., staying on task).

Although innumerable sources of information are available describing specific educational and behavioral intervention techniques (i.e., Barkley, 1990; Fiore & Becker, 1994; Swanson, 1992), the unique needs of each individual must be considered and included when implementing any behavioral or educational strategy. Arbitrarily instituting generic interventions may be counterproductive if the particular profile of the child and the situations in which problem behaviors occur are not considered. Indeed, an important component of assessing the child's functioning in the school setting should include evaluation of the setting itself. Interventions that focus on attempts to change the child's behavior without consideration of the context in which that behavior occurs may not be successful. Structuring the educational environment to prevent problem behaviors from occurring rather than reacting negatively when they do occur is an approach likely to enhance the child's functioning and to be viewed as less aversive by all involved (Horner et al., 1990).

Children with Tourette's syndrome and ADHD are at very high risk for problems in peer relations and may benefit from social skills training that focuses on enhancing children's social competencies with peers and adults (see Chapter 5 for more details on this topic). In assessing a child's need for social skills training interventions, it is critical to consider whether the child lacks particular social skills or has the skills in his or her behavioral repertoire but does not perform them because of the existence of interfering behaviors such as impulsivity or anxiety (Gresham & Elliott, 1987). The distinction is essential because it will guide the interventions that are selected for implementation. For example, if a child is able to initiate a conversation with a peer, but does not exhibit this behavior because of interfering anxiety, a social skills intervention that targets teaching the child steps to initiate a conversation will fail because it is not directed at the interfering behavior. An intervention that addresses the child's anxiety in initiating conversations directly targets the social skills problem and is more likely to be successful. A group training format that encompasses this approach can be used in school settings (Gresham & Elliott, 1993).

Because the school psychologist is in a unique position to coordinate school-based interventions with clinic- and home-based interventions, he or she should be viewed as the ideal case manager of school-based interventions for children with ADHD (Power, Atkins, Osborne, & Blum, 1994) and Tourette's syndrome (Walter & Carter, 1997). One very effective method for enhancing communication between parents and school professionals is the school-home note (Kelley, 1989; McCain & Kelley, 1993). The school-home note is a daily or weekly report that provides information to parents about the child regarding specific behaviors. Notes can be used to coordinate behavioral programs implemented in both school and home. Notes are intended to be highly individualized and should enhance communication and collaboration between parents and teachers.

Strategies for Children with Obsessive-Compulsive Disorder

Obsessive-compulsive symptoms may be silent and therefore not disruptive in the classroom. At other times, compulsive rituals can be quite disruptive and perceived as bizarre by teachers and fellow students. Adequate training of school professionals is critical to prevent misdiagnosis or misattribution of causes of the child's behavior. For example, a child with compulsive behaviors may be viewed as a behavior problem, leading to a diagnosis of oppositional defiant disorder and inappropriate placement in a class for children with severe emotional or behavioral disorders. Information provided to school professionals about the nature of obsessive-compulsive symptoms can be extremely helpful, and, in many cases, critical, to the child's successful functioning. Although not considered involuntary, the anxiety caused by intrusive thoughts or the urge to perform a compulsive habit is pressing and difficult to resist. Understanding that coping with obsessive-compulsive symptoms is not simply a matter of willpower can have a positive effect on the manner in which teachers and others respond to the child's behaviors.

If a teacher suspects the presence of obsessive-compulsive symptoms, the child's parents and the school psychologist should be alerted. Direct confrontation with the child may result in denial due to embarrassment and hence should be carefully considered before proceeding. Further, some children may initially become more anxious about their intrusive thoughts or compulsive behaviors if they suspect that their symptoms are obvious to others. As obsessive-compulsive symptoms may wax and wane, continued communication among school personnel, parents, and outside clinicians is in order. For example, teachers are in an excellent position to monitor a child's response to pharmacologic or behavioral interventions because of the daily contact they have with the child.

It is important to realize that, like tics, obsessive-compulsive behaviors are not indicative of a lack of ability or effort. A variety of modifications can be made for children with obsessive-compulsive symptoms. Children and adolescents with obsessive-compulsive disorder may need help with note taking, may need both leeway and limits regarding trips to the bathroom, and may need extra time for tests. In extreme cases, students can be given the option of completing work orally. Other strategies that may be helpful include the provision of short breaks, opportunities to switch tasks if stuck on a particular activity, and encouragement to continue working despite the presence of obsessive or compulsive symptoms. For example, a child with a rewriting compulsion may be instructed to refrain from rewriting and to wait until the urge passes. If the teacher and/or school psychologist are aware of this plan, the child will not be censured for sitting in class and not writing. Although many child experts advocate giving children choices, some children with obsessive-compulsive symptoms may have particular difficulty in making decisions; in those cases, it may be best to limit the number of options available or to make choices for the child. Some children and adolescents with obsessive-compulsive symptoms may have particular difficulty with transitions or stopping one task to proceed to a different one; they may get stuck and have difficulty ending the task because they are unable to comprehend that the task is finished. Allowing the child to return to the task at a later time may be beneficial. As with any strategy, careful consideration of the child's unique characteristics, as well as the setting in which strategies are implemented, is essential to successful intervention.

Strategies for Children with Learning Difficulties

Due to specific neuropsychological deficits, some children with Tourette's syndrome have visual-motor integration or organizational problems (Chapter 5). Therefore, tasks that require students to organize and write down material may be difficult and more time-consuming than for classmates. This problem is typically first noticed in first or second grade when teachers begin to notice poor penmanship. Deficits in visual-motor integration can also interfere with the successful or timely completion of long written assignments, neatness of written work, and copying all of the relevant information from the board or a book. Even very bright children with Tourette's, who have no trouble grasping concepts, may have difficulty completing written work or may produce sloppy work due to these visual-motor impairments. Although it may sometimes appear that a child is being lazy or avoiding work, he or she actually may be overwhelmed by the effort it takes to organize or complete a written assignment. When present, problems with visual-motor integration should be specifically targeted for remediation in the classroom. It should be noted, however, that difficulty with writing is probably a manifestation of the neurobiological underpinnings of Tourette's syndrome. Therefore, although children with Tourette's syndrome can learn to work more neatly, they are genuinely disadvantaged in this area and their sloppy or slow work must not be mistaken for lack of effort.

Children with Tourette's may have learning problems common to other children, learning problems specific to Tourette's syndrome, a combination of both, or none at all (Chapter 4; Walkup et al., 1995). Children with Tourette's syndrome and specific learning disabilities appear to benefit from the same methods and interventions as other children with learning problems. Moreover, minimal modification of strategies designed to remediate learning disabilities due to the Tourette's syndrome may be all that is necessary (Bruun, Cohen, & Leckman, 1990). There are various ways to accommodate a child with visual-spatial or psychomotor-related difficulties. Generally, the focus should be on the quality and content of a child's work rather than the quantity of written work produced. Computers can be extremely beneficial for children who evidence writing and/or spelling difficulties. Allowing a child to present a report on tape or orally, or allowing a child to dictate ideas or conceptual solutions to problems can provide alternative modes of expression. Sometimes a child may not be able to write quickly enough to get important notes or assignments down on paper. Having a teacher review assignments and a trusted classmate photocopy notes may be very helpful. When significant writing weaknesses are present, tests may be given without time restrictions, in a private room, or on a computer. Further, if tests are on scanning sheets, some children with visual-spatial difficulties may benefit from writing answers on a separate piece of paper to avoid the visual confusion caused by using the grid.

Appropriate classroom accommodations and an accepting atmosphere can make the difference between a student who feels like a failure and avoids schoolwork and one who is motivated, confident, and thriving. As discussed in Chapters 1, 8, 15, and 17, evaluations should systematically include an assessment of the child's strengths, and these should be incorporated into all behavioral and educational interventions. In addition to flexible teaching methods, a better understanding of the unique problems of children with Tourette's syndrome and learning difficulties may also prove beneficial. Encouraging self-knowledge regarding strengths and needs may help children and adolescents generalize appropriate compensatory strategies when faced with novel learning challenges. Further, helping children distinguish between aspects of their behavior that are a function of Tourette's syndrome or related conditions and their "true selves," or the person that is distinct from the illness, can promote positive self-esteem.

SUMMARY OF CHAPTER 19

Well-informed teachers working in close collaboration with parents and medical professionals are the best guarantors of success for a child with Tourette's syndrome. Interventions in the classroom may not be necessary for many children with Tourette's syndrome and related disorders. However, for those who do require them, a full range of services should be available— from simple changes in seating to special accommodations in testing—as mandated by federal and state statutes. Consideration of the unique profile and individual characteristics of each child, along with the setting in which interventions occur, is essential for success.

PREVIEW OF CHAPTER 20

Over the past two decades, pharmacological treatments have been increasingly used in the treatment of Tourette's syndrome, obsessive-compulsive disorder, and attention deficit hyperactivity disorder. Although ideal medications that safely and effectively treatment these conditions are not yet available, significant progress has been made. Drug trials are best seen as just one part of the overall treatment plan. A number of experimental treatments are also briefly covered in this chapter including the use of drugs and procedures that influence the body's immune response.

CHAPTER 20

Pharmacological and Other Somatic Approaches to Treatment

LINDA L. CARPENTER, JAMES F. LECKMAN, LAWRENCE SCAHILL, and
CHRISTOPHER J. MCDOUGLE

> Ideally, patients with mild tics who have made a good adaptation in their
> lives can avoid the use of medications.
>
> —*Roger Kurlan, 1997*

> Although beneficial for many patients, present-day treatments typically can
> only offer partial amelioration or suppression of symptoms, often at the risk
> of unacceptable side effects.
>
> —*Phillip B. Chappell, Lawrence D. Scahill, and James F. Leckman, 1997*

Contemporary assessment and treatment of Tourette's syndrome benefits
from an understanding of the phenomenology of tics and the closely related symptoms of obsessive-compulsive disorder and attention-deficit/
hyperactivity disorder (ADHD). Familiarity with the features that characterize each of these syndromes is essential in formulating an approach
to pharmacological and other interventions. As presented in earlier
chapters, the Yale approach embraces multiple treatment modalities, including education of the family, child, and school personnel, behavioral
treatment, and individual treatment. We encourage readers to review
these earlier sections before consulting this chapter.

In this chapter, we review the current approaches to pharmacotherapy
for individuals with Tourette's syndrome, obsessive-compulsive disorder,
and ADHD. We report on the use of several classes of commonly used
agents for each of the three disorders, and provide available information
about pharmacotherapy for cases where diagnostic overlap or comorbidity
occur. For the sake of completeness, we also review other somatic treatments, including immunological and neurosurgical approaches. Readers are

also referred to another recent review of this topic by members of our group (Chappell et al., 1997).

TREATMENT CONSIDERATIONS

Comorbidity is high among the three disorders described in this chapter. Symptom overlap of tic disorders, obsessive-compulsive disorder, and ADHD is impressive and can complicate diagnosis and pharmacotherapy decisions, particularly when treatment for one feature in the presenting syndrome may exacerbate another. Concurrent conduct disorders, learning disabilities and other cognitive deficits, depression, and anxiety symptoms further challenge the clinician trying to select the best and the fewest drugs for a given patient.

In light of the potential for complex presentations, it is essential to determine which symptoms are causing the greatest concern and impairment. In the case of children and adolescents, open communication with the parents and school personnel as well as the patient is usually needed to evaluate the impact of symptoms in each of several domains: (a) the patient's self-perception, (b) family functioning, (c) peer relationships, and (d) academic or occupational functioning. The Yale approach involves an initial determination of the extent to which the symptoms are causing significant distress to the patient, having an adverse effect on his or her self-esteem or ability to form friendships and interact appropriately with peers, or interfering with the performance of school- or work-related tasks (see Figure 15.1). Further, the extent to which the symptoms are causing distress to the family or impairing the parents' or siblings' ability to function in their roles effectively must be understood. A decision to intervene follows such an assessment that finds symptoms clearly related to significant difficulty in any of these areas. Unless the presenting symptoms are severe, the decision to begin medication therapy should be deferred while the individual is followed over several weeks or months and the response to initial supportive psychoeducational interventions is evaluated, as described in Chapters 15 and 18. In the case of adults, the decision to begin medications is a more private affair. Although spouses and other close family members may be consulted, it is not unusual for trials to be undertaken based on the individual's desire to see what, if any, benefits are associated with taking a specific medication.

When pharmacotherapy is indicated, we recommend identifying the most prominent and problematic symptoms and treating them in the context of the single best-fit diagnostic category (e.g., a tic disorder, obsessive-compulsive disorder, or ADHD). Monotherapy drug trials would then begin with the agents that have proven efficacy and safety for the target symptoms. The sections that follow describe treatment considerations and pharmacological approaches to each primary disorder, along with strategies for more complicated clinical presentations.

It is worth emphasizing that drug trials do not occur in isolation. At best, they are part of an overall treatment plan that emphasizes a long-term perspective and a partnership between the patient and the treatment team. We typically review with the patient and family the various treatment options—describing each medication, its likely effects and time course, as well as any common or dangerous side effects. Once a joint decision has been made to use medication, it is best to set a specific date to reevaluate the choice of medication and its effectiveness. Given the limited options available, it is also useful to avoid being too aggressive with the dosing schedule and to urge patience so that an adequate trial can be made. Finally, it is only in the most severe and refractory patients that we have undertaken trials with novel agents, particularly those associated with potentially serious side effects. Although we review the evidence in support of neurosurgical interventions in this chapter, we have generally not referred patients because of the irreversible nature of the procedures.

PHARMACOTHERAPY FOR TIC DISORDERS

The phenomenology of tic disorders is described in detail in Chapter 2. In the context of pharmacotherapy trials, however, certain features of Tourette's syndrome deserve close consideration. Specifically, it is important to remember the boutlike occurrence of tics and the ability of some patients to either unconsciously or voluntarily suppress their tics in the consulting room or during examination. Historical information from multiple sources is likely to be more reliable than the information clinicians gather from a patient's presentation in a clinic setting. Caution is also advised in deciding how aggressively to intervene with medications, as patients typically present when tics are at their worst, yet the disorder is characterized by a waxing and waning course. Indeed, many individuals are best served by waiting out the tic exacerbation without medication. Given the potential for placebo response among children, and the possibility that tics might improve regardless of what intervention is started, we recommend a conservative approach. A comprehensive review of the onset and course of the symptoms, including a reliably established baseline, is essential for determining whether to initiate a medication trial and for evaluating the effectiveness of pharmacotherapy. We encourage the regular use of empirically established rating instruments such as the Yale Global Tic Severity Scale (YGTSS) for monitoring the response to any intervention including drug trials (see Chapter 16 for additional information on the rating scales currently available).

Antidopaminergic agents and alpha-adrenergic receptor agonists have been the mainstay of monotherapy for tic disorders without significant comorbidity; alternative drugs and combination pharmacotherapy have been reserved for more complicated cases. Some of the newer atypical neuroleptic agents are the focus of recent investigation and may eventually assume a more prominent role in the pharmacotherapy of tic disorders.

Alpha-Adrenergic Receptor Agonists

Clonidine

Developed primarily as an antihypertensive agent, clonidine (Catapres®) is an imidazole derivative with action at presynaptic alpha$_2$-adrenergic autoreceptors (at low doses) and postsynaptic alpha$_2$-adrenergic receptors (at high doses). Central noradrenergic activity is dampened by stimulation of the presynaptic autoreceptors, perhaps leading to indirect mediation of activity in the dopaminergic neurons of the substantia nigra and ventral tegmental areas, implicated in Tourette's syndrome (Bunney & DeRiemer, 1982). Clonidine has provided an alternative pharmacotherapy for tics since 1979 when it was first described as useful for Tourette's syndrome patients (Chapter 1; D. Cohen et al., 1979). Subsequent efficacy studies have shown an inconsistent pattern of response: some subjects clearly benefit from clonidine (Leckman et al., 1985, 1991), but many others do not (Goetz, 1993; Goetz, Tanner, Wilson, Carroll, et al., 1987). About a quarter of Tourette's syndrome patients do well with the drug, but efforts to predict which individuals will compose the subset of clonidine responders have not yet been successful. One study suggests that motor tics are more clonidine-responsive than are phonic tics (Leckman et al., 1991). However, because clonidine has a more benign side effect profile and is not known to cause tardive dyskinesia, we typically recommend a trial of clonidine first, before turning to neuroleptic medications (Chappell, Leckman, et al., 1995).

Treatment with clonidine typically begins with a 0.025 or a 0.05 mg dose each morning, with additional doses of 0.05 mg added every three to four days, as tolerated. Multiple daily doses should be given at three- to four-hour intervals, with a total daily dose in the range of 0.15–0.25 mg in school-age children. Transdermal patch preparations of several different doses (effective for approximately five to seven days) are available for patients who have been stabilized on oral clonidine. However, in active children, the patch may fall off, and skin rashes are not uncommon at the site of the patch. Sedation is a common side effect that may limit titration to therapeutic levels, but often abates after several weeks on the medication. Irritability, insomnia, reduced salivary flow, headaches, hypotension, dizziness, sleep disturbance, and clinically insignificant EKG changes are other side effects. A mild withdrawal syndrome (anxiety, irritability, and tic exacerbation) may appear shortly before the patient is due to receive the next scheduled dose and may necessitate increases in dose after extended periods on clonidine (D. Cohen, Young, et al., 1979).

Discontinuation of clonidine should be done as a slow taper, as more severe rebound syndromes can emerge and persist when the drug is abruptly stopped (Leckman et al., 1986). Response to clonidine may not be seen until six to eight weeks after the initiation of therapy (Leckman et al., 1991).

Guanfacine

Guanfacine (Tenex®) is a newer alpha$_2$-adrenergic agonist that more selectively binds the postsynaptic 2a subtype receptors concentrated in the prefrontal cortex. Because it has activity in brain regions associated with attention and working memory (Arnsten, Cai, & Goldman-Rakic, 1988; Arnsten & Contant, 1992; Arnsten et al., 1996) and does not cause as much sedation or hypotension as clonidine (Balldin, Berggren, Eriksson, Lindstedt, & Sundkler, 1993), guanfacine offers promise as a pharmacotherapy for tic disorders. Small open-label studies have shown guanfacine is efficacious and well tolerated in ADHD (Hunt, Arnsten, & Asbell, 1995), and in a population with ADHD and comorbid Tourette's syndrome (Chappell, Riddle, et al., 1995), with transitory fatigue and headaches the most commonly reported side effects. Guanfacine was begun with initial bedtime doses of 0.5 mg, with incremental increases of 0.5 mg occurring every three to four days. Final doses ranged from 0.75–3 mg and were typically given in two or three divided doses. Larger-scale studies of guanfacine in pediatric Tourette's syndrome and ADHD populations are currently underway at Yale and elsewhere.

Typical Neuroleptics

Haloperidol

Haloperidol (Haldol®) is a high-potency butyrophenone with antagonistic effects at D$_2$ dopamine receptors that also acts as an antagonist at alpha$_1$-adrenergic receptors. The 1961 report on haloperidol by Seignot (1961) marked the beginning of the era of effective pharmacotherapy of Tourette's syndrome. FDA approval for haloperidol in the treatment of adult Tourette's syndrome was established in 1969, followed by approval for the pediatric population in 1978. Large patient surveys published in 1990 (Sandor et al., 1990) indicated it was the most commonly prescribed medication for tics, and symptom relief was reported by 70–80% of Tourette's syndrome patients receiving the drug (Erenberg et al., 1987; E. Shapiro et al., 1989). Such widespread use of haloperidol for tic disorders has highlighted the limitations of typical neuroleptic agents due to side effects; sedation, fatigue, Parkinsonian symptoms, weight gain, acute dystonic reactions, akathisia, dysphoria, and cognitive dulling are common with haloperidol and can even occur at low doses. Follow-up studies reveal up to 84% of Tourette's syndrome patients treated with haloperidol report side effects, and only 20–30% can tolerate the drug for long-term use (Erenberg et al., 1987). Furthermore, children with Tourette's syndrome may represent a population of patients with heightened vulnerability to subtle neuroleptic side effects such as depression, school phobia, aggressive outbursts, and fog states with impaired cognition (Bruun, 1988a). Finally, cases of haloperidol-induced tardive dyskinesia have been reported (Riddle et al., 1987), underscoring one of the more serious risks associated with typical neuroleptic agents. Indeed, in our experience, one of the biggest limitations associated with the use of typical neuroleptics is the difficulties individuals face in attempting to come off these medications, as the tics almost always get worse in the month or two following discontinuation. This symptom exacerbation following withdrawal can be severe and last for weeks, if not months.

Haloperidol treatment for tics is usually initiated at low doses, such as 0.25–0.5 mg/day given at bedtime, with gradual dose increase every five to seven days, until a maximum dose of 2–5 mg per day is reached. Sometimes better symptom control can be obtained by a change to a twice-daily dosing regimen. Use of the smallest dose possible for a moderate reduction in symptoms, and the addition of prophylactic anti-Parkinsonian agents, help minimize troublesome side effects (Chandler, 1990; Chappell, Leckman, et al., 1995).

Pimozide

Pimozide (Orap®) is a diphenylbutylpiperidine derivative that also blocks D_2 dopamine receptors. Unlike haloperidol, pimozide has no alpha-adrenergic activity, but does block calcium channels. It has been widely available for the past ten years but currently only carries FDA approval for treatment-refractory Tourette's syndrome. Double-blind studies have shown pimozide to be as effective as haloperidol for suppression of tic symptoms (Ross & Moldofsky, 1978; Sallee et al., 1997; E. Shapiro et al., 1989), and also suggest that pimozide has a superior side effects profile when prescribed in lower doses (Sallee & Rock, 1994). At higher doses, the two agents are very similar with regard to side effects. EKG changes (QT interval lengthening, new U waves, and T wave flattening, notching, or inversion) are also seen with pimozide and should prompt the close monitoring of serial EKG tracings at regular intervals (Regeur, Pakkenberg, Fog, & Pakkenberg, 1986).

Pimozide therapy is usually started at 0.5–1 mg in a once-daily dosing regimen. Weekly small incremental increases in dose can be made to reach a target range of 2–4 mg/day. Higher doses are unlikely to achieve better results and are associated with adverse effects (Chappell, Leckman, et al., 1995; Regeur et al., 1986).

Other Classical Neuroleptics

A third class of typical neuroleptics, the phenothiazines, may provide another option for treatment of tics when haloperidol or pimozide is poorly tolerated. Several studies have shown that fluphenazine (Prolixin®, 2–15 mg/day) is effective and may produce fewer side effects than the other two agents (Faretra, Doher, & Dowling, 1970; Goetz, Tanner, & Klawans, 1984; Regeur et al., 1986).

Atypical Neuroleptics and Other Agents That Block D$_2$ Dopamine Receptors

Risperidone

Risperidone (Risperdal®) is a benzisoxazol derivative that exhibits high affinity for both serotonin (5-HT$_2$) and dopamine (D$_2$) receptors. At low doses, it is a potent 5-HT$_2$ receptor antagonist, but at higher doses, risperidone acts like other classic antipsychotic drugs in their potent D$_2$ receptor antagonism (Leysen et al., 1988). Risperidone possesses short-acting alpha1-adrenergic and H1-histamine receptor blockade, but has little peripheral or central anticholinergic activity. It has proven effective for treatment of psychotic symptoms in schizophrenia, producing few extrapyramidal effects in the recommended dose range (4–8 mg/day; Chouinard et al., 1993; Claus, Bollen, De Cuyper, & Heylen, 1992). Risperidone does not share the risk of agranulocytosis seen with clozapine.

A role for risperidone in the treatment of chronic tic disorders has begun to be explored by several open-label studies (Bruun & Budman, 1996; Lombroso, Scahill, King, et al., 1995; Stamenkovic, Aschauer, & Kasper, 1994; van der Linden, Bruggeman, & Van Woerkom, 1994). Nine of 11 adults in the study by van der Linden and associates experienced improvement in motor and phonic tics with an average daily dose of 3.9 mg risperidone for three to four weeks. Few side effects were reported; sedation was most common and there were no extrapyramidal side effects. Lombroso and colleagues published the first data on risperidone for children and adolescents with tic disorders. All seven subjects in that 11-week, open-label series showed improvement in tic severity, with change in scores from baseline to endpoint ranging from 26% to 66%. The risperidone dose ranged from 1 to 2.5 (mean 1.5) mg/day, and was added to stable doses of clonidine or selective serotonin-reuptake inhibitor (SSRI) medications in five of the subjects. Weight gain was the most frequent adverse effect, and one patient had an acute dystonic reaction, but there were no complaints of akathisia, psychomotor retardation, or cognitive blunting. Placebo-controlled, double-blind studies are needed to establish the efficacy of risperidone for treatment of tic disorders. More time and clinical experience are also required to determine whether lower extra-pyramidal side effects (EPS) during treatment results in a lower frequency of tardive dyskinesia (TD) in the longer term. In our clinical practice at present, we typically recommend a trial with risperidone before trials with classical neuroleptics like haloperidol. Thus far we have been disappointed whenever we have tried to substitute risperidone for a classical neuroleptic, as patients have uniformly gone through a typical withdrawal reaction that appears to be barely attenuated by the risperidone. Other atypical neuroleptics with high affinity for both serotonin (5-HT$_2$) and dopamine (D$_2$) receptors, such as ziprasidone (Seeger et al., 1995), have also shown promise in the treatment of Tourette's syndrome (P. B. Chappell, personal communication, 1997).

Clozapine

Clozapine (Clozaril®) is a dibenzodiazepine compound that received FDA approval in 1990 for treatment-resistant schizophrenia. The drug has weak D_2 blocking properties; hence, its ability to block 5-HT$_{2A}$, 5-HT$_{2C}$, 5-HT$_3$, and dopamine D_1–D_4 receptors has been proposed as its mechanism of action (Meltzer, 1994). Weekly monitoring of white blood cell counts is required for all patients treated with clozapine because of the increased risk for agranulocytosis on the drug. As clozapine causes minimal extrapyramidal side effects, it was considered a reasonable candidate for investigation in the treatment of tic disorders. However, the results of one small double-blind crossover trial (Caine, Polinsky, Kartzinel, & Ebert, 1979) suggested clozapine at 150–500 mg/day for four to seven weeks was not effective for involuntary movements, and may have caused transient worsening of symptoms in four of seven Tourette's syndrome patients. Marked sedation, leukopenia, confusion, and hypotension were problematic side effects reported in that study. Although the body of information upon which to make a judgment about the efficacy of clozapine in tic disorders is meager, it seems unlikely that clozapine will offer a useful alternative to the available agents for uncomplicated Tourette's syndrome and chronic tics.

In contrast, two case reports have appeared that suggest that clozapine may be useful in the treatment of tardive Tourette's syndrome (Jaffe, Tremeau, Sharif, & Reider, 1995; Kalian, Lerner, & Goldman, 1993). Tardive Tourette's refers to the late development of motor and vocal tics following withdrawal from long-term treatment with classical neuroleptic medications. Although the relationship between tardive Tourette's and childhood-onset forms of Tourette's syndrome is obscure, supersensitivity of striatal dopamine D_2 receptors has been implicated in both disorders (Jaffe et al., 1995).

Other Agents

Sulpiride and tiapride are two substituted benzamide compounds that selectively block D_2 dopamine receptors and are reported to be favorable with regard to extrapyramidal side effects, autonomic effects, and tardive dyskinesia. Although both are currently unavailable in the United States, they have demonstrated effectiveness for Tourette's syndrome and good tolerability in controlled studies in the United Kingdom and Europe (Eggers, Rothenberger, & Berghaus, 1988; Robertson, Schnieden, & Lees, 1990).

Dopamine Agonists

Pharmaceuticals that act as full or partial agonists at dopaminergic receptors were initially developed for the treatment of Parkinson's disease and recently have been investigated as potential antipsychotics. This class of drugs includes pergolide (Permax®), which is a mixed D_2/D_1 agonist (Fuller & Clemens, 1983), and the more recently developed partial D_2 agonists talipexole, pramipexole, and teguride. Depending on their structure, these partial dopamine agonists may also bind to presynaptic D_2 autoreceptors located on nerve terminals and cell bodies (Wetzel, Hillert, Grunder, & Benkert, 1994). The net effect of these agents is determined both by their intrinsic activity and by the level of endogenous dopaminergic activity. In conditions where the endogenous dopamine tone is high, these agents may act as antagonists, but in states of low endogenous dopamine tone, they act as agonists (Gerlach, 1991; Gerlach & Peacock, 1995).

Pergolide and talipexole recently have been evaluated as potential treatments for Tourette's. Lipinski, Sallee, Jackson, and Sethuraman (1997) studied 32 patients in a six-week, open-label study, using a flexible dosing schedule. The pergolide was well tolerated, but the mean treatment dosage was significantly lower than the mean mg/day dose employed in clinical trials in Parkinson's disease. Pergolide was associated with robust decreases in tic severity and frequency in the majority of patients, with 75% of subjects experiencing a greater than 50% decrease from baseline in tic severity ratings. Pergolide was reported to be equally effective in both responders and nonresponders to previous neuroleptic treatment, and no extrapyramidal side effects were observed.

We have recently treated seven refractory Tourette's patients (age range 11–48 years) with pergolide with doses ranging from 0.15 mg to 0.75 mg in three divided doses per day (Scahill & Leckman, personal communication, 1996). Unfortunately, only one individual experienced a clinically significant improvement on pergolide. This individual was also able to wean off of haloperidol after four months of treatment without experiencing any withdrawal symptoms. The medication was typically started at 0.025 mg per day for three days, then gradually increased in 0.025 mg increments every two to three days to a maximum of 0.25 mg three times daily. Side effects were minimal.

Similar to our recent experience, Goetz, Stebbins, et al. (1987) reported negative results in a recent randomized, double-blind, placebo-controlled, crossover study of talipexole in 13 unmedicated adult men with Tourette's. In this trial, talipexole also was poorly tolerated, with significant sedation, fatigue, dizziness, and insomnia being reported.

Additional Pharmacotherapies Affecting Central Dopaminergic Tone

Tetrabenazine

A benzoquinollizine derivative, tetrabenazine, acts by reversibly depleting presynaptic dopamine storage granules and by a modest blockade of postsynaptic dopamine receptors. Like the other novel antidopaminergic agents, tetrabenazine is rarely associated with dystonic reactions and may not pose a risk for tardive dyskinesia. Tetrabenazine is available in Canada but has not been released for clinical use in the United States. Results from several open-label research protocols suggest that tetrabenazine is beneficial and well tolerated in movement disorders such as Huntington's chorea and Tourette's syndrome (Jankovic & Orman, 1988; Pakkenberg, 1968; E. Shapiro et al., 1978; Sweet et al., 1974). Doses in the 25–100 mg/day range were used, and adverse effects included Parkinsonian symptoms, sedation, depression, anxiety, insomnia, and akathisia. Tetrabenazine in combination with other typical neuroleptics may allow the use of lower doses of both medications and provide substantial relief from tic symptoms (Regeur et al., 1986).

Other Psychoactive Medications

Nicotine

Nicotine chewing gum was found to be effective in reducing tics in 8 of 10 children with Tourette's syndrome when added to ongoing treatment with haloperidol (Sanberg et al., 1989). In that study, nicotine alone produced no improvement, and the beneficial effects of the combination lasted less than one hour, with 70% of patients unable to tolerate the nicotine due to nausea or unpleasant taste. Uncontrolled open trials have investigated the potential benefits of combining transdermal nicotine patches with neuroleptics (Dursun, Reveley, Bird, & Stirton, 1994; A. Silver, Shytle, Philipp, & Sanberg, 1996), but again, the potentiation effects are usually short-lived, lasting only one to two weeks.

Benzodiazepines

A class of compounds that act principally at GABA-a receptors in the brain, benzodiazepines have been used as sedative, anticonvulsant, anxiolytic, and smooth muscle relaxing agents in adults for many years. Benzodiazepines differ with regard to pharmacokinetic properties, but all can cause dependence and tolerance. Clonazepam (Klonopin®) is a long-acting, high-potency benzodiazepine that is somewhat unusual because it also up-regulates 5-HT$_1$ receptor binding sites. A series of seven adult and adolescent Tourette's syndrome patients experienced a broad range of symptom reduction from clonazepam in combination with neuroleptics (Gonce & Barbeau, 1977), and a 50% mean reduction in tics when clonazepam was added to clonidine in children with Tourette's syndrome and ADHD (Steingard, Goldberg, Lee, & DeMaso, 1994).

Antiandrogens

Several case reports have suggested that manipulation of androgenic steroids may be helpful in the treatment of Tourette's syndrome and obsessive-compulsive disorder (Casas et al., 1986; B. Peterson, Leckman,

Scahill, et al., 1994; Sandyk, 1988). A recently completed double-blind, placebo-controlled, crossover study of the androgen receptor blocker flutamide in 13 adults with Tourette's syndrome demonstrated a significant improvement in motor tic severity (B. Peterson, Zhang, et al., in press). Although the medication was well tolerated, it demonstrated short-lived beneficial effects, which, together with the potential for serious side effects, render antiandrogen agents poor choices for treatment of tic disorders in the pediatric population.

Botulinum Toxin

Jankovic (1994) and others (Poungvarin, Devahastin, & Viriyavejakul, 1995) have reported on the beneficial effects of botulinum toxin injections in the treatment of vocal tics in Tourette's syndrome. In a majority of cases reported by Jankovic, the patients reported a decrease in the premonitory urges as well as the intensity and frequency of their tics. Based on these encouraging results, we evaluated the effects of botulinum toxin in two male patients with Tourette's syndrome (Scahill & Leckman, personal communication, 1996). Both patients exhibited forceful tics localized to specific body regions, and in both cases, the tics were preceded by intense somatosensory urges. The doses injected were similar to those reported by Jankovic, but neither patient reported any relief either of his tics or of his premonitory urges, despite clear evidence of mild weakness in the injected region. More recently, Adler, Zimmerman, Lyons, and Brin (1996) described a series of four patients with severe movement disorders, including one case of tic-induced radiculomyelopathy, who were successfully treated before and after surgery to facilitate stabilization of cervical fusion. Additional studies are needed to explore the possible benefits of botulinum toxin for individuals with refractory tic symptoms.

Antimicrobial and Immunological Interventions

As discussed in Chapter 12, Swedo, Kiessling, and their colleagues (Swedo, 1994; Swedo et al., 1994; Swedo et al., 1998) have proposed that group A beta-hemolytic streptococcal (GABHS) infections and possibly some viral infections may trigger brain-based autoimmune reactions that cause or exacerbate some cases of childhood-onset obsessive-compulsive disorder and chronic tic disorders. This hypothesis is based on the occurrence of tics and obsessive-compulsive behaviors in children with Sydenham's chorea and, conversely, of choreiform movements in children with obsessive-compulsive disorder. Prototypically, these patients are characterized by the sudden onset or exacerbation of tic and obsessive-compulsive symptoms. In some instances, there is a well-documented antecedent streptococcal pharyngitis or other upper respiratory infection. The mechanisms involved in these cases have not been identified. However, a good deal of attention has focused on the possible role of putative antineuronal antibodies that arise in response to GABHS infections and selectively cross-react with CNS neuronal antigens found in the basal ganglia and in other functionally related structures (Kiessling et al., 1993a, 1993b; Swedo et al., 1994).

Preliminary studies of treatments that affect immunological function have been undertaken in a small number of children with a sudden onset or worsening of tic or obsessive-compulsive symptoms. A. Allen et al. (1995) performed an open study of four severely affected boys. All subjects had either positive evidence of a recent GABHS infection or of a recent viral syndrome. The subjects were treated with plasmapharesis, intravenous immunoglobulin, or immunosuppressive doses of prednisone. Each of the cases was judged to have a clinically significant positive response. Swedo et al. (1994) have also reported favorable results with penicillin therapy in a small series of children with abrupt-onset obsessive-compulsive disorder who had positive throat cultures and high titers of antistreptococcal and antineuronal antibodies. Our experience has been more limited, but does support the value of penicillin prophylaxis in some cases (Tucker et al., 1996).

Currently, given the unprecedented nature of these interventions, the attendant medical risks, and the small sample sizes and unblinded nature of the preliminary studies, immunologically based therapies must be regarded as experimental. In selected cases of sudden onset of severe symptoms, it may be prudent to obtain a throat culture and titers for streptococcal antigens (antistreptolysin O and antiDNase B) and to consider a trial with antibiotics such as amoxicillin. Otherwise, the application of immunomodulatory therapies in the treatment of Tourette's and related forms of obsessive-compulsive disorder should await the outcome of ongoing controlled, double-blind studies.

Neurosurgical Procedures

As reviewed in Chapter 13, a variety of neurosurgical procedures have been performed in an effort to treat severely impaired individuals with Tourette's syndrome. With a few notable exceptions, most of these procedures involved lesioning thalamic nuclei or thalamocortical projections (Rauch et al., 1995). There are a few case reports where dramatically beneficial effects were observed, but other individuals have suffered serious and lasting adverse neurologic sequelae (Leckman, deLotbiniere, et al., 1993). Due to the irreversible nature of the lesions, we have been reluctant to consider neurosurgical interventions even in refractory cases.

PHARMACOTHERAPY FOR OBSESSIVE-COMPULSIVE DISORDER

As described in Chapters 3, 10, and 11, the association between some forms of obsessive-compulsive disorder and Tourette's syndrome is compelling. Tic disorders occur relatively more commonly in individuals with childhood-onset obsessive-compulsive disorder (Leonard et al., 1992; Riddle et al., 1990), and obsessive-compulsive disorder is found at an increased rate among relatives of Tourette's syndrome patients (Pauls, Raymond, et al., 1991). It is currently our understanding that obsessive-compulsive disorder related to Tourette's syndrome may represent a distinct biological subtype of obsessive-compulsive disorder, with special implications for treatment.

Epidemiological studies suggest that many cases of obsessive-compulsive disorder go unrecognized, are misdiagnosed, or are treated inappropriately (Flament et al., 1988). The reason for this is uncertain, but may partly be due to the wide range of symptoms and severity that present in the disorder (Rettew, Swedo, Leonard, Lenane, & Rapoport, 1992; Thomsen, 1994b, 1994c). The amount of time spent preoccupied with obsessive thoughts or engaged in ritualistic behavior can range from less than one hour to virtually the entire day, causing impaired functioning in the home, school, and social arenas. Because obsessive-compulsive disorder is often secretive, individuals may attempt to hide their symptoms. Also, in a single individual, obsessive-compulsive symptoms may vary according to setting, life stress, and even the presence of infectious disease (Swedo et al., 1994; Swedo, Rapoport, Leonard, et al., 1989).

Family involvement and education of those close to the patient are critical elements in the treatment of obsessive-compulsive disorder, which may require long-term medication and behavioral and supportive therapy (J. Rapoport, Leonard, Swedo, & Lenane, 1993; Scahill, 1996). Misperceptions or misattributions by others about the child's driven behavior due to obsessive-compulsive disorder can potentially create as much or more disruption than the symptoms themselves. The familial nature of obsessive-compulsive disorder may make it difficult for family members who have obsessive-compulsive features to acknowledge the symptoms in some cases; in other cases, symptoms may be magnified. It is not uncommon for parents to be psychologically and behaviorally entangled in their child's obsessive-compulsive symptoms, potentially compromising their ability to participate in appropriate treatment.

Proper and timely intervention is particularly important in light of reports of obsessive-compulsive disorder onset and exacerbation in the context of other central nervous system insults such as head injury, seizures, and brain tumors (Kettle & Marks, 1986; McKeon, McGuffin, & Robinson, 1984), or basal ganglia illnesses such as Huntington's disease, Tourette's syndrome, and Sydenham's chorea (Cummings & Cunningham, 1992; Hollander, Schiffman, et al., 1990; Pauls, Towbin, et al., 1986; Swedo, Rapoport, Cheslow, et al., 1989). Autoimmune inflammation of the basal ganglia triggered by a streptococcal bacterial infection may account for the sudden emergence of obsessive-compulsive disorder in some children (see Chapter 12), which may be treatable with antibiotics or plasmapheresis (Swedo et al., 1994). For the majority of cases, however, serotonin-reuptake inhibitors (SRIs), alone or in combination with cognitive-behavioral psychotherapy (March et al., 1994; Scahill et al., 1996), constitute the mainstay of treatment for pediatric obsessive-compulsive disorder. Medication trials should be 10 to 12 weeks long, followed by 9 to 12 months of maintenance therapy for those who respond (March, Leonard, & Swedo, 1995; J. Rapoport et al., 1993). Most of the work investigating pharmacotherapy for obsessive-compulsive disorder has taken place with adult subjects, but preliminary findings support the view that the same drugs may be effective in childhood and adolescent obsessive-compulsive disorder.

Early diagnosis and treatment, particularly in children with relevant positive family histories, may be useful for preventing serious developmental deficits (e.g., social avoidance; J. Rapoport et al., 1993) and possibly reactive depressive or anxiety disorders (Swedo & Rapoport, 1989). Unfortunately, follow-up studies of obsessive-compulsive disorder patients of all ages reveal that despite aggressive pharmacotherapy and clear improvements in overall functioning, approximately one-third remain moderately impaired (Leonard et al., 1992). Nevertheless, symptom control remains an important goal that appears to positively affect long-term outcome (J. Rapoport et al., 1993).

Serotonin-Reuptake Inhibitors

Clomipramine

Clomipramine (Anafranil®) is the 3-chloro analog of the tricyclic imipramine. Its major metabolite, desmethylclomipramine, exerts potent uptake blockade of both 5-HT and norepinephrine, with some weaker dopamine-blocking properties. Anecdotal reports appearing in the 1960s first suggested that clomipramine was beneficial in reducing obsessive-compulsive symptoms. Subsequent controlled trials (reviewed by Katz, de Veaugh, & Landau, 1990) and a large multicenter investigation with adult patients (Clomipramine Collaborative Study Group, 1991) confirmed its effectiveness and superiority to a host of other antidepressant medications. FDA approval for use in the pediatric obsessive-compulsive disorder population followed a multicenter study with children and adolescents (de Veaugh-Geiss et al., 1992). The results of that effort, and of the controlled trials that preceded it (Flament et al., 1985; Leonard et al., 1989), indicate that clomipramine is generally well tolerated in young obsessive-compulsive disorder patients and produces up to 40% reduction in symptoms. Dry mouth, tremor, sedation, dizziness, insomnia, and constipation are frequently occurring side effects in clomipramine trials. Although relatively rare, acute dyskinesias, seizures, heart palpitations, and hepatic enzyme elevations are among the adverse reactions reported in published trials of clomipramine in young obsessive-compulsive disorder patients (de Veaugh-Geiss et al., 1992; Flament et al., 1985).

Dosing recommendations are not straightforward because a broad range of blood levels are found when clomipramine dose is based solely on weight. How extensively one metabolizes the parent compound, which is thought to be the effective agent for obsessive-compulsive disorder, is a function of age-related changes in hepatic blood flow and genetically determined hepatic enzyme activity. Most individuals are begun on low doses (e.g., 1 mg/kg/day), with increases every three to five days guided by clinical course and side effects. Studies report beneficial responses with final doses averaging around 3 mg/kg/day. Clomipramine blood levels may be useful (a) to rule out rapid metabolism when a patient is taking the maximum dose (250 mg/day) but does not demonstrate any side effects or beneficial response, (b) when toxicity is suspected, and (c) when the addition or discontinuation of concurrent medications may alter the clomipramine level significantly. Improvement in symptoms typically begins around 3 weeks and continues until around 10 weeks on the drug (de Veaugh-Geiss et al., 1992). Cardiac effects of clinical consequence have not been reported in the large trials of childhood and adolescent obsessive-compulsive disorder, but EKG monitoring before and periodically during treatment is recommended, as increases in heart rate and conduction times (prolonged PR, QRS, and QTc intervals) are known to occur with clomipramine (Leonard et al., 1995; Oesterheld, 1996).

Selective Serotonin-Reuptake Inhibitors (SSRIs)

Fluvoxamine (Luvox®), fluoxetine (Prozac®), sertraline (Zoloft®), and paroxetine (Paxil®) are drugs that potently and selectively block reuptake of 5-HT into the presynaptic nerve terminal. Independently, and in substantial patient populations, all four agents have been demonstrated as safe, effective, and well tolerated in the treatment of adult obsessive-compulsive disorder (Greist, Chouinard, et al., 1995; Tollefson et al., 1994; Wheadon, Bushnell, & Steiner, 1993). To date, fluvoxamine, fluoxetine, and paroxetine have received formal FDA approval for use in adult obsessive-compulsive disorder, and approval for sertraline is still under consideration; none are approved for the treatment of pediatric obsessive-compulsive disorder.

Several meta-analyses of efficacy in adult obsessive-compulsive disorder (Davis, Israni, Janicak, Wang, & Holland, 1991; Greist, Jefferson, Kobak, Katzelnick, & Serlin, 1995; Piccinelli, Pini, Bellantuono, & Wilkinson, 1995) suggest the SSRIs do not significantly differ from one another and may be slightly inferior to clomipramine, but head-to-head comparisons are not available. The SSRIs as a class are thought to offer a more favorable side effect profile than tricyclic compounds like clomipramine. The more 5-HT–selective agents tend to affect the gastrointestinal (nausea, diminished appetite, diarrhea) and central nervous (anxiety, insomnia, tremor) systems, in a way that is usually transient, dose-related, and treatable. They do not share the same risk for slowed cardiac conduction, lowered seizure threshold, orthostasis, and toxicity in overdose that are problematic with clomipramine. Support for continued investigation of SSRI pharmacotherapy in pediatric obsessive-compulsive disorder follows from the notion that it may provide effective alternatives to clomipramine without the associated side effects from activity at cholinergic, adrenergic, and histaminic receptor sites. The only published data from trials of SSRIs in pediatric obsessive-compulsive disorder to date come from reports of fluoxetine and fluvoxamine.

Fluoxetine is a bicyclic compound, distinguished from the other SSRIs by its long half-life and active metabolite, norfluoxetine, which also blocks 5-HT uptake. Only a handful of published studies, most with open-label designs, have prospectively investigated the efficacy of fluoxetine in pediatric obsessive-compulsive disorder (Clarvit et al., 1994; Como & Kurlan, 1991; Kurlan, Como, Deeley, McDermott, & McDermott, 1993; Liebowitz et al., 1989; Riddle, Scahill, et al., 1992). Improvement, measured as change in Yale-Brown Obsessive Compulsive Scales (Y-BOCS) scores at endpoint, ranged from 30% to 57%. Riddle and colleagues reported results from a double-blind crossover trial of fluoxetine and placebo in children and adolescents using a fixed dose regimen (20 mg/day). The most common side effects were insomnia, motoric activation, gastrointestinal discomfort, and fatigue; there were no clinically meaningful changes in vital signs, weight, EKG, or laboratory values. Six fluoxetine-treated patients completed the entire 20-week study; the drug had to be discontinued in one subject who developed suicidal ideation. Two subjects with preexisting tic disorders demonstrated exacerbation of tic activity. Children's Y-BOCS (CY-BOCS) scores dropped 44% after the initial eight weeks of active treatment, compared with a 27% decrease after placebo. Although this difference was not statistically significant, the magnitude of improvement seen in fluoxetine-treated patients did achieve significance on the CY-BOCS and the Clinical Global Impression (CGI) scores (Guy, 1976) for global improvement. In a companion study of 14 subjects with Tourette's, the Y-BOCS scores declined 37% in subjects with obsessive-compulsive symptoms (Scahill et al., 1997). Although not yet published, preliminary findings from a placebo-controlled, double-blind study (Clarvit et al., 1994) found 67% of pediatric obsessive-compulsive disorder patients treated with fluoxetine were rated as improved by week 8, and the drug was well tolerated with no significant adverse effects reported.

Clinical experience with fluoxetine has led some investigators (March et al., 1995; Riddle, Scahill, et al., 1992) to recommend low doses (less than 20 mg daily) of fluoxetine to minimize side effects and preserve response. Alternate-day dosing, administering a portion of a capsule's contents, and prescribing liquid preparations are strategies that can be used to achieve effective daily doses as low as 2.5 mg/day. However, a recent retrospective chart-review study of 38 pediatric obsessive-compulsive disorder patients showed sustained improvement using higher doses (averaging 50 mg or 1 mg/kg daily; Geller, Biederman, Reed, Spencer, & Wilens, 1995). The sum of these data suggest that fluoxetine should be initiated at low doses, with consideration of dose escalation only if there is no response and side effects are not problematic. Fluoxetine dose adjustments should take into account the fact that steady-state concentrations of the drug are not reached for several weeks due to the long half-life of fluoxetine and its metabolite.

Fluvoxamine is another potent SSRI with little direct activity at postsynaptic receptor binding sites and no known active metabolites. Several controlled trials and a large multicenter investigation demonstrated its safety and efficacy in adult obsessive-compulsive disorder (W. Goodman, Price, Rasmussen, Mazure, Delgado, et al., 1989; Greist, Jefferson, et al., 1995; Jenike et al., 1990; Perse, Greist, Jefferson, Rosenfeld, & Dar, 1988), using doses ranging from 100 to 300 mg/day. Principal side effects reported by adults include insomnia, activation, anxiety, sedation, dizziness, tremor, nausea, and headache, similar to those experienced by adolescent inpatients with obsessive-compulsive disorder or major depression in an open-label study (Apter et al., 1994). That investigation included 14 obsessive-compulsive disorder subjects and demonstrated a modest average drop (mean 7.7, *SD* 3.7) in Y-BOCS scores, on a mean dose of 200 mg/day of fluvoxamine after six to eight weeks of treatment.

Sertraline (50–200 mg daily; Greist, Chouinard, et al., 1995) and paroxetine (40–60 mg daily; Wheadon et al., 1993) are beneficial for adults with obsessive-compulsive disorder and share similar side effects profiles with the other SSRIs. Preliminary results from a controlled trial of sertraline offer support for its application in pediatric obsessive-compulsive disorder (Cook et al., 1994). Such investigations are necessary to establish appropriate doses and explore adverse experiences that may be unique to the younger patient.

The preponderance of data indicate a minimum of 8 and up to 12 weeks of drug therapy are required for treatment of adult obsessive-compulsive disorder (W. Goodman, Rasmussen, Foa, & Price, 1994). Despite success with drugs that target the 5-HT system, as many as 40–60% of patients are clinically unchanged after an adequate trial of these agents. The results of one crossover study showing individuals had preferential drug response to either clomipramine or fluoxetine (Pigott et al., 1990), along with numerous anecdotal examples of therapeutic success with one SRI following failure with another, lead most authorities to recommend switching to a second SRI when an adequate trial of the first does not yield a response. Careful monitoring of comorbid tics is important when potentially activating medications, such as SSRIs, are prescribed for obsessive-compulsive disorder. Adding agents to ongoing SRI therapy that enhance serotonergic function, such as lithium (McDougle, Price, Goodman, Charney, & Heninger, 1991) and buspirone (McDougle, Goodman, & Price, 1993), has generally not proven useful in adults.

Benzodiazepines

Clonazepam

Several members of the benzodiazepine class have been used in the treatment of adult obsessive-compulsive disorder (Bacher, 1990; Leonard et al.,

1994; Tollefson, 1985), though no definitive role for them has been established in large controlled studies. A few open-label studies (L. Cohen & Rosenbaum, 1987; D. Ross & Piggott, 1993) and one controlled, double-blind crossover study (Hewlett, Vinogradov, & Agras, 1992) suggest that clonazepam may be useful as a monotherapy in adults with obsessive-compulsive disorder, but side effects such as ataxia, dysarthria, disinhibition, and alterations of mood indicate poor tolerability in this role. SRI augmentation with clonazepam may be a particularly helpful strategy for patients with insomnia or high levels of anxiety or when SSRI dose is limited by drug-induced activation (Jenike & Rauch, 1994). It can be added to any of the SSRIs or clomipramine, beginning at doses as low as 0.25 mg once or twice daily, with increments in dose every few days as tolerated to a maximum of 5 mg/day.

Combination of a SRI and a Neuroleptic

A second strategy for management of SRI-refractory obsessive-compulsive disorder involves targeting a second neurochemical system with the addition of dopamine receptor blocking agents. This approach grows logically from several lines of evidence from preclinical and clinical investigations that implicate dopamine in the mediation of some forms of obsessive-compulsive disorder (W. Goodman et al., 1990). Retrospective analyses of a fluvoxamine monotherapy trial in adults first revealed that the subgroup of obsessive-compulsive disorder patients with comorbid tic disorders fared significantly worse than those without tics (McDougle, Goodman, Leckman, Barr, et al., 1993). Failure to respond to fluoxetine was also seen among children with obsessive-compulsive symptoms and Tourette's syndrome in a double-blind placebo-controlled study (Kurlan et al., 1993). A follow-up study of children with obsessive-compulsive disorder found that comorbid tic disorders predicted poor long-term prognosis (Leonard et al., 1993). Several case reports (Delgado, Goodman, Price, Heninger, & Charney, 1990; Riddle, Leckman, Hardin, et al., 1988) and an open-label series (McDougle et al., 1990) suggested that this special subpopulation might benefit from a SRI-neuroleptic combination. Support for this hypothesis came from a controlled, double-blind trial of haloperidol addition to fluvoxamine in SRI-refractory adults (McDougle et al., 1994). In that study, the presence of tic-spectrum disorders was associated with response to cotherapy, a finding that was not attributable to increased blood levels of the SRI. Extrapyramidal side effects were common but treatable, and there were no serious adverse reactions in the adult subjects receiving haloperidol and fluvoxamine. Case reports (McDougle et al., 1995) and open-label studies (Saxena, Wang, Bystritsky, & Baxter, 1996) indicate the novel D_2/5-HT$_{2A}$ receptor antagonist risperidone may offer a safe and effective alternative to haloperidol as an adjunct to a SRI. Larger-scale controlled trials are underway, with encouraging preliminary results in adult populations at Yale. A recent report of risperidone augmentation of SRIs in refractory adult obsessive-compulsive disorder described a series of 21 patients openly treated with doses ranging from 0.5 to 8 mg/day (mean dose, 2.75 mg/day; Saxena et al., 1996). Five patients (24% of the sample) experienced intolerable side effects and withdrew from the study. However, 14 of 16 (87%) patients who took the drug for three weeks showed positive response. Surprisingly, individuals with tic disorders in that study had the poorest rate of response and the highest rate of akathisia.

Combination SRI–dopamine antagonist pharmacotherapy has not yet been systematically investigated in children and adolescents with refractory obsessive-compulsive disorder or comorbid tics and obsessive-compulsive disorder, but it is likely to prove beneficial for the younger population of patients. Data on tolerability and dosing are needed so that guidelines for the use of this combination pharmacotherapy can be established. Because the SSRIs differentially inhibit various cytochrome P450 hepatic isoenzymes, they are not equal in their potential for causing significant drug interactions (Ereshefsky, Riesenman, & Lam, 1996). Consideration of SRI pharmacokinetic properties in an obsessive-compulsive disorder patient who needs concurrent administration of other medications involved in hepatic metabolism may be the most important factor guiding choice of monotherapy at present.

Neurosurgical Treatments

The recognition that some obsessive-compulsive disorder patients remain severely disabled by their symptoms despite treatment trials using multiple treatment approaches (including both pharmacotherapy and behavior therapy) coupled with the advent of relatively safe neurosurgical operations has renewed interest in such interventions. In an effort to relieve obsessive-compulsive symptoms, a number of different procedures have been performed, including anterior cingulotomy (Baer et al., 1995), limbic leucotomy (Kelly, Richardson, & Mitchell-Heggs, 1973), subcaudate tractotomy (Bridges et al., 1994), and anterior capsulotomy (Mindus & Jenike, 1992). A long-term follow-up study of 33 cases confirmed the relative safety and modest efficacy of stereotactic cingulotomy for treatment of refractory obsessive-compulsive disorder (Baer et al., 1995; Jenike et al., 1991). A main complication was seizures that occurred in three cases; however, four individuals in this series committed suicide, suggesting severe comorbid depression and/or despair that this treatment of last resort failed to improve their condition. On a slightly brighter side, there is some evidence that standard treatments are more likely to be successful after neurosurgery than before (Baer et al., 1995).

At present, it is not possible to predict which patients would benefit the most from such treatments or even to know with certainty which procedure to recommend. We continue to regard these treatments as experimental and rarely will refer treatment-refractory adult cases for evaluation and possible surgery. It is hoped that the results of ongoing well-controlled prospective trials will clarify how best to proceed.

Transcranial Magnetic Stimulation

Another experimental approach in the treatment of refractory obsessive-compulsive disorder involves the use of transcranial magnetic stimulation (B. Greenberg, McCann, & Benjamin, 1997). This is an area of active investigation and it is unclear which stimulation parameters are best. Although there is a risk of seizures, the procedure is relatively safe and does not involve irreversible brain injury. It is hoped that this line of research will lead to circuit-based treatment approaches that will capitalize on our growing knowledge of the cortico-striato-thalamo-cortical loops known to be involved in obsessive-compulsive disorder (see Chapters 9 and 13 for reviews).

PHARMACOTHERAPY FOR ATTENTION-DEFICIT/ HYPERACTIVITY DISORDER

As in tic disorders and obsessive-compulsive disorder, there are no brain-imaging techniques or diagnostic tests to confirm a diagnosis of ADHD. The presentation is heterogeneous and environmentally dependent, such that symptom exacerbation often occurs in the context of stress, groups, or stimulating settings. Multimodal therapies are often needed to address the comorbidity and wide-ranging effects of behavioral problems associated with ADHD (Richters et al., 1995; Satterfield, Satterfield, & Schell, 1987).

Stimulants have played a role in the treatment of children with disruptive behaviors since 1937 (Bradley, 1937), when an account of the dramatic calming effect of benzadrine was first published. However, it was not until the 1960s that controlled investigations of amphetamines for treatment of behavioral problems were carried out (Conners, Eisenberg, & Barcai, 1967; Eisenberg, Lachman, & Molling, 1961). Since then, numerous studies have been conducted that confirm the beneficial effects of psychostimulant medications for ADHD (DuPaul & Barkley, 1990; Gittelman-Klein, 1987; Solanto, 1984). Psychostimulants have become the first-line pharmacotherapy for ADHD, repeatedly demonstrating overall response rates, safety, and efficacy outcomes superior to that seen with other classes of drugs. With these agents' increasing popularity in recent years, their limitations have been underscored, and much controversy still surrounds their use (Cowart, 1988). Popular opinion about psychostimulants varies; they have been regarded as a panacea for desperate parents, as well as dangerous street drugs that could lead to addiction and suicide. Parental concerns and attitudes about any medication can have a great impact on the success of pharmacotherapy and as such should be one of the foremost treatment considerations.

Several other classes of drugs have emerged as nonstimulant alternatives that may be appropriate choices for some patients. Accumulating data now offer some guidance in the clinical decisions related to pharmacotherapy for individuals with ADHD (Cowart, 1988; Elia, 1993; Fox & Rieder, 1993; Green, 1995; Greenhill, 1995; Werry, 1994). In uncomplicated ADHD, the most common and obvious indication for intervention with nonstimulant drugs is a scenario in which an adequate trial with stimulants yields unacceptable results. Unsatisfactory amelioration of symptoms (Green, 1991; Hunt, Capper, & O'Connell, 1990), inability to tolerate side effects (Klein & Mannuzza, 1988), loss of therapeutic effects, or unacceptable dosing requirements related to the pharmacokinetics of stimulants are all reasons for prescribing nonstimulant alternatives. Factors such as presence of significant mental retardation (Aman, Marks, Turbott, Wilsher, & Merry, 1991), high risk for abuse, presence or family history of tic disorder (Riddle, Hardin, Cho, Woolston, & Leckman, 1988; Spencer, Biederman, Kerman, Steingard, & Wilens, 1993; Spencer, Biederman, Wilens, Steingard, & Geist, 1993), and concern about inhibition of growth are considerations that might lead clinicians to favor a nonstimulant agent. Comorbid diagnoses such as pervasive developmental disorder, depression, and anxiety disorders (Biederman, Baldessarini, Wright, Knee, & Harmatz, 1989; Biederman et al., 1991a; Pliszka, 1987) are also associated with poorer outcome in stimulant-treated ADHD. In cases where both ADHD and tic symptoms are prominent, we recommend that nonstimulant medications like clonidine, guanfacine, and tricyclic antidepressants be tried first, with psychostimulants reserved for use in the subset of patients who do not respond to more conservative approaches.

Stimulants

Methylphenidate

Psychostimulants are amine compounds that resemble catecholamine neurotransmitters and have potent agonist effects at alpha- and beta-adrenergic receptor sites. The putative action of these agents in ADHD presumably lies in their ability to block the reuptake of dopamine in presynaptic nerve terminals and promote its release in striatal brain regions. Methylphenidate (MPH; Ritalin®) is one of three psychostimulants currently in use for ADHD, and is the single most widely studied and frequently prescribed drug for the disorder (Gadow, Sverd, et al., 1995; Safer & Krager, 1988). MPH, a piperidine derivative, has enjoyed increasing use in the past 10 years because it has established efficacy and safety in multiple controlled studies. MPH ameliorates many of the target symptoms of ADHD, showing large beneficial effects in measures of inhibitory control, sustained attention, gross motor activity, aggression, cognitive tasks, and compliance with adult requests (Wilens & Biederman, 1992). MPH is also a popular choice because of its rapid action, relatively low-priced generic form, wide range of tolerated doses, and low incidence of side effects (see Greenhill, 1995, for a review).

The most common side effects of MPH are shared with other drugs in its class, and include reduced appetite, insomnia, stomachaches, and headaches. Tearfulness and emotional brittleness, pallor, dizziness, and nightmares have also been reported (Greenhill, 1992a, 1992b; Wilens & Biederman, 1992). Stimulant-induced psychosis is rare (Barkley, 1977; DuPaul & Barkley, 1990; Lucas & Weiss, 1971). Reducing the dose will frequently control common side effects, which tend to abate over time on the drug. Growth retardation has been reported with longer-term use (Klein, Landa, Mattes, & Klein, 1988; Klein & Mannuzza, 1988), but compensatory or "catch-up" growth appears to occur after discontinuation of the drug (Charles, Schain, & Guthrie, 1979). Mild increases in heart rate and blood pressure are common and well tolerated, but cardiovascular effects of clinical significance are not seen with central stimulants, so routine EKG monitoring is not required. Tolerance and physiologic dependence do not generally develop with the stimulants commonly prescribed for ADHD (Safer & Allen, 1989). The emergence or worsening of movement disorders in stimulant-treated children with comorbid ADHD and tics has been described (Erenberg et al., 1985; Lowe et al., 1982; Sallee & Rock, 1994). However, recent placebo-controlled, double-blind studies suggest the overall severity of the tic disorder is not altered, in most cases, in the short term (Gadow, Sverd, et al., 1995). MPH and anticonvulsants can be safely combined in patients with seizure disorders (Feldman, Crumrine, & Handen, 1989). Children with comorbid anxiety disorders may develop more side effects than children with ADHD alone (DuPaul et al., 1994; Tannock, Ickowicz, & Schachar, 1991).

Treatment with MPH is typically started at 5 mg daily and increased every three to five days. A popular conservative approach employs a 0.3 mg/kg dose-by-weight regimen (Sprague & Sleator, 1977). There is not agreement in the literature about the dose-response effects of MPH (Gittelman-Klein, 1980), and plasma levels have been found to correlate poorly with various outcome measures (Gualtieri et al., 1982; Sebrechts et al., 1986). Specific criteria for satisfactory response remain poorly defined, making it even harder for clinicians to determine when an effective dose has been achieved. A broad acceptable range is 2.5–60 mg daily; doses higher than 1 mg/kg are rarely needed and not recommended (Barkley & DuPaul, 1993; Wilens & Biederman, 1992). MPH is typically given two or three times daily. Problematic rebound behavior may occur when MPH wears off (Malone, Kershner, & Siegel, 1988). To attenuate rebound effects, the last dose is often the lowest dose of the day. A sustained-release preparation of MPH is available in the 20 mg strength, making it possible for some patients to avoid taking the medication during school hours. Reports of the efficacy of long-acting MPH have been divergent, and we typically avoid its use. However, a review of data from controlled studies suggests equal clinical efficacy between the short-acting and long-acting forms of the drug (Greenhill, 1995). Given the continued uncertainty regarding long-term effects of stimulants, drug holidays on weekends and

392 Partnerships for Making the Best of Tourette's

summers are recommended as a strategy to minimize exposure and to assess the need for continued treatment.

Dextroamphetamine

Dextroamphetamine (Dexedrine®) exhibits a slightly more rapid onset of action than MPH and a slightly longer half-life. Comparisons of dextroamphetamine and MPH show trends for MPH to produce greater decreases in motor activity and fewer compulsive behaviors but more abnormal movements than dextroamphetamine (Borcherding, Keysor, Cooper, & Rapoport, 1989; Borcherding et al., 1990; Malone et al., 1988). The two agents are generally similar with regard to side effects, although there is some evidence that dextroamphetamine may be associated with more mood instability (Greenhill, 1995). Some individuals may respond preferentially to one stimulant over another (Elia & Rapoport, 1991; Malone et al., 1988), so trials of each agent are worthwhile. The recommended dose range maximum is 40 mg daily, or 1.5 mg/kg/day, given in two doses. The second daily dose can often be 5–10 mg less than the morning one. Sustained-release dextroamphetamine preparations (spansules) are also available in 5 mg and 10 mg strengths.

Pemoline

Pemoline (Cylert®) is a third stimulant option for the treatment of ADHD. It has been used since the mid-1970s with well-documented effects, qualitatively much the same as those seen with MPH (Conners & Taylor, 1980; Stephens, Pelham, & Skinner, 1984). Pemoline is distinguished from the other stimulants by its longer half-life (mean, 7 hours), which increases with age (Collier et al., 1985). Pemoline therapy begins with a single 37.5 mg dose, given in the morning. Weekly increments in dose can be made until improvement is noted, up to a maximum of 112.5 mg daily. Despite common beliefs that the drug has a delayed effect apparent only after three to six weeks, a placebo-controlled crossover study found pemoline as effective as the other stimulants by the third day of treatment (Pelham et al., 1990). Liver function tests should be monitored at baseline and at regular intervals in patients maintained on pemoline (Greenhill, 1989). In our experience, pemoline is the most likely of the stimulants to exacerbate tics. In our experience, pemoline is the most likely of the stimulants to exacerbate tics. Because of this side effect and the serious liver toxicity, we believe pemoline should be avoided.

Tricyclic Antidepressants

For various reasons, approximately 25% to 30% of ADHD patients do not experience a satisfactory response to psychostimulants. Many of those individuals may benefit from nonstimulant alternatives such as tricyclic antidepressants (Biederman, Baldessarini, et al., 1993; Gastfriend, Biederman, & Jellinek, 1984; Green, 1995). The mechanism of action in ADHD appears to be different from that operating in the treatment of depression, producing a more rapid onset of clinical effects at comparatively lower optimal doses and lower serum concentrations (Donnelly et al., 1986; Linnoila, Gualtieri, Jobson, & Staye, 1979) than required for antidepressant effects. Although not formally approved by the FDA for treatment of ADHD, the use of tricyclics has been well studied and clinically accepted for more than 20 years. The sum of published literature suggests that tricyclics are inferior to stimulants overall (see Green, 1995, for review), but efficacy has been clearly established for desipramine (Norpramin®; Biederman, Baldessarini, Wright, Knee, & Harmat, 1989; Donnelly et al., 1986; Greenhill, 1992a) and imipramine (Tofranil®; Quinn & Rapoport, 1975; J. Rapoport, Quinn, Bradbard, Riddle, & Brooks, 1974; Werry, Aman, & Diamond, 1980), making them solid second-line agents when stimulants have failed or are contraindicated. Nortriptyline (Pamelor®; Wilens, Biederman, Geist, Steingard, & Spencer, 1993), amitriptyline (Elavil®; Krakowski, 1965; Yepes, Balka, Winsberg, & Bialer, 1977), and clomipramine (Anafranil®; Garfinkel, Wender, Sloman, & O'Neil, 1983) have been investigated to a lesser extent, but each has modest empirical support in the treatment of ADHD.

Tricyclic monotherapy may offer a particular advantage over stimulants when comorbid depression, anxiety, or tic disorder complicates the treatment of ADHD. Desipramine improved both tics and ADHD symptoms in a retrospective study of 33 young patients (Spencer, Biederman, Kerman, et al., 1993), but no overall change in tics was noted in an earlier study (Riddle, Hardin, et al., 1988). Another retrospective investigation of 12 patients with comorbid ADHD and chronic tic disorders found good response in both areas with nortriptyline (Spencer, Biederman, Wilens, et al., 1993). The combination of desipramine and MPH showed positive response on cognitive functions in a group of children with ADHD and major depression (M. Rapport, Carlson, Kelly, & Pataki, 1993); increased side effects and elevation of tricyclic blood levels remain important considerations with those agents together (Pataki, Carlson, Kelly, Rapport, & Biancaniello, 1993).

Although tricyclic antidepressants can decrease hyperactivity and improve mood, the frequency and severity of adverse effects associated with their use in children and adolescents present significant concerns. The pharmacokinetic features that account for poor correlation between tricyclic antidepressant dose and serum levels make close monitoring for potentially serious toxicity an imperative in young patients treated with tricyclics (Biederman, Baldessarini, Wright, Knee, Harmatz, & Goldblatt, 1989). Prolonged cardiac conduction times (Leonard et al., 1995) and several cases of sudden death (Riddle, Geller, & Ryan, 1993) have been attributed to tricyclic agents in pediatric populations, so serial EKGs and serum drug levels should be followed closely (Elliott & Popper, 1990-1991; Preskorn, Jerkovich, Beber, & Widener, 1989). Sedation and other anticholinergic side effects that are common with all of the tricyclics (e.g., dry mouth, postural dizziness) may be especially problematic in child and adolescent patients, limiting dose escalation to the therapeutic range (Biederman, Baldessarini, Wright, Knee, Harmatz, & Goldblatt, 1989).

Furthermore, several reports suggest tolerance to the therapeutic effects of tricyclics may develop over time (Quinn & Rapoport, 1975; Waizer, Hoffman, Polizos, & Engelhardt, 1974).

After the appropriate baseline studies are done, tricyclic pharmacotherapy should be initiated with low doses and titrated upward gradually as tolerated until a predetermined maximum dose or serum concentration is achieved. Daily doses of 10–25 mg are appropriate for beginning treatment of ADHD with any of the tricyclics described here, but optimal dose range varies slightly among the different compounds: imipramine 1–2 mg/kg/day; desipramine 2.5–5 mg/kg/day; nortriptyline 0.4–4.5 mg/kg/day; amitriptyline 20–150 mg/day; clomipramine 3 mg/kg/day (reviewed by Green, 1995). Serum levels from 100 to 300 ng/ml of desipramine (Biederman, Baldessarini, Wright, Knee, Harmatz, & Goldblatt, 1989) and from 50 to 150 ng/ml of nortriptyline (Wilens et al., 1993) are considered therapeutic for ADHD.

Other Antidepressants

Bupropion

Bupropion hydrochloride (Wellbutrin®) is an aminoketone-class antidepressant medication that is chemically distinct from the tricyclics or other antidepressants. Four studies (Barrickman et al., 1995; Simeon, Ferguson, & Fleet, 1986), two of which were double-blind, placebo-controlled trials (Casat, Pleasants, Schroeder, & Parler, 1989; Clay, Gualtieri, Evans, & Gullion, 1988), have demonstrated bupropion's effectiveness in ADHD, with infrequent, mild, and transient side effects. Agitation, dry mouth, insomnia, headache, nausea, vomiting, constipation, and tremor were common untoward effects. Optimal doses in the published trials ranged from 50 mg/day to 250 mg/day. The increased risk for seizures, particularly at doses over 450 mg per day, renders bupropion a poor choice for patients with a known history of seizure disorder and argues in favor of alternative pharmacotherapy if higher doses are not manifestly effective. Additionally, exacerbation of tics has been reported in ADHD patients with comorbid Tourette's syndrome receiving bupropion (Spencer, Biederman, Steingard, & Wilens, 1993).

Fluoxetine

The few studies that appear in the literature describe mixed effects of fluoxetine monotherapy on ADHD (Barrickman, Noyes, Kuperman, Schumacher, & Verda, 1991; Riddle et al., 1990, 1991). However, a role for fluoxetine as an augmentation agent administered with MPH in 32 treatment-refractory ADHD patients with comorbid psychiatric diagnoses was supported by an open-label trial (Gammon & Brown, 1993). Substantial improvements in several target areas were seen, particularly among the most severely affected patients in that study. Double-blind studies are needed to explore the promising findings described by these investigators.

Monoamine Oxidase Inhibitors

Administration of MAO inhibitors like clorgyline and tranylcypromine sulfate (Parnate®), which act on "type A" substrates such as norepinephrine, 5-HT, and normetanephrine, resulted in amelioration of ADHD behaviors in a double-blind crossover study (Zametkin, Rapoport, Murphy, Linnoila, & Ismond, 1985). A "type B" MAO inhibitor, L-deprenyl, did not produce the same clinical benefits in the same patient population (Zametkin & Rapoport, 1987a). These results lend support to the hypothesis of noradrenergic dysregulation as critical in the etiology of ADHD, but MAOI drugs remain an undesirable choice of pharmacotherapy for young patients who are likely to have difficulty observing a strict tyramine-free diet. Furthermore, some MAOI agents have irreversible action and interactions between psychostimulants and MAOIs can lead to dangerous elevations in blood pressure (Zametkin et al., 1985). The newer selective MAO-B inhibitor selegiline may hold potential for use in ADHD without the complications associated with the older agents (Jankovic, 1993).

Alpha Adrenergic Receptor Agonists

Clonidine

As described above in the section on Tourette's syndrome, clonidine is an antihypertensive agent with activity at the alpha2-adrenergic receptors on the presynaptic neuron, which leads to diminished endogenous release of norepinephrine in the brain. A few studies (Hunt, 1987; Hunt, Minderaa, & Cohen, 1985) suggest that clonidine may be useful for ADHD, but the quality and magnitude of therapeutic effect is different from that observed with MPH. Clonidine may be useful for children who are extremely hyperactive, energetic, impulsive, and disinhibited (Hunt et al., 1990). A double-blind crossover study did not find clonidine better than placebo or desipramine in the treatment of ADHD with comorbid tics (Singer, Brown, & Quaskey, 1995). Children with ADHD who do appear to respond to clonidine may benefit from transdermal preparations, but extreme variation in behavior across the day may reflect fluctuations in blood levels with that form of clonidine. Dosing recommendations and side effects considerations are the same for ADHD as previously described for tic disorders.

Guanfacine

As described earlier, guanfacine holds promise as a treatment for children and adolescents who suffer from both ADHD and a tic disorder (Chappell, Riddle, et al., 1995).

Dopamine Antagonists

Older investigations of antipsychotic medications for the treatment of ADHD-equivalent disorders generally found them to be less safe and effective than stimulants (Dulcan, 1985; Gittelman-Klein, Klein, Katz,

Saraf, & Pollack, 1976; Werry, Weiss, Douglas, & Martin, 1966), so they have been regarded as last-choice agents in cases where standard pharmacotherapy has failed. However, thioridazine (Mellaril®; average daily doses 95 mg, range from 30 to 150 mg) proved better than amphetamine in a 1968 investigation of hyperkinetic syndrome in mentally retarded children (Alexandris & Lundell, 1968). Recent data also reveal that thioridazine may be an alternative pharmacotherapy without causing significant decrements in cognition (Klein, 1990/1991). Thioridazine at doses up to 2.5 mg/kg may be an especially useful monotherapy for ADHD in patients with mental retardation, who tend to show poor response to psychostimulants (Aman et al., 1991). Sedation is the principal side effect of thioridazine, and can be managed in part by administering single daily doses at bedtime.

Historically, chlorpromazine (Thorazine®) at doses up to 200 mg/d (mean, 196 mg/d) was also found superior to placebo in reducing target symptoms in hyperactive children, both acutely (Werry et al., 1966) and at follow-up five years later (G. Weiss, Kruger, Danielson, & Elman, 1975). A biphasic effect of haloperidol (Haldol®) on cognitive functions has been found in studies with hyperkinetic and aggressive children; low doses of the drug (0.025 mg/kg) were associated with improvement in symptoms, but high haloperidol doses (0.05 mg/kg) led to further impairment (Werry & Aman, 1975). Based on these findings, we typically avoid the use of haloperidol or other neuroleptics in the treatment of ADHD.

Combination pharmacotherapy is another strategy when symptoms cannot be managed with one drug alone. The addition of SRIs, stimulants, or clonidine to neuroleptics has not been systematically evaluated in children and adolescent populations, but may be helpful in ameliorating target symptoms when cautiously done with lower doses of both agents.

FUTURE DIRECTIONS

The prospects are bright for improved pharmacological approaches to Tourette's and related disorders. A number of atypical neuroleptic agents are being developed, several of which appear to be useful in the treatment of tics. More important, there is a growing recognition in the research community and the pharmaceutical industry of the need for multicenter trials that will speed the evaluation of novel agents.

However, pediatric psychopharmacology remains a neglected area with few clinical trials and limited data on long-term safety (Institute of Medicine, 1989). Recently, the National Institutes of Health have recognized these shortcomings (Vitiello & Jensen, 1997) and have begun to take steps to redress the problem. Particularly promising is the formation of several research units focused explicitly on these issues.

In considering medication trials it is also appropriate to consider the place of drugs in the overall management of these conditions. Given the waxing and waning character of Tourette's, the imperfect nature of the available drugs and their potential for harm, it is also possible that in the future more clinicians and families will elect to make do with minimal, if any, medications. However, each individual is unique, and for many patients the use of medication has made a remarkable difference in their quality of life.

Finally, we can anticipate that as pathogenic mechanisms are clarified, innovative, safe, and effective somatic treatments will emerge. Possible examples include immunologically based treatments for autoimmune forms of Tourette's and obsessive-compulsive disorder as well as circuit-based approaches using transcranial magnetic stimulation. ". . . approaches using transcranial magnetic stimulation. The discovery of vulnerability and other genes associated with Tourette's syndrome and obsessive-compulsive disorder will be able to help guide the development of biologically more 'rational' approaches to treatment. As genes and their functions are explicated, it will be possible to target treatment directly at the genetic level or at alterations in brain function and neurochemistry that are specifically part of the pathogenesis of the disorders."

SUMMARY OF CHAPTER 20

Tourette's syndrome, obsessive-compulsive disorder, and ADHD are disorders of childhood onset that hold the potential for significant disruption or impairment in every domain of the patient's development. The symptom presentations for these disorders are variable and complex, making timely and proper diagnosis a challenging but important goal. Assessment of Tourette's syndrome, obsessive-compulsive disorder, and ADHD involves understanding the larger social, academic, and familial context that surrounds the individual patient and impacts the illness. A variety of modalities of intervention are often necessary for children with these comorbid disorders. Biological approaches are centered on the use of medications targeted at the most problematic symptoms, in a closely monitored setting. Short-term efficacy has been established for a number of medications, but data documenting their safety with long-term use are rare. Comorbidity and symptom overlap among Tourette's syndrome, obsessive-compulsive disorder, and ADHD is high, and can make pharmacotherapy difficult when one constellation of symptoms worsens as a consequence of treatment for another. Combination treatments are not well studied and should be used with caution in refractory cases. The continued development and investigation of novel agents with greater efficacy and more favorable side effects profiles is clearly needed for effective treatment of complicated cases with comorbid Tourette's syndrome, obsessive-compulsive disorder, or ADHD.

PREVIEW OF CHAPTER 21

The final chapter discusses the important role of voluntary organizations, such as the Tourette Syndrome Association, in providing care and advocacy for individuals affected by this disorder. While support groups for patients, parents and siblings are important, a more holistic approach is needed that includes a broad range of endeavors that include forming collaborations with clinicians, educators, researchers, and policymakers—among others.

CHAPTER 21

Role of Voluntary Organizations in Clinical Care, Research, and Public Policy

KATHRYN A. TAUBERT

> No gain is so certain as that which proceeds from the economical use of what you already have.
>
> —*Latin proverb*

Volunteerism, an integral part of life in the United States for more than 200 years, is a demonstrably effective force for change. After a brief decline between 1982 and 1984, volunteerism and the not-for-profit sector as a whole has steadily risen (Hodgkinson & Weitzman, 1996). Presently, there are some 1.4 million not-for-profit organizations in the United States with a total budget of more than $155 billion per year (Hodgkinson & Weitzman). More impressive is the amount of time donated to such causes; in 1995, U.S. citizens donated more than 20 billion hours, with 49% of American adults volunteering (Thomas & Ericksen-Mendosa, 1996).

Volunteers gave the most time to health and humans services, religious organizations, education, and youth development. The number of equivalent full-time volunteers was 9.4 million. Total volunteer contributions to the workforce were the equivalent of $160 billion. Operating expenditures for all not-for-profit organizations were estimated to be $389.1 billion, or $1,047 for every person in the United States (Hodgkinson & Weitzman, 1996).

GOALS AND OBJECTIVES

Voluntary health organizations are some of the best known not-for-profits. These organizations raise money for research, disseminate research findings, conduct educational and medical symposia, help destigmatize the condition, provide patient care and referral, identify strategies to help constituents with educational and/or employment issues, sponsor social and family services, and represent constituents to the government on critical policy issues. Volunteers are fundamentally involved in every aspect of these efforts. Although many health organizations employ paid administrative management personnel, the ratio of paid to unpaid employees illustrates continuing dependency on volunteers. In 1990, the number of volunteers represented 40% of total employment in the not-for-profit sector (Hodgkinson & Weitzman, 1996).

Clearly, voluntary organizations are a force to consider, with substantial interest in decisions affecting constituents. Policymakers, however, should be mindful of the fact that although decisions about clinical care, research, and public policy may represent the end of the process for them, for constituents of voluntary organizations, these decisions may represent the beginning. Researchers, for example, may conclude work with the identification of medications for treatment; the patients' work may only just begin with this information. They will have to weigh possible undesirable side effects against potential benefits; furthermore, several trials with different medications may be necessary to find the most favorable. Even then, many individuals may not benefit at all.

ORIGINS AND STRENGTHS

Most major voluntary health organizations in the United States today were initiated by the efforts of a few individuals. Original efforts to locate information and services evolved, in some cases, into wide-ranging programs and services with multinational constituencies. Early success resulted in the drive to expand their scope, with some organizations virtually succeeding themselves right out of business. For example, the March of Dimes, after successful efforts to fund polio vaccine research in the 1950s, revised its mission at the request of constituents and associates worldwide. The March of Dimes Birth Defects Foundation is now dedicated to the prevention of birth defects and is among the largest voluntary health organizations in the world.

Successful voluntary organizations have four key strengths:

1. Getting people to do what needs to be done without direct financial compensation. Motivating people to perform the necessary work without salary and benefits is a cornerstone of the successful voluntary enterprise. Knowing why people volunteer and developing opportunities for them to satisfy their needs is critical to effective volunteer management.
2. Managing people within multiple lines of authority and responsibility. Voluntary organizations most often employ a matrix management

system that includes not only a multiple command structure but also related support mechanisms and an associated organizational culture and behavior (S. Davis & Lawrence, 1977). Good faith, effective negotiation, and collaboration are required.

3. Maintaining support for long-term efforts without significant, short-term results. Voluntary organizations rarely see immediate results. Cures for cancer or heart disease, equal employment opportunities, and insurance parity for the disabled are not measured by quarterly returns on investments. Leadership must be visionary, while sustaining a productive volunteer workforce with little more than meager, short-term, palliative results.

4. Successful voluntary organizations must keep client/patient needs foremost in the minds of those charged with meeting them. Derived from the marketing axiom that those who use the products and services are best able to help create and improve them, survivability in a competitive marketplace requires pervasive customer orientation.

Leaders of voluntary organizations must be proactive for their constituents' needs and unafraid to redefine missions as needs evolve. Sophisticated management methodology must be employed while maintaining a strict code of ethics unparalleled in the profit sector. Voluntary organizations' dependence on donations is subject to rigorous public scrutiny; answering to a variety of federal, state, and private mandates, reputable not-for-profits strive for rigorous standards of management and accounting not required of profit-sector business (AICPA, 1996).

THE TOURETTE SYNDROME ASSOCIATION

Education, research, and advocacy are, of course, key planks in any voluntary health agency's platform, having evolved from initial, primary purposes of mutual support. The Tourette Syndrome Association, Inc. (TSA), for example, was founded in 1972 primarily as a support group for a few families in the New York City area. Then, TSA founders believed there were only 50 or so cases of Tourette's syndrome in all recorded medical history (TSA Inc., 1996a).

In 1996, it was estimated that 1 in 200 people has some form of Tourette's syndrome; of these, over 40,000 individuals and their families avail themselves of TSA services (TSA Inc., 1996b). Presently the only national not-for-profit membership organization dedicated to identifying the cause of, cure for, and treatment of Tourette's syndrome, the TSA has 54 chapters in the United States and a presence in 30 foreign countries. TSA membership includes people with Tourette's syndrome, their relatives, and other concerned supporters. The organization publishes a quarterly newsletter with a readership of 40,000 people worldwide. TSA operates under general guidelines established by the national organization's volunteer, democratically elected, interdisciplinary board of directors. The national office employs 17 professionals and two full-time volunteers. Affiliates or local chapters of TSA are managed by volunteers with diverse personal and professional backgrounds. Several larger chapters employ a few full- or part-time administrative management and support personnel. Treatment policies and medical information are overseen by a volunteer medical advisory board. Application to the TSA research grant awards program is peer reviewed by a volunteer scientific advisory board. Since its establishment in 1984, TSA's Permanent Research Fund has provided approximately $4 million to scientists working in clinical and pre-clinical fields.

The TSA raises funds for research; collaborates with interdisciplinary scientific and medical advisory committees to set research policies and goals; provides a variety of family services; publishes educational materials; organizes workshops and symposia for scientists, clinicians, and educators; maintains databases of those diagnosed with TS; provides physician referral and other service provider lists by state; and represents its members to the government on critical policy issues.

TSA chapter volunteers organize and manage public conferences, summer camps, media campaigns, in-service programs for health and education professionals, support groups, and advocacy programs. They distribute educational materials to schools and other service providers and raise funds for national research and support. Chapters do not engage in research directly, but may assist in recruiting by informing local members about existing research projects. In addition, nationally supported research programs may exist within chapter geographical boundaries, and local volunteers often participate as study patients. TSA encourages volunteers to participate in research approved by its scientific advisory board.

OPPORTUNITIES FOR COLLABORATION

The success of participative decision making is well documented (Ouchi, 1981). Every effort should be made to ask those most affected by the outcomes of decisions to participate in making them. Legislation such as the Americans with Disabilities Act and the Health Insurance Availability and Affordability Act of 1996 argue that collaboration is essential. Many voluntary organizations routinely engage in cooperative relationships with scientific, business, and government entities at all levels (Centers for Disease Control and Prevention, 1995).

Much is made of the voluntary organizations' availability to patients, family members, and researchers as a source of assistance (National Institutes of Health, 1995). A greater role, however, awaits in contributing to substantive decisions about treatment, research goals, and public policy.

Care and Support

The needs of people with Tourette's and their families vary depending on how severe the condition is, how long they have lived with it, and when the correct diagnosis was made. At the beginning, people need education and support to manage the grief, fears, and ignorance of peers, educators, and family.

The first lines of defense for many are TSA support groups and chapter activities such as conferences and camps. Children and adults with Tourette's syndrome and their families often feel isolated, misunderstood, initially overwhelmed. Concerns about the future and difficulties over current severe episodes of tics are naturally at the forefront of everyone's mind. Being able to talk with others who understand can be invaluable. As discussed in Chapter 15, separate support groups for parents, patients, and siblings have been established by volunteers acting in conjunction with the TSA.

Society's pressure to conform falls hardest on those who believe they are alone. Being able to share experiences helps people realize they have peers. Unlike others in minority groups, children with Tourette's syndrome often have no one at home or in the neighborhood with whom they can identify. Many older adults with Tourette's syndrome may have never met another. The author, not diagnosed until age 38, successful by most societal criteria, vividly recalls her first encounter with another adult with Tourette's syndrome shortly after the diagnosis. It is a memory engraved in stone. Members of the medical community should routinely refer patients with Tourette's syndrome and their families to local TSA chapters and other advocating organizations as appropriate. As part of any treatment regimen, the benefits are real and free.

Collaborations with Educators

Collaborations with voluntary organizations need not be limited to science and research. Discussions with patients and families concerning educational accommodations may be useful for the specific situation, but may generalize to others as well. These efforts can also help sort out some of the misinformation that sometimes accompanies diagnosis for all concerned: clinicians, families, and educators, as discussed in Chapter 19.

Through pamphlets, videotapes, and direct contact with chapter representatives, the TSA helps identify appropriate educational strategies for students, develops instructional aids and tools, and resolves problems. The success of these efforts is underscored by an ever-increasing number of inquiries by parents and educators for help at the local level. Without such efforts, the writer's experience of many years ago appears, unfortunately, still relevant: in the 1950s classroom, the author was labeled stubborn for avoiding the strict seating arrangements placing her in the middle of the classroom.

With significant neck, back, and shoulder tics, her attitude and classroom performance were, at times, directly proportionate to her opportunities to sit with her back against the wall. There are clues that misunderstandings like these still occur. Many children today are diagnosed distractible or oppositional when their behavior may represent an attempt to mitigate the unpleasant social effects of Tourette's syndrome. Asking young students for insights can be enlightening; for example, at a recent TSA Educators' Conference, a young student on a panel of children with Tourette's syndrome said that being teased about the tics was worse than having them. Teachers' comments frequently include statements such as "I never knew how difficult it was for my student with Tourette's syndrome until I heard those children on that panel say what it was like for them."

Substantial anecdotal information suggests that the typical school is exceedingly restrictive to a child with a movement disorder. Bound and gagged by restrictive seating arrangements, "quiet times," codes of conduct that do not permit freedom of movement, sound, or, even thought; society may be creating new disorders of mood and conduct! More and more, "Johnny's afterschool behavior" is referred to as oppositional, his anger "episodic," the manifestation of his frustration a "rage attack." Until further, substantive studies are conducted on the societal and environmental pressures affecting these children, it is unwise to assume that their behavior is of primary biological origin. The immense frustration of living bound and gagged in a body that needs to move as much, and often as frequently, as it needs to breathe, cannot be fully understood by those who haven't experienced it firsthand. Pressured by pervasive restrictions into a pattern of disobedient, negativistic, and provocative opposition to authority figures, some children with TS in fact may be reacting appropriately to what might be perceived as inhumane treatment, considering their exacerbated need to move. Others might withdraw or become depressed.

One is struck by the similarities between epilepsy and Tourette syndrome in the evolution of society's perception of these two distinct disorders. Thomas Szasz (1995), in his book *Cruel Compassion,* cites the medical stigmatization and persecution of epileptics when they were considered "biologically disposed to engage in destructive behavior" (p. 45). Szasz notes that by the end of the nineteenth century, psychiatric dogma considered epileptics "potential criminals—specifically, that they are afflicted with an irresistible urge to commit violent acts" (p. 46). Today, of course, we know that to be false, and seizure disorders are no longer considered to be mental diseases. The term epilepsy is absent from the *Diagnostic and Statistical Manual* of the American Psychiatric Association. The current trend with TS appears, at least to this author, perilously close to replicating that which individuals with seizure disorders suffered right until the 1950s. More research on the sociological aspects of living with Tourette's syndrome, especially in children, needs to be conducted to help segregate the sociological from the biological influences on behavior. If not, the experience of patients with epilepsy may be duplicated with the creation of new disorders associated with Tourette's syndrome that have lifelong, inappropriate, stigmatizing results.

At risk also is the loss of support for those that genuinely need it. The burgeoning backlash of society against the proliferation of psychiatric coercions and excuses (Szasz, 1994b) may be seen in recent federal legislation on renewed funding for special education students, the Individuals with Disabilities Education Act of 1997. New features restrict the appropriation of services for children with disruptive behaviors not directly related to their disability. When one considers the potential consequences to educators, parents, and children of not being able to equate disruptive behavior with any underlying medical problem, the implications are staggering. The pressure, one could argue, to ensure a causal relationship will increase if services are available only to children who are neurologically impaired.

Advocacy for Full Employment

Decisions about the capacity for gainful employment should be made with full understanding of the specific abilities of disabled job applicants. Despite the presence of a disorder, an individual judged ready for work should not be barred from employment or advancement. The data suggest need for improvement in this area. Of the 13 million working-age disabled persons in the United States, only 34% work full or part time, leaving 66%, or almost 8.5 million, unemployed. Two out of three of those unemployed, however, expressed a desire to work, if employment could be found (Hudson Institute, 1988b).

A Department of Labor report (Hudson Institute, 1988a, 1988b) came to the following conclusions: (a) the overwhelming majority of employers give disabled employees "good or excellent ratings on their overall ratings of job performance and safety"; (b) "Workers who had a disability were no harder to supervise than able-bodied employees"; (c) where required at all, 80% of all employer accommodations cost less than $500; and (d) employees with disabilities "even bring extra strengths to the job as a result of their disabilities." Although Tourette's syndrome may cause disability in some cases, there is no evidence that a diagnosis of Tourette's should preclude career or lifestyle choice. Indeed, many with Tourette's syndrome lead altogether successful, productive lives. People with the disorder can be found in all disciplines and all activities, from surgery to piloting aircraft (Sacks, 1995a). However, anecdotal evidence for some people with diagnosed Tourette's suggests that unemployment may be higher than average. Greater potential exists for collaboration between employers and TSA on behalf of individuals with Tourette's. All parties would clearly benefit.

Medical Insurance

Problems regarding insurance coverage reveal the need for greater collaboration among employers, the insurance industry, and individuals with

Tourette's. The author's application for private health insurance was denied based on a Tourette's syndrome diagnosis, despite generally excellent health. Subsequent applications with more than a half dozen underwriters revealed a staggering lack of knowledge of Tourette's syndrome. One underwriter's application categorized Tourette's syndrome with the degenerative, terminal disorders of Huntington's chorea and Parkinson's disease. A *yes* to any one of the three was grounds for automatic exclusion of coverage for any medical reason.

Incidents such as these are increasing as evidenced by the number of testimonials to this issue in the Tourette's community. It is ironic that wider recognition of Tourette's syndrome has inadvertently added to this problem. Clearly, educational efforts need to be stepped up as the diagnosis of Tourette's syndrome becomes more commonplace and newly diagnosed people apply for insurance. Fueled by misunderstandings, people often find themselves in the unenviable position of having to choose between a formal diagnosis and medical insurance. For example, coprolalia, the uttering of socially unacceptable words or phrases, has been sensationalized in the media, yet it occurs in only a small percentage of individuals with Tourette's syndrome. Many people mistakenly believe that a diagnosis of Tourette's syndrome requires the presence of this symptom; of course, it does not.

Research: A Joint Commitment

Individuals with Tourette's syndrome have a vested interest in research outcomes; as noted earlier, the end of the process for researchers may represent the beginning of it for patients. Patients routinely participate in research studies and clinical trials, and securing patient involvement in decisions about new research approaches has also proven fruitful (Bliss, 1980). Voluntary organization databases can also be an effective way of recruiting subjects with a wide range of symptomatology or from specific subgroups. TSA, for example, has been instrumental in acquiring resources through its substantial client/patient database, with promising results. Twins recruited by TSA were used for National Institutes of Health studies that yielded "dramatic insight into what causes the difference in severity of tic symptoms between identical twins" (TSA Inc., 1996c, p. 1). TSA's Brain Bank Program has been responsible for acquiring tissues of deceased patients with TS for study; heretofore, these valuable tissues had been largely unavailable for research.

Public Policy

Determination of appropriate social accommodations and interventions for people with special needs is another area for collaboration. The public rights, for example, of people with disruptive tics versus others is one such issue. The threshold for tolerance of disruptive behavior will vary with the teachers', parents', and classmates' knowledge of Tourette's syndrome.

Decisions about public accommodations for people with special needs will have little meaning or impact if the individual does not participate in the process. Presently, there seems to be little discussion with policymakers outside the occasional disturbing case of litigation involving someone with Tourette's syndrome and someone outside the Tourette's community (*Cohen vs. Boston University,* 1993). This only increases the ultimate cost to society through further disenfranchisement of individuals with Tourette's syndrome.

CURRENT BARRIERS TO EFFECTIVE COLLABORATION

Resistance to Change

The attitudes of policymakers and leaders in voluntary organizations must change with the evolving needs of constituents. What may have begun as paternalistic concern for disabled children must become more collaborative as patients mature, gain self-confidence, and demand socioeconomic parity. Furthermore, the primary customer in many organizations is not always well defined. The specific needs of a single organization's multiple customer groups may conflict. For example, parents of disabled children might want resources directed primarily at a cure, yet their children's primary goals might be social and employment opportunities. Although difficult, serving as both caretaker and equal partner in health care and public policy decisions must be accomplished if organizations are to keep pace with the changing needs and demands of constituents.

Decision making and implementation at all levels should routinely include people with the disorder. This includes all aspects of the work, including settings supported by the organization while not precisely overseen by it, such as research goals and objectives. Voluntary organizations should encourage clinicians, researchers, and public policymakers to use constituents' help in efforts the organization funds and supports. For example, almost half the members of the current TSA national board of directors are individuals with Tourette's syndrome.

Research Needs to Investigate Issues of Most Relevance to Patients and Their Families

The deficiency model of patient care and research posits that all patients need and/or want to be "fixed." This, however, may not be the case (see Chapter 1). For example, most current Tourette's syndrome research focuses on finding the cause of, treatment of, and cure for Tourette's syndrome. An Internet document search for Tourette's research and medication yielded 340 documents, whereas a corresponding search for Tourette's research and self-esteem yielded only two. When medication was factored out of the latter, only a single document remained. Clearly, the current research emphasis is on medicating the individual with Tourette's syndrome.

Most adults with Tourette's syndrome, however, are not significantly disabled by their symptoms and do not require medications (TSA, 1994). Of those that do require medications, only about 50% will derive any benefit from those available (Cohen, 1990). Many people with Tourette's, frustrated by medications' side effects, seek alternative therapies, for which little hard data exist to guide them. As discussed in Chapter 20, long-term use of certain medications may have severe and potentially permanent side effects. Some within the Tourette's community wonder if dependency on these medications to control tics might result in an inability to suppress them once the medications are withdrawn. It is well known that some people with Tourette's are able, over time, to learn a measure of tic suppression and management. With the need for suppressing on one's own reduced by medication, it seems plausible that some individuals on medication might find it more difficult to learn as medications are withdrawn. Further, current research protocols typically fail to include timely feedback to study participants on results. Doing so, considering the subjects' vested interests, would likely stimulate further interest and support.

A brief time spent with members of the Tourette's community reveals that, although Tourette syndrome can be a difficult condition, not everyone wants treatment, especially until they learn precisely what else they may "lose" in the bargain (Sacks, 1985). As discussed by Leckman and Cohen in Chapters 1 and 8, there may even be some latent advantages for individuals with Tourette's. Genetic disorders may indeed be selective adaptations to changing environmental conditions. For example, "the allele implicated in sickle-cell anemia . . . confers resistance to malaria on people who inherit only one copy." These people are said to have sickle-cell trait and exhibit no symptoms of sickle-cell anemia. This resistance "is believed to be the reason the sickle-cell allele has become relatively prevalent among people native to equatorial Africa, where malaria has long been endemic" (Hubbard & Ward, 1993, p. viii).

Others suggest that the question is not what (behavior) is good or bad, but to what purpose the range of variation seems to be for. Nobel Laureate Konrad Lorenz suggests that "humanity as a species in danger, and . . . many of the dangers threatening it derive from inherited norms of behavior unique to the species—those adaptations to yesterday which, today, under greatly changed circumstances of human life, may prove harmful" (in Tiger & Fox, 1989).

In the case of Tourette's syndrome, one study performed at the Yale Child Study Center revealed that adults with this condition were able to visually bisect a line with significantly greater accuracy than control subjects (Yazgan et al., 1995). Another study suggested that Tourette's may be associated with heightened creativity (Sacks, 1992). More research of this type needs to be done to explore potential benefits associated with having Tourette's.

Some adults with Tourette's syndrome believe that overemphasis on cure supersedes a more complete definition of the disorder. For example, the 4:1 ratio of males to females suggests differences in the expression of the disorder between the sexes. However, these differences remain to be identified. In addition, there is continued controversy over what is a related disorder and what is not.

Another concern is that losses could occur in the process of "curing" Tourette's syndrome (see Chapter 8). If cognitive advantages, for example, do occur in at least some people with Tourette's syndrome, it is worthy of study to pinpoint the basic mechanisms in Tourette's syndrome or successful compensatory strategies. This information would be extremely useful for education and employment. The potential benefits to the individual's self-esteem and socioeconomic success are apparent.

As reviewed in Chapter 6, relatively little research has been devoted to helping patients resolve (without medication) the more problematic aspects of social isolation, even though this has been cited as a significant problem in Tourette's (Golden, 1990). In the writer's view, it is unlikely that this social isolation is a part of TS per se; rather, it is probably the result of the complexities of adapting to the primary symptoms of Tourette's. Many of the difficulties experienced by people with disabilities are not intrinsic to their physical or mental state, but result from societal obstacles that could be removed by appropriate social or economic measures.

In his longitudinal study of hyperactive boys, Mannuzza (Mannuzza et al., 1993) found that only 4% went on to graduate school or a profession such as accounting, law, or science, compared to 21% of normal boys. In the study, 18% of the adults who had been hyperactive as boys owned small businesses, compared with only 5% in the control group, speculating that the formerly hyperactive boys might have been less capable of holding 9–5 jobs. Furthermore, there was a significant *decrease* in the rate of mental disorder as the boys aged. One wonders at the potential socioeconomic benefits of hyperactivity in this regard, and the implication that, at least in some cases, growing up resolves specific mental disorders associated, in these cases, with hyperactivity.

A recent example of a high school student from Connecticut illustrates the extraordinary difficulties children with tics face daily in peer relations (TSA, Inc., 1997e). Ostracized because of his severe tic symptoms, this young man's life improved dramatically through the efforts of a classmate, whose research project led to her impassioned efforts to help. The result was a complete turnaround in the boy's relations with his peers, his self-esteem, and the other students' understanding of Tourette's. This inspiring story, subsequently published in the *Hartford Courant* (Hamilton, 1997) and aired on a national television talk show, demonstrates how a single, caring person can make a substantial difference in the potential outcome of another's life. It also illuminates the potential of intervention by those with greater resources than one determined, impassioned youth.

People Diagnosed with Disorders May Not Always Be Willing or Able to Provide Useful Information or Advocate for Themselves

Given the often limited ability of children to articulate their thoughts and feelings, it's little wonder their opinions may not be routinely sought. Many clinicians, educators, and parents attempt to include young patients in treatment decisions. Anecdotal information, however, obtained from people in an online Tourette's support group (Alt.support.tourette, 1997) suggests that the pressure to medicate is intense, and children are not always encouraged to participate in making the decision. The representative comments below suggest that some children (a) would choose not to medicate at all if given the choice; (b) would like to be more involved in deciding what specifically to treat; and (c) have insights into their own needs that might not be immediately apparent to adults around them. Online comments by an attorney highlighted his thwarted efforts to get a state social service agency to release a child from foster care into the custody of the mother. The agency claimed that tics developed as a result of the child's extreme "frustration and anxiety," and insisted that the child be medicated with clonidine and Mellaril, against the wishes of the child and the recommendations of a psychologist, whose independent evaluation suggested that the child's anxiety would be relieved not by medication but by discharging the child from foster care. Representative comments follow:

1. "Last night we decided to increase [my 12-year-old's] medication. . . . She . . . was quite angry with me . . . thought it should have been her decision. . . . I am going to try and work with her more carefully . . . it is sometimes a hard one to call, when parent rule comes first."
2. "My 12-year-old chose at 8 years to tic instead of medicate because she didn't want to deal with the side effects . . . especially gaining weight."
3. "My daughter has been . . . part of her treatment since she was 8. The Dr. wanted her on Ritalin, we didn't because it caused more tics. . . . We asked her which was better, to be able to pay attention better . . . or have attention problems, but less tics. She chose to keep the Ritalin, and tics. Her grades were very important to her."
4. "My feelings on the need to medicate have changed as my son grew older. From the beginning . . . I was eager to try almost anything, not really focusing on the potential side effects. But the side effects were numerous. . . . My research leads me to the conclusion that it is a very fine line . . . in order to weigh the medication benefits against the side effects . . . once the decision is made, the daily struggle continues with questioning whether or not I made the right choice for my child."

5. "The pressure placed on parents to medicate children by doctors, teachers, case managers, family friends, relatives and occasionally total strangers is horrid. When a parent is in the grief process [a recent diagnosis], it is easy to get caught up in what the professionals are telling them. . . . [Doctors] don't have time to teach a parent how to handle tics or behaviors, so they give the kid a pill."

Clinicians also face a dilemma with parents and patients, as illustrated in the comments of one prominent clinician researcher: "It is my experience that many children and families are desperate for anything that could reduce the tics. Our efforts to see families through waxing periods of tics without meds is often difficult as they simply want relief, not an 'education' about Tourette's syndrome and tics."

Parents, educators, and clinicians must take adequate steps to ensure useful feedback from all patients, including children, whenever possible. It appears that medications are sometimes used as a means of social control (Kleinman, 1988) in the classroom and elsewhere, with medication decisions made by everyone but the patient. This dilemma is exacerbated by the introduction of new medications with different side effects and outcomes. Parents and children must work as partners with professionals involved in their health, education, and welfare. It is imperative that children and adults with Tourette's syndrome not be overlooked for the valuable insights they may provide.

FUTURE PROSPECTS AND THE NEED FOR PERSEVERANCE

Given the difficult history many adults with Tourette's syndrome have experienced, requests for help by institutional policymakers may not be initially successful. Individuals will need to be reassured that (a) their input will be used to help, and not further hinder, others with education, employment, and social issues; (b) they will be treated as equal partners in making relevant policy decisions; and (c) their time and effort will result in meaningful outcomes rather than "token representation." Most adults with TS can recite personal horror stories of trying to navigate the socioeconomic–health care gauntlet on the way to proper diagnosis, treatment, and inclusion. Some may have a jaded view of health care institutions as a result. Attempts on the parts of policymakers to seek their advice after having, albeit unwittingly, contributed to their problems, may be received with suspicion and even outright hostility. This should not deter policymakers from attempting to gain the trust and support of those whom their decisions will most affect. Furthermore, both children and adults with disorders such as Tourette's that persist over the life span should be invited to participate in decisions affecting their health and welfare as symptoms and needs evolve over time.

Stephen Hawking, the physicist and author of *A Brief History of Time* (1988), severely disabled by amyotrophic lateral sclerosis, has said that, owing to a career involving primarily mental work and unfailing support from family and colleagues, "My disability hasn't been a serious handicap" (Gilkerson, as cited in Hubbard, 1988). Hawking's case is a good example of an individual's willingness to prevail over extraordinary obstacles. One wonders at the loss had he not persisted in the face of increasing debilitation that rendered him virtually immobile and without normal speech.

People with far less disabling conditions can take heart from Hawking's perseverance. Although some may not wish to risk disappointment, they must be willing to assume further courage and responsibility to reap the benefits. They should seek out opportunities for collaboration in all aspects of decisions affecting them. In this way only will they achieve what they want most: full and equitable assimilation into the entire socioeconomic fabric of society.

SUMMARY OF CHAPTER 21

Voluntary organizations represent an effective force for social change. Health organizations and their constituents have a vested interest in the outcomes of clinical care, research, and public policy decisions. Substantial opportunity exists for productive collaboration between the constituents of voluntary organizations and institutional decision makers. The strengths brought to the table by voluntary organizations are useful in a variety of ways. The Tourette Syndrome Association, Inc., is one example of the effectiveness of this approach. The evidence suggests, however, that much more needs to be done. Much is made of voluntary organizations' availability for information and treatment; more substantive participation in making policy, however, does not appear to be routine. The attitudes of leaders, constituents, and decision makers in health care and public policy must continue to evolve as needs change. A new generation of people with disabilities is making itself heard and gaining a new sense of self-respect. The enactment of legislation to ensure equitable socioeconomic parity has resulted, in part, from the efforts of these individuals. Children with disabilities and special needs are maturing, and adults are demanding socioeconomic parity. Former patients are becoming scientists, researchers, clinicians, educators, and public policy makers. The most enduring decisions will be those achieved collaboratively with policymakers who direct their health and socioeconomic fate. The power of voluntary organizations should be considered when making decisions directly affecting the lives of their constituents. Doing so is not merely charity or compliance with the law: Accessing these tremendous resources is just good business.

Yale Child Study Center Tourette's Syndrome– Obsessive-Compulsive Disorder Specialty Clinic Symptom Questionnaire

This questionnaire has been compiled by Drs. Diane B. Findley, Robert A. King, and James F. Leckman from the Yale Global Tic Severity Scale (Leckman et al., 1989); Yale-Brown Obsessive-Compulsive Scale (W. Goodman et al., 1989a; W. Goodman, Price, Rasmussen, Mazure, Delgado, et al., 1989b; Rosenfeld et al., 1991); the Tourette Syndrome and Obsessive-Compulsive Questionnaire (Cohen & Prusoff, 1980; Riddle, Leckman, & Scahill, 1988); sections of the Schedule for Tourette and Other Behavioral Disorders (Pauls & Hurst; March, 1993); the Self-Report Questionnaires (Leckman, Walker, & Cohen, 1993; Leckman, Walker et al.,1994); and the TSA Genetic Linkage Consortium's Family Self-Report Questionnaire (January, 1995).

Dear Family,

Please read this introduction first.

In this questionnaire you will be completing answers about yourself or a family member who has been referred to the Tic and Obsessive-Compulsive Disorders Clinic at Yale. Many of the questions concern tics, obsessive-compulsive symptoms, and difficulties with attention and impulsivity. If you are not sure about how to answer something or are not 100% sure of an answer, we recommend that you give it your best try and then write notes about why you are not sure or why you answered a particular question the way you did (write notes anywhere: in the margins, on the back of pages, or on an attached page). Do not worry about whether there are right or wrong answers. This is not a test. Also, feel free to call our clinic for assistance in this process.

If an answer is *never* or *no,* please mark it as such, do not leave it blank. If you leave it blank, we won't know if you meant never/no, or if you happened to skip the question. In addition to checking a category in one of our checklists, please circle or underline specific words in the examples that describe the patient's behavior. By circling or underlining the words in our examples, you are providing us with valuable information about what you or your family member has experienced in his or her lifetime.

As you go through this questionnaire, you will notice that the sections are clearly titled, and that there are directions at the beginning of each. Please take the time to refresh your memory at the beginning of each section. We have included some definitions to help you with your answers.

This form should be completed by those who know the patient well. In the case of a child, it is usually best for a parent to complete the form while an adult patient may complete the form or ask a spouse for assistance. Regardless, it can be very useful to ask other family members for help. Please feel free to ask the patient for help in answering the questions. There might be questions that only he or she could answer (for example, questions about recurrent thoughts and feelings).

We recommend using a pencil. Do not feel like you have to finish all the answers in one sitting. Work at a pace that is comfortable for you. We appreciate the hard work that is involved in filling this out.

Thank you.

DEMOGRAPHICS

Patient's name: _____   Today's date: _____
mm   dd   yy

Address: _____

City: _____ State: ____ Zip Code: _____ Soc Sec #: _____

Phone number: home (_____) _____ work (_____) _____

Sex: M F   Date of birth: _____ Age: ___ years ___ months
day/month/year

Person completing this form: _____

Relationship to patient: _____

Place of birth: _____

What hand does the patient write with? Left   Right

Race: ____   Religion: ____   Living situation: ____

1=White   1=Catholic   1=Both Biological Parents
2=African-American 2=Protestant   2=Single Parent: Mother
3=Hispanic   3=Jewish   3=Single Parent: Father
4=Asian   4=Agnostic   4=Parent & Step-Parent
5=Native-American   0=Other_____   5=Adoptive Parents
6=Pacific Islander   6=Alone
0=Other _____   7=Spouse
                                            0=Other _____

Primary language spoken at home: _____

Secondary language: _____

Who lives in the same household as the patient?

Name	Sex	Age	Birth date	Relationship to patient

If the patient is a child, please answer the following:

Father's highest education received: _____

Mother's highest education received: _____

      1=less than 7 years of schooling   5=technical school
      2=junior high school   6=partial college
      3=partial high school   7=college graduate
      4=high school graduate   8=professional degree

Father's current occupation: _____

Mother's current occupation: _____

Patient's last grade completed _____

Currently in special ed? ❑ Yes   ❑ No

Name of School: _____

If the patient is an adult, please answer the following:

Highest education received: _____

Spouse's highest education received: _____

      1=less than 7 years of schooling   5=technical school
      2=junior high school   6=partial college
      3=partial high school   7=college graduate
      4=high school graduate   8=professional degree

Current occupation: _____

Spouse's current occupation: _____

TIC SYMPTOM CHECKLIST

☞ **Note:** This section asks questions about tic symptoms. If you are completing this for your child or spouse, please do so with the patient. Even if you think he or she has never had any of these symptoms, please complete the symptom checklists that follow.

A Description of Motor Tic Symptoms

Motor tics usually begin in childhood and are characterized by sudden jerks or movements, such as forceful eye blinking or a rapid head jerk to one side or the other. The same tics seem to recur in bouts during the day and are worse during periods of fatigue and/or high emotion. Many tics occur without warning and may not even be noticed by the person doing them. Others are preceded by a subtle urge that is difficult to describe—some liken it to the urge to scratch an itch. In many cases, it is possible to voluntarily hold back the tics for brief periods of time. Although any part of the body may be affected, the face, head, neck, and shoulders are the most common areas involved. Over periods of weeks to months, motor tics wax and wane and old tics may be replaced by totally new ones. Some tics may be complex in character, such as making a facial gesture or a shoulder shrug, and could be misunderstood by other people (i.e., as if you were shrugging to say "I don't know"). Complex tics can be difficult to distinguish from compulsions; however, it is unusual to see complex tics in the absence of simple ones. Often there is a tendency to explain away the tics with elaborate explanations (e.g., "I have hay fever that has persisted" even though it is not the right time of year). Tics are usually at their worst in childhood and may virtually disappear by early adulthood, so if you are completing this form for yourself, it may be helpful to talk to your parents, an older sibling, or a relative, as you answer the following questions.

When completing this questionnaire, you may want to refer to these motor tic definitions:

- **simple motor tics:** any sudden, brief, "meaningless" movements that recur in bouts (such as excessive eye blinking or squinting).

- **complex motor tics:** any sudden, stereotyped (i.e., always done in the same manner) semi-purposeful (i.e., the movement may resemble an intentional act, but is usually involuntary and not related to what is occurring at the time) movement that involves more than one muscle group. There may often be a constellation of movements such as facial grimacing together with body movements.

- **both.**

MOTOR TIC CHECKLIST

In the boxes on the left below, please mark (X) for the tics the patient

    (1) Has EVER experienced
    (2) Is CURRENTLY experiencing (during the past week)

State AGE OF ONSET (in years) if patient has had that behavior. Also, in the tic descriptions below, please underline or underline the specific tics that the patient has experienced (circle or underline the words that apply). The "ver" column should be left blank. We use it as we review your answers after our interview with you has been completed.

[In Years]

Ever	Current	Age of onset	The patient has experienced, or others have noticed, involuntary and apparently purposeless bouts of:	Ver
			Eye movements	
			eye blinking, squinting, a quick turning of the eyes, rolling of the eyes to one side, or opening eyes wide very briefly	
			eye gestures such as looking surprised or quizzical, or looking to one side for a brief period of time, as if s/he heard a noise	
			Nose, mouth, tongue movements, or facial grimacing	
			nose twitching, biting the tongue, chewing on the lip or licking the lip, lip pouting, teeth bearing, or teeth grinding	
			broadening the nostrils as if smelling something, smiling, or other gestures involving the mouth, holding funny expressions, or sticking out the tongue	
			Head jerks/movements	
			touching the shoulder with the chin or lifting the chin up	
			throwing the head back, as if to get hair out of the eyes	
			Shoulder jerks/movements	
			jerking a shoulder	
			shrugging the shoulder as if to say "I don't know"	
			Arm or hand movements	
			quickly flexing the arms or extending them, nail biting, poking with fingers, or popping knuckles	
			passing hand through the hair in a combing-like fashion, or touching objects or others, pinching, or counting with fingers for no purpose, or writing tics, such as writing over and over the same letter or word, or pulling back on the pencil while writing	

Ever	Cur-rent	Age of onset	The patient has experienced, or others have noticed, involuntary and apparently purposeless bouts of:	Ver
			Leg, foot or toe movements	
			kicking, skipping, knee-bending, flexing or extension of the ankles; shaking, stomping or tapping the foot	
			taking a step forward and two steps backward, squatting, or deep knee-bending	
			Abdominal/trunk/pelvis movements	
			tensing the abdomen, tensing the buttocks	
			Other simple motor tics	
			Please write example(s): _____	
			Other complex motor tics	
			touching	
			tapping	
			picking	
			evening-up	
			reckless behaviors	
			stimulus-dependent tics (a tic which follows, for example, hearing a particular word or phrase, seeing a specific object, smelling a particular odor). Please write example(s): _____	
			rude/obscene gestures; obscene finger/hand gestures	
			unusual postures	
			bending or gyrating, such as bending over	
			rotating or spinning on one foot	
			copying the action of another (echopraxia)	
			sudden tic-like impulsive behaviors. Please describe: _____	
			tic-like behaviors that could injure others. Please describe: _____	

Ever	Cur-rent	Age of onset	The patient has experienced, or others have noticed, involuntary and apparently purposeless bouts of:	Ver
			self-injurious tic-like behavior(s). Please describe: _____ _____ _____ _____	

Other involuntary and apparently purposeless motor tics (that do not fit in any previous categories).

			Please describe any other patterns or sequences of motor tic behaviors: _____ _____ _____ _____	

Motor Tics:

Age of **first** motor tics? _____ years old.

Describe **first** motor tic: _____

Was tic onset sudden or gradual?   SUDDEN   GRADUAL   (Circle one)

Age of **worst** motor tics? _____ years old.

A Description of Phonic (or Vocal) Tic Symptoms

Phonic tics usually begin in childhood, typically after motor tics have already started, but can be the first tic symptoms. They are characterized by sudden utterance of sounds such as throat clearing or sniffing. The same tics seem to recur in bouts during the day and are worse during periods of fatigue and/or stress. Many tics occur without warning and may not even be noticed by the person doing them. Others are preceded by a subtle urge that is difficult to describe (some liken it to the urge to scratch an itch). In many cases it is possible to voluntarily hold back the tics for brief periods of time. Over periods of weeks to months, phonic tics wax and wane and old tics may be replaced by totally new ones. Some tics may be complex in character, such as uttering obscenities (i.e., coprolalia), or repeating over and over again what other people have said (i.e., echolalia). Complex tics can be difficult to distinguish from compulsions; however, it is unusual to see complex tics in the absence of simple ones. Often there is a tendency to explain away the tics with elaborate explanations (e.g., "I have hay fever that has persisted" even though it is not the right time of year). Tics are usually at their worst in childhood and may virtually disappear by early adulthood, so if you are completing this form for yourself, it may be helpful to talk to your parents, an older brother or sister, or older relative, as you answer the following questions.

PHONIC TIC CHECKLIST

Simple phonic tics (utterance of fast, meaningless sounds)

[In Years]

Ever	Cur-rent	Age of onset	The patient has experienced, or others have noticed, bouts of involuntary and apparently purposeless utterance of:	Ver
			coughing	
			throat clearing	
			sniffing	
			whistling	
			animal or bird noises	
			other simple phonic tics. Please list:	

Complex phonic tics (i.e., involuntary, repetitive, purposeless utterance of words, phrases or statements that are out of context, the recurrence of which may be voluntarily suppressed only for a short period of time).

			syllables. Please list:	
			words. Please list:	
			rude or obscene words or phrases. Please list:	
			repeating what someone else said, either sounds, single words or sentences; perhaps repeating what's said on TV (echolalia)	
			repeating something the patient said over and over again (palilalia)	
			other tic-like speech problems, such as sudden changes in volume or pitch. Please describe:	
			Describe any other patterns or sequences of phonic tic behaviors:	

Phonic (Vocal) Tics:

Age of **first** vocal tics? _____ years old.

Describe **first** vocal tic: _____

Was tic onset sudden or gradual?   SUDDEN   GRADUAL   (Circle one)

Age of **worst** vocal tics? _____ years old.

A Description of Multiple Tic Symptoms

Different tics may occur at the same time, either as multiple discrete tics, or in orchestrated patterns of multiple simultaneous or sequential tics (for example, an orchestrated pattern that includes a hand shake together with an eye blink accompanied by running the hand through the hair, always occurring in the same sequence). If the patient has reported, or you have noticed, either multiple discrete tics or an orchestrated pattern of inseparable tics, or both, please try to describe them.

During the **past week,** has the patient had **multiple discrete tics** occurring at the same time or **multiple sequential tics** occurring at the same time?
                    ❏ **Yes**   ❏ **No**

If "Yes," please describe:

_____
_____
_____
_____
_____
_____
_____

Does the patient have more than one cluster of tics that occur at the same time?
                    ❏ **Yes**   ❏ **No**

Please describe any of the other tic clusters: _____

_____
_____
_____
_____
_____
_____
_____
_____

Current **Severity of Tic Symptoms**. Circle one choice for each question. Rate severity **during the past week only**.

1. **During the past week, what is the longest period the patient has gone without a *MOTOR* tic** (not counting time when sleeping)?   Ver
   0 = **Always gone without.** No evidence of motor tics.
   1 = **Almost always gone without.** Motor tics occur infrequently, often not on a daily basis. Tic-free periods last for several days at a time.
   2 = **Frequently gone without.** Motor tics are usually present on a daily basis. Bouts of tics may occur on occasion, and are not sustained for more than a few minutes at a time. Tic-free intervals last for most of the day.
   3 = **Occasionally gone without.** Motor tics are present on a daily basis. Tic-free intervals as long as 3 hours are not uncommon.
   4 = **Almost never gone without.** Motor tics are present virtually every waking hour of every day, and periods of sustained tic behaviors occur regularly. Tic-free intervals are not frequent, and may last for half an hour at a time.
   5 = **Never gone without.** Motor tics are present virtually all the time. Tic-free intervals are difficult to identify and do not last longer than 5–10 minutes at most.

2. **During the past week, what is the longest period the patient has gone without a *PHONIC* tic** (not counting time when sleeping)?   Ver
   0 = **Always gone without.** No evidence of phonic tics.
   1 = **Almost always gone without.** Phonic tics occur infrequently, often not on a daily basis. Tic-free periods last for several days at a time.
   2 = **Frequently gone without.** Phonic tics are usually present on a daily basis. Bouts of tics may occur on occasion, and are not sustained for more than a few minutes at a time. Tic-free intervals last for most of the day.
   3 = **Occasionally gone without.** Phonic tics are present on a daily basis. Tic-free intervals as long as 3 hours are not uncommon.
   4 = **Almost never gone without.** Phonic tics are present virtually every waking hour of every day, and periods of sustained tic behaviors occur regularly. Tic-free intervals are not frequent, and may last for half an hour at a time.
   5 = **Never gone without.** Phonic tics are present virtually all the time. Tic-free intervals are difficult to identify and do not last longer than 5–10 minutes at most.

3. **During the past week, how forceful were the patient's *MOTOR***
   tics? Circle the relevant description for how forceful the motor tics
   have been during the past week. For example, mild tics may not be
   visible and are typically not noticed by others because of their
   minimal intensity. On the other extreme, severe tics are extremely
   forceful and exaggerated in expression, call attention to the patient
   and may result in risk of physical injury because of their forceful
   expression. In between are tics of mild, moderate, or marked
   intensity.

   Ver

   0 =   **Absent.** No evidence of motor tics.
   1 =   **Minimal forcefulness.** Tics may not be visible to others,
          and are typically not noticed by others because of their
          minimal intensity.
   2 =   **Mild forcefulness.** Tics are not more forceful than
          comparable voluntary actions and are typically not noticed
          because of their mild intensity.
   3 =   **Moderate forcefulness.** Tics are more forceful than
          comparable voluntary actions but are not outside the range of
          normal expression for comparable voluntary actions. They
          may call attention to the patient because of their forceful
          character.
   4 =   **Marked forcefulness.** Tics are more forceful than
          comparable voluntary actions and typically have an
          "exaggerated" character. Such tics frequently call attention to
          the patient because of their forceful and exaggerated
          character.
   5 =   **Severe forcefulness.** Tics are extremely forceful and
          exaggerated in expression. These tics call attention to the
          patient and may result in risk of physical injury (accidental,
          provoked, or self-inflicted) because of their forceful
          expression.

4. **During the past week, how forceful were the patient's *PHONIC***
   tics? Circle the relevant description for how loud they are. For
   example, mild tics may not be audible and are typically not noticed
   by others because of their minimal intensity. On the other extreme,
   severe tics are extremely loud and exaggerated in expression, and
   call attention to the patient. In between are tics of mild, moderate, or
   marked intensity.

   Ver

   0 =   **Absent.** No evidence of phonic tics.
   1 =   **Minimal forcefulness.** Tics may not be audible to others,
          and are typically not heard by others because of their
          minimal intensity.
   2 =   **Mild forcefulness.** Tics are not louder than comparable
          voluntary utterances and are typically not noticed because of
          their mild intensity.

3 = **Moderate forcefulness.** Tics are louder than comparable voluntary utterances but are not outside the range of normal expression. They may call attention to the patient because of their loud character.

4 = **Marked forcefulness.** Tics are louder than comparable voluntary utterances and typically have an "exaggerated" character. Such tics frequently call attention to the patient because of their loud and exaggerated character.

5 = **Severe forcefulness.** Tics are extremely loud and exaggerated in expression. These tics nearly always call attention to the patient.

5. **During the past week**, did the patient's tics **interrupt** or **disrupt**   ———
   what he or she was trying to do? Circle one response in each   Ver
   column:

MOTOR TICS ———	PHONIC TICS ———
Ver	Ver
1 - Never	1 - Never
2 - Occasionally interrupt	2 - Occasionally interrupt
3 - Frequently interrupt	3 - Frequently interrupt
4 - Occasionally disrupt	4 - Occasionally disrupt
5 - Frequently disrupt	5 - Frequently disrupt

"Worst Ever" Severity of Tic Symptoms. At what age were the tic   ———
symptoms at their worst? _____ years   Ver

Rate the *worst* severity of symptoms the patient has ever experienced in his or her life. Circle one choice for each question.

1. **During the "worst ever" tic period in the patient's life, what was   ———
   the longest period he or she went without a *MOTOR* tic** (not   Ver
   counting time when sleeping)?
   0 = **Always gone without.** No evidence of motor tics.
   1 = **Almost always gone without.** Motor tics occur infrequently, often not on a daily basis. Tic-free periods last for several days at a time.
   2 = **Frequently gone without.** Motor tics are usually present on a daily basis. Bouts of tics may occur on occasion, and are not sustained for more than a few minutes at a time. Tic-free intervals last for most of the day.
   3 = **Occasionally gone without.** Motor tics are present on a daily basis. Tic-free intervals as long as 3 hours are not uncommon.

4 = **Almost never gone without.** Motor tics are present virtually every waking hour of every day, and periods of sustained tic behaviors occur regularly. Tic-free intervals are not frequent, and may last for half an hour at a time.

5 = **Never gone without.** Motor tics are present virtually all the time. Tic-free intervals are difficult to identify and do not last longer than 5-10 minutes at most.

2. **During the "worst ever" tic period in the patient's life, what was the longest period he or she went without a *PHONIC* tic** (not counting time when sleeping)?

    Ver _____

    0 = **Always gone without.** No evidence of phonic tics.

    1 = **Almost always gone without.** Phonic tics occur infrequently, often not on a daily basis. Tic-free periods last for several days at a time.

    2 = **Frequently gone without.** Phonic tics are usually present on a daily basis. Bouts of tics may occur on occasion, and are not sustained for more than a few minutes at a time. Tic-free intervals last for most of the day.

    3 = **Occasionally gone without.** Phonic tics are present on a daily basis. Tic-free intervals as long as 3 hours are not uncommon.

    4 = **Almost never gone without.** Phonic tics are present virtually every waking hour of every day, and periods of sustained tic behaviors occur regularly. Tic-free intervals are not frequent, and may last for half an hour at a time.

    5 = **Never gone without.** Phonic tics are present virtually all the time. Tic-free intervals are difficult to identify and do not last longer than 5-10 minutes at most.

3. **During the "worst ever" tic period in the patient's life, how forceful were his or her *MOTOR* tics?** Check the relevant

    Ver _____

    description for how forceful the motor tics have been. For example, mild tics may not be visible and are typically not noticed by others because of their minimal intensity. On the other extreme, severe tics are extremely forceful and exaggerated in expression, call attention to the patient, and may result in risk of physical injury because of their forceful expression. In between are tics of mild, moderate, or marked intensity.

    0 = **Absent.** No evidence of motor tics.

    1 = **Minimal forcefulness.** Tics may not be visible to others, and are typically not noticed by others because of their minimal intensity.

    2 = **Mild forcefulness.** Tics are not more forceful than comparable voluntary actions and are typically not noticed because of their mild intensity.

3 = **Moderate forcefulness.** Tics are more forceful than comparable voluntary actions but are not outside the range of normal expression for comparable voluntary actions. They may call attention to the patient because of their forceful character.

4 = **Marked forcefulness.** Tics are more forceful than comparable voluntary actions and typically have an "exaggerated" character. Such tics frequently call attention to the patient because of their forceful and exaggerated character.

5 = **Severe forcefulness.** Tics are extremely forceful and exaggerated in expression. These tics call attention to the patient and may result in risk of physical injury (accidental, provoked, or self-inflicted) because of their forceful expression.

4. **During the "worst ever" tic period in the patient's life, how forceful were his or her *PHONIC* tics?** Check the relevant   Ver
description for how loud they are. For example, mild tics may not be audible and are typically not noticed by others because of their minimal intensity. On the other extreme, severe tics are extremely loud and exaggerated in expression, and call attention to the patient. In between are tics of mild, moderate, or marked intensity.

0 = **Absent.** No evidence of phonic tics.

1 = **Minimal forcefulness.** Tics may not be audible to others, and are typically not heard by others because of their minimal intensity.

2 = **Mild forcefulness.** Tics are not louder than comparable voluntary utterances and are typically not noticed because of their mild intensity.

3 = **Moderate forcefulness.** Tics are louder than comparable voluntary utterances but are not outside the range of normal expression. They may call attention to the patient because of their loud character.

4 = **Marked forcefulness.** Tics are louder than comparable voluntary utterances and typically have an "exaggerated" character. Such tics frequently call attention to the patient because of their loud and exaggerated character.

5 = **Severe forcefulness.** Tics are extremely loud and exaggerated in expression. These tics almost always call attention to the patient.

5. **During the "worst ever" tic period in the patient's life**, please rate how much the tics would **interrupt** or **disrupt** what he or she was trying to do. Circle one response in each column:

MOTOR TICS		PHONIC TICS	
	Ver		Ver
1 - Never		1 - Never	
2 - Occasionally interrupt		2 - Occasionally interrupt	
3 - Frequently interrupt		3 - Frequently interrupt	
4 - Occasionally disrupt		4 - Occasionally disrupt	
5 - Frequently disrupt		5 - Frequently disrupt	

Has the patient ever been **diagnosed** as having Tourette Syndrome?

❑ Yes   ❑ No

If "Yes," by whom? _____

How old was the patient? _____

Has the patient ever taken medication for Tics and/or Tourette Syndrome?

❑ Yes   ❑ No

What were the names of those medications?

1. _____   6. _____
2. _____   7. _____
3. _____   8. _____
4. _____   9. _____
5. _____   10. _____

Do the tics occur in clusters (bouts) during the course of the day?

❑ Yes   ❑ No

Do the tics typically go through periods when they are worse and then better again (a waxing and waning course)?

❑ Yes   ❑ No

Do tics vary, with some tics disappearing and new tics taking their place over time?

❑ Yes   ❑ No

Are tics more noticeable during periods of stress or emotional excitement?

❑ Yes   ❑ No

Are tics better during periods of relaxation?

❑ Yes   ❑ No

Do tics ever occur in response to some cue in the environment - certain situations or tasks will set off tics?

❑ Yes   ❑ No

If yes, please describe: _____

Can the tics be voluntarily suppressed (held back)?

❑ **Yes**   ❑ **No**

    If yes, for how long? _____ minutes

Does the patient attempt to suppress (hold back) the tics ?

❑ **Yes**   ❑ **No**

Are the tics worse after the patient has suppressed the tics for a time?

❑ **Yes**   ❑ **No**

If someone asks the patient about specific tics, are those tics likely to appear?

❑ **Yes**   ❑ **No**

Starting with the age when the patient's tics began, rate their severity, with 1 equaling the "least severe" and 5 equaling the "most severe." Do not compare the patient to others with tics, because even if you feel that the symptoms are milder than most other individual's, we want to know what periods have been most or least severe for the patient only.

| Age | Medication for Tics | | 1 | 2 | 3 | 4 | 5 |
	No	Yes	Least severe	Mild	Moderate	Severe	Most severe
2	❏	❏	❏	❏	❏	❏	❏
3	❏	❏	❏	❏	❏	❏	❏
4	❏	❏	❏	❏	❏	❏	❏
5	❏	❏	❏	❏	❏	❏	❏
6	❏	❏	❏	❏	❏	❏	❏
7	❏	❏	❏	❏	❏	❏	❏
8	❏	❏	❏	❏	❏	❏	❏
9	❏	❏	❏	❏	❏	❏	❏
10	❏	❏	❏	❏	❏	❏	❏
11	❏	❏	❏	❏	❏	❏	❏
12	❏	❏	❏	❏	❏	❏	❏
13	❏	❏	❏	❏	❏	❏	❏
14	❏	❏	❏	❏	❏	❏	❏
15	❏	❏	❏	❏	❏	❏	❏
16	❏	❏	❏	❏	❏	❏	❏
17	❏	❏	❏	❏	❏	❏	❏
18	❏	❏	❏	❏	❏	❏	❏
19	❏	❏	❏	❏	❏	❏	❏
20	❏	❏	❏	❏	❏	❏	❏
21	❏	❏	❏	❏	❏	❏	❏
22	❏	❏	❏	❏	❏	❏	❏
23	❏	❏	❏	❏	❏	❏	❏
24	❏	❏	❏	❏	❏	❏	❏
25–30	❏	❏	❏	❏	❏	❏	❏
30–35	❏	❏	❏	❏	❏	❏	❏
40–45	❏	❏	❏	❏	❏	❏	❏
45–50	❏	❏	❏	❏	❏	❏	❏
50 & over	❏	❏	❏	❏	❏	❏	❏

FEELINGS BEFORE AND AFTER TICS

If you are completing this form for someone other than yourself, ask the patient to help answer these questions.

During the **past week**, has the patient had any sensation, mental or physical awareness ("an urge," "a feeling," "an impulse," "a need") to tic?

❑ Yes   ❑ No

Is this sensation or urge more mental than physical? Check ✔ one.

❑ Mental   ❑ Somewhere in between   ❑ Physical

Has the patient **ever** had any sensation, mental or physical awareness ("an urge," "a feeling," "an impulse," "a need") to tic?

❑ Yes   ❑ No

If "Yes," please describe this sensation or awareness: _____

_____

_____

_____

_____

_____

_____

_____

How old was the patient when first aware of these sensations? _____ years old

Does the patient ever experience a sense or a feeling of **"relief"** after having a tic?

❑ Yes   ❑ No

If "Yes," please describe this feeling:

_____

_____

_____

_____

_____

_____

_____

_____

_____

_____

During the past week, where has the patient had these sensations? Please mark the location(s) with an ✘ in the figures below. Do not mark a location unless the sensation or urge is experienced *before* having a tic in that location. Circle the ✘ if there is also a feeling of "relief" after having the tic.

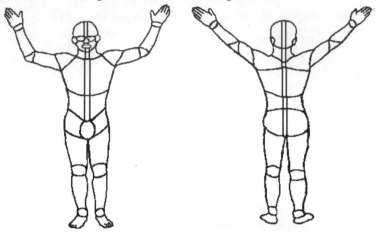

If the patient has **ever** had these sensations, where have they been located? Please mark *all* the location(s) with an ✘ on the figures below where the patient has **ever** experienced one of these sensations. Do not mark a location unless the patient has experienced either a sensation or urge *before* having a tic in that location. Circle the ✘ if a feeling of "relief" occurred after having had the tic.

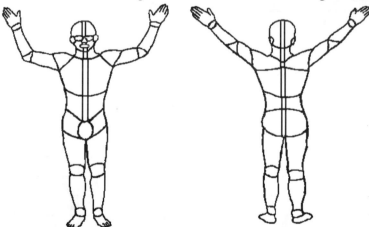

If the patient has had these sensations, **where** were they felt? Check ✔ all that apply.

❑ Muscle   ❑ Skin   ❑ Joints   ❑ Other

Please describe:

_____

_____

If the patient has had these sensations, do they help "**suppress**" the tics?

❏ Yes   ❏ No

Do medications affect the quality of the patient's pre-tic sensations or urges?

❏ Yes   ❏ No

If "Yes", please describe these effects:

_____

_____

Has medication ever increased the pre-tic sensations or urges?

❏ Yes   ❏ No

If "Yes", which medications:

_____

_____

Has medication ever decreased the pre-tic sensations or urges?

❏ Yes   ❏ No

If "Yes", which medications:

_____

_____

Are there certain tics that always occur without warning?

❏ Yes   ❏ No

If "Yes," please list: _____

_____

Does the patient consider the tics to be "**involuntary**" or "**voluntary**"? Check ✔ one.

❏ Involuntary   ❏ Mixture of voluntary & involuntary   ❏ Voluntary

OBSESSIVE COMPULSIVE SYMPTOM CHECKLIST

☞ **NOTE**: This section asks about obsessive compulsive behaviors often found associated with tics. However, even if the patient has never had any tics, **please complete the checklist that follows**.

> When completing this questionnaire, you may want to refer to the following obsessive compulsive definitions:
>
> **Obsessions** are defined as being repetitive and intrusive thoughts. Examples include a recurring concern about whether a light has been switched off or a door has been locked, and the concern continues even when the patient tries to ignore or suppress it. An example of an obsessive thought is: after hearing a tune on the radio, it keeps coming back into his or her head even when doing something else or when trying to ignore it.
>
> **Compulsions** are repetitive acts or behaviors that the patient feels he or she has to perform (e.g., checking several times that the door is locked or the light or other appliances are off).

Check ✔ only those symptoms that have bothered the patient during the **past week** or that have **ever** in the past bothered the patient. For children, parents should complete this form with the help of the child.

Past week	Ever	Age of onset	
			1. **I fear I might harm myself.** For example, fear of eating with a knife or fork, fear of handling sharp objects, fear of walking near glass windows.
			2. **I fear I might harm other people.** For example, fear of poisoning other people's food, fear of harming babies, fear of pushing someone in front of a train, fear of hurting someone's feelings, fear of being responsible by not providing assistance for some imagined catastrophe, fear of causing harm by giving wrong advice.
			3. **I have violent or horrific images in my mind.** For example, images of murders or dismembered bodies, disgusting images.
			4. **I fear that some injury or harm will befall a close family member or friend.**
			5. **I fear a separation between myself and a close family member will occur.**
			6. **I fear blurting out obscenities or insults.** For example, fear of shouting obscenities in public situations like church, fear of writing obscenities.
			7. **I fear doing something else embarrassing.** For example, fear of appearing foolish in social situations.

Past week	Ever	Age of onset	
			8. **I fear I will act on an unwanted impulse (like stabbing a friend).** For example, fear of driving car into a tree, fear of running someone over.
			9. **I fear I will steal things.** For example, fear of "cheating" cashier, fear of shoplifting inexpensive items.
			10. **I fear becoming someone else.** For example, fear of taking on the personality or behaving like someone else.
			11. **I fear that I'll harm others because I'm not careful enough (like a hit-and-run motor vehicle accident).** For example, fear of causing an accident without being aware of it.
			12. **I fear I'll be responsible for something else terrible happening (such as fire or burglary).** For example, fear of causing a fire or burglary because of not being careful in checking the house before leaving.
			13. **I am concerned or disgusted with bodily waste or secretions (like urine, feces, or saliva).** For example, fear of contracting AIDS, cancer or other diseases from public restrooms, fears of your own urine, feces, semen, or vaginal secretions.
			14. **I am concerned with dirt or germs.** For example getting germs from sitting in certain chairs, shaking hands, or touching door handles.
			15. **I am excessively concerned with environmental contaminants (like asbestos, radiation, or toxic waste).** For example, fear of being contaminated by asbestos or radon, fear of radioactive substances, fear of things associated with towns containing toxic waste sites.
			16. **I am excessively concerned with animals (like insects).** For example, fear of being contaminated by touching a dog, cat, or other animals.
			17. **I am bothered by sticky substances or residues.** For example, fear of adhesive tape and other sticky substances that may trap contaminants.
			18. **I am concerned I will get ill because of contamination.** For example, fear of getting ill as a direct result of being contaminated; beliefs about length of time until getting ill vary.
			19. **I have forbidden or perverse sexual thoughts, images, or impulses.** For example, unwanted thoughts about strangers, family, or friends.
			20. **I have sexual obsessions that involve children or incest.** For example, unwanted thoughts about sexually molesting either your own or other children.

Past week	Ever	Age of onset	
			21. **I have sexual obsessions about homosexuality.** For example, worries like "Am I a homosexual?" or "What if I suddenly become gay?" when there is no basis for these thoughts.
			22. **I have sexual obsessions about aggressive sexual behavior toward other people.** For example, unwanted images of violent sexual behavior toward adult strangers, friends, or family members.
			23. **I have obsessions about hoarding or saving things.** For example, worries about throwing unimportant things away because you might need them in the future, urges to pick up and collect useless things.
			24. **I am concerned with sacrilege and blasphemy.** For example, worries about having blasphemous thoughts, saying blasphemous things or being punished for these things.
			25. **I am excessively concerned with right or wrong (morality).** For example, worries about always doing "the right thing," worries about having told a lie or having cheated someone.
			26. **I have obsessions about symmetry or exactness.** For example, worries about papers and books being properly aligned, worries about calculations being done perfectly or handwriting being perfect.
			27. **I feel like I need to know or remember certain things.** For example, thinking you need to remember insignificant things like license plate numbers, bumper stickers or T-shirt slogans.
			28. **I fear saying certain things.** For example, fear of saying certain words because of superstitious fears, fear of saying "thirteen," fear of saying something that might be disrespectful to a dead person, fear of using words with an apostrophe (because this denotes "possession").
			29. **I fear not saying just the right thing.** For example, fear of having said the wrong thing, fear of not using the "perfect" word.
			30. **I fear losing things.** For example, worries about losing a wallet or unimportant objects like a scrap of note paper.
			31. **Intrusive (neutral) images come into my mind.** For example, random, unwanted images that come into your mind.
			32. **Intrusive nonsense sounds, words, or music come into my mind.** For example, hearing words, songs or music in your mind that you can't stop.

Past week	Ever	Age of onset	
			33. I am bothered by certain sounds or noises. For example, worries about the sounds of clocks ticking loudly, or voices in another room which may interfere with sleeping.
			34. I have lucky or unlucky numbers. For example, worries about common numbers like thirteen, having to do activities a certain "lucky" number of times, or having to start an activity only at a certain lucky hour of the day.
			35. I have colors with special significance. For example, black may be associated with death, red may be associated with blood and injury. You may avoid using objects of these colors.
			36. I have superstitious fears. For example, fear of passing a cemetery, hearse, or black cat, fear of omens associated with death.
			37. I am concerned with illness or disease. For example, worries that you have an illness like cancer, heart disease, AIDS, despite reassurance from doctors.
			38. I am excessively concerned with a part of my body or an aspect of my appearance. For example, worries that your face, ears, nose, eyes, or other part of your body is hideously ugly, despite reassurance.
			39. I have excessive or ritualized showering, bathing, tooth brushing, grooming, or toilet routines. For example, your showers, baths, and other bathroom routines may last for several hours. If the sequence of washing is interrupted, the whole process may have to be restarted.
			40. I have compulsions that involve cleaning household items or other inanimate objects. For example, excessive cleaning of faucets, toilets, floors, kitchen counters, or kitchen utensils.
			41. I do other things to prevent or remove contact with contaminants. For example, you may have family members remove insecticides, garbage, gasoline cans, raw meat, paints, varnish, drugs in the medicine cabinet, or kitty litter. If you can't avoid these things, you may wear gloves, such as when using a self-service gasoline pump.
			42. I check that I did not or will not harm others. For example, checking that you haven't hurt someone without knowing it. You may ask others for reassurance, or telephone to make sure that everything is alright.

Past week	Ever	Age of onset	
			43. **I check that I did not or will not harm myself.** For example, looking for injuries or bleeding after handling sharp or breakable objects. You may frequently go to doctors to ask for reassurance that you haven't hurt yourself.
			44. **I check that nothing terrible did happen or will happen.** For example, you may search the newspaper or listen to the radio or television for news about some catastrophe you believe you caused. You may also ask people for reassurance.
			45. **I check that I did not make mistakes.** For example, repeated checking while reading, writing, or doing simple calculations to make sure you didn't make a mistake. You can't be certain that you didn't make a mistake.
			46. **I check something related to obsessions about my body.** For example, you seek reassurance from friends or doctors that you aren't having a heart attack or getting cancer. You repeatedly take your pulse, blood pressure, or temperature. You check yourself for body odors or check your appearance in a mirror, looking for ugly features.
			47. **I re-read or re-write things.** For example, you may take hours to read a few pages in a book or to write a short letter because you get caught in a cycle of reading and re-reading. You may search for a "perfect" word or phrase, or worry that you didn't understand something you must read, or have obsessions about the shape of certain letters.
			48. **I need to repeat routine activities (like going in and out of a doorway or getting up and down from a chair).** For example, you may repeat routine activities like turning appliances on and off, combing your hair, or looking in a particular direction. You may not feel "right" unless you do these things the "right" number of times.
			49. **I have counting compulsions.** For example, you may count objects like ceiling or floor tiles, books in a book case, nails in a wall, or even grains of sand on the beach. You may also count when you repeat certain activities, like washing.
			50. **I have ordering or arranging compulsions.** For example, you may straighten paper and pens on a desktop or books in a bookcase. You may waste hours arranging things in your house in a "order," and you may become very upset if this order is disturbed.

Past week	Ever	Age of onset	
			51. **I have compulsions to hoard or collect things.** For example, you may have rooms filled with old newspapers, notes, cans, paper towels, wrappers and empty bottles—you don't throw these things away because you fear that you may one day need them. You may also pick up useless objects from the street or from garbage cans.
			52. **I have mental rituals (other than checking or counting).** For example, mental rituals are compulsions you do "in your head," like saying prayers excessively, or thinking of a "good" thought to undo a "bad" thought. These are different from obsessions because you do them intentionally to reduce anxiety or feel better.
			53. **I need to tell, ask, or confess things.** For example, you may ask other people to reassure you. You may confess to wrong behaviors you never even did. You may feel you have to tell other people certain words to feel better.
			54. **I need to touch, tap, or rub things.** For example, you may feel the urge to touch rough surfaces, like wood, or hot surfaces, like a stovetop. You may feel the urge to lightly touch other people. You might feel you have to touch an object like a telephone to prevent an illness in your family.
			55. **I take measures (other than checking) to prevent harm to myself or others, or terrible consequences.** For example, you may stay away from sharp or breakable objects. You may not handle knives or scissors, and you may stay away from fragile glass.
			56. **I have ritualized eating behaviors.** For example, you may have to arrange your food, knife, and fork in a particular order before eating. You may have to eat according to a strict ritual, or may not be able to eat until the hands of a clock are exactly on a certain time.
			57. **I have superstitious behaviors.** For example, you may not take a bus or train if its number contains an "unlucky" number like thirteen. You may not leave your house on the thirteenth of the month. You may throw away clothes you wore while passing a funeral home or cemetery.
			58. **I pull my hair out.** For example, you may pull your hair from your scalp, eyelids, eyelashes, or pubic areas. You may use your fingers or tweezers to pull your hair. You may produce bald spots on your scalp that require a wig, or pluck your eyelids or eyebrows smooth.

CURRENT SEVERITY OF OBSESSIVE-COMPULSIVE SYMPTOMS
Check ✔ one choice for each question. Rate severity during the past week only.

1. **How much of your time is occupied by obsessive thoughts?** (Or how
   frequently do the obsessive thoughts occur?)   Ver
   - ❑ 0 = **No time at all**
   - ❑ 1 = **Less than 1 hour/day;** occasional intrusion (occur no more than 5
     times a day
   - ❑ 2 = **1 to 3 hours/day;** frequent intrusion (occur more than 8 times a day,
     but most hours of the day are free of obsessions)
   - ❑ 3 = **More than 3 and up to 8 hours/day;** very frequent intrusion (occur
     more than 8 times a day and occur during most hours of the day)
   - ❑ 4 = **More than 8 hours/day;** near constant intrusion (too numerous to
     count and an hour rarely passes without several obsessions occurring)
2. **How much do your obsessive thoughts interfere with your social or work
   (or role) functioning?** (Is there anything you can't do because of them? If   Ver
   you are currently not working, how much would your performance be affected
   if you were employed?)
   - ❑ 0 = **No interference**
   - ❑ 1 = **Mild, slight interference** with social or occupational activities, but
     overall performance not impaired
   - ❑ 2 = **Moderate, definite interference** with social or occupational
     performance but still manageable
   - ❑ 3 = **Severe interference,** causes substantial impairment in social or
     occupational performance
   - ❑ 4 = **Extreme, incapacitating interference**
3. **How much distress do your obsessive thoughts cause you?** (In most cases,
   distress is equated with anxiety. Only rate anxiety that seems triggered by   Ver
   obsessions, not generalized anxiety or anxiety associated with other
   symptoms.)
   - ❑ 0 = **No distress**
   - ❑ 1 = **Mild, infrequent distress;** not disturbing
   - ❑ 2 = **Moderate, frequent, and disturbing distress;** but still manageable
   - ❑ 3 = **Severe, very frequent, and very disturbing distress**
   - ❑ 4 = **Extreme, near constant, and disabling distress**
4. **How much of an effort do you make to resist the obsessive thoughts?**
   (How often do you try to disregard or turn your attention away from these   Ver
   thoughts as they enter your mind? Only rate *effort* made to resist, not your
   success or failure in actually controlling the obsessions.)
   - ❑ 0 = **I make an effort to always resist.** Active resistance is not necessary
     because symptoms are so minimal.
   - ❑ 1 = **I try to resist most of the time.**
   - ❑ 2 = **I make some effort to resist.**
   - ❑ 3 = **I yield to all obsessions without attempting to control them,** but do
     so with some resistance.
   - ❑ 4 = **I completely and willingly yield to all obsessions.**

5. **How much control do you have over your obsessive thoughts?** (How
   successful are you in stopping or diverting your obsessive thinking?)   Ver
   - ❏ 0 = **Complete control**
   - ❏ 1 = **Much control;** usually able to stop or divert obsessions with some
     effort and concentration
   - ❏ 2 = **Moderate control;** sometimes able to stop or divert obsessions
   - ❏ 3 = **Little control;** rarely successful in stopping obsessions, can only divert
     attention with difficulty
   - ❏ 4 = **No control**; obsessions experienced as completely involuntary, rarely
     able to momentarily divert thinking

6. **How much time do you spend performing compulsive behaviors?** (How
   much longer than most people does it take to complete routine activities   Ver
   because of your rituals? or How frequently do you perform compulsions?
   Count separate occurrences of compulsive behaviors, not total number of
   repetitions, e.g., if you go into the bathroom 20 different times a day to wash
   you hands 5 times very quickly, you perform compulsions 20 times a day and
   not 100 times.)
   - ❏ 0 = **No time at all**
   - ❏ 1 = **Less than 1 hour/day** spent performing compulsions, or occasional
     performance of compulsive behaviors (no more than 8 times a day)
   - ❏ 2 = **1 to 3 hours/day** spent performing compulsions or frequent
     performance of compulsive behaviors (more than 8 times a day, but
     most hours of the day are free of compulsive behaviors)
   - ❏ 3 = **More than 3 and up to 8 hours/day** spent performing compulsions, or
     very frequent performance of compulsive behaviors (occur more than 8
     times a day and compulsions performed during most hours of the day)
   - ❏ 4 = **More than 8 hours/day** spent performing compulsions, or near
     constant performance of compulsive behaviors (too numerous to count
     and an hour rarely passes without several compulsions being
     performed)

7. **How much do your compulsive behaviors interfere with your social or
   work (or role) functioning?** (Is there anything you can't do because of them?   Ver
   If currently not employed how much would your performance be affected if
   you were employed?)
   - ❏ 0 = **No interference**
   - ❏ 1 = **Mild, slight interference** with social or occupational activities, but
     overall performance not impaired
   - ❏ 2 = **Moderate, definite interference** with social or occupational
     performance but still manageable
   - ❏ 3 = **Severe interference,** causes substantial impairment in social or
     occupational performance
   - ❏ 4 = **Extreme, incapacitating interference**

8. **How would you feel if you were prevented from performing your compulsion(s)?** (How anxious do you become? How anxious do you get while performing compulsions until you are satisfied they are completed?) Ver
   - ❑ 0 = **No increase in anxiety**
   - ❑ 1 = **Mild, slight increase in anxiety** during the performance of compulsions or if compulsions are prevented
   - ❑ 2 = **Moderate, but manageable increase in anxiety** during the performance of compulsions or if compulsions are prevented
   - ❑ 3 = **Severe, prominent and very disturbing increase in anxiety** during the performance of compulsions or if compulsions are prevented
   - ❑ 4 = **Extreme, incapacitating increase in anxiety** during the performance of compulsions or if compulsions are prevented

9. **How much of an effort do you make to resist the compulsions?** (Only rate *effort* made to resist, not your *success or failure* in actually controlling the obsessions.) Ver
   - ❑ 0 = **I make an effort to always resist.** Active resistance is not necessary because symptoms are so minimal.
   - ❑ 1 = **I try to resist most of the time.**
   - ❑ 2 = **I make some effort to resist.**
   - ❑ 3 = **I yield to all compulsions without attempting to control them,** but do so with some resistance.
   - ❑ 4 = **I completely and willingly yield to all compulsions.**

10. **How strong is the drive to perform the compulsive behavior?** (How much control do you have over the compulsions?) Ver
    - ❑ 0 = **Complete control**
    - ❑ 1 = **Much control;** experience pressure to perform the behavior, but usually able to exercise voluntary control over it
    - ❑ 2 = **Moderate control;** experience pressure to perform behavior, but can control it only with difficulty
    - ❑ 3 = **Little control;** very strong drive to perform behavior, must be carried to completion, can only delay with difficulty
    - ❑ 4 = **No control;** drive to perform behavior experienced as completely involuntary and overpowering, rarely able to even momentarily delay activity

"WORST EVER" SEVERITY OF OBSESSIVE COMPULSIVE

SYMPTOMS Check ✔ one choice for each question. Rate the worst severity of symptoms the patient has ever experienced in his/her life.

1. **How much of your time is occupied by obsessive thoughts?** (Or how
   frequently do the obsessive thoughts occur?)
   - ❏ 0 = **No time at all**
   - ❏ 1 = **Less than 1 hour/day;** occasional intrusion (occur no more than 5
     times a day
   - ❏ 2 = **1 to 3 hours/day;** frequent intrusion (occur more than 8 times a day,
     but most hours of the day are free of obsessions)
   - ❏ 3 = **More than 3 and up to 8 hours/day;** very frequent intrusion (occur
     more than 8 times a day and occur during most hours of the day)
   - ❏ 4 = **More than 8 hours/day**; near constant intrusion (too numerous to
     count and an hour rarely passes without several obsessions occurring)

   _____
   Ver

2. **How much do your obsessive thoughts interfere with your social or work
   (or role) functioning?** (Is there anything you can't do because of them? If
   you are currently not working, how much would your performance be affected
   if you were employed?)
   - ❏ 0 = **No interference**
   - ❏ 1 = **Mild, slight interference** with social or occupational activities, but
     overall performance not impaired
   - ❏ 2 = **Moderate, definite interference** with social or occupational
     performance but still manageable
   - ❏ 3 = **Severe interference,** causes substantial impairment in social or
     occupational performance
   - ❏ 4 = **Extreme, incapacitating interference**

   _____
   Ver

3. **How much distress do your obsessive thoughts cause you?** (In most cases,
   distress is equated with anxiety. Only rate anxiety that seems triggered by
   obsessions, not generalized anxiety or anxiety associated with other
   symptoms.)
   - ❏ 0 = **No distress**
   - ❏ 1 = **Mild, infrequent distress;** not disturbing
   - ❏ 2 = **Moderate, frequent, and disturbing distress;** but still manageable
   - ❏ 3 = **Severe, very frequent, and very disturbing distress**
   - ❏ 4 = **Extreme, near constant, and disabling distress**

   _____
   Ver

4. **How much of an effort do you make to resist the obsessive thoughts?**
   (How often do you try to disregard or turn your attention away from these
   thoughts as they enter your mind? Only rate _effort_ made to resist, not your
   success or failure in actually controlling the obsessions.)
   - ❏ 0 = **I make an effort to always resist.** Active resistance is not necessary
     because symptoms are so minimal.
   - ❏ 1 = **I try to resist most of the time.**
   - ❏ 2 = **I make some effort to resist.**
   - ❏ 3 = **I yield to all obsessions without attempting to control them,** but do
     so with some resistance.
   - ❏ 4 = **I completely and willingly yield to all obsessions.**

   _____
   Ver

5. **How much control do you have over your obsessive thoughts?** (How
   successful are you in stopping or diverting your obsessive thinking?)

   ❑ 0 = **Complete control**
   ❑ 1 = **Much control;** usually able to stop or divert obsessions with some
       effort and concentration
   ❑ 2 = **Moderate control;** sometimes able to stop or divert obsessions
   ❑ 3 = **Little control;** rarely successful in stopping obsessions, can only divert
       attention with difficulty
   ❑ 4 = **No control**; obsessions experienced as completely involuntary, rarely
       able to momentarily divert thinking

6. **How much time do you spend performing compulsive behaviors?** (How
   much longer than most people does it take to complete routine activities
   because of your rituals? or How frequently do you perform compulsions?
   Count separate occurrences of compulsive behaviors, not total number of
   repetitions, e.g., if you go into the bathroom 20 different times a day to wash
   you hands 5 times very quickly, you perform compulsions 20 times a day and
   not 100 times.)

   ❑ 0 = **No time at all**
   ❑ 1 = **Less than 1 hour/day** spent performing compulsions, or occasional
       performance of compulsive behaviors (no more than 8 times a day)
   ❑ 2 = **1 to 3 hours/day** spent performing compulsions or frequent
       performance of compulsive behaviors (more than 8 times a day, but
       most hours of the day are free of compulsive behaviors)
   ❑ 3 = **More than 3 and up to 8 hours/day** spent performing compulsions, or
       very frequent performance of compulsive behaviors (occur more than 8
       times a day and compulsions performed during most hours of the day)
   ❑ 4 = **More than 8 hours/day** spent performing compulsions, or near
       constant performance of compulsive behaviors (too numerous to count
       and an hour rarely passes without several compulsions being
       performed)

7. **How much do your compulsive behaviors interfere with your social or
   work (or role) functioning?** (Is there anything you can't do because of them?
   If currently not employed how much would your performance be affected if
   you were employed?)

   ❑ 0 = **No interference**
   ❑ 1 = **Mild, slight interference** with social or occupational activities, but
       overall performance not impaired
   ❑ 2 = **Moderate, definite interference** with social or occupational
       performance but still manageable
   ❑ 3 = **Severe interference,** causes substantial impairment in social or
       occupational performance
   ❑ 4 = **Extreme, incapacitating interference**

8. **How would you feel if you were prevented from performing your compulsion(s)?** (How anxious do you become? How anxious do you get while performing compulsions until you are satisfied they are completed?)
   _____
   Ver
   - ❑ 0 = **No increase in anxiety**
   - ❑ 1 = **Mild, slight increase in anxiety** during the performance of compulsions or if compulsions are prevented
   - ❑ 2 = **Moderate, but manageable increase in anxiety** during the performance of compulsions or if compulsions are prevented
   - ❑ 3 = **Severe, prominent and very disturbing increase in anxiety** during the performance of compulsions or if compulsions are prevented
   - ❑ 4 = **Extreme, incapacitating increase in anxiety** during the performance of compulsions or if compulsions are prevented

9. **How much of an effort do you make to resist the compulsions?** (Only rate _effort_ made to resist, not your _success or failure_ in actually controlling the obsessions.)
   _____
   Ver
   - ❑ 0 = **I make an effort to always resist.** Active resistance is not necessary because symptoms are so minimal.
   - ❑ 1 = **I try to resist most of the time.**
   - ❑ 2 = **I make some effort to resist.**
   - ❑ 3 = **I yield to all compulsions without attempting to control them,** but do so with some resistance.
   - ❑ 4 = **I completely and willingly yield to all compulsions.**

10. **How strong is the drive to perform the compulsive behavior?** (How much control do you have over the compulsions?)
    _____
    Ver
    - ❑ 0 = **Complete control**
    - ❑ 1 = **Much control;** experience pressure to perform the behavior, but usually able to exercise voluntary control over it
    - ❑ 2 = **Moderate control;** experience pressure to perform behavior, but can control it only with difficulty
    - ❑ 3 = **Little control;** very strong drive to perform behavior, must be carried to completion, can only delay with difficulty
    - ❑ 4 = **No control;** drive to perform behavior experienced as completely involuntary and overpowering, rarely able to even momentarily delay activity

At what **age** did you first have **obsessive** thoughts? _____ years old

At what **age** did you first have **compulsive** actions? _____ years old

At what **age** did you have your **worst ever** obsessive-compulsive symptoms?
_____ years old

Have you ever been diagnosed as having Obsessive-Compulsive Disorder?
If "Yes," by whom? _____
How old were you? _____ years old

What treatments, if any, have you received for obsessions or compulsions?
Please describe. _____
_____
_____

Starting with the age when the patient's obsessive-compulsive symptoms began, rate their severity, with 1 equaling the "least severe" and 5 equaling the "most severe." Do not compare the patient to others with obsessive-compulsive disorder, because even if you feel that the symptoms are milder than most other individuals', we want to know what periods have been most or least severe for the patient only.

| Age | Medication for OCD | | 1 | 2 | 3 | 4 | 5 |
---	No	Yes	Least severe	Mild	Moderate	Severe	Most severe
2	❑	❑	❑	❑	❑	❑	❑
3	❑	❑	❑	❑	❑	❑	❑
4	❑	❑	❑	❑	❑	❑	❑
5	❑	❑	❑	❑	❑	❑	❑
6	❑	❑	❑	❑	❑	❑	❑
7	❑	❑	❑	❑	❑	❑	❑
8	❑	❑	❑	❑	❑	❑	❑
9	❑	❑	❑	❑	❑	❑	❑
10	❑	❑	❑	❑	❑	❑	❑
11	❑	❑	❑	❑	❑	❑	❑
12	❑	❑	❑	❑	❑	❑	❑
13	❑	❑	❑	❑	❑	❑	❑
14	❑	❑	❑	❑	❑	❑	❑
15	❑	❑	❑	❑	❑	❑	❑
16	❑	❑	❑	❑	❑	❑	❑
17	❑	❑	❑	❑	❑	❑	❑
18	❑	❑	❑	❑	❑	❑	❑
19	❑	❑	❑	❑	❑	❑	❑
20	❑	❑	❑	❑	❑	❑	❑
21	❑	❑	❑	❑	❑	❑	❑
22	❑	❑	❑	❑	❑	❑	❑
23	❑	❑	❑	❑	❑	❑	❑
24	❑	❑	❑	❑	❑	❑	❑
25–30	❑	❑	❑	❑	❑	❑	❑
30–35	❑	❑	❑	❑	❑	❑	❑
40–45	❑	❑	❑	❑	❑	❑	❑
45–50	❑	❑	❑	❑	❑	❑	❑
50 & over	❑	❑	❑	❑	❑	❑	❑

During the past week, have you been aware of a need to perform compulsive acts until they are "just right"? (For example, do you need to repeat a compulsive act like checking a door or washing your hands until it "feels just right"? Other examples might include arranging objects until they "look or feel just right" or needing to repeat words or phrases until they "sound just right."

        ❏ Yes   ❏ No

Is this awareness more mental than physical? Check ✔ one.

      ❏ Mental   ❏ Somewhere in between   ❏ Physical

Have you **ever** been aware of a need to perform compulsions until they are "just right"?

        ❏ Yes   ❏ No

If "Yes," please describe this awareness in your own words: _____

_____

_____

_____

_____

How **old** were you when you **first became aware** of this need to perform compulsions until they were "just right"? _____ years old

Do perceptions (how things feel, sound, or look) ever play a role in this experience of needing to perform compulsions until they are "just right"? Check ✔ all that apply.

      ❏ How things feel   ❏ How things look   ❏ How things sound

Please describe how these perceptions relate to the "just right" feeling: _____

_____

_____

_____

_____

When do you first become aware of this need for things to be "just right"? Check ✔ all that apply.

    ❏ Before I start to do compulsions
    ❏ At the same time that I start to do compulsions
    ❏ During compulsions

How often are you able to do compulsions completely so they are "just right"? Check ✔ the best response.

      ❏ Frequently   ❏ Occasionally   ❏ Hardly ever   ❏ Never

How do you know when to **stop** performing compulsive actions? Please describe.

_____

_____

_____

_____

_____

ENVIRONMENTAL EFFECTS ON TIC AND OBSESSIVE-COMPULSIVE (OC) SYMPTOMS

At present, are the patient's symptoms affected (for better or worse)?

	No effect	Increases symptoms		Decrease symptoms		N/A
		Tics	OC	Tics	OC	
By alcohol						
By coffee						
By cigarettes						
By vitamin supplements						
By mineral supplements						
By certain kinds of foods						
By special diets						
By illness with fever						
By illness without fever						
By physical trauma (like serious accident)						
By emotional trauma (like death of a loved one)						
During menstruation						
By hot weather						
By cold weather						
By living away from home						
When sleeping						
When participating in sports						
When fatigued						
When eating						
At the doctor's office						

	No effect	Increases symptoms		Decreases symptoms		N/A
		Tics	OC	Tics	OC	
When alone						
When upset or anxious						
At social gatherings						
When studying for exams						
When reading for pleasure						
When talking to a friend						
When listening to someone else talk						
When watching TV						
When in quiet places (like the library)						
Other						

FAMILY HISTORY

Please read these instructions carefully. The following questions will help in determining whether similar symptoms run in your family.

1. Please list all relatives, *living or dead,* in each category. Be sure to put down the present age or approximate age of each relative listed. If the person has died, put down the *age of death and circle the age* so that we will know that this person has died.
2. When we ask if a person had symptoms, we wish to know if he or she *ever* did. Knowing about your relatives who had symptoms as a child and outgrew them is very important to us.
3. If you are not sure of the complete information concerning a relative, ask other family members for help. If you are not able to obtain this information from other sources, then check the "Don't Know" column.

Have any of these relatives of the patient ever had Tic or Obsessive-Compulsive (OC) Symptoms?

	No	Tics	OC	Age	Describe symptoms
1. Your spouse					
2. Your father					
Father's brother					
Father's brother					
Father's sister					
Father's sister					
3. Your mother					
Mother's brother					
Mother's brother					

	No	Tics	OC	Age	Describe symptoms
Mother's sister					
Mother's sister					
4. Your brother					
Your brother					
5. Your sister					
Your sister					
6. Your half-brother					
Your half-brother					
7. Your half-sister					
Your half-sister					
8. Your child					
Your child					
Your child					
Your child					
9. Other relatives (Specify whether maternal or paternal side)					

To the best of your knowledge, did any of the patient's relatives or ancestors ever have any of the following disorders?

	No	Don't know	Specify which relative
ADHD or Minimal Brain Dysfunction			
Rheumatic fever			
Rheumatic heart disease			
Movement disorder (chorea, dystonia, Parkinson)			
Epilepsy			
Other seizures			
Mental retardation			
Schizophrenia			
Depression			
Autism			
Phobias			
Panic attacks			
Hair pulling			

MEDICATION HISTORY

Has the patient ever been treated with any of these medications?
❑ Yes   ❑ No

If yes, please complete information in the table below. Use the following scale to indicate the benefit obtained from the medication.

Benefit Rating Scale: 0=Worsened, 1=Improved, 4=Unchanged, 9=Uncertain

Side Effects: 0=None, 1=Mild (easily tolerated), 2=Moderate, 3=Severe (could not continue to take drug)

Medications	No	Yes	Dose	Start date	Stop date	Reason drug was given	Benefit (scale above)	Side effects
Amitriptyline (Elavil)								
Bupropion (Wellbutrin)								
Clomipramine (Anafranil)								
Desipramine (Norpramin)								
Fluoxetine (Prozac)								
Fluvoxamine (Luvox)								
Imipramine (Tofranil)								
Nortriptyline (Pamelor)								
Paroxetine (Paxil)								
Sertraline (Zoloft)								
Buspirone (Buspar)								
Clonazepam (Klonopin)								
Lorazepam (Ativan)								
Benztropine (Cogentin)								
Diphenhydramine (Benadryl)								
Clozapine (Clozaril)								
Fluphenazine (Prolixin)								

Medications	No	Yes	Dose	Start date	Stop date	Reason drug was given	Benefit (scale above)	Side effects
Haloperidol (**Haldol**)								
Pimozide (**Orap**)								
Thioridazine (**Mellaril**)								
Thiothixene (**Navane**)								
Risperidone (**Risperdal**)								
Lithium								
Carbamazopine (**Tegretol**)								
Valproate (**Depakote**)								
Amphetamine (**Dexedrine**)								
Methylphenidate (**Ritalin**)								
Pemoline (**Cylert**)								
Clonidine (**Catapres**)								
Hydroxyzine (**Atarax**)								
Naltrexone								
Dilantin (**Phenytoin**)								
Guanfacine (**Tenex**)								
Other:								
Other:								
Other:								
Other:								
Other:								
Other:								
Other:								
Other:								
Other:								
Other:								
Other:								
Other:								
Other:								

APPENDIX 2

Yale Child Study Center Tourette's Syndrome– Obsessive-Compulsive Disorder Specialty Clinic Schedule for Risk and Protective Factors in Early Development

This questionnaire is a modified version of one developed by Drs. John Walkup and James Leckman (1988) and revised by Drs. Bradley Peterson and James Leckman (1993), Yale Child Study Center.

INTRODUCTION

This questionnaire consists of a series of questions about events that may have occurred in the early years of your child/children.

You will be asked for details of your pregnancy and the birth and early development of your child. In addition, you will be asked about significant life events that may have occurred during the pregnancy. You may find it helpful to consult a baby book or other records about the child's birth and early development. Thank you for taking the time to answer these questions.

Date of questionnaire completion: _____
                                       mm dd yy

Child's or young adult's name: _____

Address: _____
                        Street

_____
              City   State   Zip Code

Telephone: (   )_____

Name of person completing questionnaire: (preferably the mother)

_____

Address: _____
                        Street

_____
              City   State   Zip Code

Telephone: (   )_____

PREGNANCY

Please answer the following questions about events that may have occurred from the time your child was conceived up to the time she/he was born. If the referred individual is an adult, please contact your parents to complete as much of this form as possible.

1. How old was the child's mother when she became pregnant? ____ years

2. How old was the child's father when the mother became pregnant? ___ years

3. Were there any pregnancies prior to this one? ❑ Yes   ❑ No

4. If yes, how many? ___

How many of these pregnancies were: ___ miscarriages ___ live births ___ stillbirths ___ therapeutic abortions (initiated by a physician)

5. Length of time (in months) between the delivery of this child and the previous child: ___ months

6. Were there any special circumstances/problems involved in getting or remaining pregnant with this child?

	Yes	No
(a) Any problem in previous pregnancy	❑	❑
(b) Infertility	❑	❑
(c) Need for medication or special medical procedure to initiate or continue pregnancy	❑	❑
(d) Unplanned	❑	❑
(e) Pre-existing medical problem	❑	❑
(f) Other	❑	❑

If **Yes** to any of the above, please explain in detail.

_____

_____

_____

_____

7. During this pregnancy were there any medical problems or concerns that you recall?

_____

_____

_____

8. Did any of the following specific problems occur in the child's mother during the pregnancy? If the answer is **Yes,** please ✔ the appropriate box for the month/months in which it occurred.

	Yes	No	Don't know	1–3 mo.	4–6 mo.	7–mo. delivery
(a) Complications of a pre-existing medical problem (e.g., high blood sugar, high blood pressure, lung or heart disease)	❑	❑	❑	❑	❑	❑
(b) Illness or infections (e.g., German measles, urinary infection, genital herpes)	❑	❑	❑	❑	❑	❑
(c) Injuries to the mother's head	❑	❑	❑	❑	❑	❑
(d) Injuries to the mother's abdomen	❑	❑	❑	❑	❑	❑

	Yes	No	Don't know	1–3 mo.	4–6 mo.	7-mo. delivery
(e) Complications of pregnancy:						
(1) excess weight gain (total amount of weight gained: ____lbs.)	❑	❑	❑	❑	❑	❑
(2) inadequate weight gain (total amount of weight gained: ___ lbs.)	❑	❑	❑	❑	❑	❑
(3) severe nausea/vomiting	❑	❑	❑	❑	❑	❑
(4) severe anemia (low blood count)	❑	❑	❑	❑	❑	❑
(5) elevated blood sugar	❑	❑	❑	❑	❑	❑
(6) child born before 38 weeks	❑	❑	❑	❑	❑	❑
(7) child born after 42 weeks	❑	❑	❑	❑	❑	❑
(8) vaginal bleeding	❑	❑	❑	❑	❑	❑
(9) elevated blood pressure	❑	❑	❑	❑	❑	❑
(10) protein in urine	❑	❑	❑	❑	❑	❑
(11) swelling of face, hands & legs	❑	❑	❑	❑	❑	❑
(12) convulsions/seizures	❑	❑	❑	❑	❑	❑
(13) a diagnosis of toxemia	❑	❑	❑	❑	❑	❑
(14) placenta in the way of baby being born (placenta previa)	❑	❑	❑	❑	❑	❑
(15) placenta separated from uterus too early (abruptio placenta)	❑	❑	❑	❑	❑	❑
(16) incompatible blood (Rh factor)	❑	❑	❑	❑	❑	❑
(17) other	❑	❑	❑	❑	❑	❑

9. If **Yes** to any of the above, please explain in detail.

_____

_____

_____

10. Now focus on your experiences with **nausea** and/or **vomiting** during your pregnancy. Check ✔ the appropriate boxes in the table below.

(a)	Number of times per day		
	Occasionally	Frequently	Almost all the time
1st to 3rd Months:			
nausea alone	❑	❑	❑
nausea and vomiting	❑	❑	❑
4th to 6th Months:			
nausea alone	❑	❑	❑
nausea and vomiting	❑	❑	❑
7th Month to delivery:			
nausea alone	❑	❑	❑
nausea and vomiting	❑	❑	❑

(b) Did you lose weight during the above periods of nausea/vomiting?

❑ Yes   ❑ No

If **Yes,** please give details below.

_____

_____

(c) Were you advised to take medication for nausea or vomiting?

❑ Yes   ❑ No

If **Yes**, please complete the chart below.

Medications	Dose per day	How often did you actually take the medication?	During which months of the pregnancy did you take it?
1.			
2.			
3.			
4.			

11. Did the doctor feel the pregnancy was made complicated by a pre-existing condition? If **Yes:**

(a) What was the condition? _____

(b) How severe was the condition? ❑ life threatening   ❑ serious   ❑ mild

(c) How were you treated? _____

_____

(d) When in the pregnancy did you receive the treatment, and how long did it last? _____

_____

12. When did you start prenatal care? _____

13. How frequently did you visit the obstetrician when you were pregnant?

14. Did your doctor prescribe any medication for any of the following? If the answer is **Yes,** please ✔ and/or fill in the appropriate boxes.

	Yes	No	Medication	1–3 mo.	4–6 mo.	7-mo. delivery	Taken for how long?
(a) nausea and vomiting	❑	❑		❑	❑	❑	
(b) high blood pressure	❑	❑		❑	❑	❑	
(c) thyroid medication	❑	❑		❑	❑	❑	
(d) tranquilizer	❑	❑		❑	❑	❑	
(e) sleeping pills	❑	❑		❑	❑	❑	
(f) pain medication	❑	❑		❑	❑	❑	
(g) antibiotics	❑	❑		❑	❑	❑	
(h) antihistamines (e.g., benadryl)	❑	❑		❑	❑	❑	

	Yes	No	Medication	1–3 mo.	4–6 mo.	7-mo. delivery	Taken for how long?
(i) anti-inflammatory agents	❑	❑		❑	❑	❑	
(j) steroids (e.g., cortisone)	❑	❑		❑	❑	❑	
(k) insulin	❑	❑		❑	❑	❑	
(l) diuretics ("water pills")	❑	❑		❑	❑	❑	
(m) medication to prevent miscarriage	❑	❑		❑	❑	❑	
(n) hormones	❑	❑		❑	❑	❑	
(o) vitamins	❑	❑		❑	❑	❑	
(p) iron	❑	❑		❑	❑	❑	
(q) medication for controlling convulsions/seizures	❑	❑		❑	❑	❑	

(r) name and location of the doctor who prescribed the medication: _____

15. Did the doctor do any diagnostic tests? (X-ray, ultrasound, amniocentesis, other)

❑ Yes   ❑ No

If **Yes,** please specify what trimester:
❑ 1st–3rd mos.   ❑ 4th–6th mos.   ❑ 7th–delivery

(a) Type: _____
(b) Reason: _____
(c) Complications: _____

16. Did the doctor want you to change your activity level or life style in any way during the pregnancy? (e.g. bed rest, hospitalization, reduce caffeine, alcohol, nicotine, or other drug use)   ❑ Yes   ❑ No
(a) What was recommended? _____
(b) Reason: _____
(c) What did you do? _____

17. During the pregnancy did you. . .

	Yes	No	Occasionally	Every month	Every 2 weeks	Every week	Almost daily	Daily	1–3 mo.	4–6 mo.	7-mo. deliv.
Drink more than 3 cups coffee/tea in 24 hours?	❑	❑	❑	❑	❑	❑	❑	❑	❑	❑	❑
On average smoke more than 10 cigarettes in 24 hours?	❑	❑	❑	❑	❑	❑	❑	❑	❑	❑	❑
Drink more than 2 drinks alcohol in 24 hours?	❑	❑	❑	❑	❑	❑	❑	❑	❑	❑	❑
Smoke marijuana?	❑	❑	❑	❑	❑	❑	❑	❑	❑	❑	❑

(Frequency columns; Period of pregnancy: 1–3 mo., 4–6 mo., 7-mo. deliv.)

					Frequency				Period of pregnancy		
	Yes	No	Occasion-ally	Every month	Every 2 weeks	Every week	Almost daily	Daily	1–3 mo.	4–6 mo.	7-mo. deliv.
Use narcotic-type drugs? which type? specify:	❑	❑	❑	❑	❑	❑	❑	❑	❑	❑	❑
Use speed and/or stimulants?	❑	❑	❑	❑	❑	❑	❑	❑	❑	❑	❑
Use cocaine?	❑	❑	❑	❑	❑	❑	❑	❑	❑	❑	❑
Use any other prescription pain killers?	❑	❑	❑	❑	❑	❑	❑	❑	❑	❑	❑
Other street drugs? which type? specify:	❑	❑	❑	❑	❑	❑	❑	❑	❑	❑	❑

*A reminder: the information you provide here will be kept in strict confidence.

Up to this point, you have been asked specifically about you and your baby during pregnancy. Now you will be asked about significant **life events** that occurred to **you or your family** during this same time period.

18. Think about your pregnancy and describe the following life circumstances during that time period:

    (a) Your place of residence (where you were living at the time): _____

    _____

    (b) Your marital status (describe): _____

    _____

    (c) Your and your spouse's employment status (describe): _____

    _____

    (d) Your financial situation: _____

    _____

    (e) Your emotional support system: _____

    _____

    (f) Mental health problems: _____

    _____

19. Were there any changes with regard to **employment** for you or for any member of your family during pregnancy? If so, please indicate who made the changes and whether these changes were voluntary or involuntary and for the better or for the worse.

	Yes	No	N/A	If yes, who?	Voluntary?	Involuntary?	Better?	Worse?
(a) change in amount of work								
(1) increase	❑	❑	❑		❑	❑	❑	❑
(2) decrease	❑	❑	❑		❑	❑	❑	❑
(b) change in work schedule	❑	❑	❑		❑	❑	❑	❑
(c) change in level of responsibility	❑	❑	❑		❑	❑	❑	❑

	Yes	No	N/A	If yes, who?	Voluntary?	Involuntary?	Better?	Worse?
(d) began a new job	❏	❏	❏		❏	❏	❏	❏
(e) quit a particular job	❏	❏	❏		❏	❏	❏	❏
(f) period of unemployment	❏	❏	❏		❏	❏	❏	❏
(g) particularly stressful type of job	❏	❏	❏		❏	❏	❏	❏
(h) other (describe below)	❏	❏	❏		❏	❏	❏	❏

_____

_____

_____

_____

To what extent was your family able to cope with these events?
❏ N/A   ❏ Completely   ❏ To a great extent   ❏ Mild
❏ Only some   ❏ Not at all

How much impact did these changes/events have on the family?
❏ N/A   ❏ Completely   ❏ To a great extent   ❏ Mild
❏ Only some   ❏ Not at all

20. Were there any **financial** changes for you or a member of your family? If so, please indicate who made the changes and whether these changes were voluntary or involuntary and for the better or for the worse.

	Yes	No	N/A	If yes, who?	Voluntary?	Involuntary?	Better?	Worse?
(a) change in financial status (incl. change in source of income)	❏	❏	❏		❏	❏	❏	❏
(b) change in amount of financial obligation/ responsibility	❏	❏	❏		❏	❏	❏	❏

To what extent was your family able to cope with these events?
❏ N/A   ❏ Completely   ❏ To a great extent   ❏ Mild
❏ Only some   ❏ Not at all

How much impact did these changes/events have on the family?
❏ N/A   ❏ Completely   ❏ To a great extent   ❏ Mild
❏ Only some   ❏ Not at all

21. Were there any significant changes or problems in the **marriage** or in the **family?** If so, please indicate who made the changes and whether these changes were voluntary or involuntary and for the better or for the worse.

	Yes	No	N/A	If yes, who?	Voluntary?	Involuntary?	Better?	Worse?
(a) marital conflict	❏	❏	❏		❏	❏	❏	❏
(b) physical/sexual abuse	❏	❏	❏		❏	❏	❏	❏
(c) separation	❏	❏	❏		❏	❏	❏	❏

	Yes	No	N/A	If yes, who?	Voluntary?	Involuntary?	Better?	Worse?
(d) reconciliation	☐	☐	☐		☐	☐	☐	☐
(e) divorce	☐	☐	☐		☐	☐	☐	☐
(f) new relationship/affair	☐	☐	☐		☐	☐	☐	☐
(g) marriage	☐	☐	☐		☐	☐	☐	☐
(h) other (describe below)	☐	☐	☐		☐	☐	☐	☐

To what extent was your family able to cope with these events?
☐ N/A   ☐ Completely   ☐ To a great extent   ☐ Mild
☐ Only some   ☐ Not at all

How much impact did these changes/events have on the family?
☐ N/A   ☐ Completely   ☐ To a great extent   ☐ Mild
☐ Only some   ☐ Not at all

22. Were there any changes in the **physical** or **personal environment** for you or any other family member? If so, please indicate who made the changes and whether these changes were voluntary or involuntary and for the better or for the worse.

	Yes	No	N/A	If yes, who?	Voluntary?	Involuntary?	Better?	Worse?
(a) move to a different residence	☐	☐	☐		☐	☐	☐	☐
(b) loss of a family member (including a pet)	☐	☐	☐		☐	☐	☐	☐
(c) gain of a family member (including a pet)	☐	☐	☐		☐	☐	☐	☐
(d) change in social network	☐	☐	☐		☐	☐	☐	☐
(e) other (describe below)	☐	☐	☐		☐	☐	☐	☐

To what extent was your family able to cope with these events?
☐ N/A   ☐ Completely   ☐ To a great extent   ☐ Mild
☐ Only some   ☐ Not at all

How much impact did these changes/events have on the family?
☐ N/A   ☐ Completely   ☐ To a great extent   ☐ Mild
☐ Only some   ☐ Not at all

23. Were there any major changes in the **health** of you or any member of your family? If so, please indicate who made the changes and whether these changes were voluntary or involuntary and for the better or for the worse.

	Yes	No	N/A	If yes, who?	Voluntary?	Involuntary?	Better?	Worse?
(a) illness	❑	❑	❑		❑	❑	❑	❑
(b) injury	❑	❑	❑		❑	❑	❑	❑
(c) hospitalization	❑	❑	❑		❑	❑	❑	❑
(d) other (describe below)	❑	❑	❑		❑	❑	❑	❑

To what extent was your family able to cope with these events?
❑ N/A   ❑ Completely   ❑ To a great extent   ❑ Mild
❑ Only some   ❑ Not at all

How much impact did these changes/events have on the family?
❑ N/A   ❑ Completely   ❑ To a great extent   ❑ Mild
❑ Only some   ❑ Not at all

24. Did you or any member of your family experience any **emotional/ psychiatric** or **substance abuse** problem during the pregnancy? If so, please indicate who had the problem and whether these changes were voluntary or involuntary and for the better or for the worse.

	Yes	No	N/A	If yes, who?	Voluntary?	Involuntary?	Better?	Worse?
(a) emotional	❑	❑	❑		❑	❑	❑	❑
(b) substance abuse	❑	❑	❑		❑	❑	❑	❑

If **Yes** to emotional problem, please specify:

	Yes	No	N/A	Details
(a) anxiety	❑	❑	❑	
(b) depression	❑	❑	❑	
(c) Obsessive-Compulsive Disorder	❑	❑	❑	
(d) any treatment	❑	❑	❑	
(e) other (describe below)	❑	❑	❑	

To what extent was your family able to cope with these events?
❑ N/A   ❑ Completely   ❑ To a great extent   ❑ Mild
❑ Only some   ❑ Not at all

How much impact did these changes/events have on the family?
❑ N/A   ❑ Completely   ❑ To a great extent   ❑ Mild
❑ Only some   ❑ Not at all

25. Did you or any member of your family experience any **legal** problems? If so, please indicate who had the problem and whether these changes were voluntary or involuntary and for the better or for the worse.

	Yes	No	N/A	If yes, who?	Voluntary?	Involuntary?	Better?	Worse?
(a) civil	❑	❑	❑		❑	❑	❑	❑
(b) criminal	❑	❑	❑		❑	❑	❑	❑

To what extent was your family able to cope with these events?
  ❑ N/A   ❑ Completely   ❑ To a great extent   ❑ Mild
          ❑ Only some   ❑ Not at all

How much impact did these changes/events have on the family?
  ❑ N/A   ❑ Completely   ❑ To a great extent   ❑ Mild
          ❑ Only some   ❑ Not at all

26. Would you tell me about your **support system** during pregnancy? How helpful was (were) your:

	N/A	Not at all	Mildly	Moderately	Very	Extremely
(a) spouse	❑	❑	❑	❑	❑	❑
(b) parents	❑	❑	❑	❑	❑	❑
(c) relatives	❑	❑	❑	❑	❑	❑
(d) friends	❑	❑	❑	❑	❑	❑
(e) clergy/church	❑	❑	❑	❑	❑	❑
(f) social agencies	❑	❑	❑	❑	❑	❑
(g) other (describe below)	❑	❑	❑	❑	❑	❑

_____

_____

Please characterize the adequacy of your support system:

	Inadequate	Adequate	More than adequate
first three months	❑	❑	❑
second three months	❑	❑	❑
third three months	❑	❑	❑

Labor and Delivery

27. How long was your labor? _____ hours
   Please describe your labor: _____

   _____

28. How much time occurred between the time your membranes ruptured and your child was born? _____ hours

29. Did your membranes rupture naturally? ❑ Yes   ❑ No

30. Do you remember any special concerns or complications with the delivery of this child? ❑ Yes   ❑ No

Please explain: _____

_____

How much pain did you experience?

❑ none   ❑ hardly any pain   ❑ some pain
❑ an average amount of pain ❑ more than expected   ❑ severe pain
❑ extreme pain   ❑ extreme pain for a protracted period > 2–3 hr.

31. Did the doctor use any medication to?

	Yes	No
(a) induce labor	❑	❑
(b) slow labor	❑	❑
(c) relieve pain during labor/delivery	❑	❑
(d) other	❑	❑

If **Yes** to any of the above, describe **type of medication, dosage,** and **why** it was given. _____

_____

32. Did the doctor do any special tests during labor?

	Yes	No
(a) X-rays	❑	❑
(b) ultrasound	❑	❑
(c) fetal monitor (for heart rate of the baby)	❑	❑
(1) internal (inside the birth canal)	❑	❑
(2) external (on the mother's belly)	❑	❑
(d) any other tests	❑	❑

33. Was the delivery a vaginal delivery? ❑ Yes   ❑ No
Did the doctor intervene in any way during the vaginal delivery (like forceps)? ❑ Yes   ❑ No   ❑ Don't know
Describe: _____

_____

34. Did the doctor do a C-section? ❑ Yes   ❑ No
If **Yes:**
(a) Reason for C-section? _____
(b) Was it planned? ❑ Yes   ❑ No
(c) Was it an emergency? ❑ Yes   ❑ No
If **Yes,** please give reason. _____

_____

35. Were there any of the following?

	Yes	No
(a) prolonged labor	❑	❑
(b) unusual presentation (buttocks, face, foot presenting first)	❑	❑
(c) cord prolapse (appearance of the cord outside the birth canal with the baby still inside)	❑	❑
(d) cord around the baby's neck	❑	❑
(e) knotted cord	❑	❑

If **Yes** to any of the questions above, please explain. _____
_____
_____

36. (a) What was the child's birth weight? ____lbs.   ____oz.
    (b) What was his or her length? ____inches

37. Was the baby premature (i.e., more than 2 weeks early)? ❑ Yes   ❑ No
    How many weeks early? ____weeks

38. On the day of birth, did the child appear to be:
              ❑ Happy   ❑ Sad   ❑ Angry   ❑ Other? ____

39. Was the baby born late (i.e., more than 2 weeks late)? ❑ Yes   ❑ No
    How many weeks late? ____weeks

40. Was this a multiple pregnancy (twins, triplets, quadruplets)? ❑ Yes   ❑ No
    If **Yes,** what was the birth order? _____
    _____

41. Were there any special concerns or complications immediately after this child's birth?   ❑ Yes   ❑ No

42. Was there any concern about the baby's appearance?

	Yes	No	Don't know
(a) birth defect	❑	❑	❑
(b) blue in color	❑	❑	❑
(c) low level of activity	❑	❑	❑
(d) floppiness of muscles	❑	❑	❑
(e) decreased response to stimuli (spank)	❑	❑	❑
(f) other (please describe)			

If **Yes** to any of the above, please give details. _____
_____

43. Was there any concern about the baby's breathing/crying?

	Yes	No	Don't know
(a) delay in breathing	❑	❑	❑
(b) delay in cry	❑	❑	❑
(c) weak/abnormal cry	❑	❑	❑
(d) breathing in fluids (aspiration)	❑	❑	❑

(e) other (please describe)

44. Was there any concern that the baby was delivered in distress?

	Yes	No	Don't know
(a) dark or stained (meconium) fluid	❑	❑	❑
(b) decreased or increased fetal heart rate	❑	❑	❑

(c) other (please describe)

If **Yes** to any of the above, please give details. _____

_____

_____

_____

45. Did the doctor or nursing staff intervene in any special way immediately after the baby's birth?

	Yes	No	Don't know
(a) oxygen therapy	❑	❑	❑
(b) suctioning	❑	❑	❑
(c) medication	❑	❑	❑
(d) incubator	❑	❑	❑
(e) intensive care unit (ICU)	❑	❑	❑
(f) surgery	❑	❑	❑
(g) ventilator, blood transfusion	❑	❑	❑

(h) other (please describe)

If **Yes** to any of the above, please give details. _____

_____

_____

_____

46. Was there any particular problem that directly affected the mother's health during the delivery?

	Yes	No	Don't know
(a) blood loss	❏	❏	❏
(b) infection	❏	❏	❏
(c) complication of anesthesia	❏	❏	❏

(d) other (please describe) _____

If **Yes** to any of the above, please give details. _____

_____

_____

47. When did the child have her/his first feed?

	Yes	No	Don't know
(a) within 48 hours	❏	❏	❏
(b) more than 48 hours	❏	❏	❏

48. During the first two weeks of the child's life, were there any medical problems?

	Yes	No	Don't know
(a) thyroid problems	❏	❏	❏
(b) metabolic problems	❏	❏	❏
(c) dehydration	❏	❏	❏
(d) jaundice	❏	❏	❏
(e) low sugar	❏	❏	❏
(f) convulsions	❏	❏	❏
(g) fever	❏	❏	❏
(h) bleeding in head	❏	❏	❏
(i) problems maintaining temperature	❏	❏	❏
(j) low blood pressure	❏	❏	❏

(k) other (please describe) _____

If **Yes** to any of the above, please give details. _____

_____

_____

_____

_____

_____

_____

49. Did any problems require medical intervention, such as:

	Yes	No	Don't know
(a) special nursery care	❑	❑	❑
(b) prolonged hospital stay	❑	❑	❑
(c) medications	❑	❑	❑
(d) surgery	❑	❑	❑

(e) other (please describe) _____

If **Yes** to any of the above, please give details. _____

_____

_____

50. Did the mother develop any medical/emotional problem that interfered with her ability to care for the baby during the first two weeks?

	Yes	No	Don't know
(a) infection	❑	❑	❑
(b) bleeding	❑	❑	❑
(c) special medical care (specify: _____)	❑	❑	❑
(d) isolation from others	❑	❑	❑
(e) depression	❑	❑	❑
(f) infant feeding problem	❑	❑	❑

(g) other (please describe) _____

If **Yes** to any of the above, please give details. _____

_____

_____

51. Please summarize the mother's emotional reaction to the individual trimesters (3 month periods) of your pregnancy. Place a number (from 1 to 5) beside each 3-month period according to the following scale:

1	2	3	4	5
Very negative	Generally negative	Normal	Generally positive	Very positive

1–3 months: _____   **1–4 months:** _____   **7 mo.–delivery:** _____

Please provide any comments you may have about each of these 3-month periods: _____

_____

_____

_____

_____

52. Please summarize the mother's emotional reaction to labor and delivery. (Check one) ❏ Very negative ❏ Generally negative ❏ Normal ❏ Generally positive ❏ Very positive

Please describe: _____

_____

_____

_____

_____

53. Would you summarize the mother's reaction to the first two weeks of the child's life? (Check one) ❏ Very negative ❏ Generally negative ❏ Normal ❏ Generally positive ❏ Very positive

Please describe: _____

_____

_____

_____

_____

First Year of Child's Life

Now please focus on the **first year** of your child's life and answer the following questions:

54. Please describe your child during the *first year* of life.

	Always	Sometimes	Never
(a) happy, contented	❏	❏	❏
(b) cranky, irritable	❏	❏	❏
(c) aloof, passive	❏	❏	❏
(d) alert, active	❏	❏	❏
(e) withdrawn	❏	❏	❏
(f) easily comforted	❏	❏	❏

55. Were there any problems with:

	Always	Sometimes	Never
(a) feeding	❏	❏	❏
(b) sleeping	❏	❏	❏
(c) weight gain	❏	❏	❏
(d) growth	❏	❏	❏
(e) bowel or bladder	❏	❏	❏
(f) motor development (strength, coordination, physical skills)	❏	❏	❏
(g) health	❏	❏	❏
(h) hearing or seeing	❏	❏	❏

	Always	Sometimes	Never
(i) injury to head with loss of consciousness	❑	❑	❑
(j) surgery	❑	❑	❑
(k) convulsions/seizures	❑	❑	❑
(l) birth defects (head, face, neck, body, limbs, heart, lungs, gut)	❑	❑	❑
(m) floppiness of muscles	❑	❑	❑

If **Yes** to any of the above, please give details. _____

_____

_____

_____

56. What was your child's treatment history in the first year? (If you check **Yes,** please fill in the appropriate boxes.)

	Yes	No	Type	Reason	Child's age	Duration (weeks)	Effect
(a) medical help	❑	❑					
(b) medication	❑	❑					
(c) outpatient treatment for an illness	❑	❑					
(d) hospitalization	❑	❑					
(e) psychiatric help	❑	❑					
(f) family support	❑	❑					
(g) other	❑	❑					

If **Yes** to any of the above, please give details. _____

_____

_____

_____

57. Would you summarize the mother's emotional reaction to the first year of your child's life? (Check one) ❑ Very negative   ❑ Generally negative   ❑ Normal   ❑ Generally positive   ❑ Very positive

Please elaborate: _____

_____

_____

_____

_____

_____

_____

1–5 Years of Child's Life

Now I want you to change your focus to the period spanning the years 1–5 of your child's life (i.e., prior to going to school).

58. Would you describe your child's temperament/behavior as:

	Always	Sometimes	Never
(a) happy, contented	❑	❑	❑
(b) cranky, irritable	❑	❑	❑
(c) aloof, passive	❑	❑	❑
(d) alert, active	❑	❑	❑
(e) withdrawn, loner	❑	❑	❑
(f) sad, depressed	❑	❑	❑
(g) anxious	❑	❑	❑
(h) excessive worry	❑	❑	❑
(i) temper tantrums	❑	❑	❑
(j) had repeated, intrusive thoughts	❑	❑	❑

59. Did your child have any problems with the following? If you check **Yes,** please fill in the appropriate boxes.

	Yes	No	Age noticed	Duration
(a) speech	❑	❑		
(b) attention	❑	❑		
(c) overactivity	❑	❑		
(d) excess aggression	❑	❑		
(e) impulsivity	❑	❑		
(f) unusual fearfulness	❑	❑		
(g) inability to separate from mother or primary caretaker	❑	❑		
(h) difficulty managing behavior	❑	❑		
(i) getting along with peers	❑	❑		
(j) sleeping	❑	❑		
(k) eating	❑	❑		
(l) bowel training	❑	❑		
(m) bladder training	❑	❑		

60. How would you summarize your emotional reaction to the years 1–5 of your child's life? (Check one) ❑ Very negative   ❑ Generally negative
❑ Normal   ❑ Generally positive   ❑ Very positive

Please elaborate: _____

_____

_____

_____

_____

Pediatric History (Ages 1–18)

61. **During the ages of 1–18,** did your child have any medical problems, such as:

	Yes	No	Age of onset	Onset before tics?	Onset before OC?
(a) seizures, convulsions	❏	❏			
(b) diabetes	❏	❏			
(c) head injuries with loss of consciousness, bleeding through ear/nose, or convulsions	❏	❏			
(d) encephalitis	❏	❏			
(e) meningitis	❏	❏			
(f) high blood pressure	❏	❏			
(g) migraine headaches	❏	❏			
(h) thyroid:	❏	❏			
• overactive	❏	❏			
• underactive	❏	❏			
• enlarged	❏	❏			
(i) heart disease, other	❏	❏			
(j) arthritis	❏	❏			
(k) autoimmune disorder	❏	❏			
(l) blood disorder	❏	❏			
(m) cancer	❏	❏			
(n) hepatitis	❏	❏			
(o) kidney disease	❏	❏			
(p) liver disease	❏	❏			
(q) chicken pox	❏	❏			
(r) measles	❏	❏			
(s) mumps	❏	❏			
(t) polio	❏	❏			
(u) rubella	❏	❏			
(v) tonsillitis	❏	❏			
(w) roseola	❏	❏			
(x) whooping cough	❏	❏			
(y) tremors	❏	❏			
(z) anemia	❏	❏			
(aa) eczema	❏	❏			
(bb) gout	❏	❏			
(cc) jaundice	❏	❏			
(dd) psoriasis	❏	❏			
(ee) pneumonia	❏	❏			
(ff) low blood pressure	❏	❏			

(gg) Other (please describe)

If **Yes** to any of the above, please give details. _____

_____

_____

62. During the ages of 1–18, did your child have **ear infections?**

❑ None at all   ❑ Fewer than most children   ❑ About the same as most
❑ More than most children ❑ A lot more than most children   children

If your child had ear infections, how was it usually treated?
           ❑ Antibiotics   ❑ Decongestants

Was your child ever on these medications for as long as 3 months at a time?
         ❑ Yes (how many times? ____)   ❑ No

Were tubes put in? ❑ Yes   ❑ No

63. During the ages of 1–18, did your child have **strep infections?**
         ❑ Yes   ❑ No

If **Yes,** complete the chart below.

Age of strep infection	Treatment?	Any complications?

64. During the ages of 1–18, did your child have **rheumatic fever?**
         ❑ Yes   ❑ No

If **Yes,** complete the chart below.

Age of rheumatic fever	Treatment?	Any complications?

65. During the ages of 1–18, did your child have **asthma?**
         ❑ Yes (age of onset: ___)   ❑ No
What **asthma treatments** has your child had?
❑ pills (names) _____
❑ inhalants (names) _____
❑ steroids (names) _____

How many times has your child been to the emergency room for asthma? ___

How many times has your child been hospitalized for asthma? ___

Was your child's asthma ever life threatening? ❑ Yes   ❑ No

Does the child's family have a history of asthma? ❑ Yes   ❑ No

If **Yes,** complete the chart below.

Family member	No asthma	Mild asthma	Moderate asthma	Severe asthma
Mother	❑	❑	❑	❑
Father	❑	❑	❑	❑
Brother	❑	❑	❑	❑
Sister	❑	❑	❑	❑

66. During the ages of 1–18, did your child have **allergies?** ❑ Yes   ❑ No

If **Yes,** please list the allergies: _____

_____

_____

_____

Has your child ever received shots or other treatments for allergies?
❑ Yes   ❑ No

If **Yes,** please give details: _____

_____

67. Did you seek help for any of the above problems? ❑ Yes   ❑ No

If **Yes,** state the effect of the help on the problem by completing the chart below.

	Yes	No	Child's age	Duration	Effect
(a) medical help	❑	❑			
• medications	❑	❑			
• outpatient treatment	❑	❑			
• hospitalization	❑	❑			
(b) psychiatric help	❑	❑			
• outpatient	❑	❑			
• inpatient	❑	❑			
(c) family support	❑	❑			
• friend	❑	❑			
• family	❑	❑			
• church	❑	❑			
• social service agency	❑	❑			
• special educational facility	❑	❑			

If **Yes** to any of the above, please give details. _____

_____

68. Developmental milestones. At what age did your child:

	Months
(a) sit	
(b) walk	

(c) have a toilet–trained bladder in the
    daytime
    night time

(d) have toilet–trained bowels in the
    daytime
    night time

(e) say "mama"

(f) say "daddy"

(g) first complete a sentence

(h) Did people outside of the family understand your
    child's speech?   ❑ Yes   ❑ No

69. Generally speaking, in comparison with other children of your child's age,
how was your child's development overall? (check one)
    ❑ Average   ❑ Above average   ❑ Below average

70. Was your child involved in any preschool program? ❑ Yes   ❑ No

If **Yes,** what were the child's ages of participation? _____

What was the nature of that experience? (check one)
    ❑ Very negative   ❑ Generally negative   ❑ Normal
    ❑ Generally positive   ❑ Very positive

71. Would you say that your child's overall intelligence is
    ❑ Average   ❑ Above average   ❑ Below average

72. How would you summarize your emotional reaction to the **years 6–18** or
your child's life? (check one)
    ❑ Very negative   ❑ Generally negative   ❑ Normal
    ❑ Generally positive   ❑ Very positive

Please elaborate: _____
_____
_____
_____

73. Please tell us briefly about your son or daughter (how would you describe
them to a friend?). _____
_____
_____
_____
_____

References

Abbruzzese, M., Ferri, S., & Scarone, S. (1995). Wisconsin Card Sorting Test performance in obsessive compulsive disorder: No evidence for involvement of dorsolateral prefrontal cortex. *Psychiatry Research, 58,* 37–43.

Abidin, R. R. (1983). *Parenting stress inventory.* Charlottesville, VA: Pediatric Psychology Press.

Abikoff, H., Gittelman, R., & Klein, D. F. (1980). Classroom observation code for hyperactive children: A replication of validity. *Journal of Consulting Clinical Psychology, 48,* 555–565.

Abwender, D. A., Como, P. G., Kurlan, R., Parry, K., Fett, K., Cui, A. L., Plumb, S., & Deeley, C. (1996). School problems in Tourette's syndrome. *Archives of Neurology, 53,* 509–511.

Achenbach, T. M. (1991a). *Integrative guide for the 1991 CBCL/4-18vYSR and TRF Profiles.* Burlington: University of Vermont Press.

Achenbach, T. M. (1991b). *Manual for the child behavior checklist/4-18 and 1991 profile.* Burlington: University of Vermont Department of Psychiatry.

Achenbach, T. M. (1995). Developmental issues in assessment, taxonomy, and diagnosis of child and adolescent psychopathology. In D. Cichetti & D. J. Cohen (Eds.), *Developmental psychopathology* (Vol. 1). New York: Wiley.

Achenbach, T. M., & Edelbrock, A. (1978). The classification of child psycholopathology: A review and analysis of empirical efforts. *Psychology Bulletin, 85,* 1275–1301.

Achenbach, T. M., & Edelbrock, C. S. (1981). Behavioral problems and competencies reported by parents of normal and disturbed children aged four to sixteen. *Monographs of the Society for Research in Child Development, 46.*

Achenbach, T. M., & Edelbrock, C. S. (1983). *Manual for the child behavior checklist and revised child behavior profile.* Burlington: University of Vermont Department of Psychology.

Adler, C. H., Zimmerman, R. S., Lyons, M. K., & Brin, M. F. (1996). Perioperative use of botulinumtoxin for movement disorder-induced cervical spine disease. *Movement Disorders, 11,* 79–81.

Adler, T., & Furman, W. (1988). A model for children's relationships and peer dysfunctions. In S. W. Duck (Ed.), *Handbook of personal relationships: Theory, research, and interventions* (pp. 99–116). London: Wiley.

Agostini, E., Collette, A., Orlando, G., & Tredici, G. (1983). Apraxia in deep cerebral lesion. *Journal of Neurology, Neurosurgery and Psychiatry, 46,* 804–808.

AICPA Audit and Accounting Guide. (1996). *Not-for-profit organizations.*

Akbari, H. M., Anderson, G. M., Pollack, E. S., Chatterjee, D., Leckman, J. F., Riddle, M. A., & Cohen, D. J. (1993). Serotonin receptor binding and tissue indoles in postmortem cortex of Tourette's syndrome individuals. *Society for Neuroscience Abstracts, 19,* 838.

Albano, A. M., Marten, P. A., Holt, C. S., Heimberg, R. G., & Barlow, D. H. (1995). Cognitive-behavioral group treatment for social phobia in adolescents. A preliminary study. *Journal of Nervous Mental Disorders, 183,* 649–656.

Albin, R. L., Reiner, A., Anderson, K. D., Dure, L. S., IV, Handelin, B., Balfour, R., Whetsell, W. O., Jr., Penney, J. B., & Young, A. B. (1992). Preferential loss of striato-external pallidal projection neurons in presymptomatic Huntington's disease. *Annals of Neurology, 31,* 425–430.

Albin, R. L., Young, A. B., & Penney, J. B. (1989). The functional anatomy of basal ganglia disorders. *Trends in Neuroscience, 12,* 366–375.

Albin, R. L., Young, A. B., & Penney, J. B. (1995). The functional anatomy of basal ganglia disorders. *Trends in Neuroscience, 18,* 63–64.

Alexander, G. E., Crutcher, M., & DeLong, M. (1990). Basal ganglia-thalamo-cortical circuits: Parallel substrates for motor, oculomotor, "prefrontal," and "limbic" functions. *Progress in Brain Research, 85,* 119–146.

Alexander, G. E., & Delong, M. R. (1985). Microstimulation of the primate neostriatum: II. Somatotopic organization of striatal microexcitable zones and their relation to neuronal response properties. *Journal of Neurophysiology, 53,* 1417–1430.

Alexander, G. E., DeLong, M. R., & Strick, P. L. (1986). Parallel organization of functionally segregated circuits linking basal ganglia and cortex. *Annual Review of Neuroscience, 9,* 357–381.

Alexandris, A., & Lundell, F. W. (1968). Effect of thioridazine, amphetamine and placebo on the hyperkinetic syndrome and cognitive area in mentally deficient children. *Canadian Medical Association Journal, 98,* 92–96.

Allen, A. J., Leonard, H. L., & Swedo, S. E. (1995). Case study: New infection-triggered, auto immune subtype of pediatric OCD and Tourette's syndrome. *Journal of the American Academy of Child & Adolescent Psychiatry, 34,* 307–311.

Allen, R. P., Singer, H. S., Brown, J. E., & Salam, M. M. (1992). Sleep disorders in Tourette syndrome: A primary or unrelated problem? *Pediatric Neurology, 8,* 275–280.

Alsobrook, J. P., II. (1996). *A family and molecular genetics study of obsessive-compulsive disorder.* Doctoral thesis, Yale University, New Haven, CT.

Alsobrook, J. P., II, & Pauls, D. L. (1997). The genetics of obsessive compulsive disorder. In M. A. Jenike, L. Baer, & W. E. Minichiello (Eds.), *Obsessive-compulsive disorders: Theory and management: A guide for clinicians, patients and families* (3rd ed.). Littleton, MA: Year Book Medical.

Altemus, M., Pigott, T., Kalogeras, K. T., Demitrack, M., Dubbert, B., Murphy, D. L., & Gold, P. W. (1992). Abnormalities in the regulation of vasopressin and corticotropin releasing factor secretion in obsessive-compulsive disorder. *Archives of General Psychiatry, 49,* 9–20.

Alt.support.tourette. (1997). The Internet Newsgroup devoted to on-line support for TS.

Aman, M. G., Marks, R. E., Turbott, S. H., Wilsher, C. P., & Merry, S. N. (1991). Methylphenidate and thioridazine in the treatment of intellectually subaverage children: Effects on cognitive-motor performance. *Journal of the American Academy of Child & Adolescent Psychiatry, 30,* 816–824.

American Academy of Child & Adolescent Psychiatry. (1989). *Report of the task force on scientific affairs.* Washington, DC: Author.

American Psychiatric Association. (1968). *Diagnostic and statistical manual of mental disorders* (2nd ed.). Washington, DC: Author.

American Psychiatric Association. (1980). *Diagnostic and statistical manual of mental disorders* (3rd ed.). Washington, DC: Author.

American Psychiatric Association. (1987). *Diagnostic and statistical manual of mental disorders* (3rd ed. rev.). Washington, DC: Author.

American Psychiatric Association. (1994). *Diagnostic and statistical manual of mental disorders* (4th ed.). Washington, DC: Author.

Andersen, R. A. (1987). Inferior parietal lobule function in spatial perception and visuomotor integration. In F. Plum, V. B. Mountcastle, & S. R. Geiger (Eds.), *The handbook of physiology, Section 1: The nervous system, Vol. V. Higher functions of the brain* (pp. 483–518). Bethesda, MD: American Physiological Society.

Andersen, R. A., Brotchie, P. R., & Mazzoni, P. (1992). Evidence for the lateral intra parietal area as the parietal eye field. *Current Opinion in Neurobiology, 2,* 840–846.

Andersen, R. A., & Zipser, D. (1988). The role of the posterior parietal cortex in coordinate transformations for visual-motor integration. *Canadian Journal of Physiological Pharmacology, 66,* 488–501.

Anderson, B. J., & Steinmetz, J. E. (1994). Cerebellar and brainstem circuits involved in classical eyeblink conditioning. *Reviews in the Neurosciences, 5,* 251–73.

Anderson, G. M. (1993). Review of the role of serotonin in disruptive behavior [Editorial]. *Journal of Child and Adolescent Psychopharmacology, 3,* vii–ix.

Anderson, G. M., & Cohen, D. J. (1996). Developmental aspects of neurochemistry. In M. Lewis (Ed.), *Child and adolescent psychiatry: A comprehensive textbook* (pp. 30–39). Baltimore: Williams & Wilkins.

Anderson, G. M., Pollak, E. S., Chatterjee, D., Leckman, J. F., Riddle, M. A., & Cohen, D. J. (1992a). Postmortem analyses of brain monoamines and amino acids in Tourette's syndrome: A preliminary study of subcortical regions. *Archives of General Psychiatry, 49,* 584–586.

Anderson, G. M., Pollak, E. S., Chatterjee, D., Leckman, J. F., Riddle, M. A., & Cohen, D. J. (1992b). Postmortem analysis of subcortical monoamines and amino acids in Tourette syndrome. In T. N. Chase, A. J. Friedhoff & D. J. Cohen (Eds.), *Advances in neurology: Vol. 58. Tourette syndrome: Genetics, neurobiology and treatment* (pp. 123–133). New York: Raven Press.

Anderson, J. C., Williams, S., McGee, R., & Silva, P. A. (1987). *DSM-III* disorders in pre-adolescent children: Prevalence in a large sample from the general population. *Archives of General Psychiatry, 44,* 69–76.

Andrews, G., Stewart, G., Allen, R., & Henderson, A. S. (1990). The genetics of six neurotic disorders: A twin study. *Journal of Affective Disorders, 19,* 23–29.

Ang, A., Borison, R., Dysken, M., & Davis, J. M. (1982). Reduced excretion of MHPG in tourette's syndrome. In A. J. Friedhoff & T. N. Chase (Eds.), *Advances in neurology: Vol. 35. Gilles de la Tourette syndrome* (pp. 171–175). New York: Raven Press.

Angelini, L., Mazzucchi, A., Picciotto, F., Nardocci, N., & Broggi, G. (1980). Focal lesion of the right cingulum: A case report in a child. *Journal of Neurology, Neurosurgery and Psychiatry, 43,* 355–357.

Angold, A., Prendergast, M., Cox, A., Harrington, E., Simonoff, E., & Rutter, M. (1995). The child & adolescent psychiatric assessment (CAPA). *Psychological Medicine, 25,* 739–753.

Angst, J. (1994). The epidemiology of obsessive compulsive disorder. In E. Hollander, J. Zohar, D. Marazziti, & B. Olivier (Eds.), *Current insights in obsessive compulsive disorder* (pp. 93–104). New York: Wiley.

Aosaki, T., Graybiel, A. M., & Kimura, M. (1994). Effects of nigrostriatal dopamine on acquired neural responses in the striatum of behaving monkey. *Science, 265,* 412–415.

Aosaki, T., Kimura, M., & Graybiel, A. M. (1995). Temporal and spatial characteristics of tonically active neurons of the primate's striatum. *Journal of Neurophysiology, 73,* 1234–1252.

Apter, A., Bernhout, E., & Tyano, S. (1984). Severe obsessive compulsive disorder in adolescence: A report of eight cases. *Journal of Adolescence, 7,* 349–358.

Apter, A., Fallon, T. J., King, R. A., Ratzoni, G., Weizman, A., Leckman, J. F., Pauls, D. L., Kron, S., & Cohen, D. J. (1996). Obsessive compulsive characteristics: From symptoms to syndrome. *Journal of the American Academy of Child & Adolescent Psychiatry, 35,* 907–912.

Apter, A., Pauls, D. L., Bleich, A., Zohar, A. H., Kron, S., Ratzoni, G., Dycian, A., Kotler, M., Weizman, A., & Cohen, D. J. (1992). A population-based epidemiological study of Tourette syndrome among adolescents in Israel. In T. N. Chase, A. J. Friedhoff & D. J. Cohen (Eds.), *Advances in Neurology: Vol. 58. Tourette syndrome: Genetics, neurobiology and treatment* (pp. 61–65). New York: Raven Press.

Apter, A., Pauls, D. L., Bleich, A., Zohar, A. H., Kron, S., Ratzoni, G., Dycian, A., Kotler, M., Weizman, A., Gadot, N., & Cohen, D. J. (1993). An epidemiological study of Gilles de la Tourette's syndrome in Israel. *Archives of General Psychiatry, 50,* 734–738.

Apter, A., Ratzioni, G., King, R., Weizman, A., Iancu, I., Binder, M., & Riddle, M. A. (1994). Fluvoxamine open-label treatment of adolescent inpatients with obsessive-compulsive disorder or depression. *Journal of the American Academy of Child & Adolescent Psychiatry, 33,* 342–348.

Apter, A., Zohar, A., Ratzoni, G., King, R. A., Dycian, A., Binder, M., Weizman, A., Leckman, J. F., Pauls, D. L., Cohen, D. J., & Kron, S. (in press). An epidemiological study of anxiety disorders and some related conditions in a community based sample of adolescents. Manuscript submitted for publication.

Arkowitz, H., & Messer, S. B. (1984). *Psychoanalytic therapy and behavior therapy: Is integration possible?* New York: Plenum Press.

Arnsten, A., Cai, J. X., & Goldman-Rakic, P. S. (1988). The alpha-2 adrenergic agonist, guanfacine improves memory in aged monkeys without sedative or hypotensive side effects: Evidence for alpha-2 receptor subtypes. *Journal of Neuroscience, 8,* 4287–4298.

Arnsten, A., & Contant, T. A. (1992). Alpha-2 adrenergic agonists decrease distractibility in aged monkeys performing the delayed response task. *Psychopharmacology, 108,* 159–169.

Arnsten, A., Steere, J., & Hunt, R. (1996). The contribution of alpha 2-noradrenergic mechanisms of prefrontal cortical cognitive function. Potential significance for attention-deficit hyperactivity disorder. *Archives of General Psychiatry, 53,* 448–455.

Aronowitz, B. R., Hollander, E., DeCaria, C., Cohen, L., Saoud, J. B., Stein, D., Liebowitz, M. R., & Rosen, W. G. (1994). Neuropsychology of obsessive-compulsive disorder: Preliminary findings. *Neuropsychiatry, Neuropsychology and Behavioral Neurology, 7,* 81–86.

Arregui, A., Hollingsworth, Z., Penney, J. B., & Young, A. B. (1994). Auto radiographic evidence for increased dopamine uptake sites in striatum of hypoxic mice. *Neuroscience Letters, 167,* 195–197.

Asam, U. (1982). A follow-up study of Tourette syndrome. In A. Friedhoff & T. N. Chase (Eds.), *Advances in neurology: Vol. 35. Gilles de la Tourette syndrome* (pp. 285–286). New York: Raven Press.

Aston-Jones, G., & Bloom, F. E. (1981). Activity of norepinephrine-containing locus coeruleus neurons in behaving rats anticipates fluctuations in the sleep-waking cycle. *Journal of Neuroscience, 1,* 876–886.

Atkins, M. S., & Pelham, W. E. (1991). School-based assessment of attention deficit hyperactivity disorder. *Journal of Learning Disabilities, 24,* 197–204.

Atkins, M. S., Pelham, W. E., & Licht, M. H. (1989). The differential validity of teacher ratings of inattention/overactivity and aggression. *Journal of Abnormal Child Psychology, 17,* 423–435.

August, G. J., & Garfinkel, B. D. (1993). The nosology of attention-hyperactivity disorder. *Journal of the American Academy of Child & Adolescent Psychiatry, 32,* 155–165.

Aylward, E. H., Harris, G. J., Hoehn-Saric, R., Barta, P. E., Machlin, S. R., & Pearlson, G. D. (1996). Normal caudate nucleus in obsessive-compulsive disorder assessed by quantitative neuroimaging. *Archives of General Psychiatry, 53,* 577–584.

Azrin, N. H., & Nunn, R. G. (1973). Habit reversal: A method of eliminating nervous habits and tics. *Behavior Research and Therapy, 11,* 619–628.

Azrin, N. H., & Peterson, A. L. (1988a). Behavior therapy for Tourette's syndrome and tic disorders. In D. J. Cohen, J. F. Leckman, & R. D. Bruun (Eds.), *Tourette syndrome and tic disorders: Clinical understanding and treatment* (pp. 237–255). New York: Wiley.

Azrin, N. H., & Peterson, A. L. (1988b). Habit reversal for the treatment of Tourette syndrome. *Behavior Research and Therapy, 26,* 347–351.

Azrin, N. H., & Peterson, A. L. (1990). Treatment of Tourette syndrome by habit reversal: A waiting-list control group comparison. *Behavior Therapy, 21,* 305–318.

Bacher, N. M. (1990). Clonazepam treatment of obsessive compulsive disorder [Letter to the editor]. *Journal of Clinical Psychiatry, 51,* 168–169.

Bacon. (1994). *The advancement of learning: With a brief memoir of the author.* New York: Kessinger. (Original work published 1605)

Baer, L. (1992). Behavior therapy for obsessive-compulsive disorder and trichotillomania. Implications for Tourette syndrome. In T. N. Chase, A. J. Friedhoff & D. J. Cohen (Eds.), *Advances in neurology: Vol. 58. Tourette syndrome: Genetics, neurobiology and treatment* (pp. 333–334). New York: Raven Press.

Baer, L. (1994). Factor analysis of symptom subtypes of obsessive compulsive disorder and their relation to personality and tic disorders. *Journal of Clinical Psychiatry, 55,* 18–23.

Baer, L., Breiter, H. C., Goodman, W. K., Rasmussen, S. A., Eisen, J. L., Barr, L., Shera, D., & Jenike, M. A. (in press). Identifying subtypes in obsessive-compulsive disorder and their relationship to Tourette and tic disorder: A factor analytic study. *Journal of Abnormal Psychology.*

Baer, L., Rauch, S. L., Ballantine, H. T., Martuza, R., Cosgrove, R., Cassem, E., Giriunas, I., Manzo, P. A., Dimino, C., & Jenike, M. A. (1995). Cingulotomy for intractable obsessive-compulsive disorder. *Archives of General Psychiatry, 52,* 384–392.

Baker, G. B., Bornstein, R. A., Douglass, A. B., Carroll, A., & King, G. (1990). Urinary excretion of metabolites of norepinephrine in Tourette's syndrome. *Molecular & Chemical Neuropathology, 13,* 225–232.

Baldwin, M., Frost, L. L., & Wood, C. D. (1954). Investigation of the primate amygdala. Movements of the face and jaws. *Neurology, 4,* 596–598.

Balldin, J., Berggren, U., Eriksson, E., Lindstedt, G., & Sundkler, A. (1993). Guanfacine as an alpha-2-agonist inducer of growth hormone secretion—a comparison with clonidine. *Psychoneuroendocrinology, 18,* 45–55.

Balthazar, K. (1956). über das anatomisehe substrat der generalisierten tic-krankeit (maladie des tics, Gilles de la Tourette): Entwicklungshemmung des corpus striatum. *Arch fur Psychiatrie und Nervenkrankheiten, 195,* 531–539.

Barkley, R. A. (1977). A review of stimulant drug research with hyperactive children. *Journal of Child Psychology & Psychiatry, 18,* 137–165.

Barkley, R. A. (1981). Hyperactivity. In E. Mash & L. Terdal (Eds.), *Behavioral assessment of childhood disorders* (pp. 127–184). New York: Guilford Press.

Barkley, R. A. (1990). *Attention deficit hyperactivity disorder: A handbook for diagnosis and treatment.* New York: Guilford Press.

Barkley, R. A. (1995). *Taking charge of ADHD: The complete authoritative guide for parents.* New York: Guilford Press.

Barkley, R. A. (1997). Behavioral inhibition, sustained attention, and executive functions: Constructing a unifying theory of ADHD. *Psychological Bulletin, 121,* 65–94.

Barkley, R. A., & DuPaul, C. A. (1993). Stimulants. In J. S. Werry & M. G. Aman (Eds.), *Practitioners guide to psychoactive drugs for children and adolescents* (pp. 206–238). New York: Plenum Press.

Barkley, R. A., DuPaul, G. J., & McMurray, M. B. (1990). A comprehensive evaluation of attention deficit disorder with and without hyperactivity defined by research criteria. *Journal of Consulting and Clinical Psychology, 58,* 775–789.

Barkley, R. A., DuPaul, G. J., & McMurray, M. B. (1991). Attention deficit disorder with and without hyperactivity: Clinical response to three dose levels on methylphenidate. *Pediatrics, 87,* 519–531.

Barkley, R. A., Fischer, M., Edelbrock, C. S., & Smallish, L. (1990). The adolescent outcome of hyperactive children diagnosed research criteria-I. An 8 year prospective follow-up study. *Journal of the American Academy of Child & Adolescent Psychiatry, 29,* 546–557.

Barkley, R. A., Fischer, M., Edelbrock, C. S., & Smallish, L. (1991). The adolescent outcome of hyperactive children diagnosed by research criteria–III. Mother-child interactions, family conflicts and maternal psychopathology. *Journal of Child Psychology & Psychiatry, 32,* 233–255.

Barkley, R. A., Fischer, M., Newby, R., & Breen, M. (1988). Development of a multi-method clinical protocol for assessing stimulant drug responses in ADHD children. *Journal of Clinical Child Psychology, 17,* 14–24.

Barkley, R. A., Grodzinsky, G., & DuPaul, G. J. (1992). Frontal lobe functions in attention deficit disorder with and without hyperactivity: A review and research report. *Journal of Abnormal Child Psychology, 20,* 163–188.

Baron-Cohen, S., Cross, P., Crowson, M., & Robertson, M. (1994). Can children with Gilles de la Tourette syndrome edit their intentions? *Psychological Medicine, 24,* 29–40.

Baron-Cohen, S., Tager-Flusberg, H., & Cohen, D. J. (Eds.). (1993). *Understanding other minds: Perspectives from autism.* London: Oxford University Press.

Barr, C. L., Livingston, J., Williamson, R., Sandor, P., Kidd, K. K., Pauls, D., & Tsui, L. C. (1994). Genome scan for linkage to Gilles de la Tourette syndrome. *American Journal of Human Genetics, 55,* 345.

Barr, C. L., Wigg, K. G., Zovko, E., Sandor, P., & Tsui, L. C. (1996). No evidence for a major gene effect of the dopamine D4 receptor gene in the susceptibility to Gilles de la Tourette syndrome in five Canadian families. *American Journal of Medical Genetics, 67,* 301–305.

Barrickman, L., Noyes, R., Kuperman, S., Schumacher, E., & Verda, M. (1991). Treatment of ADHD with fluoxetine: A preliminary trial. *Journal of the American Academy of Child & Adolescent Psychiatry, 30,* 762–767.

Barrickman, L., Perry, P., Allen, A., Kuperman, S., Arndt, S., Herrmann, K., & Schumacher, E. (1995). Buproprion versus methylphenidate in the treatment of attention-deficit hyperactivity disorder. *Journal of the American Academy of Child & Adolescent Psychiatry, 34,* 649–657.

Bates, J. F., & Goldman-Rakic, P. S. (1993). Prefrontal connections of medial motor areas in the rhesus monkey. *Journal of Comparative Neurology, 336,* 211–228.

Baumgardner, T. L., Singer, H. S., Denckla, M. B., Rubin, M. A., Abrams, M. T., Colli, M. J., & Reiss, A. L. (1996). Corpus callosum morphology in children with Tourette syndrome and attention deficit hyperactivity disorder. *Neurology, 47,* 477–482.

Baxter, L. R., Phelps, J. M., Mazziotta, J. C., Guze, B. H., & Schwartz, J. M. (1987). Local cerebral glucose metabolic rates in obsessive-compulsive disorder: A comparison with rates in unipolar depression and normal controls. *Archives of General Psychiatry, 44,* 211–218.

Baxter, L. R., Schwartz, J. M., Bergman, K. S., Szuba, M. P., Guze, B. H., Mazziotta, J. C., Alazraki, A., Selin, C. E., Ferng, H. K., Munford, P., & Phelps, M. E. (1992). Caudate glucose metabolic rate changes with both drug and behavior therapy for obsessive-compulsive disorder. *Archives of General Psychiatry, 49,* 681–689.

Baxter, L. R., Schwartz, J. M., Guze, B. H., Bergman, K., & Szuba, M. P. (1990). PET imaging in obsessive compulsive disorder with and without depression. *Journal of Clinical Psychiatry, 51,* 61–69.

Baxter, L. R., Schwartz, J. M., Mazziotta, J., Phelps, M. E., Pahl, J. J., Buze, B. E., & Fairbanks, L. (1988). Cerebral glucose metabolic rates in nondepressed patients with obsessive-compulsive disorder. *American Journal of Psychiatry, 145,* 1560–1563.

Beery, K., & Buktenica, N. (1989). *The developmental test of visual-motor integration.* Toronto: Modern Curriculum Press.

Behar, D., Rapoport, J. L., Berg, C. J., Denckla, M. B., Mann, L., Cox, C., Fedio, P., Zahn, T., & Wolfman, M. G. (1984). Computerized tomography and neuropsychological test measures in children with obsessive-compulsive disorder. *American Journal of Psychiatry, 141,* 363–369.

Bellodi, L., Sciuto, G., Diaferia, G., Ronchi, P., & Smeraldi, E. (1992). Psychiatric disorders in the families of patients with obsessive-compulsive disorder. *Psychiatry Research, 42,*111–120.

Bender, L. (1938). A visual motor gestalt test and its clinical use. *American Orthopsychiatric Association Research Monographs, 3.*

Benkelfat, C., Nordahl, T. E., Semple, W. E., King, A. C., Murphy, D. L., & Cohen, R. M. (1990). Local cerebral glucose metabolic rates in obsessive-compulsive disorder. Patients treated with clomipramine. *Archives General Psychiatry, 47,* 840–848.

Benson, D. F. (1991). The role of frontal dysfunction in attention deficit hyperactivity disorder. *Journal of Child Neurology, 6,* 9–12.

Benton, A. L. (1994). *Judgment of line orientation.* Los Angeles: Western Psychological Services.

Benton, A. L., Hannay, H. J., & Varney, N. R. (1975). Visual perception of line direction in patients with unilateral brain disease. *Neurology, 25,* 907–910.

Benton, A. L., Varney, N. R., & Hamsher, K. (1978). Visuospatial judgment. A clinical test. *Archives of Neurology, 35,* 364–367.

Berg, C. J., Rapoport, J. L., & Flament, M. (1986). The Leyton Obsessional Inventory-Child Version. *Journal of the American Academy of Child & Adolescent Psychiatry, 25,* 84–91.

Berg, C. J., Rapoport, J. L., Whitaker, A., & Davies, M. (1989). Childhood obsessive-compulsive disorder: A two-year prospective follow-up of a community sample. *Journal of the American Academy of Child & Adolescent Psychiatry, 28,* 528–533.

Berg, C. J., Whitaker, A., Davies, M., Flament, M. F., & Rapoport, J. L. (1988). The survey form of the Leyton Obsessional Inventory-Child Version: Norms from an epidemiological study. *Journal of the American Academy Child & Adolescent Psychiatry, 27,* 759–763.

Berger, M., Yule, W., & Rutter, M. (1975). Attainment and adjustment in two geographical areas: I. The prevalence of specific reading retardation. *British Journal of Psychiatry, 126,* 510 –526.

Berkson, J. (1946). Limitations of the application of fourfold table analysis to hospital data. *Biometrics, 2,* 47–51.

Berthier, M. L., Kulisevsky, J., & Campos, V. M. (1998). Bipolar disorder in adult patients with Tourette's syndrome: A clinical study. *Biological Psychiatry, 43*(5), 364–370.

Bhatia, K., & Marsden, C. (1994). The behavioral and motor consequences of focal lesions of the basal ganglia in man. *Brain, 117,* 859–876.

Biederman, J., Baldessarini, R. J., Wright, V., Keenan, K., & Faraone, S. (1993). A double-blind placebo-controlled study of desipramine in the treatment of ADD: III. Lack of impact of comorbidity and family history factors on clinical response. *Journal of the American Academy of Child & Adolescent Psychiatry, 32,* 199–204.

Biederman, J., Baldessarini, R. J., Wright, V., Knee, D., & Harmatz, J. S. (1989). A double-blind placebo controlled study of desipramine in the treatment of ADD: I. Efficacy. *Journal of the American Academy of Child & Adolescent Psychiatry, 28,* 777–784.

Biederman, J., Baldessarini, R. J., Wright, V., Knee, D., Harmatz, J. S., & Goldblatt, A. (1989). A double-blind placebo controlled study of desipramine in the treatment of ADD: II. Serum drug levels and cardiovascular findings. *Journal of the American Academy of Child & Adolescent Psychiatry, 28,* 903–911.

Biederman, J., Faraone, S. V., Doyle, A., Lehman, B. K., Kraus, I., Perrin, J., & Tsuang, M. T. (1993). Convergence of the child behavior checklist with structured interview-based psychiatric diagnoses of ADHD children with and without hyperactivity. *Journal of Child Psychology & Psychiatry, 34,* 1241–1251.

Biederman, J., Faraone, S. V., Keenan, K., Benjamin, J., Krifcher, B., Moore, C., Sprich-Buckminster, S., Ugaglia, K., Jellinek, M. S., Steingard, R., Spencer, T., Norman, D., Kolodny, R., Kraus, I., Perrin, J., Keller, M. B., & Tsuang, M. T. (1992). Further evidence for family genetic risk factors in attention deficit hyperactivity disorder: Patterns of comorbidity in probands and relatives in psychiatrically and pediatrically referred samples. *Archives of General Psychiatry, 49,* 728–738.

Biederman, J., Faraone, S. V., Keenan, K., Steingard, R., & Tsuang, M. T. (1991). Familial association between attention deficit disorder (ADD) and anxiety disorder. *American Journal of Psychiatry, 148,* 251–256.

Biederman, J., Faraone, S. V., Keenan, K., & Tsuang, M. T. (1991). Evidence of familial association between attention deficit disorder and major affective disorders. *Archives of General Psychiatry, 48,* 633–642.

Biederman, J., Faraone, S. V., Mick, E., Spencer, T., Wilens, T., Kiely, K., Guite, J., Ablon, J. S., Reed, E., & Warburton, R. (1995). High risk for ADHD in children of parents with childhood onset ADHD: A pilot study. *American Journal of Psychiatry, 152,* 431–435.

Biederman, J., Faraone, S. V., Milberger, S., Guite, J., Mick, E., Chen, L., Mennin, D., Marrs, A., Ouellette, D., Moore, P., Spencer, T., Norman, D., Wilens, T., Kraus, I., & Perrin, J. (1996). A prospective 4-year follow-up study of attention-deficit hyperactivity and related disorders. *Archives of General Psychiatry, 53,* 437–446.

Biederman, J., Milberger, S., Faraone, S., Kiely, K., Guite, J., Mick, E., Ablon, S., Warburton, R., & Reed, E. (1995). Family-environment risk factors for attention-deficit hyperactivity disorder. A test of Rutter's indicators of adversity. *Archives of General Psychiatry, 52,* 464–470.

Biederman, J., Munir, K., Knee, D., Habelow, W., Armentano, M., Autor, S., Hoge, S. K., & Waternaux, C. (1986). A family study of patients with attention deficit disorder and normal controls. *Journal of Psychiatry Research, 20,* 263–274.

Biederman, J., Newcorn, J., & Sprich, S. (1991a). Comorbidity of attention deficit hyperactivity disorder with conduct, depressive, anxiety, and other disorders. *American Journal of Psychiatry, 148,* 564–577.

Biederman, J., Newcorn, J., & Sprich, S. (1991b). Comorbidity in child psychopathology: Concepts, issues, and research strategies. *Journal of Child Psychology and Psychiatry, 32,* 1063–1080.

Bierman, K. L. (1986). The relation between social aggression and peer rejection in middle childhood. In R. J. Prinz (Ed.), *Advances in behavioral assessment of children and families* (Vol. 2, pp. 151–178). Greenwich, CT: JAI Press.

Billings, A. (1978). Self-monitoring in the treatment of tics: A single-subject analysis. *Journal of Behavior Therapy and Experimental Psychiatry, 9,* 339–342.

Bird, H. R., Canino, G., Rubio-Stipec, M., Gould, M. S., Ribera, J., Sesman, M., Woodbury, M., Huertas-Goldman, S., Pagan, A., Sanchez-Lacay, A., & Moscoso, M. (1988). Estimates of the prevalence of childhood maladjustment in a community survey in Puerto Rico. *Archives of General Psychiatry, 45,* 1120–1126.

Black, D. W., Noyes, R., Jr., Goldstein, R. B., & Blum, N. (1992). A family study of obsessive-compulsive disorder. *Archives of General Psychiatry, 49,* 362–368.

Bliss, J. (1980). Sensory experiences of Gilles de la Tourette syndrome. *Archives of General Psychiatry, 37,* 1343–1347.

Bolton, D., Collins, S., & Steinberg, D. (1983). The treatment of obsessive-compulsive disorder in adolescence: A report of fifteen cases. *British Journal of Psychiatry, 142,* 456–464.

Bonda, E., Petrides, M., Frey, S., & Evans, A. (1995). Neural correlates of mental transformations of the body-in-space. *Proceedings of the National Academy of Science USA, 92,* 11180–11184.

Bonnet, K. A. (1982). Neurobiological dissection of Tourette syndrome: A neurochemical focus on a human neuroanatomical model. In A. J. Friedhoff & T. N. Chase (Eds.), *Advances in neurology: Vol. 35. Gilles de la Tourette syndrome* (pp. 77–82). New York: Raven Press.

Boone, K. B., Ananth, J., Philpott, L., Kaur, A., & Djenderedjian, A. (1991). Neuropsychological characteristics of nondepressed adults with obsessive-compulsive disorder. *Neuropsychiatry, Neuropsychology and Behavioral Neurology, 4,* 96–109.

Borcherding, B. G., Keysor, C. S., Cooper, T. B., & Rapoport, J. L. (1989). Differential effects of methylphenidate and dextroamphetamine on the motor activity level of hyperactive children. *Neuropsychopharmacology, 2,* 253–263.

Borcherding, B. G., Keysor, C. S., Rapoport, J. L., Elia, J., & Amass, J. (1990). Motor/vocal tics and compulsive behaviors on stimulant drugs: Is there a common vulnerability? *Psychiatric Research, 33,* 83–94.

Bornstein, R. A. (1990). Neuropsychological performance in children with Tourette syndrome. *Psychiatric Research, 33,* 73–81.

Bornstein, R. A. (1991a). Neuropsychological correlates of obsessive characteristics in Tourette's syndrome. *Journal of Neuropsychiatry and Clinical Neurosciences, 3,* 157–162.

Bornstein, R. A. (1991b). Neuropsychological performance in adults with Tourette's syndrome. *Psychiatric Research, 37,* 229–236.

Bornstein, R. A., & Baker, G. B. (1988). Neuropsychological correlates of urinary amine metabolites in Tourette's syndrome. *International Journal of Neuroscience, 42,* 113–120.

Bornstein, R. A., & Baker, G. B. (1992). Urinary indoleamines in Tourette syndrome patients with obsessive-compulsive characteristics. *Psychiatry Research, 41,* 267–274.

Bornstein, R. A., Baker, G. B., Bazylewich, T., & Douglas, A. B. (1991). Tourette syndrome and neuropsychological performance. *Acta Psychiatrica Scandinavica, 84,* 212–216.

Bornstein, R. A., Carroll, A., & King, G. (1985). Relationship of age to neuropsychological deficit in Tourette syndrome. *Developmental and Behavioral Pediatrics, 6,* 284–286.

Bornstein, R. A., King, G., & Carroll, A. (1983). Neuropsychological abnormalities in Gilles de la Tourette's syndrome. *Journal of Nervous and Mental Disease, 171,* 497–502.

Bornstein, R. A., Stefl, M. E., & Hammond, L. (1990). A survey of Tourette syndrome patients and their families: The 1987 Ohio Tourette survey. *Journal of Neuropsychiatry and Clinical Neurosciences, 2,* 275–281.

Bornstein, R. A., & Yang, V. (1991). Neurological performance in medicated and unmedicated patients with Tourette's disorder. *American Journal of Psychiatry, 148,* 468–471.

Bowlby, J. (1969). *Attachment and loss: Attachment* (Vol. 1). New York: Basic Books.

Boyle, M. H., Offord, D. R., Racine, Y., Sanford, M., Szatmari, P., Fleming, J. E., & Price-Munn, N. (1993). Evaluation of the diagnostic interview for children and adolescents for use in general population samples. *Journal of Abnormal Child Psychology, 21,* 663–681.

Bradley, C. (1937). The behavior of children receiving benzedrine. *American Journal of Psychiatry, 94,* 577–585.

Braun, A. R., Stoetter, B., Randolph, C., Hsiao, J. K., Vladar, K., Gernert, J., Carson, R. E., Herscovitch, P., & Chase, T. N. (1993). The functional neuroanatomy of Tourette's syndrome: An FDG-PET study: I. Regional changes in cerebral glucose metabolism differentiating patients and controls. *Neuropsychopharmacology, 9,* 277–291.

Breiter, H. C., Rauch, S. L., Kwong, K. K., Baker, J. R., Weisskoff, R. M., Kennedy, D. N., Kendrick, A. D., Davis, T. L., Jiang, A., Cohen, M. S., Stern, C. E., Belliveau, J. W., Baer, L., O'Sullivan, R. L., Savage, C. R., Jenike, M. A., & Rosen, B. R. (1996). Functional magnetic resonance imaging of symptom provocation in obsessive-compulsive disorder. *Archives of General Psychiatry, 53,* 595–606.

Breslau, N., Brown, G. G., Deldotto, J. E., & Kumar, S. (1996). Psychiatric sequelae of low birth weight at 6 years of age. *Journal of Abnormal Child Psychology, 24,* 385–400.

Bridges, P. K., Barlett, J. R., Hale, A. S., Poynton, A. M., Malizia, A. L., & Hodgkiss, A. D. (1994). Psychosurgery: Stereotactic subcaudate tractomy. An indispensable procedure. *British Journal of Psychiatry, 165,* 599–611.

Brigham, T. A. (1989). *Self-management for adolescents: A skills training program.* New York: Guilford Press.

Brody, N. (1992). *Intelligence.* New York: Academic Press.

Bronze, M. S., & Dale, J. B. (1993). Epitopes of streptococcal M proteins that evoke antibodies that cross-react with human brain. *Journal of Immunology, 151,* 2820–2828.

Brookshire, B. L., Butler, I. J., Ewing-Cobbs, L., & Fletcher, J. M. (1994). Neuropsychological characteristics of children with Tourette syndrome: Evidence for a nonverbal learning disability? *Journal of Clinical and Experimental Neuropsychology, 16,* 289–302.

Brown, P., & Marsden, C. D. (1992). Myoclonus. In H. L. Klawans, C. G. Goetz, & C. M. Tanner (Eds.), *Textbook of clinical neuropharmacology and therapeutics* (2nd ed., pp. 75–82). New York: Raven Press.

Brown, R., & Jahanshahi, M. (1995). Depression in Parkinson's disease: A psychosocial viewpoint. In W. J. Weiner & A. E. Lang (Eds.), *Advances in neurology: Vol. 65. Behavioral neurology of movement disorders* (pp. 61–84). New York: Raven Press.

Bruun, R. D. (1984). Gilles de la Tourette's syndrome: An overview of clinical experience. *Journal of the American Academy of Child Psychiatry, 2,* 126–133.

Bruun, R. D. (1988a). The natural history of Tourette's syndrome. In D. J. Cohen, R. D. Bruun, & J. F. Leckman (Eds.), *Tourette's syndrome and tic disorders: Clinical understanding and treatment* (pp. 21–39). New York: Wiley.

Bruun, R. D. (1988b). Subtle and under recognized side effects of neuroleptic treatment in children with Tourette's disorder. *American Journal of Psychiatry, 145,* 621–624.

Bruun, R. D., & Budman, C. L. (1996). Risperidone as a treatment for Tourette's syndrome. *Journal of Clinical Psychiatry, 57,* 29–31.

Bruun, R. D., Cohen, D. J., & Leckman, J. (1990). *Guide to the diagnosis and treatment of Tourette syndrome.* New York: Tourette Syndrome Association.

Bruun, R. D., Shapiro, A. K., & Shapiro, E. (1976). A follow-up of eighty patients with Tourette's syndrome. *Psychopharmacology Bulletin, 12,* 15–17.

Buetow, K. H., Weber, J. L., Ludwigsen, S., Scherpbier-Heddema, T., Duyk, G. M., Sheffield, V. C., Wang, Z., & Murray, J. C. (1994). Integrated human genome-wide maps constructed using CEPH reference panel. *Nature Genetics, 6,* 391–393.

Bullen, J. G., & Helmsley, D. R. (1983). Sensory experience as a trigger in Gilles de la Tourette's syndrome. *Journal of Behavior Therapy and Experimental Psychiatry, 14,* 197–201.

Bunney, B., & DeRiemer, S. (1982). Effect of clonidine on dopaminergic neuron activity in the substantia nigra: Possible indirect mediation by noradrenergic regulation of the serotonergic system. In A. J. Friedhoff & T. N. Chase (Eds.), *Advances in Neurology: Vol. 35. Gilles de la Tourette Syndrome* (pp. 99–105). New York: Raven Press.

Burd, L., Kauffman, D. W., & Kerbeshian, J. (1992). Tourette syndrome and learning disabilities. *Journal of Learning Disabilities, 25,* 598–604.

Burd, L., Kerbeshian, J., Wiknheiser, M., & Fisher, W. (1986a). Prevalence of Gilles de la Tourette syndrome in North Dakota adults. *American Journal of Psychiatry, 143,* 787–788.

Burd, L., Kerbeshian, J., Wiknheiser, M., & Fisher, W. (1986b). Prevalence of Gilles de la Tourette syndrome in North Dakota school-age children. *Journal of the American Academy of Child &Adolescent Psychiatry, 25,* 552–553.

Butler, I. J., Koslow, S. H., Seifert, W. E., Jr., Caprioli, R. M., & Singer, H. S. (1979). Biogenic amine metabolism in Tourette syndrome. *Annals of Neurology, 6,* 37–39.

Butter, C. M. (1969). Perseveration in extinction and in discrimination reversal tasks following selective frontal ablations in Macaca mulatta. *Physiology & Behavior, 4,* 163–171.

Butters, N., & Rosvold, H. E. (1968). Effect of caudate and septal nuclei lesions on resistance to extinction and delayed alternation. *Journal of Comparative Physiology and Psychology, 65,* 397–403.

Caine, E. D., McBride, M. C., Chiverton, P., Bamford, K. A., Redliess, S., & Shiao, J. (1988). Tourette's syndrome in Monroe county school children. *Neurology, 38,* 472–475.

Caine, E. D., Polinsky, R. J., Kartzinel, R., & Ebert, M. H. (1979). The trial use of clozapine for abnormal involuntary disorders. *American Journal of Psychiatry, 136,* 317–320.

Calvocoressi, L., Lewis, B., Harris, M., Trufan, S. J., Goodman, W. K., McDougle, C. J., & Price, L. H. (1995). Family accommodation in obsessive-compulsive disorder. *American Journal of Psychiatry, 152,* 441–443.

Campbell, S. B., & Werry, J. S. (1986). Attention deficit disorder (hyperactivity). In H. C. Quay & J. S. Werry (Eds.), *Psychopathological disorders of childhood* (3rd ed., pp. 111–155). New York: Wiley.

Cannon, T. D., Mednick, S. A., Parnas, J., Schulsinger, F., Praestholm, J., & Vestergaard, A. (1993). Developmental brain abnormalities in the offspring of schizophrenic mothers: I. Contributions of genetic and perinatal factors. *Archives of General Psychiatry, 50,* 551–564.

Cannon, T. D., Mednick, S. A., Parnas, J., Schulsinger, F., Praestholm, J., & Vestergaard, A. (1994). Developmental brain abnormalities in the offspring of schizophrenic mothers: II. Structural brain characteristics of schizophrenia and schizotypal personality disorder. *Archives of General Psychiatry, 51,* 955–962.

Cantwell, D. P. (1975). Genetics of hyperactivity. *Journal of Child Psychology and Psychiatry, 16,* 262–264.

Cantwell, D. P., & Baker, L. (1991). Association between attention deficit-hyperactivity disorder and learning disorders. *Journal of Learning Disabilities, 24,* 88–95.

Caparulo, B. K., Cohen, D. J., Rothman, S. L., Young, J. G., Katz, J. D., Shaywitz, S. E., & Shaywitz, B. A. (1981). Computed tomographic brain scanning in children with developmental neuropsychiatric disorders. *Journal of the American Academy of Child & Adolescent Psychiatry, 20,* 338–357.

Caplan, L. R., Schmahmann, J. D., Kase, C. S., Feldman, D., Baquis, G., Greenberg, J. P., Gorelick, P. B., Helgason, C., & Hier, D. B. (1990). Caudate infarcts. *Archives of Neurology, 49,* 1187–1194.

Capstick, N., & Seldrup, J. (1977). Obsessional states: A study in the relationship between abnormalities occurring at the time of birth and the subsequent development of obsessional symptoms. *Acta Psychiatrica Scandinavica, 56,* 427–431.

Carey, G., & Gottesman, I. I. (1981). Twin and family studies of anxiety, phobic and obsessive disorders. In D. F. Klein & J. Rabkin (Eds.), *Anxiety: New research and changing concepts* (pp. 117–136). New York: Raven Press.

Carlesimo, G. A., Fadda, L., & Caltagirone, C. (1993). Basic mechanisms of constructional apraxia in unilateral brain-damaged patients. Role of visuoperceptual and executive disorders. *Journal of Clinical and Experimental Neuropsychology, 15,* 342–358.

Carr, J. E. (1995). Competing responses for the treatment of Tourette syndrome and tic disorders. *Behavior Research and Therapy, 33,* 455–456.

Carr, J. E., & Bailey, J. S. (1996). A brief behavior therapy protocol for Tourette syndrome. *Journal of Behavior Therapy and Experimental Psychiatry, 27,* 33–40.

Carr, J. E., Taylor, C. C., Wallander, R. J., & Reiss, M. L. (1996). A functional-analytic approach to the diagnosis of a transient tic disorder. *Journal of Behavior Therapy and Experimental Psychiatry, 27,* 291–297.

Carter, A. S., Lidsky, I., Scahill, L., Schultz, R. J., & Pauls, D. L. (1997). *Socioemotional function in children with Tourette's syndrome with and without ADHD.* Unpublished manuscript.

Carter, A. S., Pauls, D. L., Leckman, J. F., & Cohen, D. J. (1994). A prospective longitudinal study of Gilles de la Tourette's syndrome. *Journal of the American Academy of Child & Adolescent Psychiatry, 33,* 377–385.

Cartwright, R. D., & Wood, E. (1991). Adjustment disorders of sleep: The sleep effects of a major stressful event and its resolution. *Psychiatry Research, 39,* 199–209.

Casas, M., Alvarez, E., Duro, P., Garcia-Ribera, C., Udina, C., Velat, A., Abella, D., Rodriguez-Espinosa, J., Salva, P., & Jane, F. (1986). Antiandrogenic treatment of obsessive-compulsive neurosis. *Acta Psychiatrica Scandinavica, 73,* 221–222.

Casat, C. D., Pleasants, D. Z., Schroeder, D. H., & Parler, D. W. (1989). Bupropion in children with attention deficit disorder. *Psychopharmacology Bulletin, 25,* 198–201.

Cassens, G., Inglis, A. K., Appelbaum, P. S., & Gutheil, T. G. (1990). Neuroleptics: Effects on neuropsychological function in chronic schizophrenic patients. *Schizophrenia Bulletin, 16,* 477–499.

Castellanos, F. X., Giedd, J. N., Eckburg, P., Marsh, W. L., Vaituzis, A. C., Kaysen, D., Hamburger, S. D., & Rapoport, J. L. (1994). Quantitative morphology of the caudate nucleus in attention deficit hyperactivity disorder. *American Journal of Psychiatry, 151,* 1791–1796.

Castellanos, F. X., Giedd, J. N., March, W. L., Hamburger, S. D., Vaituzis, A. C., Dickstein, D. P., Sarfatti, S. E., Vauss, Y. C., Snell, J. W., Lange, J., Kaysen, D., Krain, A. L., Ritchie, G. F., Rajapakse, J. C., & Rapoport, J. L. (1996). Quantitative brain magnetic resonance imaging in attention deficit hyperactivity disorder. *Archives of General Psychiatry, 53,* 607–616.

Catalano, M., Sciuto, G., DiBella, D., Novelli, E., Nobile, M., & Bellodi, L. (1994). Lack of association between obsessive-compulsive disorder and the dopamine D3 receptor gene. *American Journal of Medical Genetics, 54,* 253–255.

Centers for Disease Control and Prevention. (1995, April). *General considerations regarding health education and risk reduction activities.* http://wonder.cdc.gov:80/TD/RHER3702.PCW.html.

Chambers, W., Puig-Antich, J., Hirsch, M., Paez, P., Ambrosini, P. J., Tabrizi, M. A., & Davies, M. (1985). The assessment of affective disorders in children and adolescents by semistructured interview. *Archives of General Psychiatry, 42,* 696–702.

Chandler, J. D. (1990). Propranolol treatment of akathisia in Tourette's syndrome. *Journal of the American Academy of Child & Adolescent Psychiatry, 29,* 475–477.

Channon, S., Flynn, D., & Robertson, M. M. (1992). Attentional deficits in Gilles de la Tourette syndrome. *Neuropsychiatry, Neuropsychology and Behavioral Neurology, 5,* 170–177.

Chappell, P. B. (1994). Sequential use of opioid antagonists and agonists in Tourette's syndrome [Comment]. *Lancet, 343,* 556.

Chappell, P. B., Anderson, G. M., Goodman, W. K., Price, L. H., Hall, L. M., Cohen, D. J., & Leckman, J. F. (1995). Kynurenine pathway metabolites in CSF and plasma of Tourette syndrome patients. *Society for Neuroscience Abstracts, 21,* 1111.

Chappell, P. B., Leckman, J. F., Goodman, W. K., Bissette, G., Pauls, D. L., Anderson, G. M., Riddle, M., Scahill, L., McDougle, C. J., & Cohen, D. J. (1996). Elevated cerebrospinal fluid corticotopin-releasing factor in Tourette's patients: Comparison to obsessive-compulsive disorder and normal controls. *Biological Psychiatry, 39,* 776–783.

Chappell, P. B., Leckman, J. F., Pauls, D. L., & Cohen, D. J. (1990). Biochemical and genetic analyses of Tourette's syndrome. In S. I. Deutsch, A. Weizman, & R. Weizman (Eds.), *Application of basic neuroscience to child psychiatry* (pp. 241–260). New York: Plenum Medical Book.

Chappell, P. B., Leckman, J. F., & Riddle, M. A. (1995). The pharmacologic treatment of tic disorders. In M. Lewis & M. Riddle (Eds.), *Child and adolescent psychiatric clinics of North America: Pediatric psychopharmacology* (Vol. 4, pp. 197–215). Philadelphia: Saunders.

Chappell, P. B., Leckman, J. F., Riddle, M. A., Anderson, G. M., Listwak, S. J., Ort, S. I., Hardin, M. T., & Cohen, D. J. (1992). Neuroendocrine and behavioral effects of naloxone in Tourette's syndrome. In A. J. Friedhoff & T. N. Chase (Eds.), *Advances in neurology: Vol. 35. Gilles de la Tourette syndrome* (pp. 253–262). New York: Raven Press.

Chappell, P. B., Leckman, J. F., Scahill, L., Hardin, M. T., Anderson, G. M., & Cohen, D. J. (1993). Neuroendocrine and behavioral effects of the selective kappa agonist spiradoline (U-62066E) in Tourette's syndrome. *Psychiatry Research, 47,* 267–280.

Chappell, P. B., McSwiggan-Hardin, M. T., Scahill, L., Rubenstein, M., Walker, D., Cohen, D. J., & Leckman, J. F. (1994). The role of videotape tic counts in the assessment of Tourette syndrome: Stability, reliability, and validity. *Journal of the American Academy of Child & Adolescent Psychiatry, 33,* 386–393.

Chappell, P. B., Riddle, M., Anderson, G., Scahill, L., Hardin, M., Walker, D., Cohen, D., & Leckman J. (1994). Enhanced stress responsivity of Tourette syndrome patients undergoing lumbar puncture. *Biological Psychiatry, 36,* 35–43.

Chappell, P. B., Riddle, M. A., Scahill, L., Lynch, K. A., Schultz, R., Arnsten, A., Leckman, J. F., & Cohen, D. J. (1995). Guanfacine treatment of comorbid attention-deficit hyperactivity disorder in Tourette's syndrome: Preliminary clinical experience. *Journal of the American Academy of Child & Adolescent Psychiatry, 34,* 1140–1146.

Chappell, P. B., Scahill, L. D., & Leckman, J. F. (1997). Future therapies of Tourette syndrome. *Neurological Clinics of North America, 15,* 429–450.

Charles, L., Schain, R. J., & Guthrie, D. (1979). Long term use and discontinuation of methylphenidate on hyperactive children's ability to sustain attention. *Pediatrics, 64,* 412–418.

Chase, T. N., Friedhoff, A. J., Cohen, D. J. (Eds.). (1992). *Advances in neurology: Vol. 58. Tourette syndrome: Genetics, neurobiology and treatment.* New York: Raven Press.

Chase, T. N., Geoffrey, V., Gillespie, M., & Burrows, G. H. (1986). Structural and functional studies of Gilles de la Tourette syndrome. *Revue Neurologique, 142,* 851–855.

Choi, Y. C., Lee, M. S., & Choi, I. S. (1993). Delayed-onset focal dystonia after diffuse cerebral hypoxia—two case reports. *Journal of Korean Medical Science, 8,* 476–481.

Chokka, P. R., Baker, G. B., Bornstein, R. A., & de Groot, C. M. (1995). The biochemistry of Tourette's syndrome. *Metabolic Brain Disease, 10,*107–124.

Chouinard, G., Jones, B., Remington, G., Bloom, D., Addington, D., MacEwan G. W., Labelle, A., Beauclair, L., & Arnott, W. (1993). A Canadian multicenter placebo-controlled study of fixed doses of risperidone and haloperidol in the treatment of chronic schizophrenic patients. *Journal of Clinical Psychopharmacology, 13,* 25–40.

Christensen, K. J., Kim, S. W., Dysken, M. W., & Hoover, K. M. (1992). Neuropsychological performance in obsessive-compulsive disorder. *Biological Psychiatry, 31,* 4–18.

Christie, M. J., Williams, J. T., Osborne, P. B., & Bellchambers, C. E. (1997). Where is the locus in opioid withdrawal? *Trends in Pharmacological Sciences, 18,* 134–140.

Cicchetti, D., & Cohen, D. J. (Eds.). (1995a). *Developmental psychopathology: Vol. 1. Theory and method & Vol. 2. Risk, disorder and adaptation.* New York: Wiley.

Cicchetti, D., & Cohen, D. J. (1995b). Perspectives on developmental psychopathology. In D. Cicchetti & D. J. Cohen (Eds.), *Developmental psychopathology: Vol. 1. Theory and method* (pp. 3–20). New York: Wiley.

Cicchetti, D., & Tucker, D. (1994). Development and self-regulatory structures of the mind. *Developmental Psychopathology, 6,* 533–549.

Clarvit, S. R., Graae, F., Piacentini, J., Tancer, N., Gitow, A., DelBene, D., Davies, S., Jaffer, M., & Liebowitz, M. (1994). Double-blind, placebo-controlled study of fluoxetine for child and adolescent obsessive-compulsive disorder. *American Academy of Child & Adolescent Psychiatry Abstracts, 10*(No. NR-65), 56.

Claus, A., Bollen, J., De Cuyper, H., & Heylen, L. E. (1992). Risperidone versus haloperidol in the treatment of chronic schizophrenic inpatients: A multicentre double-blind comparative study. *Acta Psychiatrica Scandinavica, 85,* 295–305.

Clay, T. H., Gualtieri, C. T., Evans, R. W., & Gullion, C. M. (1988). Clinical and neuropsychological effects of the novel antidepressant bupropion. *Psychopharmacology Bulletin, 24,* 143–148.

Clements, S. (1966). *Minimal brain dysfunction in children* (NINBD Monograph No. 3). Washington, DC: U.S. Public Health Service.

Clomipramine Collaborative Study Group. (1991). Clomipramine in the treatment of patients with obsessive-compulsive disorder. *Archives of General Psychiatry, 48,* 730–738.

Coffey, B. J. (1993). Anxiety disorders in Tourette's syndrome. *Child & Adolescent Psychiatry Clinics of North America, 2,* 709–725.

Coffey, B. J., Frazier, J., & Chen, S. (1992). Comorbidity, Tourette syndrome, and anxiety disorders. In T. N. Chase, A. J. Friedhoff & D. J. Cohen (Eds.), *Advances in neurology: Vol. 58. Tourette syndrome: Genetics, neurobiology and treatment* (pp. 95–104). New York: Raven Press.

Coffey, B. J., & Park, K. S. (1997). Behavioral and emotional aspects of Tourette syndrome. *Neurologic Clinics of North America, 15,* 277–289.

Cohen, A., & Leckman, J. F. (1992). Sensory phenomena associated with Gilles de la Tourette syndrome. *Journal of Clinical Psychiatry, 5*(3), 19–323.

Cohen, D. J. (1974). Competence and biology: Methodology in studies of infants, twins, psychosomatic disease, and psychosis. In E. J. Anthony & C. Koupernik (Eds.), *The child in his family: Children at psychiatric risk* (pp. 361–394). New York: Wiley.

Cohen, D. J. (1980). The pathology of the self in primary childhood autism and Gilles de la Tourette syndrome. In B. Blinder (Ed.), *Psychiatric Clinics of North America, Vol. 3* (pp. 383–402). Philadelphia: W. B. Saunders Co.

Cohen, D. J. (1990). *Tourette's syndrome: Developmental psychopathology of a model psychiatric disorder of childhood.* The 27th Annual Institute of Pennsylvania Hospital Award Lecture in Memory of Edward A. Strecker.

Cohen D. J. (1991a). Finding meaning in one's self and others: Clinical studies of children with autism and Tourette's syndrome. In F. Kessel, M. Bornstein, & A. Sameroff (Eds.), *Contemporary constructions of the child: Essays in honor of William Kessen* (pp. 159–175). Hillsdale, N.J.: Erlbaum.

Cohen, D. J. (1991b). Tourette's syndrome: A model disorder for integrating psychoanalytic and biological perspectives. *International Review of Psychoanalysis, 18,* 195–209.

Cohen, D. J. (1995). Psychosocial therapies for children and adolescents: Overview and future directions. *Journal of Abnormal Child Psychology, 23,* 141–156.

Cohen, D. J., Bruun, R. D., & Leckman, J. F. (1988). *Tourette's syndrome and tic disorder: Clinical understanding and treatment.* New York: Wiley.

Cohen, D. J., Detlor, J., Shaywitz, B. A., & Leckman, J. F. (1982). Interaction of biological and psychological factors in the natural history of Tourette's syndrome: A model of childhood neuropsychiatric disorders. In T. N. Chase, A. J. Friedhoff, & D. J. Cohen (Eds.), *Advances in neurology: Vol. 58. Tourette syndrome: Genetics, neurobiology and treatment.* (pp. 31–40). New York: Raven Press.

Cohen, D. J., Detlor, J., Young, J. G., & Shaywitz, B. A. (1980). Clonidine ameliorates Gilles de la Tourette syndrome. *Archives of General Psychiatry, 37,* 1350–1357.

Cohen, D. J., Friedhoff, A. J., Leckman, J. F., & Chase, T. N. (1992). Tourette syndrome: Extending basic research to clinical care. In T. N. Chase, A. J. Friedhoff & D. J. Cohen (Eds.), *Advances in neurology: Vol. 58. Tourette syndrome: Genetics, neurobiology and treatment* (pp. 341–362). New York: Raven Press.

Cohen, D. J., & Leckman, J. F. (1989). Commentary on the treatment of Tourette's syndrome with CNS stimulants. *Journal of the American Academy of Child & Adolescent Psychiatry, 28,* 580–582.

Cohen, D. J., & Leckman, J. F. (1994). Developmental psychopathology and neurobiology of Tourette's syndrome. *Journal of the American Academy of Child & Adolescent Psychiatry, 33,* 2–15.

Cohen, D. J., Leckman, J. F., & Shaywitz, B. A. (1984). The Tourette's syndrome and other tics. In D. Shaffer, A. A. Ehrhardt, & L. Greenhill (Eds.), *Diagnosis and treatment in pediatric psychiatry* (pp. 3–28). New York: Macmillan Free Press.

Cohen, D. J., Ort, S. I., Caruso, K. A., Anderson, G. M., Hunt, R. D., Shaywitz, B. A., Kreminitzer, M., & Leckman, J. F. (1987). Parotid gland salivary secretion in Tourette's syndrome and attention deficit disorder: A model system for the study of neurochemical regulation. *Journal of the American Academy of Child Psychiatry, 26,* 65–68.

Cohen, D. J., Riddle, M. A., & Leckman, J. F. (1992). Pharmacotherapy of Tourette's syndrome and associated disorders. *Psychiatric Clinics of North America, 15,* 109–129.

Cohen, D. J., Shaywitz, B. A., Caparulo, B., Young, J. G., & Bowers, M. B., Jr. (1978). Chronic, multiple tics of Gilles de la Tourette's disease. CSF acid monoamine metabolites after probenecid administration. *Archives of General Psychiatry, 35,* 245–250.

Cohen, D. J., Shaywitz, B. A., Young, J. G., & Bowers, M. B., Jr. (1980). Cerebrospinal fluid monoamine metabolites in neuropsychiatric disorders of childhood. In J. H. Wood (Ed.), *Neurobiology of cerebrospinal fluid: Vol. 1* (pp. 665–683). New York: Plenum Publishing Corporation.

Cohen, D. J., Shaywitz, B. A., Young, J. G., Carbonari, C. M., Nathanson, J. A., Lieberman, D., Bowers, M. B., Jr., & Maas, J. W. (1979). Central biogenic amine metabolism in children with the syndrome of chronic multiple tics of Gilles de la Tourette: Norepinephrine, serotonin, and dopamine. *Journal of the American Academy of Child Psychiatry, 18,* 320–341.

Cohen, D. J., Towbin, K. E., & Leckman, J. F. (1992). Tourette's syndrome: A model developmental neuropsychiatric disorder. In C. Chiland & J. G. Young (Eds.), *New approaches to mental health from birth to adolescence* (pp. 121–152). New Haven, CT: Yale University Press.

Cohen, D. J., Young, J. G., Nathanson, J. A., & Shaywitz, B. A. (1979). Clonidine in Tourette's syndrome. *Lancet, 2,* 551–553.

Cohen, J. L., Hollander, E., DeCaria, C. M., Stein, D. J., Simeon, D., Liebowitz, M. R., & Aronowitz, B. R. (1996). Specificity of neuropsychological impairment in obsessive compulsive disorder: A comparison with social phobic and normal control subjects. *Journal of Neuroscience & Clinical Neurosciences, 8,* 82–85.

Cohen, L. S., & Rosenbaum, J. F. (1987). Clonazepam: New uses and potential problems. *Journal of Clinical Psychiatry, 48*(10, Suppl.), 50–55.

Cohen, P., Velez, N., Kohn, M., Schwab-Stone, M., & Johnson, J. (1987). Child psychiatric diagnosis by computer algorithm: Theoretical issues and empirical tests. *Journal of the American Academy of Child & Adolescent Psychiatry, 26,* 631–638.

Cohen v. Boston University. (1993). A graduate student refused re-admission because of a TS diagnosis.

Coie, J. D., & Dodge, K. A. (1983). Continuinities and changes in children's social status: A five-year longitudinal study. *Merrill-Palmer Quarterly, 29,* 261–281.

Coie, J. D., Dodge, K. A., & Coppotelli, H. (1982). Dimensions and types of social status: A cross-age perspective. *Developmental Psychology, 18,* 557–570.

Collier, C. P., Soldin, S. J., Swanson, J. M., MacLeod, S. M., Weinberg, F., & Rochefort, J. G. (1985). Pemoline pharmacokinetics and long term therapy in children with attention deficit disorder and hyperactivity. *Clinical Pharmacokinetics, 10,* 269–286.

Comings, D. E. (1990). Blood serotonin and tryptophan in Tourette syndrome. *American Journal of Medical Genetics, 36,* 418–430.

Comings, D. E. (1995a). Tourette's syndrome: A behavioral spectrum disorder. In W. J. Weiner & A. E. Lang (Eds.), *Advances in neurology: Vol. 65. Behavioral neurology of movement disorders* (pp. 293–303). New York: Raven Press.

Comings, D. E. (1995b). Tourette syndrome: A hereditary neuropsychiatric spectrum disorder. *Annals of Clinical Psychiatry, 6,* 235–247.

Comings, D. E., & Comings, B. G. (1984). Tourette's syndrome and attention deficit disorder with hyperactivity: Are they genetically related? *Journal of the American Academy of Child Psychiatry, 23,* 138–146.

Comings, D. E., & Comings, B. G. (1985). Tourette syndrome: Clinical and psychological aspects of 250 cases. *American Journal of Human Genetics, 35,* 435–450.

Comings, D. E., & Comings, B. G. (1987a). A controlled study of Tourette syndrome: I. Attention-deficit learning disorders, and school problems. *American Journal of Human Genetics, 41,* 701–741.

Comings, D. E., & Comings, B. G. (1987b). A controlled study of Tourette syndrome: II. Conduct. *American Journal of Human Genetics, 41,* 742–760.

Comings, D. E., & Comings, B. G. (1987c). A controlled study of Tourette syndrome: III. Phobias and panic attacks. *American Journal of Human Genetics, 41,* 761–781.

Comings, D. E., & Comings, B. G. (1987d). A controlled study of Tourette syndrome: IV. Obsessions, compulsions, and schizoid behaviors. *American Journal of Human Genetics, 41,* 782–803.

Comings, D. E., & Comings, B. G. (1987e). A controlled study of Tourette syndrome: V. Depression and mania. *American Journal of Human Genetics, 41,* 804–821.

Comings, D. E., & Comings, B. G. (1987f). A controlled study of Tourette syndrome: VI. Early development, sleep problems, allergies, and handedness. *American Journal of Human Genetics, 41,* 822–838.

Comings, D. E., & Comings, B. G. (1987g). A controlled study of Tourette's syndrome: VII. Summary: A Common genetic disorder causing disinhibition in the limbic system. *American Journal of Human Genetics, 41,* 839–866.

Comings, D. E., & Comings, B. G. (1987h). Tourette syndrome and attention deficit disorder with hyperactivity. *Archives of General Psychiatry, 44,* 1023–1026.

Comings, D. E., Comings, B. G., Devor, E. J., & Cloninger, C. R. (1984). Detection of a major gene for Gilles de la Tourette syndrome. *American Journal of Human Genetics, 36,* 586–600.

Comings, D. E., Comings, B. G., Muhleman, D., Dietz, G., Shahbahrami, B., Tast, D., Knell, E., Kocsis, P., Baumgarten, R., Kovacs, B. W., Levy, D. L., Smith, M., Borison, R. L., Evans, D., Klein, D. N., MacMurray, J., Tosk, J. M., Sverd, J., Gysin, R., & Flanagan, S. D. (1991). The dopamine D2 receptor locus as a modifying gene in neuropsychiatric disorders. *Journal of the American Medical Association, 266,* 1793–1800.

Comings, D. E., Goetz, I. E., Holden, J., & Holtz, J. (1981). Huntington disease and Tourette syndrome: II. Uptake of glutamic acid and other amino acids by fibroblasts. *American Journal of Human Genetics, 33,* 175–186.

Comings, D. E., Himes, J. A., & Comings, B. G. (1990). An epidemiological study of Tourette's syndrome in a single school district. *Journal of Clinical Psychiatry, 51,* 463–469.

Comings, D. E., Wu, S., Chiu, C., Ring, R. H., Gade, R., Ahn, C., MacMurray, J. P., Dietz, G., & Muhleman, D. (1996). Polygenic inheritance of Tourette syndrome, stuttering, attention deficit hyperactivity, conduct, and oppositional defiant disorder: The additive and subtractive effect of the three dopaminergic genes—DRD2, D beta H, and DAT1. *American Journal of Medical Genetics, 67,* 264–288.

Como, P. G. (1993). Neuropsychological testing. In R. Kurlan (Ed.), *Handbook of Tourette's syndrome and related tic and behavioral disorders* (pp. 221–243). New York: Marcel Dekker.

Como, P. G., & Kurlan, R. (1991). An open-label trial of fluoxetine for obsessive-compulsive disorder in Gilles de la Tourette's syndrome. *Neurology, 41,* 872–874.

Conners, C. K. (1969). A teacher rating scale for use in drug studies in children. *American Journal of Psychiatry, 126,* 884–888.

Conners, C. K. (1989). *Conners' Rating Scales Manual.* North Tonowanda, NY: Multi-Health Systems.

Conners, C. K. (1994). *The Connors Continuous Performance Test (CPT): Computer program* (Version 3.0). North Tonawanda, NY: Multi-Health Systems.

Conners, C. K., & Barkley, R. A. (1985). Rating scales and checklists for child psychopathology. *Psychopharmacology Bulletin, 21,* 809–816.

Conners, C. K., Eisenberg, L., & Barcai, A. (1967). Effect of dextroamphetamine on children: Studies on subjects with learning disabilities and school behavior problems. *Archives of General Psychiatry, 17,* 478–485.

Conners, C. K., & Taylor, E. (1980). Pemoline, methylphenidate, and placebo in children with minimal brain dysfunction. *Archives of General Psychiatry, 37,* 922–930.

Cook, E. H., Jr., Charak, D. A., Trapani, C., Zelko, F. A. J., Arida, J., Kieffer, J. E., Jaselskis, C. A., & Leventhal, B. L. (1994). Sertraline treatment of obsessive-compulsive disorder in children and adolescents: Preliminary findings. *American Academy of Child & Adolescent Psychiatry Abstracts, 10*(No. NR-71), 57.

Cook, E. H., Stein, M. A., Krasowski, M. D., Cox, N. J., Olkon, D. M., Kieffer, J. E., & Leventhal, B. L. (1995). Association of attention-deficit disorder and the dopamine transporter gene. *American Journal of Human Genetics, 56,* 993–998.

Cooper, I. S. (1969). *Involuntary movement disorders.* New York: Harper & Row.

Cooper, J. (1970). The Leyton Obsessional Inventory. *Psychological Medicine, 1,* 48–64.

Corbett, J. A., Mathews, A. M., Connell, P. H., & Shapiro, D. A. (1969). Tics and Gilles de la Tourette's syndrome: A follow-up study and critical review. *British Journal of Psychiatry, 115,* 1229–1241.

Cosgrove, G. R., & Rauch, S. L. (1995). *Psychosurgery and Neurosurgery Clinic of North America, 6,* 167–176.

Costello, E. J., & Angold, A. (1988). Scales to assess child and adolescent depression: Checklists, screens, and nets. *Journal of the American Academy of Child & Adolescent Psychiatry, 27,* 726–737.

Costello, E. J., Angold, A., Burns, B. J., Stangl, D. K., Tweed, D. L., & Erkanli, A. (1996). The Great Smokey Mountains study of youth: Functional impairment and serious emotional disturbance. *Archives of General Psychiatry, 53,* 1137–1143.

Costello, E. J., Angold, A., Burns, B. J., Stangl, D. K., Tweed, D. L., Erkanli, A., & Worthman, C. M. (1996). The Great Smoky Mountains study of youth, goals, design, and the prevalence of *DSM-III-R* disorders. *Archives of General Psychiatry, 53,* 1129–1136.

Costello, E. J., Costello, A. J., Edelbrock, C., Burns, B. J., Dulcan, M. K., Brent, D., & Janiszewski, S. (1988). Psychiatric diagnoses in pediatric primary care: Prevalence and risk factors. *Archives of General Psychiatry, 45,* 1107–1116.

Cottraux, J., Mollard, E., Bouvard, M., & Marks, I. (1993). Exposure therapy, fluvoxamine, or combination treatment in obsessive-compulsive disorder: One year followup. *Psychiatry Research, 49,* 63–75.

Courchesne, E., Townsend, J. P., Akshoomoff, N. A., Yeung-Courchesne, R., Press, G. A., Murakami, J. W., Lincoln, A. J., James, H. E., Saitoh, O., Egaas, B., Haas, R. H., & Schreibman, L. (1993). A new finding: Impairment in shifting attention in autistic patients. In S. H. Broman & J. Grafman (Eds.), *Atypical cognitive deficits in developmental disorders: Implications for brain function* (pp. 101–137). Washington, DC: Erlbaum.

Cowart, V. S. (1988). The Ritalin controversy: What's made this drug's opponents hyperactive? *Journal of the American Medical Association, 259,* 2521–2523.

Crosley, C. J. (1979). Decreased serotonergic activity in Tourette syndrome. *Annals of Neurology, 5,* 596.

Crum, R. M., & Anthony, J. C. (1993). Cocaine use and other suspected risk factors for obsessive-compulsive disorder: A prospective study with data from the epidemiologic catchment area surveys. *Drug and Alcohol Dependence, 31,* 281–295.

Cuffe, S. P., McCullough, E. L., & Pumariega, A. J. (1994). Comorbidity of attention deficit hyperactivity disorder and post traumatic stress disorder. *Journal of Child and Family Studies, 3,* 327–336.

Cummings, J. L. (1995). Behavioral and psychiatric symptoms associated with Huntington's disease. In W. J. Weiner & A. E. Lang (Eds.), *Advances in neurology: Vol. 65. Behavioral neurology of movement disorders* (pp. 179–181). New York: Raven Press.

Cummings, J. L., & Cunningham, K. (1992). Obsessive-compulsive disorder in Huntington's disease. *Biologic Psychiatry, 31,* 236–270.

Dale, J. B., & Beachey, E. H. (1985). Multiple heart cross-reactive epitopes of streptococcal M protein. *Journal of Experimental Medicine, 161,* 113–122.

Damasio, A. R. (1985). Disorders of complex visual processing: Agnosias, achromatopsia, Balint's syndrome, and related difficulties of orientation and construction. In M. M. Mesulam (Ed.), *Principles of behavioral neurology* (pp. 259–288). Philadelphia: Davis.

Damasio, A. R. (1994). *Descartes' error: Emotion, reason and the human brain.* New York: Putnam.

Damasio, A. R., Damasio, H., & Chui, H. (1980). Neglect following damage to frontal lobe or basal ganglia. *Neuropsychologia, 18,* 123–132.

Damasio, A. R., Tranel, D., & Damasio, H. (1990). Individuals with sociopathic behavior caused by frontal damage fail to respond autonomically to social stimuli. *Behavioural Brain Research, 41,* 81–94.

Darwin, C. (1859). *On the origin of species by means of natural selection or the preservation of favored races in the struggle for life.* London: Murray.

Davis, J., Israni, T., Janicak, P., Wang, Z., & Holland, D. (1991). A meta-analysis of drug efficacy studies in obsessive compulsive disorder. *Biological Psychiatry, 29,* 444S.

Davis, S. M., & Lawrence, P. R. (1977). *Matrix.* Reading, MA: Addison-Wesley.

Dawkins, R. (1976). *The selfish gene.* Oxford, England: Oxford University Press.

Dawkins, R. (1987). *The blind watchmaker. Why the evidence of evolution reveals a universe without design.* New York: Norton.

de Boer, J. A., & Westenberg, H. G. M. (1992). Oxytocin in obsessive compulsive disorder. *Peptides, 13,* 1083–1085.

de Divitiis, E., D'Errico, A., & Cerillo, A. (1977). Stereotactic surgery in Gilles de la Tourette syndrome. *Acta Neurochirurgica, 24,* 73.

de Groot, C. M., Bornstein, R. A., Janus, M. D., & Mavissakalian, M. R. (1995). Patterns of obsessive compulsive symptoms in Tourette subjects are independent of severity. *Anxiety, 1,* 268–274.

de Groot, C. M., Janus, M. D., & Bornstein, R. A. (1995). Clinical predictors of psychopathology in children and adolescents with Tourette's syndrome. *Journal of Psychiatric Research, 29,* 59–70.

Delgado, P. L., Goodman, W. K., Price, L. H., Heninger, G. R., & Charney, D. S. (1990). Fluvoxamine/pimozide treatment of concurrent Tourette's and obsessive compulsive disorder. *British Journal of Psychiatry, 157,* 762–765.

Denckla, M. B., Harris, E. L., Aylward, E. H., Singer, H. S., Reiss, A. L., Reader, M. J., Bryan, R. N., & Chase, G. A. (1991). Executive functions and volume of the basal ganglia in children with Tourette's syndrome and attention deficit hyperactivity disorder. *Annals of Neurology, 30,* 476.

Department of Health and Human Services. (1990). *The national plan for research on child and adolescent disorders* (DHHS Publication No. ADM 90–1683). Washington, DC: U.S. Government Printing Office.

DeRosier, M. E., Kupersmidt, J. B., & Patterson, C. J. (1994). Children's academic and behavioral adjustment as a function of the chronicity and proximity of peer rejection. *Child Development, 65,* 1799–1813.

Deutsch, C. K., Matthysse, S., Swanson, J. M., & Farkas, L. G. (1990). Genetic latent structure analysis of dysmorphology in attention deficit disorder. *Journal of the American Academy of Child & Adolescent Psychiatry, 29,* 189–194.

deVeaugh-Geiss, J., Moroz, G., Biederman, J., Cantwell, D., Fontaine, R., Greist, J. H., Reichler, R., Katz, R., & Landau, P. (1992). Clomipramine hydrochloride in childhood and adolescent obsessive-compulsive disorder: A multicenter trial. *Journal of the American Academy of Child & Adolescent Psychiatry, 31,* 45–49.

Devinsky, O. (1983). Neuroanatomy of Gilles de la Tourette's syndrome. Possible midbrain involvement [Review]. *Archives of Neurology, 40,* 508–514.

Devinsky, O., Morrell, M. J., & Vogt, B. A. (1995). Contributions of anterior cingulate cortex to behavior. *Brain, 118,* 279–306.

Devor, E. J. (1984). Complex segregation analysis of Gilles de la Tourette syndrome: Further evidence for a major locus mode of transmission. *American Journal of Human Genetics, 36,* 704–709.

deVries, G. J., Best, W., & Sluiter, A. A. (1983). The influence of androgens on the development of a sex difference in the vasopressinergic innervation of the rat lateral septum. *Developmental Brain Research, 8,* 377–380.

deVries, G. J., Buijs, R. M., van Leeuwen, F. W., Caffe, A. R., & Swaab, D. F. (1985). The vasopressinergic innervation of the brain in normal and castrated rats. *Journal of Comparative Neurology, 233,* 236–254.

Diamond, A., & Goldman-Rakic, P. S. (1989). Comparison of human infants and rhesus monkeys on Piaget's AB task: Evidence for dependence on dorsolateral prefrontal cortex. *Experimental Brain Research, 74,* 24–40.

Diamond, M. C. (1991). Hormonal effects on the development of cerebral lateralization. *Psychoneuroendocrinology, 16,* 121–129.

Divac, I., Rosvold, H., & Szwarcbart, M. (1967). Behavioral effects of selective ablation of the caudate nucleus. *Journal of Comparative Physiology and Psychology, 63,* 184–190.

Doleys, D. M., & Kurtz, P. S. (1974). A behavioral treatment program for the Gilles de la Tourette syndrome. *Psychological Reports, 35,* 43–48.

Donnelly, M., Zametkin, A. J., Rapoport, J. L., Ismond, D. R., Weingartner, H., Lane, E., Oliver, J., Linnoila, M., & Potter, W. Z. (1986). Treatment of childhood hyperactivity with desipramine: Plasma drug concentration, cardiovascular effects, plasma and urinary catecholamine levels, and clinical response. *Clinical Pharmacology Therapy, 39,* 72–81.

Douglas, V. I. (1988). Cognitive deficits in children with attention deficit disorder with hyperactivity. In L. M. Bloomingdale & J. Sergeant (Eds.), *Attention deficit disorder: Criteria, cognition, intervention* (pp. 65–81). New York: Plenum Press.

Douglass, H. M., Moffitt, T. E., Dar, R., McGee, R., & Silva, P. (1995). Obsessive-compulsive disorder in a birth cohort of 18 year olds: Prevalence and predictors. *Journal of the American Academy of Child & Adolescent Psychiatry, 34,* 1424–1431.

Drewe, E. (1975). Go-no-go learning after frontal lobe lesions in humans. *Cortex, 11,* 8–16.

Dulcan, M. K. (1985). Attention deficit disorder: Evaluation and treatment. *Pediatric Annals, 14,* 383–400.

DuPaul, G. J. (1991). Parent and teacher ratings of ADHD symptoms: Psychometric properties in a community based sample. *Journal of Clinical Child Psychology, 20,* 245–253.

DuPaul, G. J., & Barkley, R. A. (1990). Medication therapy. In R. A. Barkley (Ed.), *Attention deficit hyperactivity disorder: A handbook for diagnosis and treatment* (2nd ed.). New York: Guilford Press.

DuPaul, G. J., Barkley, R. A., & McMurray, M. B. (1994). Response of children with ADHD to methylphenidate: Interaction with internalizing symptoms. *Journal of the American Academy of Child & Adolescent Psychiatry, 33,* 894–903.

Dursun, S. M., Farrar, G., Handley, S. L., Rickards, H., Betts, T., & Corbett, J. A. (1994). Elevated plasma kynurenine in Tourette syndrome. *Molecular & Chemical Neuropathology, 21,* 55–60.

Dursun, S. M., Hewitt, S., King, A. L., & Reveley, M. (1996). Treatment of blepharospasm with nicotine nasal spray. *Lancet, 348,* 60.

Dursun, S. M., Reveley, M. A., Bird, R., & Stirton, F. (1994). Long lasting improvement of Tourette's syndrome with transdermal nicotine [Letter]. *Lancet, 344,* 1577.

Dykens, E., Leckman, J. F., Riddle, M. A., Hardin, M. T., Schwartz, S., & Cohen, D. (1990). Intellectual, academic, and adaptive functioning of Tourette syndrome children with and without attention deficit disorder. *Journal of Abnormal Child Psychology, 18,* 607–615.

Eapen, V., Pauls, D. L., & Robertson, M. M. (1993). Evidence for autosomal dominant transmission in Tourette's syndrome–United Kingdom Cohort Study. *British Journal of Psychiatry, 162,* 593–596.

Eapen, V., Robertson, M. M., Alsobrook, J. P., II, & Pauls, D. L. (1997). Obsessive compulsive symptoms in Gilles de la Tourette's syndrome and obsessive compulsive disorder: Differences by diagnosis and family history. *American Journal of Medical Genetics, 74,* 432–438.

Eaves, L., Silberg, J., Hewitt, J., Meyer, J., Rutter, M., Simonoff, E., Neale, M., & Pickles, A. (1993). Genes, personality, and psychopathology: A latent class analysis of liability to symptoms of attention-deficit hyperactivity disorder in twins. In R. Plomin & G. McLearn (Eds.), *Nature, nurture, and psychology* (pp.). Washington, DC: American Psychological Association.

Ebaugh, F. G. (1923). Neuropsychiatric sequelae of acute epidemic encephalitis in children. *American Journal of Diseases of Childhood, 25,* 89–97.

Eblen, F., & Graybiel, A. M. (1995). Highly restricted origin of prefrontal cortical inputs to striosomes in the macque monkey. *Journal of Neuroscience, 15,* 5999–6013.

Edelbrock, C., & Achenbach, T. (1984). The teacher version of the Child Behavior Checklist: Boys aged 6 to 11. *Journal of Consulting and Clinical Psychology, 52,* 207–217.

Edelbrock, C., & Costello, A. J. (1988). Convergence between statistically derived behavior problem syndromes and child psychiatric diagnosis. *Journal of Abnormal Child Psychology, 16,* 219–231.

Edell, B. H., & Motta, R. W. (1989). The emotional adjustment of children with Tourette's syndrome. *Journal of Psychology, 123,* 1–57.

Edelman, G. M. (1987). *Neural darwinism—The theory of neuronal group selection.* New York: Basic Books.

Edelman, G. M., & Tononi, G. (1995). Neural darwinism—The brain as a selectional system. In J. Cornwell (Ed.), *Nature's imagination: The frontiers of scientific thought.* New York: Oxford University Press.

Eggers, C. H., Rothenberger, A., & Berghaus, U. (1988). Clinical and neurobiological findings in children suffering from tic disease following treatment with tiapride. *European Archives of Psychiatry & Neurological Science, 237,* 223–229.

Eisenberg, L., Lachman, R., & Molling, P. (1961). A psychopharmacologic experiment in a training school for delinquent boys. Methods, problems and findings. *American Journal of Orthopsychiatry, 33,* 431–447.

Eldridge, R., Sweet, R., Lake, R., Ziegler, M., & Shapiro, A. K. (1977). Gilles de la Tourette's syndrome: Clinical, genetic, psychologic, and biochemical aspects in 21 selected families. *Neurology, 27,* 115–124.

Elia, J. (1993). Drug treatment for hyperactive children. Therapeutic guidelines. *Drugs, 46,* 863–871.

Elia, J., & Rapoport, J. (1991). Methylphenidate versus dextroamphetamine: Why both should be tried. In B. Osman & L. L. Greenhill (Eds.), *Ritalin: Theory and patient management* (pp. 243–265). New York: Mary Ann Liebert.

Elliott, G. R., & Popper, C. W. (1990/1991). Tricyclic antidepressants: The QT interval and other cardiovascular parameters [Editorial]. *Journal of Child & Adolescent Psychopharmacology, 1,* 187–189.

Erenberg, G., Cruse, R. P., & Rothner, A. D. (1985). Gilles de la Tourette's syndrome: Effects of stimulant drugs. *Neurology, 35,* 1346–1348.

Erenberg, G., Cruse, R. P., & Rothner, A. D. (1986). Tourette syndrome. *Cleveland Clinic Quarterly, 53,* 127–131.

Erenberg, G., Cruse, R. P., & Rothner. A. D. (1987). The natural history of Tourette syndrome: A follow-up study. *Annals of Neurology, 22,* 383–385.

Ereshefsky, L., Riesenman, C., & Lam, Y. W. F. (1996). Serotonin selective reuptake inhibitor drug interactions and the cytochrome P450 system. *Journal of Clinical Psychiatry, 57,* 17–24.

Evans, D. W., Leckman, J. F., Carter, A., Reznick, J. S., Henshaw, D., & Pauls, D. L. (1997). Ritual, habit, and perfectionism: The prevalence and development of compulsive like behavior in normal young children. *Child Development, 68,* 58–68.

Evers, R. A. F., & van de Wetering, B. J. M. (1994). A treatment model for motor tics based on a specific tension-reduction technique. *Journal of Behavior Therapy and Experimental Psychiatry, 25,* 255–260.

Ewens, W. J., & Spielman, R. S. (1995). The transmission/disequilibrium test: History, subdivision, and admixture. *American Journal of Human Genetics, 57,* 455–464.

Fahn, S. (1993). Motor and vocal tics. In R. Kurlan (Ed.), *The handbook of Tourette's syndrome and related tic and behavioral disorders* (pp. 3–17). New York: Marcel Dekker.

Fahn, S., & Erenberg, G. (1988). Differential diagnosis of tic phenomena: A neurological perspective. In D. J. Cohen, R. D. Bruun, & J. F. Leckman (Eds.), *Tourette's syndrome and tic disorders: Clinical understanding and treatment* (pp. 41–54). New York: Wiley.

Falk, C. T., & Rubinstein, P. (1987). Haplotype relative risks: An easy reliable way to construct a proper control sample for risk calculations. *Annals of Human Genetics, 51,* 227–233.

Fallon, T., Jr., & Schwab-Stone, M. (1994). Determinants of reliability in psychiatric surveys of children aged 6 to 12. *Journal of Child Psychology & Psychiatry, 35,* 1391–1408.

Faraone, S. V., & Biederman, J. (1994). Genetics of attention-deficit hyperactivity disorder. *Child & Adolescent Psychiatric Clinics of North America,* 285–302.

Faraone, S. V., Biederman, J., Chen, W. J., Krifcher, B., Keenan, K., Moore, C., Sprich, S., & Tsuang, M. (1992). Segregation analysis of attention deficit hyperactivity disorder: Evidence for single gene transmission. *Psychiatric Genetics, 2,* 257–275.

Faraone, S. V., Biederman, J., Keenan, K., & Tsuang, M. T. (1991). A family-genetic study of girls with *DSM-III* attention deficit disorder. *American Journal of Psychiatry, 48,* 112–117.

Faraone, S. V., Biederman, J., Krifcher, B., Lehman, B., Spencer, T., Lehman, B., Spencer, T., Norman, D., Seidman, L. J., Kraus, I., Perrin, J., Chen, W. J., & Tsuang, M. T. (1993). Intellectual performance and school failure in children with attention deficit hyperactivity disorder and their siblings. *Journal of Abnormal Psychology, 102,* 616–623.

Faraone, S. V., Biederman, J., & Milberger, S. (1995). How reliable are maternal reports of their children's psychopathology? One-year recall of psychiatric diagnoses of ADHD children. *Journal of the American Academy Child & Adolescent Psychiatry, 34,* 1001–1008.

Faraone, S. V., Biederman, J., Sprich-Buckminster, S., Chen, W., & Tsuang, M. (1993). Efficiency of diagnostic criteria for attention deficit disorder: Toward an empirical approach to designing and validating diagnostic algorithms. *Journal of the American Academy of Child & Adolescent Psychiatry, 32,* 166–174.

Faretra, G., Doher, L., & Dowling, J. (1970). Comparison of haloperidol and fluphenazine in disturbed children. *American Journal of Psychiatry, 126,* 1670–1673.

Feighner, J. P., Robins, E., & Guze, S. B. (1972). Diagnostic criteria for use in psychiatric research. *Archives of General Psychiatry, 26,* 57–63.

Feldman, H., Crumrine, P., & Handen, B. L. (1989). Methylphenidate in children with seizures and attention-deficit disorder. *American Journal of Disabled Children, 143,*

Fernando, S. J. M. (1967). Gilles de la Tourette syndrome: A report on four cases and a review of published case reports. *British Journal of Psychiatry, 113,* 607–617.

Ferrari, M., Matthews, W. S., & Barabas, G. (1984). Children with Tourette syndrome: Results of psychological tests given prior to drug treatment. *Developmental and Behavioral Pediatrics, 5,* 116–119.

Ferrier, D. (1886). *The function of the brain* (2nd ed.). London: Smith, Elder.

Ferrier, D. (1890). *The Croonian lectures on cerebral localisation.* London: Smith, Elder.

Finney, J. W., Rapoff, M. A., Hall, C. L., & Christophersen, E. R. (1983). Replication and social validation of habit reversal treatment for tics. *Behavior Therapy, 14,* 116–126.

Fiore, T. A., & Becker, E. A. (1994). *Promising classroom interventions for students with attention deficit disorder.* Washington, DC: U.S. Department of Education.

Flament, M. F., Koby, E., Rapoport, J. L., Berg, C. J., Zahn, T., Cox, C., Denckla, M., & Lenane, M. (1990). Childhood obsessive-compulsive disorder: A prospective follow-up study. *Journal of Child Psychology & Psychiatry, 31,* 363–380.

Flament, M. F., Rapoport, J. L., Berg, C. J., Sceery, W., Kitts, C., Mellstrom, B., & Linnoila, M. (1985). Clomipramine treatment of childhood obsessive compulsive disorder: A double-blind controlled study. *Archives of General Psychiatry, 42,* 977–983.

Flament, M. F., Whitaker, A., Rapoport, J. L., Davies, M., Berg, C. Z., Kalikow, K., Sceery, W., & Schaffer, D. (1988). Obsessive-compulsive disorder in adolescence: An epidemiological study. *Journal of the American Academy of Child & Adolescent Psychiatry, 27,* 764–771.

Fleming, B., Anderson, R., Rhees, R., Kinghorn, E., & Bakaitis, J. (1986). Effects of prenatal stress on sexually dimorphic 21 in the cerebral cortex of the rat. *Brain Research Bulletin, 16,* 395–398.

Foa, E. B., & Emmelkamp, P. M. G. (1983). *Failures in behavior therapy.* New York: Wiley.

Foa, E. B., Steketee, G., Grayson, J. B., Turner, R. M., & Latimer, P. R. (1984). Deliberate exposure and blocking of obsessive-compulsive rituals: Immediate and long-term effects. *Behavior Therapy, 15,* 450–472.

Fox, A. M., & Rieder, M. J. (1993). Risks and benefits of drugs used in the management of the hyperactive child. *Drug Safety, 9,* 38–50.

Frank, M. S., Sieg, K. G., & Gaffney, G. R. (1991). Somatic complaints in childhood tic disorders. *Psychosomatics, 32,* 396–399.

Frankel, M., Cummings, J. L., Robertson, M. M., Trimble, M. R., Hill, M. A., & Benson, D. F. (1986). Obsessions and compulsions in Gilles de la Tourette's syndrome. *Neurology, 36,* 378–382.

Freud, S. (1953a). Case 2, Frau Emmy von N. In J. Strachey (Ed.), *The standard edition of the complete psychological works of Sigmund Freud* (Vol. II, pp. 48–105). London: Hogarth Press.

Freud, S. (1953b). Three essays on the theory of sexuality. In J. Strachey (Ed.), *The standard edition of the complete psychological works of Sigmund Freud* (Vol. VII, pp. 123–245). London: Hogarth Press.

Freud, S. (1953c). Repression. In J. Strachey (Ed.), *The standard edition of the complete psychological works of Sigmund Freud* (Vol. XIV). London: Hogarth Press.

Fride, E., & Weinstock, M. (1988). Prenatal stress increases anxiety related behavior and alters cerebral lateralization of dopamine activity. *Life Sciences, 42,* 1059–1065.

Fride, E., & Weinstock, M. (1989). Alterations in behavioral and striatal dopamine asymmetries induced by prenatal stress. *Pharmacology Biochemistry and Behavior, 32,* 425–430.

Fried, I., Katz, A., McCarthy, G., Sass, K., Spencer, S., & Spencer, D. (1991). Functional organization of human supplementary motor cortex studies by electrical stimulation. *Journal of Neuroscience, 11,* 3656–3666.

Friedhoff, A. J., & Chase, T. N. (Eds.). (1982). *Advances in neurology: Vol. 35. Gilles de la Tourette's syndrome.* New York: Raven Press.

Frost, L. A., Moffitt, T. E., & McGee, R. (1989). Neuropsychological correlates of psychopathology in an unselected cohort of young adolescents. *Journal of Abnormal Psychology, 98,* 307–313.

Fulker, D. W., Cardon, L. R., DeFries, J. C., Kimberling, W. J., Pennington, B. F., & Smith, S. D. (1991). Multiple regression analysis of sib-pair on reading to detect quantitative trait loci. *Reading and Writing Interdisciplinary Journal, 3,* 299–313.

Fuller, R. W., & Clemens, J. A. (1991). Pergolide: A dopamine agonist at both D_1 and D_2 receptors. *Life Science, 49,* 925–930.

Fuster, J. M. (1995). *Memory in the cerebral cortex.* Cambridge, MA: MIT Press.

Gadow, K. D., Nolan, E., Sprafkin, J., & Sverd, J. (1995). School observations of children with attention-deficit hyperactivity disorder and comorbid tic disorder: Effects of methylphenidate treatment. *Developmental Behavioural Pediatrics, 16,* 167–176.

Gadow, K. D., Sverd, J., Sprafkin, J., Nolan, E. E., & Ezor, S. N. (1995). Efficacy of methylphenidate for attention-deficit hyperactivity disorder in children with tic disorder. *Archives of General Psychiatry, 52,* 444–455.

Gainotti, G. (1985). Constructional apraxia. In P. J. Vinken, G. W. Bruyn, & H. L. Klawans (Eds.), *Handbook of clinical neurology* (pp. 491–505). Amsterdam, The Netherlands: Elsevier Science.

Gainotti, G., & Tiacci, C. (1970). Patterns of drawing disability in right and left hemispheric patients. *Neuropsychologia, 8,* 379–384.

Galderisi, S., Mucci, A., Catapano, F., D'Amato, A. C., & Maj, M. (1995). Neuropsychological slowness in obsessive-compulsive patients. Is it confined to tests involving the fronto-subcortical systems? *British Journal of Psychiatry, 167,* 394–398.

Gamble, W. C., & McHale, S. M. (1989). Coping with stress in sibling relationships: A comparison of children with disabled and nondisabled siblings. *Journal of Applied Developmental Psychology, 10,* 353–373.

Gammon, G. D., & Brown, T. E. (1993). Fluoxetine and methylphenidate in combination for treatment of attention deficit disorder and comorbid depressive disorder. *Journal of Child & Adolescent Psychopharmacology, 3,* 1–10.

Gao, J.-H., Parson, L. M., Bower, J. M., Xiong, J., Li, J., & Fox, P. T. (1996). Cerebellum implicated in sensory acquisition and discrimination rather than motor control. *Science, 272,* 545–547.

Garfinkel, B. D., Wender, P. H., Sloman, L., & O'Neil, I. (1983). Tricyclic antidepressant and methylphenidate treatment of attention deficit disorder in children. *Journal of American Academy of Child & Adolescent Psychiatry, 22,* 343–348.

Garland, E. J., & Weiss, M. (1996). Case study: Obsessive difficult temperament and its response to serotonergic medication. *Journal of the American Academy of Child & Adolescent Psychiatry, 35,* 916–920.

Gastfriend, D. R., Biederman, J., & Jellinek, M. S. (1984). Desipramine in the treatment of adolescents with attention deficit disorder. *American Journal of Psychiatry, 141,* 906–908.

Gelernter, J., & Freimer, M. (1994). PstI STS RFLP at serotonin transporter protein (SERT) locus. *Human Molecular Genetics, 3,* 383.

Gelernter, J., Grandy, D. K., Bunzow, J., Pakstis, A. J., Civelli, O., Retief, A. E., Litt, M., & Kidd, K. K. (1989). D2 dopamine receptor locus (probe hD2G1) maps close to D11S29 (probe L7) and is also linked to PBGD (probe PBGD0.9) and D11S84 (probe p2-7-ID6) on 11q. *Cytogenetic and Cell Genetics, 51,* 1002.

Gelernter, J., Kennedy, J., Grandy, D., Zhou, Q.-Y., Civelli, O., Pauls, D. L., Pakstis, A., Kurlan, R., Sunahara, R., Niznik, H., O'Dowd, B., Seeman, P., & Kidd, K. K. (1993). Exclusion of close linkage of Tourette's syndrome to D1-dopamine receptor. *American Journal of Psychiatry, 150,* 449–453.

Gelernter, J., Pakstis, A. J., & Kidd, K. K. (1995). Linkage mapping of serotonin transporter protein gene SLC6A4 on chromosome 17. *Human Genetics, 95,* 677–680.

Gelernter, J., Pakstis, A. J., Pauls, D. L., Kurlan, R., Gancher, S., Civelli, O., Grandy, D., & Kidd, K. K. (1990). Gilles de la Tourette syndrome not linked to D2-dopamine receptor. *Archives of General Psychiatry, 47,* 1073–1077.

Gelernter, J., Pauls, D. L., Leckman, J. F., Kidd, K. K., & Kurlan, R. (1994). D2 dopamine receptor (DRD2) alleles do not influence severity of Tourette syndrome in four large kindreds. *Archives of Neurology, 51,* 397–400.

Geller, D. A., Biederman, J., Reed, E. D., Spencer, T., & Wilens, T. E. (1995). Similarities in response to fluoxetine in the treatment of children and adolescents with obsessive-compulsive disorder. *Journal of the American Academy of Child & Adolescent Psychiatry, 34,* 36–44.

George, M. S., Ketter, T. A., Parekh, P. I., Rosinsky, N., Ring, H., Casey, B. J., Trimble, M. R., Horwitz, B., Herscovitch, P., & Post, R. M. (1994). Regional brain activity when selecting a response despite interference: An H2^{15}O PET study of the Stroop and an emotional Stroop. *Human Brain Map, 1,* 194–209.

George, M. S., Robertson, M. M., Costa, D. C., Ell, P. J., Trimble, M. R., Pilowsky, L., & Verhoeff, N. G. (1994). Dopamine receptor availability in Tourette's syndrome. *Psychiatry Research: Neuroimaging, 55,* 193–203.

George, M. S., Trimble, M. R., Costa, D. C., Robertson, M. M., Ring, H. A., & Ell, P. J. (1992). Elevated frontal cerebral blood flow in Gilles de la Tourette syndrome: A 99Tcm-HMPAO SPECT study. *Psychiatry Research, 45,* 143–151.

George, M. S., Trimble, M. R., Ring, H. A., Sallee, F. R., & Robertson, M. M. (1993). Obsessions in obsessive-compulsive disorder with and without Gilles de la Tourette's syndrome. *American Journal of Psychiatry, 150,* 93–97.

Georgiou, N., Bradshaw, J. L., Phillips, J. G., & Chiu, E. (1996). The effect of Huntington's disease and Gilles de la Tourette's syndrome on the ability to hold and shift attention. *Neuropsychologia, 34,* 843–851.

Gerlach, J. (1991). New antipsychotics: Classification, efficacy, and adverse effects. *Schizophrenia Bulletin, 17,* 289–309.

Gerlach, J., & Peacock, L. (1995). New antipsychotics: The present status. *International Clinical Psychopharmacology, 10,* 39–48.

Gevins, A., Smith, M. E., Leong, H., McEvoy, L., Whitfield, S., Du, R., & Rush, G. (1998). Monitoring working memory load during computer-based asks with EEG pattern recognition methods. *Human Factors, 40,* 79–91.

Giedd, J. N., Castellanos, F. X., Casey, B. J., Kozuch, P., King, A. C., Hamburger, S. D., & Rapoport J. L. (1994). Quantitative morphology of the corpus callosum in attention deficit hyperactivity disorder. *American Journal of Psychiatry, 151,* 665–669.

Giedd, J. N., Rapoport, J. L., Kruesi, M. J. P., Parker, C., Schapiro, M. B., Allen, A. J., Leonard, H. L., Kaysen, D., Dickstein, D. P., Marsh, W. L., Kozuch, P. L., Vaituzis, A. C., Hamburger, S. D., & Swedo, S. E. (1995). Sydenham's chorea: Magnetic resonance imaging of the basal ganglia. *Neurology, 45,* 2199–2202.

Gilles de la Tourette, G. (C. G. Goetz & H. L. Klawans [Trans.]). (1982). Étude sur une affection nerveuse caractérisée par de l'incoordination motrice accompagnée d'echolalie et de coprolalie [Study of a neurologic condition characterized by motor incoordination accompanied by echolalia and coprolalia]. In A. J. Friedhoff & T. N. Chase (Eds.), *Advances in neurology: Vol. 35. Gilles de la Tourette syndrome* (pp. 1–16). New York: Raven Press.

Gillman, S., Dauth, D. W., Frey, K. A., & Penny, J. B. (1987). Experimental hemiplegia in the monkey: Basal ganglia glucose activity during recovery. *Annals of Neurology, 22,* 370 –376.

Gittelman-Klein, R. (1980). The role of psychological tests for differential diagnosis in child psychiatry. *Journal of the American Academy of Child & Adolescent Psychiatry, 19,* 413–437.

Gittelman-Klein, R. (1987). Pharmacotherapy of childhood hyperactivity: An update. In H. Y. Meltzer (Ed.), *Psychopharmacology: The third generation of progress* (3rd ed., pp. 1215–1224). New York: Raven Press.

Gittelman-Klein, R., Klein, D. F., Katz, S., Saraf, K., & Pollack, E. (1976). Comparative effects of methylphenidate and thioridazine in hyperkinetic children: I. Clinical results. *Archives of General of Psychiatry, 33,* 1217–1231.

Gittelman-Klein, R., Mannuzza, S., Shenker, R., & Bonagura, N. (1985). Hyperactive boys almost grown up: I. Psychiatric status. *Archives of General Psychiatry, 42,* 937–947.

Glaze, D. G., Frost, J. D., & Jankovic, J. (1983). Sleep in Gilles de la Tourette's syndrome: Disorder of arousal. *Neurology, 33,* 586–592.

Goeth, J. W. (1994). *Collected works in twelve volumes.* Princeton: Princeton University Press.

Goetz, C. G. (1993). Clonidine. In R. Kurlan (Ed.), *Handbook of Tourette's syndrome and related tic and behavioral disorders* (pp. 377–388). New York: Marcel Dekker.

Goetz, C. G., & Bennett, D. A. (1992). Pharmacology of paroxysmal dyskinesias. In H. L. Klawans, C. G. Goetz, & C. M. Tanner (Eds.), *Textbook of clinical neuropharmacology and therapeutics* (2nd ed., pp. 207–214). New York: Raven Press.

Goetz, C. G., & Klawans, H. L. (1992). Gilles de la Tourette on Tourette's syndrome. In A. J. Friedhoff, T. N. Chase, & D. J. Cohen (Eds.), *Advances in neurology: Vol. 35. Gilles de la Tourette's syndrome* (pp. 1–16). New York: Raven Press.

Goetz, C. G., Stebbins, G. T., & Thelen, J. A. (1987). Talipexole and adult Gilles de la Tourette's syndrome: Double-blind, placebo-controlled clinical trial. *Movement Disorders, 9,* 315–317.

Goetz, C. G., Tanner, C. M., & Klawans, H. L. (1984). Fluphenazine and multifocal tic disorders. *Archives of Neurology, 41,* 271–272.

Goetz, C. G., Tanner, C. M., Stebbins, G. T., Leipzig, G., & Carr, W. C. (1992). Adult tics in Gilles de la Tourette's syndrome. Description and risk factors. *Neurology, 42,* 784–788.

Goetz, C. G., Tanner, C. M., Wilson, R. S., Carroll, V. S., Como, P. G., & Shannon, K. M. (1987). Clonidine and Gilles de la Tourette syndrome: Double-blind study using objective rating methods. *Annals of Neurology, 21,* 307–310.

Goetz, C. G., Tanner, C. M., Wilson, R. S., & Shannon, K. M. (1987). A rating scale for Gilles de la Tourette's syndrome: Description, reliability, and validity. *Neurology, 37,* 1542–1544.

Golden, G. S. (1974). Gilles de la Tourette's syndrome following methylphenidate administration. *Developmental Medicine and Child Neurology, 16,* 76–78.

Golden, G. S. (1984). Psychologic and neuropsychologic aspects of Tourette's syndrome. *Neurologic Clinics, 2,* 91–102.

Golden, G. S. (1990). Tourette syndrome: Recent advances. *Neurologic Clinics, 8,* 3.

Goldman-Rakic, P. (1987). Circuitry of primate prefrontal cortex and regulation of behavior by representational memory. In V. Mountcastle, F. Plum, & S. Geiger (Eds.), *Handbook of physiology. The nervous system* (pp. 373–416). Bethesda, MD: American Physiological Society.

Goldman-Rakic, P. (1988). Topography of cognition: Parallel distributed networks in primate association cortex. *Annual Review of Neurosciences, 11,* 137–156.

Goldman-Rakic, P., & Selemon, L. (1990). New frontiers in basal ganglia research. *Trends in Neorscience, 13,* 241–243.

Gonce, M., & Barbeau, A. (1977). Seven cases of Gilles de la Tourette's syndrome: Partial relief with clonazepam: A pilot study. *Canadian Journal of Neurology of Science, 3,* 279–283.

Goodman, R., & Stevenson, J. (1989). A twin study of hyperactivity: I. An examination of hyperactivity scores and categories derived from Rutter teacher and parent questionnaires. *Journal of Child Psychology & Psychiatry, 30,* 671–689.

Goodman, W. K., McDougle, C. J., Price, L. H., Riddle, M. A., Pauls, D. L., & Leckman, J. F. (1990). Beyond the serotonin hypothesis: A role for dopamine in some forms of obsessive compulsive disorder? *Journal of Clinical Psychiatry, 51*(Suppl.), 36–43.

Goodman, W. K., Price, L. H., Rasmussen, S. A., Delgado, P. L., Heninger, G. R., & Charney, D. S. (1989). Efficacy of fluvoxamine in obsessive-compulsive disorder: A double-blind comparison with placebo. *Archives of General Psychiatry, 46,* 36–43.

Goodman, W. K., Price, L. H., Rasmussen, S. A., Mazure, C., Delgado, P., Heninger, G. R., & Charney, D. S. (1989). The Yale-Brown Obsessive Compulsive Scale: Validity. *Archives of General Psychiatry, 46,* 1012–1016.

Goodman, W. K., Price, L. H., Rasmussen, S. A., Mazure, C., Fleischmann, R. L., Hill, C. L., Heninger, G. R., & Charney, D. S. (1989). The Yale-Brown Obsessive Compulsive Scale: Development, use and reliability. *Archives of General Psychiatry, 46,* 1006–1011.

Goodman, W. K., Rasmussen, S. A., Foa, E., & Price, L. H. (1994). Obsessive compulsive disorder. In R. F. Prien & D. S. Robinson (Eds.), *Clinical evaluation of psychotropic drugs: Principles and guidelines* (pp. 431–466). New York: Raven Press.

Gottesman, I. I., & Shields, J. A. (1982). *Schizophrenia: The epigenetic puzzle.* Cambridge, England: Cambridge University Press.

Goyette, C. H., Conners, C. K., & Ulrich, R. F. (1978). Normative data on revised Conners' Parent and Teacher Rating Scales. *Journal of Abnormal Child Psychology, 6,* 221–236.

Grad, L. R., Pelcovitz, D., Olson, M., Matthews, M., & Grad, G. J. (1984). Obsessive-compulsive symptomology in children with Tourette's syndrome. *Journal of the American Academy of Child Psychiatry, 26,* 9–74.

Graybiel, A. M. (1990). Neurotransmitters and neuromodulators in the basal ganglia. *Trends in Neuroscience, 13,* 244–254.

Graybiel, A. M. (1995). Building action repertoires: Memory and learning functions of the basal ganglia. *Current Opinions in Neurobiology, 5,* 733–741.

Graybiel, A. M. (1996). Basal ganglia: New therapeutic approaches to Parkinson's disease. *Current Biology, 6,* 368–371.

Graybiel, A. M., Aosaki, T., Flaherty, A. W., & Kimura, M. (1994). The basal ganglia and adaptive motor control. *Science, 265,* 1826–1831.

Green, W. H. (1991). *Child and adolescent clinical psychopharmacology.* Baltimore: Williams & Wilkins.

Green, W. H. (1995). The treatment of attention-deficit hyperactivity disorder with nonstimulant medications. *Child and Adolescent Psychiatric Clinics of North America, 4,* 169.

Greenberg, B. D., McCann, U. D., & Benjamin, J. (1997). Repetitive TMS as a probe in anxiety disorders: Theoretical considerations and case reports. *CNS Spectrums, 2,* 47–52.

Greenberg, D. A. (1992). There is more than one way to collect data for linkage analysis. What a study of epilepsy can tell us about linkage strategy for psychiatric disease. *Archives of General Psychiatry, 49,* 745–750.

Greenfield, G., & Wolfsohn, J. (1922). The pathology of Sydenham's chorea. *Lancet, 2,* 603–607.

Greenhill, L. L. (1989). Treatment issues in children with attention-deficit hyperactivity disorder. *Psychiatry Annals, 119,* 604–613.

Greenhill, L. L. (1992a). Pharmacologic treatment of attention deficit hyperactivity disorder. *Psychiatric Clinics of North America, 15,* 1–28.

Greenhill, L. L. (1992b). Pharmacotherapy: Stimulants. *Child and Adolescent Psychiatric Clinics of North America. Pediatric Psychopharmacology, 1,* 411–417.

Greenhill, L. L. (1995). Attention-deficit hyperactivity disorder: The stimulants. *Child and Adolescent Psychiatric Clinics of North America. Pediatric Psychopharmacology, 4,* 123-.

Greist, J. H. (1992). *Fluvoxamine in OCD: A multicenter parallel design double-blind placebo-controlled trial.* Poster presented at the 18th CINP Congress.

Greist, J. H., Chouinard, G., DuBoff, E., Halaris, A., Kim, S. W., Koran, L., Liebowitz, M., Lydiard, R. B., Rasmussen, S., White, K., & Sikes, C. (1995). Double-blind parallel comparison of three dosages of sertraline and placebo in outpatients with obsessive-compulsive disorder. *Archives of General Psychiatry, 52,* 289–295.

Greist, J. H., Jefferson, J. W., Kobak, K. A., Katzelnick, D. J., & Serlin, R. C. (1995). Efficacy and tolerability of serotonin transport inhibitors in obsessive-compulsive disorder. *Archives of General Psychiatry, 52,* 53–60.

Gresham, F. M., & Elliott, S. N. (1987). Social skills deficits of learning-disabled students: Issues of definition, classification, and assessment. *Journal of Reading, Writing, & Learning Disabilities International, 3,* 131–148.

Gresham, F. M., & Elliott, S. N. (1993). Social skills intervention guide: Systematic approaches to social skills training. *Special Services in the Schools, 8,* 137–158.

Grice, D. E., Leckman, J. F., Pauls, D. L., Kurlan, R., Kidd, K. K., Pakstis, A. J., Chang, F. M., Cohen, D. J., & Gelernter, J. (1996). Linkage disequilibrium between an allele at the dopamine D4 receptor locus with Tourette's syndrome by the transmission disequilibrium test. *American Journal of Human Genetics, 59,* 644–652.

Grimshaw, L. (1964). Obsessional disorder and neurological illness. *Journal of Neurology, Neurosurgery, & Psychiatry, 27,* 229–231.

Gross, J., Lun, A., & Berndt, C. (1993). Early postnatal hypoxia induces long-term changes in the dopamine system in rats. *Journal of Neural Transmission. General Section, 93,* 103–121.

Grossman, A., Moult, P. J., Cunnah, D., & Besser, M. (1986). Different opioid mechanisms are involved in the modulation of ACTH and gonadotrophin release in man. *Neuroendocrinology, 42,* 357–360.

Grossman, H. Y., Mostofsky, D. I., & Harrison, R. H. (1986). Psychological aspects of Gilles de la Tourette syndrome. *Journal of Clinical Psychology, 42,* 228–235.

Gruart, A., & Delgado-Garcia, J. M. (1994). Discharge of identified deep cerebellar nuclei neurons related to eye blinks in the alert cat. *Neuroscience, 61,* 665–681.

Gualtieri, C. T., Wargin, W., Kanoy, R., Patrick, K., Shen, C. D., Youngblood, W., Mueller, R. A., & Breese, G. R. (1982). Clinical studies of methylphenidate serum levels in children and adults. *Journal of the American Academy of Child & Adolescent Psychiatry, 21,* 19–26.

Guy, W. (1976). *ECDEU Assessment Manual for Psychopharmacology* (Publication 76-338). Washington, DC: U.S. Department of Health, Education, and Welfare.

Gyapay, G., Morissette, J., Vignal, Dib, C., Fizames, C., Millasseau, P., Marc, S., Bernardi, G., Lathrop, M., & Weissenbach, J. (1994). The 1993–1994 Genethon human genetic linkage map. *Nature Genetics, 7,* 246–339.

Haber, S. N. (1986). Neurotransmitters in the human and nonhuman primate basal ganglia. *Human Neurobiology, 5,* 159–168.

Haber, S. N., Kowall, N., Vonsattel, J., Bird, E., & Richardson, E. J. (1986). Gilles de la Tourette's syndrome: A postmortem neuropathological and immunohistochemical study. *Journal of Neurological Sciences, 75,* 225–241.

Haber, S. N., & Wolfer, D. (1992). Basal ganglia peptidergic staining in Tourette syndrome. A follow-up study. In T. N. Chase, A. J. Friedhoff & D. J. Cohen (Eds.), *Advances in neurology: Vol. 58. Tourette syndrome: Genetics, neurobiology and treatment* (pp. 145–150). New York: Raven Press.

Hagin, R. A., Beecher, R., Pagano, G., & Kreeger, H. (1982). Effects of Tourette syndrome on learning. *Advances in Neurology, 35,* 323–328.

Hamilton, A. M. (1959). The assessment of anxiety states by rating. *British Journal of Medical Psychology, 32,* 50–55.

Hamilton, A. M. (1997, February 13). From taunts to tolerance of Tourette's. *The Hartford Courant,* pp. A1–A10.

Hamlett, K. W., Pellegrini, D. S., & Katz, K. S. (1992). Childhood chronic illness as a family stressor. *Journal of Pediatric Psychology, 17,* 33–47.

Hanin, I., Merikangas, J. R., Merikangas, K. R., & Kopp, U. (1979). Red-cell choline and Gilles de la Tourette syndrome. *New England Journal of Medicine, 301,* 661–662.

Hanna, G. L. (1995). Demographic and clinical features of obsessive-compulsive disorder in children and adolescents. *Journal of the American Academy of Child & Adolescent Psychiatry, 34,* 19–27.

Hanna, G. L., McCracken, J. T., & Cantwell, D. P. (1991). Prolactin in childhood obsessive-compulsive disorder: Clinical correlates and response to clomipramine. *Journal of American Academy of Child & Adolescent Psychiatry, 30,* 173–178.

Harcherik, D. F., Cohen, D. J., Paul, R., Ort, S., Shaywitz, B. A., Volkmar, F. R., Rothman, S., & Leckman, J. F. (1985). Computed tomographic brain scanning in four neuropsychiatric disorders of childhood: Attention deficit disorder, autism, language disorder, and Tourette's disorder. *American Journal of Psychiatry, 142,* 731–734.

Harcherik, D. F., Leckman, J. F., Detlor, J., & Cohen, D. J. (1984). A new instrument for clinical studies of Tourette's syndrome. *Journal of the American Academy of Child & Adolescent Psychiatry, 23,* 153–160.

Harrington, R., Fudge, H., Rutter, M., Pickles, A., & Hill, J. (1990). Adult outcomes of childhood and adolescent depression: I. Psychiatric status. *Archives of General Psychiatry, 47,* 465–473.

Harris, E. L., Schuerholz, L., Singer, H. S., Reader, M. J., Brown, J. E., Cox, C., Mohr, J., Chase, G. A., & Denkla, M. B. (1995). Executive function in children with Tourette syndrome and/or attention deficit hyperactivity disorder. *Journal of International Neuropsychological Society, 1,* 511–516.

Hassler, R., & Dieckmann, G. (1970). Stereotaxic treatment of tics and inarticulate cries or coprolalia considered as motor obsessional phenomena in Gilles de la Tourette's disease. *Revue Neurologique, 123,* 89–100.

Hasstedt, S. J., Leppert, M., Filloux, F., van de Wetering, B. J. M., & McMahon, W. M. (1995). Intermediate inheritance of Tourette syndrome, assuming assortative mating. *American Journal of Human Genetics, 57,* 682–689.

Haviland, M. G., Dial, T. H., & Pincus, H. A. (1988). Characteristics of senior medical students planning to subspecialize in child psychiatry. *Journal of the American Academy of Child & Adolescent Psychiatry, 27,* 404–407.

Hawker, K., & Lang, A. E. (1990). Hypoxic-ischemic damage to basal ganglia. Case reports and a review of the literature. *Movement Disorders, 5,* 219–224.

Hawking, S. W. (1988). *A brief history of time.* New York: Bantam Books.

Hays, R. B. (1988). Friendship. In S. W. Duck (Ed.), *Handbook of personal relationships: Theory, research, and interventions* (pp. 391–408). London: Wiley.

Hazrati, L.-N., & Parent, A. (1991). Contralateral pallidothalamic and pallidotegmental projections in primates: An anterograde and retrograde labeling study. *Brain Research, 567,* 212–223.

Head, D., Bolton, D., & Hymas, N. (1989). Deficit in cognitive shifting ability with obsessive-compulsive disorder. *Biological Psychiatry, 25,* 929–937.

Hebebrand, J., Klug, B., Fimmers, R., Seuchter, S. A., Wettke-Schäfer, R., Deget, F., Camps, A., Lisch, S., Hebebrand, K., von Gontard, A., Lehmkuhl, G., Poustka, F., Schmidt, M., Baur, M. P., & Remschmidt, H. (1997). Rates of tic disorders and obsessive compulsive symptomatology in families of children and adolescents with Gilles de la Tourette syndrome. *Journal of Psychiatric Research, 31,* 519–530.

Hechtman, L., Weiss, G., Perlman, T., & Amsel, R. (1984). Hyperactives as young adults: Initial predictors of adult outcome. *Journal of the American Academy of Child & Adolescent Psychiatry, 25,* 250–260.

Heilman, K. M., Voeller, K. K. S., & Nadeau, S. E. (1991). A possible pathophysiologic substrate of attention deficit hyperactivity disorder. *Journal of Child Neurology, 6,* S74–S79.

Henry, C., Guegant, G., Cador, M., Arnauld, E., Arsaut, J., Le Moal, M., & Demotes-Mainart, J. (1995). Prenatal stress in rats facilitates amphetamine-induced sensitization and induces long-lasting changes in dopamine receptors in the nucleus accumbens. *Brain Research, 685,* 179–186.

Henry, C., Kabbaj, M., Simon, H., Le Moal, M., & Maccari, S. (1994). Prenatal stress increases the hypothalamo-pituitary-adrenal axis response in young and adult rats. *Journal of Neuroendocrinology, 6,* 341–345.

Herman, J. P., & Cullinan, W. E. (1997). Neurocircuitry of stress: Central control of the hypothalamo-pituitary-adrenocortical axis. *Trends in Neuroscience, 20,* 78–84.

Heutink, P. (1993). *Gene mapping of complex disorders.* Unpublished doctoral thesis, Erasmus University, Rotterdam, The Netherlands.

Hewlett, W. A., Vinogradov, S., & Agras, W. S. (1992). Clomipramine, clonazepam, and clonidine treatment of obsessive-compulsive disorder. *Journal of Clinical Psychopharmacology, 12,* 420–430.

Hibbs, E. D., Hamburger, S. D., Lenane, M., Rapoport, J. L., Kruesi, M. J., Keysor, C. S., & Goldstein, M. J. (1991). Determinants of expressed emotion in families of disturbed and normal children. *Journal of Child Psychology & Psychiatry, 32,* 757–770.

Hill, J. C., & Schoener, E. P. (1996). Age dependent decline of attention deficit hyperactivity disorder. *American Journal of Psychiatry, 153,*1143–1146.

Hinshaw, S. P. (1994). *Attention deficits and hyperactivity in children.* London: Sage.

Hodges, K. (1993). Structured interviews for assessing children. *Journal of Child Psychology & Psychiatry, 34,* 49–68.

Hodges, K., McKnew, D., Burbach, D. J., & Roebuck, L. (1987). Diagnostic concordance between the child assessment schedule (CAS) and the schedule for affective disorder and schizophrenia for school-age children (K-SADS) in an outpatient sample using lay interviews. *Journal of the American Academy of Child & Adolescent Psychiatry, 26,* 654–661.

Hodges, K., McKnew, D., Cytryn, L., Stern, L., & Kline, J. (1982). The child assessment schedule (CAS) diagnostic interview: A report on reliability and validity. *Journal of the American Academy of Child & Adolescent Psychiatry, 21,* 468–473.

Hodgkinson, V. A., & Weitzman, M. S. (1996). *The independent sector and its place in the economy.* Williamsburg, VA: Philanthropic Research. (http://www.guidestar.org/philanthropy2.shtml)

Hoehn-Saric, R., Pearlson, G., Harris, G., Machlin, S., & Camargo, E. (1991). Effects of fluoxetine on regional cerebral blood flow in obsessive-compulsive patients. *American Journal of Psychiatry, 148,* 1243–1245.

Hollander, E., Cohen, L., Richards, M., Mullen, L., DeCaria, C., & Stern, Y. (1993). A pilot study of the neuropsychology of obsessive-compulsive disorder and Parkinson's disease: Basal ganglia disorders. *Journal of Neuropsychiatry & Clinical Neurosciences, 5,* 104–107.

Hollander, E., DeCaria, C. M., Schneier, F. R., Schneier, H. A., Liebowitz, M. R., & Klein, D. F. (1990). Fenfluramine augmentation of serotonin reuptake blockade antiobsessional treatment. *Journal of Clinical Psychiatry, 51,* 119–123.

Hollander, E., Schiffman, E., Cohen, B., Rivera–Stein, M. A., Rosen, W., Gorman, J. M., Fyer, A. J., Papp, L., & Liebowitz, M. R. (1990). Signs of central nervous system dysfunction in obsessive–compulsive disorder. *Archives of General Psychiatry, 47,* 27–32.

Hollander, E., & Wong, C. M. (1996). The relationship between executive impairment and serotongergic sensitivity in obsessive-compulsive disorder. *Neuropsychiatry, Neuropsychology and Behavioral Neurology, 9,* 230–233.

Holzer, J. C., Goodman, W. K., Price, L. H., Bear, L., Leckman, J. F., & Heninger, G. R. (1994). Obsessive compulsive disorder with and without a chronic tic disorder: A comparison of symptoms in 70 patients. *British Journal of Psychiatry, 164,* 469–473.

Honjo, S., Hirano, C., Murase, S., Kaneko, T., Sugiyama, T., Ohtaka, K., Aoyama, T., Takei, Y., Ionoko, K., & Wakabayashi, S. (1989). Obsessive-compulsive symptoms in childhood and adolescence. *Acta Psychiatrica Scandinavica, 80,* 83–91.

Horner, R. H., Dunlap, G., Koegel, R. L., Carr, E. G., Sailor, W., Anderson, J., Albin, R. W., & O'Neill, R. E. (1990). Toward a technology of "nonaversive" behavioral support. *Journal of the Association for Persons with Severe Handicaps, 15,* 125–132.

Hubbard, R., & Ward, E. (1993). Exploding the gene myth. *Beacon Press,* p. 24.

Hubble, J. P., & Koller, W. C. (1995). The Parkinsonian personality. In W. J. Weiner & A. E. Lang (Eds.), *Advances in neurology: Vol. 65. Behavioral neurology of movement disorders* (pp. 43–48). New York: Raven Press.

Hudizak, J. J., & Todd, R. D. (1993). Familial subtyping attention deficit hyperactivity. *Current Opinions in Psychiatry, 6,* 489–493.

Hudson Institute. (1988a, September). *Opportunity 2000, creative affirmative strategies for a changing workforce, Indianapolis, IN.* Prepared for the U.S. Dept. of Labor, Employment Standards Administration. From U.S. Census Bureau, "Current Population Survey," pp. 100–103. Publisher by Hudson Institute.

Hudson Institute. (1988b, September). "A study of accommodations provided to handicapped employees by federal contractors" (Final report, U.S. Department of Labor). *Opportunity 2000,* pp. 118.

Hunt, R. D. (1987). Treatment effects of oral and transdermal clonidine in relation to methylphenidate: An open pilot study in ADD-H. *Psychopharmacologic Bulletin, 23,* 111–114.

Hunt, R. D., Capper, L., & O'Connell, P. (1990). Clonidine in child and adolescent psychiatry. *Journal of Child and Adolescent Psychopharmacology, 1,* 87–102.

Hunt, R. D., Minderaa, R. B., & Cohen, D. J. (1985). Clonidine benefits children with attention deficit disorder and hyperactivity: Report of a double-blind placebo-crossover therapeutic trial. *Journal of the American Academy Child & Adolescent Psychiatry, 24,* 617–629.

Husby, G., van de Rijn, I., Zabriskie, J. B., Abdin, Z. H., & William, R. C. (1976). Antibodies reacting with cytoplasm of subthalamic and caudate nuclei neurons in chorea and acute rheumatic fever. *Journal of Experimental Medicine, 144,* 1094–1110.

Hutt, M. L. (1977). *The Hutt adaptation of the Bender-Gestalt test* (3rd ed.). New York: Grune and Stratton.

Hutzell, R. R., Platzek, D., & Logue, P. E. (1974). Control of symptoms of Gilles de la Tourette's syndrome by self-monitoring. *Journal of Behavior Therapy and Experimental Psychiatry, 5,* 71–76.

Hyde, T. M., Aaronson, B. A., Randolph, C., Rickler, K. C., & Weinberger, D. R. (1992). Relationship of birth weight to the phenotypic expression of Gilles de la Tourette's syndrome in monozygotic twins. *Neurology, 42,* 652–658.

Hyde, T. M., Emsellem, H. A., Randolph, C., Rickler, K. C., & Weinberger, D. R. (1994). Electroencephalographic abnormalities in monozygotic twins with Tourette's syndrome. *British Journal of Psychiatry, 164,* 811–817.

Hyde, T. M., Stacey, M., Coppola, R., Handel, S., Rickler, K., & Weinberger, D. (1995). Cerebral morphometric abnormalities in Tourette's syndrome: A quantitative MRI study of monozygotic twins. *Neurology, 45,* 1176–1182.

Hymas, N., Lees, A., Bolton, D., Epps, K., & Head, D. (1991). The neurology of obsessional slowness. *Brain, 114,* 2203–2233.

Hynd, G. W., Hern, K. L., Novey, E. S., Eliopulos, D., Marshall, R., Gonzalez, J. J., & Voeller, K. K. (1993). Attention deficit-hyperactivity disorder and asymmetry of the caudate nucleus. *Journal of Child Neurology, 8,* 339–347.

Hynd, G. W., Semrud-Clikeman, M., Lorys, A. R., Novey, E. S., Eliopulos, D., & Lyytinen, H. (1991). Corpus callosum morphology in attention deficit-hyperactivity disorder: Morphometric analysis of MRI. *Journal of Learning Disabilities, 24,* 141–146.

Hyvärinen, J. (1982). *The parietal cortex of monkey and man.* Berlin: Springer-Verlag.

Incagnoli, T., & Kane, R. (1983). Developmental perspective of the Gilles de la Tourette syndrome. *Perceptual and Motor Skills, 57,* 1271–1281.

Incagnoli, T., & Kane, R. L. (1981). Neuropsychological functioning in Gilles de la Tourette's syndrome. *Journal of Clinical Neuropsychology, 3,*167–171.

Insel, T. R. (1992a). A neuropeptide for affiliation: Evidence from behavioral, receptor, auto radiographic and comparative studies. *Psychoneuroendocrinology, 17,* 3–35.

Insel, T. R. (1992b). Toward a neuroanatomy of obsessive compulsive disorder. *Archives of General Psychiatry, 49,* 739–745.

Insel, T. R. (1997). A neurobiological basis of social attachment. *American Journal of Psychiatry, 154,* 726–735.

Insel, T. R., Gillin, J. C., Moore, A., Mendelson, W. B., Loewenstein, R. J., & Murphy, D. L. (1982). The sleep of patients with obsessive-compulsive disorder. *Archives of General Psychiatry, 39,* 1372–1377.

Insel, T. R., Kinsley, C. H., Mann, P. E., & Bridges, R. S. (1990). Prenatal stress has long-term effects on brain opiate receptors. *Brain Research, 511,* 93–97.

Institute of Medicine. (1989). *Research on children and adolescents with mental, behavioral, and developmental disorders* (Division of mental health and behavioral medicine). Washington, DC: National Academy Press.

Itard, J. M. G. (1825). Mémoire sur quelques fonctions involontaires des appareils de la locomotion, de la préhension et de la voix. *Archives of General Medicine, 8,* 385–407.

Iverson, S., & Mishkin, M. (1970). Perseverative interference in monkeys following selective lesions of the inferior prefrontal cortex. *Experimental Brain Research, 11,* 376–386.

Jadresic, D. (1992). The role of the amygdaloid complex in Gilles de la Tourette's syndrome. *British Journal of Psychiatry, 161,* 532–534.

Jaffe, E., Tremeau, F., Sharif, Z., & Reider, R. (1995). Clozapine in tardive Tourette syndrome. *Biologic Psychiatry, 38,* 196–197.

Jagger, J., Prusoff, B., Cohen, D. J., Kidd, K. K., Carbonari, C. M., & John, K. (1982). The epidemiology of Tourette's syndrome: A pilot study. *Schizophrenia Bulletin, 8,* 267–277.

James, W. (1995). In G. H. Bird (Ed.), *Selected writings.* New York: Everymans Library.

Jankovic, J. (1993). Deprenyl in attention deficit associated with Tourette's disorder. *Archives of Neurology, 50,* 286–288.

Jankovic, J. (1994). Botulinum toxin in the treatment of dystonic tics. *Movement Disorders, 9,* 347–349.

Jankovic, J. (1997). Phenomenology and classification of tic disorders. *Neurologic Clinics of North America, 15,* 267–276.

Jankovic, J., Glaze, D. G., & Frost, J., Jr. (1984). Effect of tetrabenazine on tics and sleep of Gilles de la Tourette's syndrome. *Neurology, 34,* 688–692.

Jankovic, J., & Orman, J. (1988). Tetrabenazine therapy of dystonia, chorea, tics, and other dyskinesias. *Neurology, 38,* 391–394.

Jaspers, K. (1968). *General psychopathology.* Chicago: Chicago University Press.

Jenike, M. A., Baer, L., Ballantine, H. T., Martuza, J. L., Tynes, S., Giriunas, I., Buttolph, M. L., & Cassem, N. H. (1991). Cingulatomy for refractory obsessive-compulsive disorder: A long-term follow-up of 33 patients. *Archives of General Psychiatry, 48,* 548–555.

Jenike, M. A., Breiter, H. C., Baer, L., Kennedy, D. N., Savage, C. R., Olivares, M. J., O'Sullivan, R. L., Shera, D. M., Rauch, S. L., Keuthen, N., Rosen, B. R., Caviness, V. S., & Filipek, P. A. (1996). Cerebral structural abnormalities in obsessive-compulsive disorder. *Archives of General Psychiatry, 53,* 625–632.

Jenike, M. A., Hyman, S., Baer, L., Holland, A., Minichiello, W. E., Buttolph, L., Summergrad, P., Seymour, R., & Ricciardi, J. (1990). A controlled trial of fluvoxamine in obsessive-compulsive disorder: Implications for a serotonergic theory. *American Journal of Psychiatry, 147,* 1209–1215.

Jenike, M. A., & Rauch, S. L. (1994). Managing the patient with treatment-resistant obsessive compulsive disorder: Current strategies. *Journal of Clinical Psychiatry, 55*(Suppl.), 11–17.

Jenike, M. A., Rauch, S. L., Cummings, J. L., Savage, C. R., & Goodman, W. K. (1996). Recent developments in neurobiology of obsessive-compulsive disorder. *Journal of Clinical Psychiatry, 57,* 492–503.

Jensen, P. S., Salzberg, A. D., Richters, J. E., & Watanabe, H. K. (1993). Scales, diagnoses and child psychopathology: 1. CBCL and DISC relationships. *Journal of the American Academy of Child & Adolescent Psychiatry, 32,* 397–406.

Jensen, P. S., Traylor, J., Xenakis, S. N., & Davis, H. (1988). Child psychopathology rating scales and interrater agreement: Parents' gender and psychiatric symptoms. *Journal of the American Academy of Child & Adolescent Psychiatry, 27,* 442–450.

Jensen, P. S., Watanabe, H. K., Richters, J. E., Cortes, R., Roper, M., & Liu, S. (1995). Prevalence of mental disorder in military children and adolescents: Findings from a two-stage community survey. *Journal of the American Academy of Child & Adolescent Psychiatry, 34,* 1514–1524.

Johnson, M. R., & Lydiard, R. B. (1995). The neurobiology of anxiety disorders. *Psychiatric Clinics of North America, 18,* 681–725.

Johnston, C. (1996). Parent characteristics and parent-child interactions in families of nonproblem children and ADHD children with higher and lower levels of oppositional-defiant behavior. *Journal of Abnormal Child Psychology, 24,* 85–104.

Jones, S. R., Jaber, M., Giros, B., Wightman, R. M., & Caron, M. G. (1996). Dopamine dynamics and psychostimulant effects in dopamine transporter knockout mice. *Social Neuroscience Abstracts, 22,* 620.2.

Kahn, E., & Cohn, L. H. (1934). Organic driveness: A brainstem syndrome and an experience. *New England Journal of Medicine, 210,* 748–756.

Kalian, M., Lerner, V., & Goldman, M. (1993). Atypical variants of tardive dyskinesia, treated by a combination of clozapine with propranolol and clozapine with tetrabenazine. *Journal of Nervous Mental Disease, 181,* 649–651.

Kane, M. J. (1994). Premonitory urges as "attentional tics" in Tourette's syndrome. *Journal of the American Academy of Child & Adolescent Psychiatry, 33,* 805–808.

Karno, M., Golding, J. M., Sorenson, S. B., & Burnam, M. A. (1988). The epidemiology of obsessive-compulsive disorder in five U.S. communities. *Archives of General Psychiatry, 45,* 1094–1099.

Katz, R. J., deVeaugh, G. J., & Landau, P. (1990). Clomipramine in obsessive-compulsive disorder. *Biologic Psychiatry, 28,* 401–414.

Kaufman, A. S., & Kaufman, N. L. (1985). *Kaufman test of educational achievement: Brief form manual.* Circle Pines, MN: American Guidance Service.

Kaufman, A. S., & Kaufman, N. L. (1990). *Kaufman Brief Intelligence Test.* Circle Pines, MN: American Guidance Service.

Kaufman, J., Birmaher, B., Brent, D., Rao, U., Flynn, C., Moreci, P., Williamson, D., & Ryan, N. (1997). Schedule for affective disorders and schizophrenia for school-age children—present and lifetime version (K-SADS-PL): Initial reliability and validity data. *Journal of the American Academy of Child & Adolescent Psychiatry, 36,*980–988.

Kazdin, A. E. (1988). *Child psychotherapy: Developing and identifying effective treatments.* New York: Pergamon Press.

Kazdin, A. E. (1989). Identifying depression in children: A comparison of alternative selection criteria. *Journal of Abnormal Child Psychology, 17,* 437–454.

Kazdin, A. E. (1993). Treatment of conduct disorder: Progress and directions in psychotherapy research. *Development and Psychopathology, 5,* 277–310.

Kelley, A. E., Lang, C. G., & Gauthier, A. M. (1988). Induction of oral stereotypy following amphetamine microinjection into a discrete subregion of the striatum. *Psychopharmacology, 95,* 556–559.

Kelley, M. L. (1989). *School-home notes: A behavioral intervention for parents and teachers.* New York: Guilford Press.

Kellner, C. H., Jolley, R. R., Holgate, R. C., Austin, L., Lydiard, R. B., Laraia, M., & Ballenger, J. C. (1991). Brain MRI in obsessive-compulsive disorder. *Psychiatry Research, 36,* 45–49.

Kelly, P., Richardson, A., & Mitchell-Heggs, N. (1973). Stereotactic limbic leukotomy: Neurophysiological aspects and operative technique. *British Journal of Psychiatry, 123,* 133–140.

Kerbeshian, J. B., Burd, L., & Klug, M. (1995). Comorbid Tourette's disorder and bipolar disorder: An etiologic perspective. *American Journal of Psychiatry, 152,* 1646–1651.

Kertesz, A., Ferro, J., & Black, S. (1986). Subcortical neglect: Anatomic, behavioral and recovery aspects. *Neurology, 36,* 132.

Kettle, P. A., & Marks, M. (1986). Neurological factors in obsessive compulsive disorder: Two case reports and a review of the literature. *British Journal of Psychiatry, 149,* 315–319.

Kidd, K. K., & Pauls, D. L. (1982). Genetic hypotheses for Tourette syndrome. In A. J. Friedhoff & T. N. Chase (Eds.), *Advances in neurology: Vol. 35. Gilles de la Tourette syndrome* (pp. 243–250). New York: Raven Press.

Kidd, K. K., Prusoff, B. A., & Cohen. D. J. (1980). Familial pattern of Gilles de la Tourette syndrome. *Archives of General Psychiatry, 37,* 1336–1339.

Kiessling, L. S., Marcotte, A. C., Benson, M., Kuhn, C. III, & Wrenn, D. (1993). Relationship between GABHS and childhood movement disorders. *Pediatric Research, 33,* 12A.

Kiessling, L. S., Marcotte, A. C., & Culpepper L. (1993a). Antineuronal antibodies in movement disorders. *Pediatrics, 92,* 39–43.

Kiessling, L. S., Marcotte, A. C., & Culpepper, L. (1993b). Antineuronal antibodies: Tics and obsessive compulsive symptoms. *Journal of Developmental and Behavioral Pediatrics, 14,* 281–282.

Kim, S. W., Dysken, M. W., & Kuskowski, M. (1990). The Yale Brown Obsessive Compulsive Scale: A reliability and validity study. *Psychiatry Research, 34,* 99–106.

King, D. J. (1990). The effect of neuroleptics on cognitive and psychomotor function. *British Journal of Psychiatry, 157,* 799–811.

King, R. A., & Cohen, D. J. (1994). Psychotherapy in the neuropsychiatric disorders of childhood: ADHD, OCD, and Tourette's syndrome. In *Annual review of psychiatry* (Vol. 13, pp. 519–530). Washington, DC: American Psychiatric Press.

King, R. A., Leckman, J. F., & Cohen, D. J. (1991). Movement disorders. In J. Weiner (Ed.), *The comprehensive textbook of child and adolescent psychiatry.* Washington, DC: American Psychiatric Press.

King, R. A., Leonard, H. L., & March, J. S. (1998). Work group on quality issues. Practice parameters on the assessment and treatment of children and adolescents with obsessive-compulsive disorder. *Journal of the American Academy of Child & Adolescent Psychiatry, 37*(Suppl.).

King, R. A., Riddle, M. A., Chappell, P. B., Hardin, M. T., Anderson, G. M., Lombroso, P., & Scahill, L. (1991). Emergence of self-destructive phenomena in children and adolescents during fluoxetine treatment. *Journal of the American Academy of Child & Adolescent Psychiatry, 30,* 179–186.

King, R. A., Scahill, L., Vitulano, L. A., Schwab-Stone, M., Terciak, K., & Riddle, M. A. (1995). Childhood trichotillomania: Clinical phenomenology, comorbidity, and family genetics. *Journal of the American Academy of Child & Adolescent Psychiatry, 34,* 1451–1459.

King, R. A., Segman, R. H., & Anderson, G. M. (1994). Serotonin and suicidality: The impact of acute fluoxetine administration: 1. Serotonin and suicide. *Israel Journal of Psychiatry and Related Sciences, 31,* 271–279.

Kinomura, S., Larsson, J., Gulyas, B., & Roland, P. E. (1996). Activation by attention of the human reticular formation and thalamic intralaminar nuclei. *Science, 271,* 512–515.

Kirk, A., & Kertesz, A. (1989). Hemispheric contributions to drawing. *Neuropsychologia, 27,* 881–886.

Kisher, K., & Cunningham, M. (1985). A link between streptococci and heart. *Science,* 413–415.

Kita, H., & Kitai, S. T. (1991). Intracellular study of rat globus pallidus neurons: Membrane properties and responses to neostriatal, subthalamic and nigral stimulation. *Brain Research, 564,* 296–305.

Klawans, H. L., Falk, D. K., Nausieda, P. A., & Weiner, W. J. (1978). Gilles de la Tourette syndrome after long-term chlorpromazine therapy. *Neurology, 28,* 1064–1068.

Klein, R. G. (1990/1991). Thioridazine effects on the cognitive performance of children with attention-deficit hyperactivity disorder. *Journal of Child & Adolescent Psychopharmacology, 1,* 263–270.

Klein, R. G., Landa, B., Mattes, J. A., & Klein, D. F. (1988). Methylphenidate and growth in hyperactive children: A controlled withdrawal study. *Archives of General Psychiatry, 45*(12), 1127–1130.

Klein, R. G., & Mannuzza, S. (1988). Hyperactive boys almost grown up; III: methylphenidate effects on ultimate height. *Archives of General Psychiatry, 45,* 1131–1134.

Kleinman, A. (1988). *Rethinking psychiatry: From cultural category to personal experience.* New York: Macmillan.

Klempel, K. (1974). Gilles de la Tourette's symptoms induced by L-dopa. *South African Medical Journal, 48,* 1379–1380.

Knowlton, B. J., Mangels, J. A., & Squire, L. R. (1996). A neostriatal habit learning system in humans. *Science, 273,* 1399–1402.

Knox, L., Albano, A., & Barlow, D. (1996). Parental involvement in the treatment of childhood compulsive disorder: A multiple-baseline examination incorporating parents. *Behavior Therapy, 27,* 93–114.

Kochenow, N. K. (1990). Normal pregnancy and prenatal care. In J. R. Scott, P. J. DiSaia, C. B. Hammond, & W. N. Spellacy (Eds.), *Danforth's obstetrics and gynecology* (6th ed., pp. 123–159). Philadelphia: Lippincott.

König, P., & Enge, A. K. (1995). Correlated firing in sensory-motor systems. *Current Opinions in Neurobiology, 5,* 511–519.

Korzen, A. V., Pushkov, V. V., Kharitonov, R. A., & Shustin, V. A. (1991). Stereotaxic thalamotomy in the combined treatment of Gilles de la Tourette's disease. *Zhurnal Neuropatologii i Psikhiatrii, 91,* 100–101.

Kovacs, M. (1985). The Children's Depression Inventory (CDI). *Psychopharmacology, 21,* 995–1000.

Krakowski, A. J. (1965). Amitriptyline in treatment of hyperkinetic children. *Psychosomatics, 6,* 355–360.

Kramer, P. L., Pauls, D. L., Price, R. A., & Kidd, K. K. (1989). Estimation of segregation and linkage parameters in simulated data: 1. Segregation analysis with different ascertainment schemes. *American Journal of Human Genetics, 45,* 83–94.

Kruglyak, L., & Lander, E. S. (1995). Complete multipoint sib-pair analysis of qualitative and quantitative traits. *American Journal of Human Genetics, 57,* 439–454.

Kurlan, R. (1989). Tourette syndrome: Current concepts. *Neurology, 39,* 1625–1630.

Kurlan, R. (1997). Treatment of tics. *Neurologic Clinics of North America, 15,* 403–409.

Kurlan, R., Como, P. G., Deeley, C., McDermot, M., & McDermott, M. P. (1993). A pilot controlled study of fluoxetine for obsessive-compulsive symptoms in children with Tourette's syndrome. *Clinical Neuropharmacology, 16,* 167–172.

Kurlan, R., Daragjati, C., Como, P. G., McDermott, M. P., Trinidad, K. S., Roddy, S., Brower, C. A., & Robertson, M. M. (1996). Non-obscene complex socially inappropriate behavior in Tourette's syndrome. *Journal of Neuropsychiatry and Clinical Neurosciences, 8,* 311–317.

Kurlan, R., Kersun, J., Ballantine, H., Jr., & Caine, E. D. (1990). Neurosurgical treatment of severe obsessive-compulsive disorder associated with Tourette's syndrome. *Movement Disorders, 5,* 152–155.

Kurlan, R., Lichter, D., & Hewitt, D. (1989). Sensory tics in Tourette's syndrome. *Neurology, 39,* 731–734.

Kurlan, R., Majumdar, L., Deeleym, C., Mudholkar, G. S., Plumb, S., & Como, P. G. (1991). A controlled trial of propoxyphene and naltrexone in patients with Tourette's syndrome. *Annals of Neurology, 30,* 19–23.

Kurlan, R., & McDermott, M. P. (1993). Rating tic severity. In R. Kurlan (Ed.), *Handbook of Tourette's syndrome and related tic and behavioral disorders* (pp. 199–220). New York: Marcel Dekker.

Kurlan, R., Whitmore, D., Irvine, C., McDermott, M. P., & Como, P. G. (1994). Tourette's syndrome in a special education population: A pilot study involving a single school district. *Neurology, 44,* 699–702.

Kuskowski, M. A., Malone, S. M., Kim, S. W., Dysken, M. W., Okaya, A. J., & Christensen, K. J. (1993). Quantitative EEG in obsessive-compulsive disorder. *Biological Psychiatry, 33,* 423–430.

Lahey, B. B., Piacentini, J. C., McBurnett, K., Stone, P., Hartdagen, S., & Hynd, G. (1988). Psychopathology in the parents of children with conduct disorder and hyperactivity. *Journal of the American Academy of Child & Adolescent Psychiatry, 27,* 163–170.

Lake, C. R., Ziegler, M. G., Eldridge, R., & Murphy, D. L. (1977). Catecholamine metabolism in Gilles de la Tourette's syndrome. *American Journal of Psychiatry, 134,* 257–260.

Lakke, J. P., & Wilmink, J. T. (1985). A case of Gilles de la Tourette's syndrome with midbrain involvement. *Journal of Neurology, Neurosurgery and Psychiatry, 48,* 1293–1296.

Lalouel, J. M., Rao, D. C., Morton, N. E., & Elston, R. C. (1983). A unified model for complex segregation analysis. *American Journal of Human Genetics, 35,* 816–826.

Landau, S., & Moore, L. A. (1990). Social skills deficits in children with attention-deficit hyperactive disorder. *School Psychology Review, 20,* 235–251.

Lander, E. S., & Schork, N. J. (1994). Genetic dissection of complex traits. *Science, 265,* 2037–2048.

Lang, A. E. (1992). Clinical phenomenology of tic disorders: Selected aspects. In T. N. Chase, A. J. Friedhoff & D. J. Cohen (Eds.), *Advances in neurology: Vol. 58. Tourette syndrome: Genetics, neurobiology and treatment* (pp. 25–32). New York: Raven Press.

Lanser, J. B. K., Van Santen, W. H. C., Jennekens-Schinkel, A., & Roos, R. A. C. (1993). Tourette's syndrome and right hemisphere dysfunction. *British Journal of Psychiatry, 163,* 116–118.

Laplane, D., Levasseur, M., Pillon, B., Dubois, B., Baulac, M., Mazoyer, B., Tran Dinh, S., Sette, G., Danze, F., & Baron, J. C. (1989). Obsessive compulsive and other behavioral changes with bilateral basal ganglia lesions: A neuropsychological, magnetic resonance imaging, and positron tomographic study. *Brain, 112,* 699–725.

Lapouse, R., & Monk, M. A. (1964). Behavior deviations in a representative sample of children. *American Journal of Orthopsychiatry, 34,* 436–446.

Larumbe, R., Vaamonde, J., Artieda, J., Zubieta, J. L., & Obeso, J. A. (1993). Reflex blepharospasm associated with bilateral basal ganglia lesion. *Movement Disorders, 8,* 198–200.

Lavigne, J. V., & Ryan, M. (1979). Psychologic adjustment of siblings of children with chronic illness. *Pediatrics, 63,* 616–627.

Lawrence, M., & Redmond, D. (1985). MPTP lesions and dopaminergic drugs alter eye blink rate in African green monkeys. *Pharmacology, Biochemistry and Behavior, 38,* 869–874.

Lazar, R. M., Weiner, M., Wald, H. S., & Kula, R. W. (1995). Visuoconstructional deficit following infarction in the right basal ganglia: A case report and some experimental data. *Archives of Clinical Neuropsychology, 10,* 543–553.

Leckman, J. F. (1997). What genes confer vulnerability to Gilles de la Tourette's syndrome? *Psychiatric Annals, 27,* 1–4.

Leckman, J. F., Anderson, G. M., Cohen, D. J., Ort, S. I., Harcherik, D. F., Hoder, E. L., & Shaywitz, B. A. (1984). Whole blood serotonin and tryptophan levels in Tourette's disorder: Effects of acute and chronic clonidine treatment. *Life Sciences, 35,* 2497–2503.

Leckman, J. F., Cohen, D. J., Gertner, J. M., Ort, S., & Harcherik, D. (1984). Growth hormone response to clonidine in children ages 4 to 17: Tourette's syndrome vs. children with short stature. *Journal of the American Academy of Child & Adolescent Psychiatry, 23,* 174–181.

Leckman, J. F., Cohen, D. J., Price, R. A., Riddle, M. A., Minderaa, R. B., Anderson, G. M., & Pauls, D. L. (1986). The pathogenesis of Gilles de la Tourette's syndrome: A review of data and hypotheses. In N. S. Shah & N. B. Shah (Eds.), *Movement disorders* (pp. 257–272). New York: Plenum Press.

Leckman, J. F., deLotbiniere, A. J., Marek, K., Gracco, C., Scahill, L., & Cohen, D. J. (1993). Severe disturbances in speech, swallowing, and gait following stereotactic infrathalamic lesions in Gilles de la Tourette's syndrome. *Neurology, 43,* 890–894.

Leckman, J. F., Detlor, J., Harcherik, D. F., Ort, S., Shaywitz, B. A., & Cohen, D. J. (1985). Short- and long-term treatment of Tourette's syndrome with clonidine: A clinical perspective. *Neurology, 35,* 343–351.

Leckman, J. F., Detlor, J., Harcherik, D. F., Young, J. G., Anderson, G. M., Shaywitz, B. A., & Cohen, D. J. (1983). Acute and chronic clonidine treatment in Tourette's syndrome: A preliminary report on clinical response and effect on plasma and urinary catecholamine metabolites, growth hormone, and blood pressure. *Journal of the American Academy of Child Psychiatry, 2,* 433–440.

Leckman, J. F., Dolnansky, E. S., Hardin, M. T., Clubb, M., Walkup, J. T., Stevenson, J., & Pauls, D. L. (1990). Perinatal factors in the expression of Tourette's syndrome: An exploratory study. *Journal of the American Academy of Child & Adolescent Psychiatry, 29,* 220–226.

Leckman, J. F., Goodman, W. K., Anderson, G. M., Riddle, M. A., Chappell, P. B., McSwiggan-Hardin, M. T., Walker, D. E., Scahill, L. D., Ort, S. I., Pauls, D. L., Cohen, D. J., & Price, L. H. (1995). CSF biogenic amines in obsessive compulsive disorder and Tourette's syndrome. *Neuropsychopharmacology, 12,* 73–86.

Leckman, J. F., Goodman, W. K., North, W. G., Chappell, P. B., Price, L. H., Pauls, D. L., Anderson, G. M., Riddle, M. A., McSwiggan-Hardin, M. T., McDougle, C. J., Barr, L. C., & Cohen, D. J. (1994a). Elevated levels of cerebrospinal fluid levels oxytocin in obsessive compulsive disorder: Comparison with Tourette's syndrome and healthy controls. *Archives of General Psychiatry, 51,* 782–92.

Leckman, J. F., Goodman, W. K., North, W. G., Chappell, P. B., Price, L. H., Pauls, D. L., Anderson, G. M., Riddle, M. A., McSwiggan-Hardin, M. T., McDougle, C. J., Barr, L. C., & Cohen, D. J. (1994b). The role of central oxytocin in obsessive compulsive disorder and related normal behavior. *Psychoneuroendocrinology, 19,* 723–749.

Leckman, J. F., Grice, D. E., Barr, L. C., deVries, A. L. C., Martin, C., Cohen, D. J., Goodman, W. K., & Rasmussen, S. A. (1995). Tic-related vs. non-tic related obsessive compulsive disorder. *Anxiety, 1,* 208–215.

Leckman, J. F., Grice, D. E., Boardman, J., Zhang, H., Vitale, A., Bondi, C., Alsobrook, J., Peterson, B. S., Cohen, D. J., Rasmussen, S. A., Goodman, W. K., McDougle, C. J., & Pauls, D. L. (1997). Symptoms of obsessive-compulsive disorder. *American Journal of Psychiatry, 154,* 911–917.

Leckman, J. F., Hardin, M. T., Riddle, M. A., Stevenson, J., Ort, S. I., & Cohen, D. J. (1991). Clonidine treatment of Gilles de la Tourette's syndrome. *Archives of General Psychiatry, 48,* 324–328.

Leckman, J. F., & Mayes, L. C. (in press-a). Maladies of love—An evolutionary perspective on some forms of obsessive-compulsive disorder. In D. M. Hann, L. Huffman, I. Lederhendler, & D. Meinecke (Eds.), *Advancing research in developmental plasticity: Integrating the behavioral science and neuroscience of mental health.* Rockville, MD: NIMH, US Department of Health and Human Services.

Leckman, J. F., & Mayes, L. C. (in press-b). Understanding developmental psychopathology: Are evolutionary accounts useful? *Journal of the American Academy of Child & Adolescent Psychiatry.*

Leckman, J. F., McDougle, C. J., Pauls D. L., Peterson, B. S., Grice, D. E., & King, R. A. (in press). Tic-related vs. non-tic-related obsessive-compulsive disorder. In W. K. Goodman & J. Mazur (Eds.), *Treatment challenges in obsessive-complusive disorder.* Hillsdale, NJ: Erlbaum.

Leckman, J. F., Ort, S., Cohen, D. J., Caruso, K. A., Anderson, G. M., & Riddle, M. A. (1986). Rebound phenomena in Tourette's syndrome after abrupt withdrawal of clonidine: Behavioral, cardiovascular, and neurochemical effects. *Archives of General Psychiatry, 43,* 1168–1176.

Leckman, J. F., Pauls, D. L., & Cohen, D. J. (1995). Tic disorders. In F. E. Bloom & D. J. Kupfer (Eds.), *Psychopharmacology: The fourth generation of progress.* New York: Raven Press.

Leckman, J. F., Pauls, D. L., Peterson, B. S., Riddle, M. A., Anderson, G. M., & Cohen, D. J. (1992). Pathogenesis of Tourette syndrome: Clues form the clinical phenotype and natural history. In T. N. Chase, A. J. Friedhoff & D. J. Cohen (Eds.), *Advances in neurology: Vol. 58. Tourette syndrome: Genetics, neurobiology and treatment* (pp. 15–24). New York: Raven Press.

Leckman, J. F., & Peterson, B. S. (1993). The pathogenesis of Tourette's syndrome: Role of epigenetic factors active in early CNS development. *Biological Psychiatry, 34,* 425–427.

Leckman, J. F., Peterson, B. S., Anderson, G. M., Arnsten, A. F., Pauls, D. L., & Cohen, D. J. (1997). Pathogenesis of Tourette's syndrome. *Journal of Child Psychology and Psychiatry, 38,* 119–142.

Leckman, J. F., Price, R. A., Walkup, J. T., Ort, S., Pauls, D. L., & Cohen, D. J. (1987). Nongenetic factors in Gilles de la Tourette's syndrome [letter]. *Archives of General Psychiatry, 44,* 100.

Leckman, J. F., Riddle, M. A., Berrettini, W. H., Anderson, G. M., Hardin, M. T., Chappell, P. B., Bissette, G., Nemeroff, C. B., Goodman, W. K., & Cohen, D. J. (1988). Elevated CSF levels of dynorphin A[1–8] in Tourette's syndrome. *Life Sciences, 43,* 2015–2023.

Leckman, J. F., Riddle, M. A., Hardin, M. T., Ort, S. I., Swartz, K. L., Stevenson, J., & Cohen, D. J. (1989). The Yale Global Tic Severity Scale (YGTSS): Initial testing of a clinical-rated scale of tic severity. *Journal of the American Academy of Child & Adolescent Psychiatry, 28,* 566–573.

Leckman, J. F., & Scahill, L. (1990). Possible exacerbation of tics by androgenic steroids [letter]. *New England Journal of Medicine, 322,* 1674.

Leckman, J. F., Sholomskas, D., Thompson, W. D., Belanger, A., & Weissman, M. M. (1982). Best estimate of lifetime psychiatric diagnosis. *Archives of General Psychiatry, 39,* 879–883.

Leckman, J. F., Walker, D. E., & Cohen, D. J. (1993). Premonitory urges in Tourette's syndrome. *American Journal of Psychiatry, 150,* 98–102.

Leckman, J. F., Walker, D. E., Goodman, W. K., Pauls, D. L., & Cohen, D. J. (1994). "Just right" perceptions associated with compulsive behaviors in Tourette's syndrome. *American Journal of Psychiatry, 151,* 675–680.

Leckman, J. F., Zhang, H., Vitale, A., Lahnin, F., Lynch, K., Bondi, C., Kim, Y.-S., & Peterson, B. S. (1998). Trajectories of tic severity in Tourette's syndrome: The first two decades. *Pediatrics, 102,* 14–19.

Lees, A. J. (1985). *Tics and related disorders.* New York: Churchill Livingstone.

Lees, A. J., Robertson, M., Trimble, M. R., & Murray, N. F. F. (1984). A clinical study of Gilles de la Tourette syndrome in the United Kingdom. *Journal of Neurology, Neurosurgery and Psychiatry, 47,* 1–8.

Lenane, M. C., Swedo, S. E., Leonard, H., Pauls, D. L., Sceery, W., & Rapoport, J. (1990). Psychiatric disorders in first degree relatives of children and adolescents with obsessive-compulsive disorder. *Journal of the American Academy of Child & Adolescent Psychiatry, 29,* 407–412.

Leonard, H. L., Goldberger, E. L., Rapoport, J. L., Cheslow, D. L., & Swedo, S. E. (1990). Childhood rituals: Normal development or obsessive-compulsive symptoms? *Journal of the American Academy of Child & Adolescent Psychiatry, 29,* 17–23.

Leonard, H. L., Lenane, M. C., Swedo, S. E., Rettew, D. C., Gershon, E. S., & Rapoport, J. L. (1992). Tics and Tourette's syndrome: A two to seven year follow-up of 54 obsessive compulsive children. *American Journal of Psychiatry, 149,* 1244–1251.

Leonard, H. L., Meyer, M. C., Swedo, S. E., Richter, D., Hamburger, S. D., Allen, A. J., Rapoport J. L., & Tucker, E. (1995). Electrocardiographic changes during desipramine and clomipramine treatment in children and adolescents. *Journal of the American Academy of Child & Adolescent Psychiatry, 34,* 1460–1468.

Leonard, H. L., Swedo, S. E., Lenane, M. C., Rettew, D. C., Hamburger, S., Barko, J. J., & Rapoport, J. L. (1993). A two to seven year follow-up study of 54 obsessive-compulsive children and adolescents. *Archives of General Psychiatry, 50,* 429–439.

Leonard, H. L., Swedo, S. E., Rapoport, J. L., Koby, E. V., Lenane, M. C., Cheslow, D. L., & Hamburger, S. D. (1989). Treatment of childhood obsessive compulsive disorder with clomipramine and desipramine: A double-blind crossover comparison. *Archives of General Psychiatry, 46,* 1088–1092.

Leonard, H. L., Topol, D., Bukstein, O., Hindmarsh, D., Allen, A. J., & Swedo, S. E. (1994). Clonazepam as an augmenting agent in the treatment of childhood-onset obsessive-compulsive disorder. *Journal of the American Academy of Child & Adolescent Psychiatry, 33*, 792–794.

Lerer, R. J. (1987). Motor tics, Tourette syndrome and learning disabilities. *Journal of Leaning Disabilities, 20*, 266–267.

Leysen, J. E., Gommeren, W., Eens, A., De Chaffoy, De Courcelles, D., Stoof, J. C., & Janssen, P. A. J. (1988). Biochemical profile of risperidone, a new antipsychotic. *Journal of Pharmacology Experimental Therapy, 247*, 661–670.

Liebowitz, M. R., Hollander, E., Schneier, F., Campeas, R., Hatterer, J., Papp, L., Fairbanks, J., Sandberg, D., Davies, S., & Stein, M. (1989). Fluoxetine treatment of obsessive-compulsive disorder: An open clinical trial. *Journal of Clinical Psychopharmacology, 9*, 423–427.

Lim, S. H., Dinner, D. S., Pillay, P. K., Luders, H., Morris, H. H., Klem, G., Wyllie, E., & Awad, I. A. (1994). Functional anatomy of the human supplementary sensorimotor area: Results of extraoperative electrical stimulation. *Electroencephalography and Clinical Neurophysiology, 91*, 179–193.

Lin, X., Swaroop, A., Vaccarino, F. M., Murtha, M. T., Ruddle, F. H., & Leckman, J. F. (1996). Characterization and sequence analysis of the human homeobox-containing gene, *GBX2. Genomics, 31*, 335–342.

Linnoila, M., Gualtieri, C. T., Jobson, K., & Staye, J. (1979). Characteristics of the therapeutic response to imipramine in hyperactive children. *American Journal of Psychiatry, 136*, 1201–1203.

Lipinski, J. F., Salle, F. R., Jackson, C., & Sethuraman, G. (1997). Dopamine agonist treatment of Tourette disorder in children: Results of an open-label trial of pergolide. *Movement Disorders, 12*, 402–407.

Lipkin, P. H., Goldstein, I. J., & Adesman, A. R. (1994). Tics and dyskinesias associated with stimulant treatment in attention-deficit hyperactivity disorder. *Archives of Pediatric and Adolescent Medicine, 148*, 859–861.

Lombroso, P. J., Mack, G., Scahill, L., King, R. A., & Leckman, J. F. (1991). Exacerbation of Tourette's syndrome associated with thermal stress: A family study. *Neurology, 41*, 1984–1987.

Lombroso, P. J., Scahill, L. D., Chappell, P. B., Pauls, D. L., Cohen, D. J., & Leckman, J. F. (1995). Tourette's syndrome: A multigenerational, neuropsychiatric disorder. In W. J. Weiner & A. E. Lang (Eds.), *Advances in neurology: Vol. 65. Behavioral neurology of movement disorders* (pp. 305–318). New York: Raven Press.

Lombroso, P. J., Scahill, L. D., King, R. A., Lynch, K. A., Chappel, P. B., Peterson, B. S., McDougle, C. J., & Leckman, J. F., (1995). Risperidone treatment of children and adolescents with chronic tic disorders: A preliminary report. *Journal of the American Academy of Child & Adolescent Psychiatry, 34*, 1147–1152.

Loney, J., & Milich, R. (1982). Hyperactivity, inattention and aggression in clinical practice. In M. Wolraich & D. K. Routh (Eds.), *Advances in behavioral pediatrics* (Vol. 2, pp. 113–147). Greenwich, CT: JAI Press.

Loong, J. W. K. (1991). *The continuous performance test.* San Luis O'Bispo, CA: Wang Neuropsychological Laboratory.

Lopez, R. E. (1965). Hyperactivity in twins. *Canadian Psychiatry Association Journal, 10*, 421–426.

Lopez-Villegas, D., Kulisevsky, J., Deus, J., Junque, C., Pujol, J., Guardia, E., & Grau, J. M. (1996). Neuropsychological alterations in patients with computed tomography-detected basal ganglia calcification. *Archives of Neurology, 53,* 252–256.

Lou, H. C., Henriksen, L., Bruhn, P., Borner, H., & Nielsen, J. B. (1989). Striatal dysfunction in attention deficit and hyperkinetic disorder. *Archives of Neurology, 46,* 48–52.

Lowe, T. L., Cohen, D. J., Detlor, J., Kremenitzer, M. W., & Shaywitz, B. A. (1982). Stimulant medications precipitate Tourette's syndrome. *Journal American Medical Association, 247,* 1168–1169.

Lucas, A. R., Beard, C. M., Raiput, A. H., & Kurland, L. T. (1982). Tourette syndrome in Rochester Minnesota, 1968–1979. In A. J. Friedhoff & T. N. Chase (Eds.), *Advances in neurology: Vol. 35. Gilles de la Tourette syndrome* (pp. 267–269). New York: Raven Press.

Lucas, A. R., Kauffman, P. E., & Morris, E. M. (1967). Gilles de la Tourette disease: A clinical study of fifteen cases. *Journal of the American Academy of Child & Adolescent Psychiatry, 6,* 700–722.

Lucas, A. R., & Weiss, M., (1971). Methylphenidate hallucinosis. *Journal of the American Medical Association, 217,* 1079–1081.

Luria, A. R. (1980). *Higher cortical functions in man.* New York: Basic Books.

Luxenberg, J. S., Swedo, S. E., Flament, M. F., Friedland, R. P., Rapoport, J., & Rapoport, S. I. (1988). Neuroanatomical abnormalities in obsessive-compulsive disorder detected with quantitative X-ray computed tomography. *American Journal of Psychiatry, 145,* 1089–1093.

Lydiard, R. B., Brawman-Mintzer, O., & Ballenger, J. C. (1996). Recent developments in the psychopharmacology of anxiety disorders. *Journal of Consulting & Clinical Psychology, 64,* 660–668.

Machlin, S. R., Harris, G. J., Pearlson, G. D., Hoehn-Saric, R., Jeffery, P., & Camargo, E. E. (1991). Elevated medial-frontal cerebral blood flow in obsessive-compulsive patients: A SPECT study. *American Journal of Psychiatry, 148,* 1240–1242.

MacLean, P. D., & Delgado, J. M. R. (1953). Electrical and chemical stimulation of frontotemporal portion of limbic system in the waking animal. *Electroencephalography and Clinical Neurophysiology, 5,* 91–100.

Mahler, M. S., & Luke, J. A. (1946). Outcome of the tic syndrome. *Journal of Nervous and Mental Disease, 103,* 433–445.

Mak, F. L., Chung, S. Y., Lee, P., & Chen, S. (1982). Tourette syndrome in the Chinese: A follow-up of 15 cases. In A. J. Friedhoff & T. N. Chase (Eds.), *Advances in neurology: Vol. 35. Gilles de la Tourette syndrome* (pp. 281–283). New York: Raven Press.

Malison, R. T., McDougle, C. J., van Dyck, C. H., Scahill, L., Baldwin, R. M., Seibyl, J. P., Price, L. H., Leckman, J. F., & Innis, L. B. (1995). [^{123}I]Beta-CIT SPECT imaging demonstrates increased striatal dopamine transporter binding in Tourette's syndrome. *American Journal of Psychiatry, 152,* 1359–1361.

Malloy, P. (1987). Frontal lobe dysfunction in obsessive-compulsive disorder. In E. Perceman (Ed.), *The frontal lobe revisited* (pp. 207–233). New York: IRBN Press.

Malone, M. A., Kershner, J. R., & Siegel, L. (1988). The effects of methylphenidate on levels of processing and laterality in children with attention deficit disorder. *Journal of Abnormal Child Psychology, 16,* 379–395.

Manjula, B. N., & Fichetti, V. A. (1980). Tropomyosin-like seven residue periodicity in three immunologically distinct streptococcal M proteins and its implications for the antiphagocytic property of the molecule. *Journal of Experimental Medicine, 151,* 695–701.

Mannuzza, S., Gittelman-Klein, R., Bonagura, N., Konig, P. H., & Shenker, R. (1988). Hyperactive boys almost grown up. II: Status of subjects without a mental disorder. *Archives of General Psychiatry, 45,* 13–18.

Mannuzza, S., Gittelman-Klein, R., Horowitz-Konig, P., & Giampino, T. L. (1989). Hyperactive boys almost grown up: Criminality and its relationship to psychiatric status. *Archives of General Psychiatry, 46,* 1073–1079.

Mannuzza, S., Klein, R. G., Bessler, A., Malloy, P., & LaPadula, M. (1993). Adult outcome of hyperactive boys: Educational achievement, occupational rank, and psychiatric status. *Archives of General Psychiatry, 50,* 565–576.

March, J. S. (1995). Cognitive-behavioral psychotherapy for children and adolescents with OCD: A review and recommendations for treatment. *Journal of the American Academy of Child & Adolescent Psychiatry, 34,* 7–18.

March, J. S., Leonard, H. L., & Swedo, S. E. (1995). Pharmacotherapy of obsessive-compulsive disorder. In M. Lewis & M. Riddle (Eds.), *Child and adolescent psychiatric clinics of North America: Pediatric psychopharmacology* (Vol. 4, p. 217). Philadelphia: Saunders.

March, J. S., & Mulle, K. (1995). Manualized cognitive-behavioral psychotherapy for obsessive-compulsive disorder in childhood: A preliminary single case study. *Journal of Anxiety Disorders, 9,* 175–184.

March, J. S., Mulle, K., & Herbel, B. (1994). Behavioral psychotherapy for children and adolescents with obsessive-compulsive disorder: An open trial of a new protocol-driven treatment package. *Journal of the American Academy of Child & Adolescent Psychiatry, 33,* 333–341.

Marcus, J., Hans, S. L., Auerbach, J. G., & Auerbach, A. G. (1993). Children at risk for schizophrenia: The Jerusalem infant development study. *Archives of General Psychiatry, 50,* 797–809.

Marks, I. M. (1987). *Fears, phobias, and rituals.* New York: Oxford University Press.

Marshall, R. S., Lazar, R. M., Binder, J. R., Desmond, D. W., Drucker, P. M., & Mohr, J. P. (1994). Interhemispheric localization of drawing dysfunction. *Neuropsychologia, 32,* 493–501.

Martin, A., Pigott, T. A., Lalonde, F. M., Dalton, I., Dubbert, B., & Murphy, D. L. (1993). Lack of evidence for Huntington's disease-like cognitive dysfunction in obsessive-compulsive disorder. *Biological Psychiatry, 33,* 345–353.

Martinot, J. L., Allilaire, J. F., Mazoyer, B. M., Hantouche, E., Huret, J. D., Legaut-Demare, F., Deslauriers, A. G., Hardy, P., Pappata, S., Baron, J. C., & Syrota, A. (1990). Obsessive-compulsive disorder: A clinical, neuropsychological and positron emission tomography study. *Acta Psychiatrica Scandinavica, 82,* 233–242.

Masten, A. S., & Coatsworth, J. D. (1995). Competence, resilience, and psychopathology. In D. Cicchetti & D. J. Cohen (Eds.), *Developmental psychopathology: Vol. 2. Risk, disorder, and adaptation* (pp. 715–752). New York: Wiley.

Matarazzo, J. D. (1990). Psychological assessment versus psychological testing. *American Psychologist, 45,* 999–1017.

Mayberg, H. S., & Solomon, D. H. (1995). Depression in Parkinson's disease: A biochemical and organic viewpoint. In W. J. Weiner & A. E. Lang (Eds.), *Advances in neurology: Vol. 65. Behavioral neurology of movement disorders* (pp. 49–60). New York: Raven Press.

Mayes, L. C., & Cohen, D. J. (1995). Constitution. In B. E. Moore & B. D. Fine (Eds.), *Psychoanalysis: The major concepts* (pp. 271–292). New Haven: Yale University Press.

Mayes, L. C., & Cohen, D. J. (1996a). Children's developing theory of mind. *Journal of the American Psychoanalytic Association, 44,* 117–142.

Mayes, L. C., & Cohen, D. J. (1996b). Anna Freud and developmental psychoanalytic psychology. *Psychoanalytic Study of the Child, 51,* 117–141.

McCain, A. P., & Kelley, M. L. (1993). Managing the classroom behavior of an ADHD preschooler: The efficacy of a school-home note intervention. *Child and Family Behavior Therapy, 15,* 33–44.

McConville, B. J., Fogelson, M. H., Norman, A. B., Klykylo, W. M., Manderscheid, P. Z., Parker, K. W., & Sandberg, P. R. (1991). Nicotine potentiation of haloperidol in reducing tic frequency in Tourette's disorder. *American Journal of Psychiatry, 148,* 793–794.

McConville, B. J., Norman, A. B., Fogelson, M. H., & Erenberg, G. (1994). Sequential use of opioid antagonists and agonists in Tourette's syndrome. *Lancet, 343,* 601.

McConville, B. J., Sandberg, P. R., Fogelson, M. H., King, J., Cirino, P., Parker, K. W., & Norman, A. B. (1992). The effects of nicotine plus haloperidol compared to nicotine only and placebo nicotine only in reducing tic severity and frequency in Tourette's disorder. *Biological Psychiatry, 15,* 832–840.

McCracken, J. T. (1991). A two-part model of stimulant action on attention deficit hyperactivity disorder in children. *Journal of Neuropsychiatry, 3,* 219–225.

McCubbin, H. I., McCubbin, M. A., Nevin, R. S., & Cauble, E. (1983). *Coping-health inventory for parents: Family health program.* Madison, WI: The University of Wisconsin-Madison.

McCubbin, H.I & Patterson, J. M. (1991). FILE: Family Inventory of Life Events and Changes. In H. I. McCubbin & A. I.Thompson (Eds.), *Family Assessment Inventories for Research and Practice.* Madison: University of Wisconsin-Madison.

McDougle, C. J., Fleischmann, R. L., Epperson, C. N., Wasylink, S., Leckman, J. F., & Price L. H. (1995). Risperidone addition in fluvoxamine-refractory obsessive compulsive disorder: Three cases. *Journal of Clinical Psychiatry, 56,* 526–528.

McDougle, C. J., Goodman, W. K., Leckman, J. F., Barr, L. C., Heninger, G. R., & Price, L. H. (1993). The efficacy of fluvoxamine in obsessive compulsive disorder: Effects of comorbid chronic tic disorder. *Journal of Clinical Psychopharmacology, 13,* 354–358.

McDougle, C. J., Goodman, W. K., Leckman, J. F., Lee, N. C., Heninger, G. R., & Price, L. H. (1994). Haloperidol addition in fluvoxamine-refractory obsessive compulsive disorder: A double blind placebo-controlled study in patients with and without tics. *Archives of General Psychiatry, 51,* 302–308.

McDougle, C. J., Goodman, W. K., Leckman, J. F., & Price, L. H. (1993). The psychopharmacology of obsessive compulsive disorder: Implications for treatment and pathogenesis. *Psychiatric Clinics of North America, 16,* 749–766.

McDougle, C. J., Goodman, W. K., & Price, L. H. (1993). The pharmacotherapy of obsessive compulsive disorder. *Pharmacopsychiatry, 26*(Suppl.), 24–29.

McDougle, C. J., Goodman, W. K., Price, L. H., Delgado, P. L., Krystal, J. H., Charney, D. S., & Heninger, G. R. (1990). Neuroleptic addition in fluvoxamine-refractory obsessive-compulsive disorder. *American Journal of Psychiatry, 147,* 652–654.

McDougle, C. J., Price, L. H., Goodman, W. K., Charney, D. S., & Heninger, G. R. (1991). A controlled trial of lithium augmentation in fluvoxamine-refractory obsessive compulsive disorder: Lack of efficacy. *Journal of Clinical Psychopharmacology, 11,* 175–184.

McFie, J., & Zangwill, O. L. (1960). Visual-constructive disabilities associated with lesions of the left cerebral hemisphere. *Brain, 83,* 243–260.

McGuire, P. K., Bates, J. F., & Goldman-Rakic, P. S. (1991). Interhemispheric integration: 2. Symmetry and convergence of the corticostriatal projections of the left and the right principal sulcus (PS) and the left and the right supplementary motor area (SMA) of the rhesus monkey. *Cerebral Cortex, 1,* 408–417.

McIntosh, D. E., Mulkins, R. S., & Dean, R. S. (1995). Utilization of maternal perinatal risk indicators in the differential diagnosis of ADHD and UADD children. *International Journal of Neuroscience, 81,* 35–46.

McKeever, P. (1983). Siblings of chronically ill children: A literature review with implications for research and practice. *American Journal of Orthopsychiatry, 53*(2), 209–218.

McKeever, W. F., Seitz, K. S., Hoff, A. L., Marino, M. F., & Diehl, J. A. (1983). Interacting sex and familial sinistrality characteristics influence both language lateralization and spatial ability in right handers. *Neuropsychologia, 21,* 661–668.

McKeon, J., McGuffin, P., & Robinson, P. (1984). Obsessive-compulsive neurosis following a head injury: A report of four cases. *British Journal of Psychiatry, 144,* 190–192.

McKeon, P., & Murray, R. (1987). Familial aspects of obsessive-compulsive neurosis. *British Journal of Psychiatry, 151,* 528–534.

Mednick, S. A., Machon, R. A., Huttunen, M. O., & Bonett, D. (1988). Adult schizophrenia following prenatal exposure to an influenza epidemic. *Archives of General Psychiatry, 5,* 189–192.

Meltzer, H. (1994). An overview of the mechanism of action of clozapine. *Journal of Clinical Psychiatry, 55* (Suppl. B), 47–52.

Melville, H. (1947). *Moby Dick.* New York: Oxford University Press. (Original work published 1851)

Mendelson, W. B., Caine, E. D., Goyer, P., Ebert, M., & Gillin, J. C. (1980). Sleep in Gilles de la Tourette syndrome. *Biologic Psychiatry, 15,* 339–43.

Mercadante, M. T., Prado, L. P. G., Campos, M. D., Shavitt, R. G., Kiss, M. H., Marques-Dias, M. J., Valle, R. C., Lombroso, P., Leckman, J. F., & Miguel, E. C. (1997). Sintomas obsessivo-compulsivos e tiques vocais em pacientes com coreia de Sydenham: Dado preliminares. *Informaço Psiquiátrica, 16*(Suppl.), 16–19.

Merry, S. N., & Andrews, L. K. (1994). Psychiatric status of sexually abused children 12 months after disclosure of abuse. *Journal of the American Academy of Child & Adolescent Psychiatry, 337,* 939–994.

Messiha, F. S., Knopp, W., Vanecko, S., O'Brien, V., & Corson, S. A. (1971). Haloperidol therapy in Tourette's syndrome: Neurophysiological, biochemical and behavioral correlates. *Life Sciences, 10,* 449–57.

Meuldijk, R., & Colon, E. J. (1992). Methadone treatment of Tourette's disorder. *American Journal of Psychiatry, 149,* 139–140.

Miguel, E. C., Baer, L., Rauch, S. L., Coffey, B. J., Savage, C. R., O'Sullivan, R. L., Philips, K., Moretti, C., Leckman, J. F., & Jenike, M. A. (1997). Repetitive motor behaviors in obsessive-compulsive disorder and Tourette's syndrome: Phenomenological differences. *British Journal of Psychiatry, 170,* 140–145.

Miguel, E. C., Coffey, B. J., Baer, L., Savage, C. R., Rauch, S. L., & Jenike, M. A. (1995). Phenomenology of intentional repetitive behaviors in obsessive-compulsive disorder and Tourette's disorder. *Journal of Clinical Psychiatry, 56,* 246–255.

Mikkelsen, E. J., Deltor, J., & Cohen, D. J. (1981). School avoidance and school phobia triggered by haloperidol in patients with Tourette's disorder. *American Journal of Psychiatry, 138,* 1572–1576.

Miklos, G. L. G., & Rubin, G. M. (1996). The role of the genome project in determining functional insights from model organisms. *Cell, 86,* 521–529.

Milberger, S., Biederman, J., Faraone, S. V., Chen, L., & Jones, J. (1996). Is maternal smoking during pregnancy a risk factor for attention deficit hyperactive disorder in children? *American Journal of Psychiatry, 153,* 1138–1142.

Miller, A. L. (1970). Treatment of a child with Gilles de la Tourette's syndrome using behaviour modification techniques. *Journal of Behavior Therapy and Experimental Psychiatry, 1,* 319–321.

Miltenberger, R. G., & Fuqua, R. W. (1985). A comparison of contingent vs. noncontingent competing response practice in the treatment of nervous habits. *Journal of Behavior Therapy and Experimental Psychiatry, 16,* 195–200.

Miltenberger, R. G., Fuqua, R. W., & McKinley, T. (1985). Habit reversal with muscle tics: Replication and component analysis. *Behavior Therapy, 16,* 39–50.

Mindus, P., & Jenike, M. A. (1992). Neurosurgical treatments of malignant obsessive-compulsive disorder. *Psychiatric Clininics of North America, 15,* 921–938.

Mishkin, M., & Manning, F. (1978). Nonspatial memory after selective prefrontal lesions in monkeys. *Brain Research, 143,* 313–323.

Mishkin, M., Vest, B., Waxler, M., & Rosvold, H. E. (1969). A re-examination of the effects of frontal lesions on object alternation. *Neuropsychologia, 7,* 357–363.

Modell, J., Mountz, J., Curtis, G., & Green, J. (1989). Neruophysiologic dysfunction in basal ganglia/limbic striatal and thatlmocortical circuits as a pathogenetic mechanism of obsessive-compulsive disorder. *Journal of Neuropsychiatry, 1,* 27–36.

Mondrup, K., Dupont, E., & Braendgaard, H. (1985). Progabide in the treatment of hyperkinetic extrapyramidal movement disorders. *Acta Neurologica Scandinavica, 72,* 341–343.

Montgomery, M. A., Clayton, P. C., & Friedhoff, A. J. (1982). Psychiatric illness in Tourette syndrome patients and first-degree relatives. In A. J. Friedhoff & T. N. Chase (Eds.), *Advances in neurology: Vol. 35. Gilles de la Tourette syndrome* (pp. 335–339). New York: Raven Press.

Moos, R. H., & Moos, B. M. (1976a). *Family environment scale: Manual.* Palo Alto, CA: Consulting Psychologists Press.

Moos, R. H., & Moos, B. S. (1976b). A typology of family social environments. *Family Process, 15,* 357–371.

Morecraft, R. J., Geula, C., & Mesulam, M. M. (1992). Cytoarchitecture and neural afferents of orbitofrontal cortex in the brain of the monkey. *Journal of Comparative Neurology, 323,* 341–358.

Moriarty, J., Campos Costa, D., Schmitz, B., Trimble, M. R., Ell, P. J., & Robertson, M. M. (1995). Brain perfusion abnormalities in Gilles de la Tourette's syndrome. *British Journal of Psychiatry, 167,* 249–254.

Morphew, J. A., & Sim, M. (1969). Gilles de la Tourette syndrome: A clinical and psychopathological study. *British Journal of Medical Psychology, 42,* 293–301.

Morrison, J. R., & Stewart, M. A. (1973). The psychiatric status of the legal families of adopted hyperactive children. *Archives of General Psychiatry, 28,* 888–891.

Mountcastle, V. B., Lynch, J. C., Georgopoulos, A., Sakata, H., & Acuña, C. (1975). Posterior parietal association cortex of the monkey: Command function for operations within exterpersonal space. *Journal of Neurophysiology, 38,* 871–908.

Muller, N., Putz, A., Klages, E., Hofschuster, E., Straube, A., & Ackenheil, M. (1994). Blunted growth hormone response to clonidine in Tourette syndrome. *Psychoneuroendocrinology, 19,* 335–341.

Murray, T. J. (1982). Doctor Samuel Johnson's abnormal movements. In A. J. Friedhoff & T. N. Chase (Eds.), *Advances in neurology: Vol. 35. Gilles de la Tourette syndrome* (pp. 25–30). New York: Raven Press.

National Institutes of Health. (1995). Voluntary organizations. In NINDS *Guide to health information about neurobiological disorders.*

Naugle, R. I., Chelune, G. J., & Tucker, G. (1993). Validity of the Kaufman Brief Intelligence Test. *Psychological Assessment, 5,* 182–186.

Nee, L. E., Caine, E. D., Polinsky, R. J., Eldgridge, R., & Ebert, M. H. (1980). Gilles de la Tourette syndrome: Clinical and family study of 50 cases. *Annals of Neurology, 7,* 41–49.

Nee, L. E., Polinsky, R. J., & Ebert, M. H. (1982). Tourette syndrome: Clinical and family studies. In A. J. Friedhoff & T. N. Chase (Eds.), *Advances in neurology: Vol. 35. Gilles de la Tourette syndrome* (pp. 291–295). New York: Raven Press.

Nelson, K. B. (1991). Prenatal and perinatal factors in the etiology of autism. *Pediatrics, 87,* 761–766.

Newcomb, A. F., & Bukowski, W. M. (1983). Social impact and social preference as determinants of children's peer group status. *Developmental Psychology, 19,* 856–867.

Nichols, P. L., & Chen, T.-C. (1981a). Demographics and maternal characteristics. In *Minimal brain dysfunction: A prospective study* (pp. 76–105). Hillsdale, NJ: Erlbaum.

Nichols, P. L., & Chen, T.-C. (1981b). Pregnancy and delivery complications. In *Minimal brain dysfunction: A prospective study* (pp. 107–119). Hillsdale, NJ: Erlbaum.

Nicolini, H., Hanna, G., Baxter, L., Schwartz, J., & Weissbacker, K., & Spence, M. A. (1991). Segregation analysis of obsessive compulsive and associated disorders. Preliminary results. *Ursus Med, 1,* 25–28.

Nieuwenhuys, R. (1985). *Survey of chemically defined cell groups and pathways. Chemoarchitecture of the brain.* New York: Springer-Verlag.

Nieuwenhuys, R., & Voogd, J. C. (1988). Olfactory and limbic systems. *The human central nervous system* (3rd ed.). New York: Springer-Verlag.

Nolan, E. E., Gadow, K. D., & Sverd, J. (1994). Observations and ratings of tics in school settings. *Journal of Abnormal Child Psychology, 22,* 579–593.

Nolan, E. E., Sverd, J., Gadow, K. D., Sprafkin, J., & Ezor, S. N. (1996). Associated psychopathology in children with both ADHD and chronic tic disorder. *Journal of the American Academy of Child & Adolescent Psychiatry, 35,* 1622–1626.

Nomura, Y., Kita, M., & Segawa, M. (1992). Social adaptation of Tourette syndrome families in Japan. In T. N. Chase, A. J. Friedhoff & D. J. Cohen (Eds.), *Advances in neurology: Vol. 58. Tourette syndrome: Genetics, neurobiology and treatment* (pp. 323–332). New York: Raven Press.

Novelli, E., Nobile, M., Diferia, G., Sciuto, G., & Catalano, M. (1994). A molecular investigation suggests no relationship between obsessive-compulsive disorder and the dopamine D2 receptor. *Neuropsychobiology, 29,* 61–63.

O'Brien, J. S., & Brennan, J. H. (1979). The elimination of a severe long term facial tic and vocal distortion with multi-facet behavior therapy. *Journal of Behavior Therapy and Experimental Psychiatry, 10,* 257–261.

Oesterheld, J. (1996). TCA cardiotoxicity: The latest [Letter]. *Journal of the American Academy of Child & Adolescent Psychiatry, 35,* 701–702.

Office of Education. (1990). *Individuals with disabilities education act (IDEA).* 20 U.S.C. 1401 (1) (15).

Ollendick, T. H. (1981). Self-monitoring and self-administered overcorrection: The modification of nervous tics in children. *Behavior Modification, 5,* 75–84.

Orvaschel, H., & Puig-Antich, J. (1987). *Schedule for affective disorders and schizophrenia for school-age children (K-SADS)* (4th ed.). Pittsburgh, PA: Western Psychiatric Institute and Clinic.

Osterreith, P. A. (1944). Le test de copie d'une figure complexe. *Archives de Psychologie, 30,* 206–356.

Ouchi, W. (1981). *Theory Z.* Addison-Wesley.

Ozonoff, S., Strayer, D. L., McMahon, W. M., & Filloux, F. (1994). Executive function abilities in autism and Tourette syndrome: An information processing approach. *Journal of Child Psychology & Psychiatry, 35,* 1015–1032.

Packer, L. E. (1997). Social and educational resources for patients with TS. *Neurologic Clinics of North America, 15,* 457–471.

Pakkenberg, H. (1968). The effect of tetrabenazine in some hyperkinetic syndromes. *Acta Neurologica Scandinavica, 44,* 391–393.

Pakstis, A. J., Heutink, P., Pauls, D. L., Kurlan, R., van de Wetering, B. J. M., Leckman, J. F., Sandkuyl, L. A., Kidd, J. R., Breedveld, G. J., Castiglione, C. M., Weber, J., Sparkes, R. S., Cohen, D. J., Kidd, K. K., & Oostra, B. A. (1991). Progress in the search for genetic linkage with Tourette syndrome: An exclusion map covering more than 50% of the autosomal genome. *American Journal of Human Genetics, 48,* 281–294.

Palumbo, D., Maughan, A., & Kurlan, R. (1997). Tourette syndrome is only one of several causes of a developmental basal ganglia syndrome. *Archives of Neurology, 54,* 475–483.

Pardo, J. V., Pardo, P. J., Janer, K. W., & Raichle, M. E. (1990). The anterior cingulate cortex mediates processing selection in the Stroop attentional conflict paradigm. *Proceedings of the National Academy of Sciences (USA), 87,* 256–259.

Parent, A. (1990). Serotonergic innervation of the basal ganglia. *Journal of Comparative Neurology, 299,* 1–16.

Parent, A., & Hazrati, L.-N. (1995a). Functional anatomy of the basal ganglia: 1. The cortico-basal ganglia-thalamo-cortical loop. *Brain Research Review, 20,* 91–127.

Parent, A., & Hazrati, L.-N. (1995b). Functional anatomy of the basal ganglia: 2. The place of subthalamic nucleus and external pallidum in basal ganglia circuitry. *Brain Research Review, 20,* 128–154.

Park, S., Como, P. G., Cui, L., & Kurlan, R. (1993). The early course of the Tourette's syndrome clinical spectrum. *Neurology, 43,* 1712–1715.

Parker, J. G., & Asher, S. R. (1993). Friendship and friendship quality in middle childhood: Links with peer group acceptance and feelings of loneliness and social dissatisfaction. *Developmental Psychology, 29,* 611–621.

Parker, J. G., & Gottman, M. (1989). Social and emotional development in a relational context: Links with peer group acceptance and feelings of loneliness from early childhood to adolescence. In T. J. Berndt & G. W. Ladd (Eds.), *Peer relations in child development* (pp. 95–131). New York: Wiley.

Parker, J. G., Rubin, K. H., Price, J. M., & DeRosier, M. E. (1995). Peer relationships, child development and adjustment: A developmental psychopathology perspective. In D. Cicchetti & D. J. Cohen (Eds.), *Developmental psychopathology: Vol. 2. Risk, disorder and adaptation* (pp. 96–161). New York: Wiley.

Parker, K. W., & Sanberg, P. R. (1991). Nicotine potentiation of haloperidol in reducing tic frequency in Tourette's. *American Journal of Psychiatry, 148,* 793–794.

Parraga, H. C., & McDonald, H. G. (1996). Etiology of Tourette's disorder. *Journal of the American Academy of Child & Adolescent Psychiatry, 35,* 2–3.

Pasamanick, B., & Kawi, A. (1956). A study of the association of prenatal and perinatal factors in the development of tics in children. *Journal of Pediatrics, 48,* 596–602.

Passingham, R. E. (1972). Non-reversal shifts after selective prefrontal ablations in monkeys (Macaca mulatta). *Neuropsychologia, 10,* 41–46.

Pataki, C. S., Carlson, G. A., Kelly, K. L., Rapport, M. D., & Biancaniello, T. M. (1993). Side effects of methylphenidate and desipramine alone and in combination in children. *Journal of the American Academy of Child & Adolescent Psychiatry, 32,* 1065–1072.

Pato, M. T., Murphy, D. L., & DeVabe, C. L. (1991). Sustained plasma concentrations of fluoxetine and/or norfluoxetine four and eight weeks after fluoxetine discontinuation. *Journal of Clinical Psychopharmacology, 11,* 224–225.

Pato, M. T., Zohar-Kadouch, R., Zohar, J., & Murphy, D. L. (1988). Return of symptoms after discontinuation of clomipramine in patients with obsessive-compulsive disorder. *American Journal of Psychology, 145,* 1521–1525.

Pauls, D. L. (1990). Emerging genetic markers and their role in potential preventive intervention strategies. In P. Muehrer (Ed.), *Conceptual research models for preventing mental disorders* (pp). Rockville, MD: NIMH.

Pauls, D. L. (1993). Behavioural disorders: Lessons in linkage. *Nature Genetics, 3,* 4–5.

Pauls, D. L., Alsobrook, J. P., II, Almasy, L., Leckman, J. F., & Cohen, D. J. (1991). Genetic and epidemiological analyses of the Yale Tourette's syndrome family study data. *Psychiatric Genetics, 2,* 28.

Pauls, D. L., Alsobrook, J. P., II, Goodman, W., Rasmussen, S., & Leckman, J. F. (1995). A family study of obsessive compulsive disorder. *American Journal of Psychiatry, 152,* 76–84.

Pauls, D. L., Cohen, D. J., Heimbuch, R., Detlor, J., & Kidd, K. K. (1981). Familial pattern and transmission of Gilles de la Tourette syndrome and multiple tics. *Archives of General Psychiatry, 38,*1091–1093.

Pauls, D. L., Hurst, C. R., Kruger, S. D., Leckman, J. F., Kidd, K. K., & Cohen, D. J. (1986). Evidence against a genetic relationship between Tourette syndrome and attention deficit disorder. *Archives of General Psychiatry, 43,* 1177–1179.

Pauls, D. L., & Leckman, J. F. (1986). The inheritance of Gilles de la Tourette syndrome and associated behaviors: Evidence for an autosomal dominant transmission. *New England Journal of Medicine, 315,* 993–997.

Pauls, D. L., Leckman, J. F., & Cohen D. J. (1993). Familial relationship between Gilles de la Tourette syndrome, attention deficit disorder, learning disabilities, speech disorders, and stuttering. *Journal of the American Academy of Child & Adolescent Psychiatry, 32,* 1044–1050.

Pauls, D. L., Leckman, J. F., & Cohen D. J. (1994). Evidence against a relationship between Tourette's syndrome and anxiety, depression, panic and phobic disorders. *British Journal of Psychiatry, 164,* 215–221.

Pauls, D. L., Pakstis, A. J., Kurlan, R., Kidd, K. K., Leckman, J. F., Cohen, D. J., Kidd, J. R., Como, P., & Sparkes, R. (1990). Segregation and linkage analyses of Gilles de la Tourette's syndrome and related disorders. *Journal of the American Academy of Child & Adolescent Psychiatry, 29,* 195–203.

Pauls, D. L., Raymond, C. L., Leckman, J. F., & Stevenson, J. M. (1991). A family study of Tourette's syndrome. *American Journal of Human Genetics, 48,* 154–163.

Pauls, D. L., Towbin, K. E., Leckman, J. F., Zahner, G. E. P., & Cohen, D. J. (1986). Gilles de la Tourette's syndrome and obsessive-compulsive disorder: Evidence supporting a genetic relationship. *Archives of General Psychiatry, 43,* 1180–1182.

Pekarik, G., Prinz, R. J., Liebert, D. E., Weintraub, S., & Neale, J. M. (1976). The Pupil Evaluation Inventory: A sociometric technique for assessing children's social behavior. *Journal of Abnormal Child Psychology, 4,* 83–97.

Pelham, W. E., & Bender, M. E. (1982). Peer relations in hyperactive children: Description and treatment. In K. Gadow & I. Bialer (Eds.), *Advances in learning and behavioral disabilities* (pp. 365–436). Greenwich, CT: JAI Press.

Pelham, W. E., Gnagy, E. M., Greenslade, K. E., & Milich, R. (1992). Teacher ratings of *DSM-III-R* symptoms for the disruptive behavior disorders. *Journal of the American Academy of Child & Adolescent Psychiatry, 31,* 210–218.

Pelham,W. E., Greenslade, K. E., Vodde-Hamilton, M., Murphy, D. A., Greenstein, J. J., Gnagy, E. M., Guthrie, K. J., Hoover, M. D., & Dahl, R. E. (1990). Relative efficacy of long-acting stimulants on ADHD children: A comparison of standard methylphenidate, Ritalin SR-20, Dexedrine Spansule, and Pemoline. *Pediatrics, 86,* 226–237.

Pennington, B. F. (1991). *Diagnosing learning disorders.* New York: Guilford Press.

Perse, T. L., Greist, J. H., Jefferson, J. W., Rosenfeld, R., & Dar, D. (1988). Fluvoxamine treatment of obsessive compulsive disorder. *American Journal of Psychiatry, 144,* 1543–1548.

Peters, D. A. V. (1982). Prenatal stress: Effects on brain biogenic amine and plasma corticosterone levels. *Pharmacology, Biochemistry and Behavior, 17,* 721–725.

Peters, D. A. V. (1990). Maternal stress increases fetal brain and neonatal cerebral cortex 5-hydroxytryptamine synthesis in rats: A possible mechanism by which stress influences brain development. *Pharmacology, Biochemistry and Behavior, 35,* 943–947.

Petersen, S. E., Shulman, G. L., Buckner, R. L., Corbetta, M., Miezin, F. M., & Raichle, M. E. (1996). *Consistent blood flow increases during active visual tasks occur in subcortical areas but not cortex* [abstract]. Boston, MA.

Peterson, A. A., & Azrin, N. H. (1992). An evaluation of behavioral treatments for Tourette syndrome. *Behavior Research and Therapy, 30,* 167–174.

Peterson, A. A., Campise, R. L., & Azrin, N. H. (1994). Behavioral and pharmacological treatments for tic and habit disorders: A review. *Journal of Developmental and Behavioral Pediatrics, 15,* 430–441.

Peterson, B. S., Bronen, R. A., & Duncan, C. C. (1996). Three cases of Gilles de la Tourette's syndrome and obsessive-compulsive disorder symptom change associated with pediatric cerebral malignancies. *Journal of Neurology, Neurosurgery and Psychiatry, 61,* 497–505.

Peterson, B. S., & Cohen, D. J. (1998). The treatment of Tourette's syndrome: Multimodal developmental intervention. *Journal of Clinical Psychiatry, 59*(Suppl. 1), 62–72.

Peterson, B. S., Gore, J. C., Riddle, M. A., Cohen, D. J., & Leckman, J. F. (1994). Abnormal magnetic resonance imaging T2 relaxation time asymmetries in Tourette's syndrome. *Psychiatry Research: Neuroimaging, 55,* 205–221.

Peterson, B. S., & Klein, J. E. (1997). Neuroimaging of Tourette's syndrome neurobiologic substrate. *Neuroimaging, 6,* 343–364.

Peterson, B. S., & Leckman, J. F. (in press). Temporal characterization of tics in Gilles de la Tourette's syndrome. *Biological Psychiatry.*

Peterson, B. S., Leckman, J. F., & Cohen, D. J. (1995). Tourette's syndrome: A genetically predisposed and an environmentally specified developmental psychopathology. In D. Cicchetti & D. J. Cohen (Eds.), *Developmental psychopathology: Risk, disorder and adaptation,* Vol. 2 (pp. 213–242). New York: Wiley.

Peterson, B. S., Leckman, J. F., Duncan, J. S., Wetzles, R., Riddlem, M. A., Hardin, M., & Cohen, D. J. (1994). Corpus callosum morphology from magnetic resonance images in Tourette's syndrome. *Psychiatry Research: Neuroimaging, 55,* 85–99.

Peterson, B. S., Leckman, J. F., Scahill, L., Naftolin, F., Keefe, D., Charest, N. J., & Cohen, D. J. (1992). Steroid hormones and CNS sexual dimorphisms modulate symptom expression in Tourette's syndrome. *Psychoneuroendocrinology, 17,* 553–563.

Peterson, B. S., Leckman, J. F., Scahill, L., Naftolin, F., Keefe, D., Charest, N. J., King, R. A., Hardin, M. T., & Cohen, D. J. (1994). Steroid hormones and Tourette's syndrome: Early experience with antiandrogen therapy. *Journal of Clinical Psychopharmacology, 14,* 131–135.

Peterson, B. S., Riddle, M. A., Cohen, D. J., Katz, L. D., Smith, J. C., Hardin, M. T., & Leckman, J. F. (1993). Reduced basal ganglia volumes in Tourette's syndrome using three-dimensional reconstruction techniques from magnetic resonance images. *Neurology, 43,* 941–949.

Peterson, B. S., Riddle, M. A., Cohen, D. J., Katz, L. D., Smith, J. C., & Leckman, J. F. (1993). Human basal ganglia volume asymmetries on magnetic resonance images. *Magnetic Resonance Imaging, 11,* 493–498.

Peterson, B. S., Skudlarski, P., Anderson, A. W., Zhang, H., Gatenby, J. C., Lacadie, C. M., Leckman, J. F., & Gore, J. C. (1998). Tourette's syndrome: A failure of subcortical inhibition. *Archives of General Psychiatry, 55,* 326–333.

Peterson, B. S., Zhang, Z., Bondi, C., Anderson, G. A., Naftolin, F., & Leckman, J. F. (in press). A double-blind, placebo-controlled, crossover trial of an antiandrogen in the treatment of Tourette's syndrome. *Journal of Clinical Psychopharmacology.*

Pfiffner, L. J., & Barkley, R. A. (1990). Educational placement and classroom management. In R. A. Barkley (Ed.), *Hyperactive children: A handbook for diagnosis and treatment* (2nd ed., pp. 498–539). New York: Guilford Press.

Piacentini, J., Gitow, A., Jaffer, M., Graae, F., & Whitaker, A. (1994). Outpatient behavioral treatment of child and adolescent obsessive compulsive disorder. *Journal of Anxiety Disorders, 8,* 277–289.

Piacentini, J., Shaffer, D., Fisher, P., Schwab-Stone, M., Davies, M., & Gioia, P. (1993). The diagnostic interview schedule for children-revised version (DISC-R): 3. Concurrent criterion validity. *Journal of the American Academy of Child & Adolescent Psychiatry, 32,* 658–665.

Piccinelli, M., Pini, S., Bellantuono, C., & Wilkinson, G. (1995). Efficacy of drug treatment in obsessive-compulsive disorder. A meta-analytic review. *British Journal of Psychiatry, 166,* 424–443.

Piercy, M., Hécaen, H., & Ajuriaguerra, J. (1960). *Constructional apraxia associated with unilateral cerebral lesions.*

Pigott, T. A., Pato, M. T., Bernstein, S. E., Grover, G. N., Hill, J. L., Tolliver, T. J., & Murphy, D. L. (1990). Controlled comparisons of clomipramine and fluoxetine in the treatment of obsessive-compulsive disorder: Behavioral and biological results. *Archives of General Psychiatry, 47,* 926–993.

Pitman, R. K. (1993). Posttraumatic obsessive-compulsive disorder: A case study. *Comparative Psychiatry, 34,* 102–107.

Pitman, R. K., Green, R. C., Jenike, M. A., & Mesulam, M. M. (1987). Clinical comparison of Tourette's disorder and obsessive-compulsive disorder. *American Journal of Psychiatry, 144,* 1166–1171.

Planck, M. W. (1981). In J. Murphy (Ed.), *Where is science going?* New York: Ox Bow.

Pliszka, S. R. (1987). Tricyclic antidepressants in the treatment of children with attention deficit disorder. *Journal of the American Academy of Child & Adolescent Psychiatry, 26,* 127–132.

Plutarch. (1992). Sertorius. In J. Dryden & A. H. Cough (Eds.), *Lives of noble Grecians and Romans.* New York: Random House.

Popper, K. R. (1959). *The logic of scientific discovery.* New York: Basic Books.

Poungvarin, N., Devahastin, V., & Viriyavejakul, A. (1995). Treatment of various movement disorders with botulinum A toxin injection: An experience of 900 patients. *Journal of the Medical Association of Thailand, 78,* 281–288.

Power, T. J., Atkins, M. S., Osborne, M. L., & Blum, N. J. (1994). The school psychologist as manager of programming for ADHD. *School Psychology Review, 23,* 279–291.

Preskorn, S. H., Jerkovich, G. S., Beber, J. H., & Widener, P. (1989). Therapeutic drug monitoring of tricyclic antidepressants: A standard of care issue. *Psychopharmacology Bulletin, 25,* 281–284.

Price, R. A., Kidd, K. K., Cohen, D. J., Pauls, D. L., & Leckman, J. F. (1985). A twin study of Tourette syndrome. *Archives of General Psychiatry, 42,* 815–820.

Price, R. A., Kramer, P. L., Pauls, D. L., & Kidd, K. K. (1989). Estimation of segregation and linkage parameters in simulated data: 2. Simultaneous estimation with one linked marker. *American Journal of Human Genetics, 45,* 95–105.

Price, R. A., Leckman, J. F., & Pauls, D. L. (1986). Tics and central nervous system stimulants in twins and non-twins with Tourette syndrome. *Neurology, 36,* 232–237.

Price, R. A., Pauls, D. L., Kruger, S. D., & Caine, E. D. (1988). Family data support a dominant major gene for Tourette syndrome. *Psychiatry Research, 24,* 251–261.

Prien, R. F., & Robinson, D. S. (Eds.). (1994). *Clinical evaluation of psychotropic drugs: Principles and guidelines.* New York: Raven Press.

Quinn, P. O., & Rapoport, J. L. (1975). One-year follow-up of hyperactive boys treated with imipramine or methylphenidate. *Archives of General Psychiatry, 132,* 241–245.

Quintana, J., & Fuster, J. M. (1993). Spatial and temporal factors in the role of prefrontal and parietal cortex in visuomotor integration. *Cerebral Cortex, 3,* 122–132.

Rabey, J. M., Lewis, A., Graff, E., & Korczyn, A. D. (1992). Decreased (^{3}H) quinuclidinyl benzilate binding to lymphocytes in Gilles de la Tourette syndrome. *Biological Psychiatry, 31,* 889–895.

Rabey, J. M., Oberman, Z., Graff, E., & Korczyn, A. D. (1995). Decreased dopamine uptake into platelet storage granules in Gilles de la Tourette disease. *Biological Psychiatry, 38,* 112–115.

Rachman, S. (1993). Obsessions, responsibility and guilt. *Behavior Research and Therapy, 31,* 149–154.

Rachman, S., & de Silva, P. (1978). Abnormal and normal obsessions. *Behavior Research and Therapy, 16,* 233–248.

Rachman, S., de Silva, P., & Röper, G. (1976). The spontaneous decay of compulsive urges. *Behavior Research and Therapy, 14,* 445–453.

Rachman, S., & Hodgson, R. J. (Eds.). (1980). *Obsessions and compulsions.* NJ: Prentice-Hall.

Randolph, C., Hyde, T. M., Gold, J. M., Goldberg, T. E., & Weinberger, D. R. (1993). Tourette's syndrome in monozygotic twins: Relationship of tic severity to neuropsychological function. *Archives of Neurology, 50,* 725–728.

Rapoport, J. L., Buchsbaum, M. S., Weingartner, H., Zhan, T. P., Ludlow, C., & Mikkelsen, E. J. (1980). Dextroamphetamine: Its cognitive and behavioral effects in normal and hyperactive boys and normal men. *Archives of General Psychiatry, 37,* 933–943.

Rapoport, J. L., Leonard, H. L., Swedo, S. E., & Lenane, M. C. (1993). Obsessive compulsive disorder in children and adolescents: Issues in management. *Journal of Clinical Psychiatry, 54,* 27–29.

Rapoport, J. L., Quinn, P. O., Bradbard, G., Riddle, K. D., & Brooks, E. (1974). Imipramine and methylphenidate treatment of hyperactive boys. *Archives of General Psychiatry, 30,* 789–798.

Rapport, M. D., Carlson, G. A., Kelly, K. L., & Pataki, C. (1993). Methylphenidate and desipramine in hospitalized children: 1. Separate and combined effects on cognitive function. *Journal of the American Academy of Child & Adolescent Psychiatry, 32,* 333–342.

Rasmussen, S. A. (1994). Genetic studies of obsessive compulsive disorder. In E. Hollander, J. Zohar, D. Marazziti, & B. Olivier (Eds.), *Current insights in obsessive compulsive disorder* (pp. 105–114). New York: Wiley.

Rasmussen, S. A., & Eisen, J. L. (1988). Clinical and epidemiological findings of significance to neuropharmacologic trials in OCD. *Psychopharmacology Bulletin, 24,* 466–470.

Rasmussen, S. A., & Eisen, J. L. (1991). Phenomenology of OCD: Clinical subtypes, heterogeneity and coexistence. In J. Zohar, T. Insel, & S. Rasmussen (Eds.), *The psychobiology of obsessive-compulsive disorder* (pp. 13–43). New York: Springer.

Rasmussen, S. A., & Tsuang, M. T. (1986). Clinical characteristics and family history in *DSM-III* obsessive-compulsive disorder. *American Journal of Psychiatry, 143,* 317–322.

Rasmusson, A. M., Anderson, G. M., Lynch, K. A., McSwiggaan-Hardin, M., Scahill, L. D., Mazure, C. M., Goodman, W. R., Price, L. H., Cohen, D. J., & Leckman, J. F. (1997). A preliminary study of tryptophan depletion on tics, obsessive compulsive symptoms, and mood in Tourette's syndrome. *Biologic Psychiatry, 41,* 117–121.

Rauch, S. L., Baer, L., Cosgrove, G. R., & Jenike, M. A. (1995). Neurosurgical treatment of Tourette's syndrome: A critical review. *Comprehensive Psychiatry, 36,* 141–156.

Rauch, S. L., Jenike, M. A., Alpert, N. M., Baer, L., Breiter, H. C., Savage, C. R., & Fischman, A. J. (1994). Regional cerebral blood flow measured during symptom provocation in obsessive-compulsive disorder using oxygen 15-labeled carbon dioxide and positron emission tomography. *Archives of General Psychiatry, 51,* 62–70.

Raymond, J. L., Lisberger, S. G., & Mauk, M. D. (1996). The cerebellum: A neuronal learning machine. *Science, 272,* 1126–1131.

Regeur, L., Pakkenberg, B., Fog, R., & Pakkenberg, H. (1986). Clinical features and long-term treatment with pimozide in 65 patients with Gilles de la Tourette's syndrome. *Journal of Neurology, Neurosurgery and Psychiatry, 49,* 791–795.

Reitan, R. M., & Davison, L. A. (1974). *Clinical neuropsychology: Current status and applications.* Washington, DC: Winston.

Rettew, D. C., Swedo, S. E., Leonard, H. L., Lenane, M. C., & Rapoport, J. L. (1992). Obsessions and compulsions across time in 79 children and adolescents with obsessive-compulsive disorder. *Journal of the American Academy of Child & Adolescent Psychiatry, 31,* 1050–1056.

Rey, A. (1941). L'examen psychologique dans les cas d'encéphalopathie traumatique. *Archives de Psychologie, 28,* 286–340.

Reynolds, C. R., & Kamphaus, R. W. (1992). *Behavior assessment system for children (BASC) manual.* Circle Pines, MN: American Guidance Service.

Richardson, E. P. (1982). Neuropathological studies of Tourette syndrome. In A. J. Friedhoff & T. N. Chase (Eds.), *Advances in neurology: Vol. 35. Gilles de la Tourette syndrome* (pp. 83–87). New York: Raven Press.

Richters, J., Arnold, L., Jensen, P., Abikoff, H., Conners, C., Greenhill, L., Hechtman, L., Hinshaw, S., Pelham, W., & Swanson, J. (1995). NIMH collaborative multisite multimodal treatment study of children with ADHD: 1. Background and rationale. *Journal of the American Academy of Child & Adolescent Psychiatry, 34,* 987–1000.

Rickards, H., Dursun, S. M., Farrar, G., Betts, T., Corbett, J. A., & Handley, S. L. (1996). Increased plasma kynurenine and its relationship to neopterin and tryptophan in Tourette's syndrome. *Psychological Medicine, 26,* 857–862.

Riddle, M. A., Geller, B., & Ryan, N. (1993). Another sudden death in a child treated with desipramine. *Journal of the American Academy of Child & Adolescent Psychiatry, 32,* 792–797.

Riddle, M. A., Hardin, M. T., Cho, S. C., Woolston, J. L., & Leckman, J. F. (1988). Desipramine treatment of boys with attention-deficit hyperactivity disorder and tics: Preliminary clinical experiences. *Journal of the American Academy of Child & Adolescent Psychiatry, 27,* 811–814.

Riddle, M. A., Hardin, M. T., Towbin, K. E., Leckman, J. F., & Cohen, D. J. (1987). Tardive dyskinesia following haloperidol treatment for Tourette's syndrome. *Archives of General Psychiatry, 44,* 98–99.

Riddle, M. A., Jatlow, P. I., Anderson, G. M., Cho, S. C., Hardin, M. T., Cohen, D. J., & Leckman, J. F. (1989). Plasma debrisoquin levels in the assessment of plasma homovanillic acid. The debrisoquin method. *Neuropsychopharmacology, 2,* 123–129.

Riddle, M. A., King, R. A., Hardin, M. T., Scahill, L., Ort, S. I., & Leckman, J. F. (1991). Behavioral side effects of fluoxetine in children and adolescents. *Journal of Child & Adolescent Psychopharmacology, 3,* 193–198.

Riddle, M. A., Leckman, J. F., Anderson, G. M., Hardin, M. T., Ort, S. I., Stevenson, J., & Cohen, D. J. (1988). Tourette's syndrome and associated disorders: Clinical and neurochemical correlates. *Journal of the American Academy of Child and Adolescent Psychiatry, 27,* 409–412.

Riddle, M. A., Leckman, J. F., Anderson, G. M., Ort, S. I., Hardin, M. T., Stevenson, J., & Cohen, D. J. (1988). Plasma MHPG: Within- and across-day stability in children and adults with Tourette's syndrome. *Biological Psychiatry, 24,* 391–398.

Riddle, M. A., Leckman, J. F., Hardin, M. T., Anderson, G. M., & Cohen, D. J. (1988). Fluoxetine treatment of obsessions and compulsions in patients with Tourette's syndrome. *American Journal of Psychiatry, 145,* 1173–1174.

Riddle, M. A., Lynch, K. A., Scahill, L., deVries, A. L., Cohen, D. J., & Leckman, J. F. (1995). Methylphenidate discontinuation and re-initiation during long-term treatment of children with Tourette's disorder and attention-deficit hyperactivity disorder. *Journal of Child & Adolescent Psychopharmacology, 5,* 205–214.

Riddle, M. A., Rasmusson, A. M., Woods, S. W., & Hoffer, P. B. (1992). SPECT imaging of cerebral blood flow in Tourette syndrome. In T. N. Chase, A. J. Friedhoff & D. J. Cohen (Eds.), *Advances in neurology: Vol. 58. Tourette syndrome: Genetics, neurobiology and treatment* (pp. 207–211). New York: Raven Press.

Riddle, M. A., Scahill, L., King, R. A., Hardin, M. T., Anderson, G. M., Ort, S. I., Smith, J. C., Leckman, J. F., & Cohen, D. J. (1992). Double-blind, crossover trial of fluoxetine and placebo in children and adolescents with obsessive compulsive disorder. *Journal of the American Academy of Child & Adolescent Psychiatry, 31,* 1062–1069.

Riddle, M. A., Scahill, L., King, R. A., Hardin, M. T., Towbin, K. E., Ort, S. I., Leckman, J. F., & Cohen, D. J. (1990). Obsessive compulsive disorder in children and adolescents: Phenomenology and family history. *Journal of the American Academy of Child & Adolescent Psychiatry, 29,* 766–772.

Rimbaud, A. (1976). Aube. In P. Schmidt (Ed.), *Complete works.* New York: HarperCollins.

Risch, N., & Zhang, H. P. (1995). Extreme discordant sib-pairs for mapping quantitative trait loci in humans. *Science, 268,* 1584–1589.

Robertson, M. M. (1989). The Gilles de la Tourette syndrome: The current status. *British Journal of Psychiatry, 154,* 147–169.

Robertson, M. M., Channon, S., Baker, J., & Flynn, D. (1993). The psychopathology of Gilles de la Tourette's syndrome. A controlled study. *British Journal of Psychiatry, 162,* 114–117.

Robertson, M. M., Doran, M., Trimble, M., & Lees, A. J. (1990). The treatment of Gilles de la Tourette syndrome by limbic leucotomy. *Journal of Neurology, Neurosurgery and Psychiatry, 53,* 691–694.

Robertson, M. M., & Eapen, V. (1995). *Movement and allied disorders in childhood.* Chichester, England: Wiley.

Robertson, M. M., Schnieden, V., & Lees, A. J. (1990). Management of Gilles de la Tourette syndrome using sulpiride. *Clinical Neuropharmacology, 3,* 229–235.

Robertson, M. M., Trimble, M. R., & Lees, A. J. (1988a). The neurobiology of obsessive-compulsive disorder. *Journal of the American Medical Association, 260,* 2888–2890.

Robertson, M. M., Trimble, M. R., & Lees, A. J. (1988b). The psychopathology of the Gilles de la Tourette: A phenomenological analysis. *British Journal of Psychiatry, 152,* 383–390.

Robertson, M. M., Verrill, M., Mercer, M., James, B., & Pauls, D. L. (1994). Tourette's syndrome in New Zealand: A postal survey. *British Journal of Psychiatry, 164,* 263–266.

Robertson, M. M., & Yakeley, J. W. (1993). Obsessive-compulsive disorder and self-injurious behavior. In R. Kurlan (Ed.), *Handbook of Tourette's syndrome and related tic and behavioral disorders* (pp. 45–87). New York: Marcel Dekker.

Robins, L. N. (1995). How to choose among the riches: Selecting a diagnostic instrument. In M. T. Tsuang, M. Tohen, & G. E. P. Zahner (Eds.), *Textbook in psychiatric epidemiology* (pp. 243–252). New York: Wiley.

Robinson, D., Wu, H., Munne, R. A., Ashtari, M., Alvir, J. M. J., Lerner, G., Koreen, A., Cole, K., & Bogerts, B. (1995). Reduced caudate nucleus volume in obsessive-compulsive disorder. *Archives of General Psychiatry, 52,* 393–398.

Rogeness, G. A., Javors, M. A., & Pliszka, S. R. (1992). Neurochemistry and child and adolescent psychiatry. *Journal of the American Academy of Child and Adolescent Psychiatry, 31,* 765–781.

Rolls, E. T., Thorpe, S. I., & Maddison, S. P. (1983). Responses of striatal neurons in the behaving monkey: 1. Head of caudate nucleus. *Behavioral Brain Research, 7,* 179–210.

Röper, G., & Rachman, S. (1976). Obsessional checking: Experimental replication and development. *Behaviour Research and Therapy, 14,* 25–32.

Röper, G., Rachman, S., & Hodgson, R. (1973). An experiment on obsessional checking. *Behaviour Research and Therapy, 11,* 271–277.

Rosenberg, D. R., Dick, E. L., Ohearn, K. M., & Sweeney, J. A. (1997). Response inhibition deficits in obsessive-compulsive disorder—An indicator of dysfunction in frontostriatal circuits. *Journal of Psychiatry & Neuroscience, 22,* 29–38.

Rosenberg, G. S., & Davis, K. L. (1982). The use of cholinergic precursors in neuropsychiatric diseases. *American Journal of Clinical Nutrition, 36,* 709–720.

Rosenberg, L. A., Brown, J., & Singer, H. S. (1994). Self-reporting of behavior problems in patients with tic disorders. *Psychological Reports, 74,* 653–654.

Rosenberg, L. A., Brown, J., & Singer, H. S. (1995). Behavioral problems and severity of tics. *Journal of Clinical Psychology, 51,* 760–767.

Rosenberg, L. A., Harris, J. C., & Singer, H. S. (1984). Relationship of the child behavior checklist to an independent measure of psychopathology. *Psychological Reports, 54,* 427–430.

Rosenfeld, R., Dar, R., Anderson, D., Kobak, K. A., & Greist, J. H. (1992). A computer-administered version of the Yale-Brown Obsessive-Compulsive Scale. *Psychological Assessment, 4,* 329–332.

Ross, D. C., & Piggott, L. R. (1993). Clonazepam for OCD [letter]. *Journal of the American Academy of Child & Adolescent Psychiatry, 32,* 470.

Ross, G., Lipper, E., & Auld, P. A. (1992). Hand preference, prematurity and developmental outcome at school age. *Neuropsychologia, 30,* 483–494.

Ross, M. S., & Moldofsky, H. (1978). A comparison of pimozide and haloperidol in the treatment of Gilles de la Tourette syndrome. *American Journal of Psychiatry, 135,* 585–587.

Rosvold, H., & Mishkin, M. (1961). Nonsensory effects of frontal lesions on discrimination learning and performance. In J. Delafresnaye (Ed.), *Brain mechanisms and learning.* Oxford, England: Blackwell.

Roth, B. L., Craigo, S. C., Choudhary, M. S., Uluer, A., Monsma, F. J., Shen, Y., Meltzer, H. Y., & Sibley, D. R. (1994). Binding of typical and atypical antipsychotic agents to 5-hydroxytryptamine-6 and 5-hydroxytryptamine-7 receptors. *Journal of Pharmacology and Experimental Therapeutics, 268,* 1403–1410.

Rubin, K. H., Chen, X., & Hymel, S. (1993). Socioemotional characteristics of withdrawn and aggressive children. *Merrill-Palmer Quarterly, 39,* 518–534.

Rubin, R. T., Ananth, J., Villanueva-Meyer, J., Trajmar, P. G., & Mena, I. (1995). Regional [133] Xenon cerebral blood flow and cerebral ^{99m}Tc-HMPAO uptake in patients with obsessive-compulsive disorder before and during treatment. *Biological Psychiatry, 38,* 429–437.

Rubin, R. T., Villanueva-Meyer, J., Ananth, J., Trajmar, P. G., & Mena, I. (1992). Regional xenon 133 cerebral blood flow and cerebral technetium 99m HMPAO uptake in unmedicated patients with obsessive-compulsive disorder and matched normal control subjects. Determination by high-resolution single-photon emission computed tomography. *Archives of General Psychiatry, 49,* 695–702.

Rutter, M., Cox, A., Tupling, C., Berger, M., & Yule, W. (1975). Attainment and adjustment in two geographical areas: 1. The prevalence of psychiatric disorders. *British Journal of Psychiatry, 126,* 493–506.

Rutter, M., & Gould, M. (1985). Classification. In M. Rutter & L. Hersov (Eds.), *Child and adolescent psychiatry: Modern approaches* (pp. 304–321). Oxford, England: Blackwell Scientific.

Rutter, M., Tizard, J., & Whitmore, K. (1970). *Education health and behavior.* London: Hamilton.

Rutter, M., Tuma, A. H., & Lann, I. L. (1989). *Assessment and diagnosis in child psychopathology.* New York: Guilford Press.

Sacks, O. (1985). *The man who mistook his wife for a hat and other clinical tales* (pp. 92–100). New York: Harper & Row.

Sacks, O. (1992). Tourette's syndrome and creativity. *British Medical Journal, 305,* 1515–1516.

Sacks, O. (1995). *An anthropologist on Mars.* New York: Knopf.

Sadovnick, D., & Kurlan, R. (1997). The increasingly complex genetics of Tourette's syndrome. *Neurology, 48,* 801–802.

Safer, D. J., & Allen, R. P. (1989). Absence of tolerance to the behavioral effects of methylphenidate in hyperactive and inattentive children. *Journal of Pediatrics, 115,* 1003–1008.

Safer, D. J., & Krager, J. M. (1988). A survey of medication treatment for hyperactive/inattentive students. *Journal of the American Medical Association, 260,* 2256–2258.

Saint-Cyr, J. A., Taylor, A. E., & Nicholson, K. (1995). Behavior and the basal ganglia. In W. J. Weiner & A. E. Lang (Eds.), *Advances in neurology: Vol. 65. Behavioral neurology of movement disorders* (pp. 1–25). New York: Raven Press.

Sallee, F. R., Kopp, U., & Hanin, I. (1992). Controlled study of erythrocyte choline in Tourette syndrome. *Biological Psychiatry, 31,* 1204–1212.

Sallee, F. R., & Rock, C. M. (1994). Effects of pimozide on cognition in children with Tourette syndrome: Interaction with comorbid attention-deficit hyperactivity disorder. *Acta Psychiatrica Scandinavica, 90,* 4–9.

Sameroff, A. J. (1987). The social context of development. In N. Eisenberg (Ed.), *Contemporary topics in child development* (pp. 273–291). New York: Wiley.

Sanberg, P. R., McConville, B. J., Fogelson, H. M., Manderscheid, P. Z., Parker, K. W., Blythe, M. M., Klykylo, W. M., & Norman, A. B. (1989). Nicotine potentiates the effects of haloperidol in animals and in patients with Tourette syndrome. *Biomedical Pharmacotherapy, 43,* 19–23.

Sandor, P., Musisi, S., Moldofsky, H., & Lang, A. (1990). Tourette syndrome: A follow-up study. *Journal of Clinical Psychopharmacology, 10,* 197–199.

Sandyk, R. (1985). The effect of naloxone in Tourette's syndrome. *Annals of Neurology, 18,* 367–368.

Sandyk, R. (1988). Clomiphene citrate in Tourette's syndrome. *International Journal of Neuroscience, 43,* 103–106.

Sandyk, R. (1989). Abnormal opiate receptor functions in Tourette's syndrome. *International Journal of Neuroscience, 44,* 209–214.

Santangelo, S. L., Pauls, D. L., Goldstein, J. M., Faraone, S. V., Tsuang, M. T., & Leckman, J. F. (1994). Tourette's syndrome: What are the influences of gender and comorbid obsessive-compulsive disorder? *Journal of the American Academy of Child & Adolescent Psychiatry, 33,* 795–804.

Santangelo, S. L., Pauls, D. L., Lavoi, P. W., Faraone, S. V., & Tsuang, M. T. (1996). Assessing risk for the Tourette spectrum of disorders among 1st degree relatives of probands with Tourette syndrome. *American Journal of Medical Genetics, 67,* 107–116.

Sargent, J. R., Sahler, O. J. Z., Roghmann, K. J., Mulhern, R. K., Barbarian, O. A., Carpenter, P. J., Copeland, D. R., Dolgin, M. J., & Zeltzer, L. K. (1995). Sibling adaptation to childhood cancer collaborative study: Siblings' perceptions of the cancer experience. *Journal of Pediatric Psychology, 20,* 151–164.

Satterfield, J. H., Satterfield, B. I., & Schell, A. E. (1987). Therapeutic interventions to prevent delinquency in hyperactive boys. *Journal of the American Academy of Child & Adolescent Psychiatry, 26,* 56–64.

Savage, C. R., Keuthen, N. J., Jenike, M. A., Brown, H. D., Baer, L., Kendrick, A. D., Miguel, E. C., Rauch, S. L., & Albert, M. S. (1996). Recall and recognition memory in obsessive-compulsive disorder. *Journal of Neuropsychiatry and Clinical Neuroscience, 8,* 99–103.

Saxena, S., Wang, D., Bystritsky, A., & Baxter, L. R., Jr. (1996). Risperidone augmentation of SRI treatment for refractory obsessive-compulsive disorder. *Journal of Clinical Psychiatry, 57,* 303–306.

Scahill, L. (1996). Contemporary approaches to pharmacotherapy in Tourette's syndrome and obsessive-compulsive disorder. *Journal of Child & Adolescent Psychiatric Nursing, 9,* 27–43.

Scahill, L., Leckman, J. F., & Marek, K. L. (1995). Sensory phenomena in Tourette's syndrome. In W. J. Weiner & A. E. Lang (Eds.), *Advances in neurology: Vol. 65. Behavioral neurology of movement disorders* (pp. 273–280). New York: Raven Press.

Scahill, L., Lynch, K. A., & Ort, S. I. (1995). Tourette syndrome: Update and review. *Journal of School Nursing, 11,* 24–32.

Scahill, L., & Ort, S. I. (1995). Clinical ratings in child psychiatric nursing. *Journal of Child & Adolescent Psychiatric Nursing, 8,*33–41.

Scahill, L., Ort, S. I., & Hardin, M. T. (1993a). Tourette's syndrome, Part I: Definition and diagnosis. *Archives of Psychiatric Nursing, 7,* 203–208.

Scahill, L., Ort, S. I., & Hardin, M. T. (1993b). Tourette's syndrome, Part II: Contemporary approaches to assessment and treatment. *Archives of Psychiatric Nursing, 7,* 209–216.

Scahill, L., Riddle, M. A., McSwiggin-Hardin, M., Ort, S. I., King, R. A., Goodman, W. K., Cicchetti, D., & Leckman, J. F. (1997). Children's Yale-Brown obsessive compulsive scale: Reliability and validity. *Journal of the American Academy of Child & Adolescent Psychiatry, 65,* 844–853.

Scahill, L., Vitulano, L. A., Brenner, E., Lynch, K. A., & King, R. A. (1996). Behavioral therapy in children and adolescents with obsessive-compulsive disorder: A pilot study. *Journal of Child & Adolescent Psychopharmacology, 6,* 191–202.

Scahill, L., Walker, R., Lechner, S. N., & Tynan, K. E. (1993). Inpatient treatment of obsessive compulsive disorder: A case study. *Journal of Child & Adolescent Psychiatric Nursing, 6,* 5–14.

Scarone, S., Colombo, C., Livian, S., Abbruzzese, M., Ronchi, P., Locatelli, M., Scotti, G., & Smeraldi, E. (1992). Increased right caudate nucleus size in obsessive-compulsive disorder: Detection with magnetic resonance imaging. *Psychiatry Research, 45,* 115–121.

Schuerholz, L. J., Baumgardner, T. L., Singer, H. S., Reiss, A. L., & Denckla, M. B. (1996). Neuropsychological status of children with Tourette's syndrome with and without attention deficit hyperactivity disorder. *Neurology, 46,* 958–965.

Schulman, M. (1974). Control of tics by maternal reinforcement. *Journal of Behavior Therapy and Experimental Psychiatry, 5,* 95–96.

Schultz, R. T., Carter, A. S., Gladstone, M., Scahill, L., Leckman, J. F., Peterson, B. S., Zhang, H., Cohen, D. J., & Pauls, D. (1998). Visual-motor, visuoperceptual and fine motor functioning in children with Tourette syndrome. *Neuropsychology, 12,* 134–145.

Schwab-Stone, M., Fallon, T., Briggs, M., & Crowther, B. (1994). Reliability of diagnostic reporting for children aged 6–11 years: A test-retest study of the diagnostic interview schedule for children–revised. *American Journal of Psychiatry, 151,* 1048–1054.

Schwab-Stone, M. E., Shaffer, D., Fisher, P., Dulcan, M. K., Jensen, P. S., Bird, H. R., Goodman, S. H., Lahey, B. B., Lichtman, J. H., Canino, G., Rubio-Stipec, M., & Rae, D. S. (1996). Criterion validity of the NIMH diagnostic interview schedule for children version 2.3 (DISC-2.3): Description, acceptability, prevalence rates, and performance in the MECA study. *Journal of the American Academy of Child & Adolescent Psychiatry, 35,* 878–888.

Schwabe, M. J., & Konkol, R. J. (1992). Menstrual cycle-related fluctuations of tics in Tourette syndrome. *Pediatric Neurology, 8,* 43–46.

Schwartz, J. M. (1996). *Brain lock.* New York: HarperCollins.

Schwartz, J. M., Stoessel, P. W., Baxter, L. R., Martin, K. M., & Phelps, M. E. (1996). Systematic changes in cerebral glucose metabolic rate after successful behavior modification treatment of obsessive-compulsive disorder. *Archives of General Psychiatry, 53,* 109–113.

Scott, B. L., & Jankovic, J. (1996). Delayed-onset progressive movement disorders after static brain lesions. *Neurology, 46,* 68–74.

Sebrechts, M. M., Shaywitz, S. E., Shaywitz, B. A., Jatlow, P., Anderson, G. M., & Cohen, D. J. (1986). Components of attention, methylphenidate dosage, and blood levels in children with attention deficit disorder. *Journal of Pediatrics, 77,* 222–228.

Seeger, T. F., Seymour, P. A., Schmidt, A. W., Zorn, S. H., Schulz, D. W., Lebel, L. A., McLean, S., Guanowsky, V., Howard, H. R., & Lowe, J. A. (1995). Ziprasidone (CP-88,059): A new antipsychotic with combined dopamine and serotonin antagonist activity. *Journal of Pharmacology and Experimental Therapeutics, 275,* 101–113.

Seeman, P., Bzowej, N. H., Guan, H. C., Bergeron, C., Becker, L. E., Reynolds, G. P., Bird, E. D., Riederer, P., Jellinger, K., & Watanabe, S. (1987). Human brain dopamine receptors in children and aging adults. *Synapse, 1,* 399–404.

Seignot, M. J. N. (1961). Un cas de maladie des tics de Gilles de al Tourette guéeri par le R-1625. *Annals of Medical Psychology, 119,* 578–579.

Selinger, D., Cohen, D. J., Ort, S. I., Anderson, G. M., & Leckman, J. F. (1984). Parotid salivary response to clonidine in Tourette's syndrome: Indicators of noradrenergic responsivity. *Journal of the American Academy of Child Psychiatry, 23,* 392–398.

Semrud-Clikeman, M. S., Biederman, J., Sprich, S., Krifcher, B., Norman, D., & Faraone, S. (1992). Comorbidity between ADHD and learning disability: A review and report in a clinically referred sample. *Journal of the American Academy of Child & Adolescent Psychiatry, 31,* 439–448.

Semrud-Clikeman, M. S., Filipek, P. A., Biederman, J., Steingard, R., Kennedy, D., Renshaw, P., & Bekken, K. (1994). Attention-deficit hyperactivity disorder: Magnetic resonance imaging morphometric analysis of the corpus callosum. *Journal of the American Academy of Child & Adolescent Psychiatry, 33,* 875–881.

Shady, G. A., Fulton, W. A., & Champion, L. M. (1988). Tourette syndrome and educational problems in Canada. *Neuroscience and Biobehavioral Reviews, 12,* 263–265.

Shaffer, D., Fisher, P., Dulcan, M. K., Davies, M., Piacentini, J., Schwab-Stone, M. E., Lahey, B. B., Bourdon, K., Jensen, P. S., Bird, H. R., Canino, G., & Regier, D. A. (1996). The NIMH diagnostic interview schedule for children version 2.3 (DISC-2.3): Description, acceptability, prevalence rates, and performance in the MECA study. Methods for the epidemiology of child and adolescent mental disorders study. *Journal of the American Academy of Child & Adolescent Psychiatry, 35,* 865–877.

Sham, P. C., O'Callaghan, E., Takei, N., Murray, G. K., Hare, E. H., & Murray, R. M. (1992). Schizophrenia following pre-natal exposure to influenza epidemics between 1939 and 1960. *British Journal of Psychiatry, 160,* 461–466.

Shapiro, A. K., Baron, M., Shapiro, E., & Levitt, M. (1984). Enzyme activity in Tourette's syndrome. *Archives of Neurology, 41,* 282–285.

Shapiro, A. K., & Shapiro, E. (1968). Treatment of Gilles de la Tourette's syndrome. *British Journal of Psychiatry, 114,* 345–350.

Shapiro, A. K., & Shapiro, E. S. (1984). Controlled study of pimozide vs. placebo in Tourette syndrome. *Journal of the American Academy of Child & Adolescent Psychiatry, 23,* 161–173.

Shapiro, A. K., Shapiro, E. S., Bruun, R. D., & Sweet, R. D. (1978). *Gilles de la Tourette syndrome.* New York: Raven Press.

Shapiro, A. K., Shapiro, E. S., Young, J. G., & Feinberg, T. (1988). *Gilles de la Tourette syndrome* (2nd ed.). New York: Raven Press.

Shapiro, E. S., Shapiro, A. K., & Clarkin, J. (1974). Clinical psychological testing in Tourette's syndrome. *Journal of Personality Assessment, 38,* 464–478.

Shapiro, E. S., Shapiro, A. K., Fulop, G., Hubbard, M., Mandeli, J., Nordlie, J., & Phillips, R. (1989). Controlled study of haloperidol, pimozide, and placebo for the treatment of GTS. *Archives of General Psychiatry, 46,* 722–730.

Sharenow, E. L., Fuqua, R. W., & Miltenberger, R. G. (1989). The treatment of muscle tics with dissimilar competing response practice. *Journal of Applied Behavior Analysis, 22,* 35–42.

Shaywitz, B., Fletcher, B., & Shaywitz, S. (1995). Defining and classifying LD and AD/HD. *Journal of Child Neurology, 1*(Suppl.), 550–557.

Shucard, D. W., Benedict, R. H. B., Tekokkilic, A., & Lichter, D. G. (1997). Slowed reaction time during a continuous performance test in children with Tourette's syndrome. *Neuropsychology, 11,* 147–155.

Silbersweig, D. A., Stern, E., Chee, K., Trimble, M. R., Robertson, M. M., & Dolan, R. J. (1995). Functional neuroanatomical correlates of tics in Tourette's syndrome. In *New research program and abstracts: 148th annual meeting of American Psychiatric Association* (p. 96). Washington, DC: American Psychiatric Press.

Silva, R. R., Munoz, D. M., Barickman, J., & Friedhoff, A. J. (1995). Environmental factors and related fluctuation of symptoms in children and adolescents with Tourette's disorder. *Journal of Child Psychology & Psychiatry & Applied Disciplines, 36,* 305–312.

Silver, A. A., & Sanberg, P. R. (1993). Transdermal nicotine patch and potentiation of haloperidol in Tourette's syndrome. *Lancet, 342,*182.

Silver, A. A., Shytle, R. D., Philipp, M. K., & Sanberg, P. R. (1996). Case study: Long-term potentiation of neuroleptics with transdermal nicotine in Tourette's syndrome. *Journal of the American Academy of Child & Adolescent Psychiatry, 35,* 1631–1636.

Silver, L. (1992). Diagnosis of attention deficit hyperactivity disorder in adult life. *Child & Adolescent Psychiatry Clinics of North America, 1,* 325–334.

Silverstein, F., Smith, C. B., & Johnstone, M. V. (1985). Effect of clonidine on platelet alpha 2-adrenoreceptors and plasma norepinephrine of children with Tourette syndrome. *Developmental Medicine and Child Neurology, 27,* 793–799.

Silverstein, M. S., Como, P. G., Palumbo, D. R., West, L. L., & Osborn, L. M. (1995). Multiple sources of attentional dysfunction in adults with Tourette's syndrome: Comparison with attention deficit-hyperactivity disorder. *Neuropsychology, 2,* 157–164.

Simeon, J. G., Ferguson, H. B., & Fleet, J. V. W. (1986). Bupropion effects in attention deficit and conduct disorder. *Canadian Journal of Psychiatry, 31,* 581–585.

Simerly, R. B., Swanson, L. W., & Gorski, R. A. (1985). Reversal of the sexually dimorphic distribution of serotonin-immunoreactive fibers in the medial preoptic nucleus by treatment with perinatal androgen. *Brain Research, 340,* 91–98.

Singer, H. S. (1981). Transient Gilles de la Tourette's syndrome after chronic neuroleptic withdrawal. *Developmental Medicine and Child Neurology, 23,* 518–530.

Singer, H. S., Brown, J., & Quaskey, S. (1995). The treatment of attention-deficit hyeractivity disorder in Tourette's syndrome: A double-blind placebo-controlled study with clonidine and desipramine. *Pediatrics, 95,* 74–81.

Singer, H. S., Butler, I. J., Tune, L. E., Seifert, W. E., Jr., & Coyle, J. T. (1982). Dopaminergic dysfunction in Tourette syndrome. *Annals of Neurology, 12,* 361–366.

Singer, H. S., Hahn, I. H., Krowiak, E., Nelson, E., & Moran, T. (1990). Tourette syndrome: A neurochemical analysis of postmortem brain tissue. *Annales of Neurology, 27,* 443–446.

Singer, H. S., Hahn, I. H., & Moran, T. H. (1991). Abnormal dopamine uptake sites in postmortem striatum from patients with Tourette's syndrome. *Annals of Neurology, 30,* 558–562.

Singer, H. S., Oshida, L., & Coyle, J. T. (1984). CSF cholinesterase activity in Gilles de la Tourette's syndrome. *Archives of Neurology, 41,* 756–757.

Singer, H. S., Reiss, A. L., Brown, R. N., Aylward, E. H., Shih, B. A., Chee, E., Harris, E. L., Reader, M. J., Chase, G. A., Bryan, R. N., & Denckla, M. B. (1993). Volumetric MRI changes in basal ganglia of children with Tourette's syndrome. *Neurology, 43,* 950–956.

Singer, H. S., & Rosenberg, L. A. (1989). Development of behavioral and emotional problems in Tourette syndrome. *Pediatric Neurology, 5,* 41–44.

Singer, H. S., Schuerholz, L. J., & Denckla, M. B. (1995). Learning difficulties in children with Tourette syndrome. *Journal of Child Neurology, 10,* s58–s61.

Singer, H. S., Tune, L. E., Butler, I. J., Zaczek, R., & Coyle, J. T. (1982). Clinical symptomatology, CSF neurotransmitter metabolites, and serum haldol levels in Tourette syndrome. In A. J. Friedhoff & T. N. Chase (Eds.), *Advances in neurology: Vol. 35. Gilles de la Tourette syndrome* (pp. 177–183). New York: Raven Press.

Singer, H. S., Wong, D. F., Brown, J. E., Brandt, J., Krafft, L., Shaya, E., Dannals, R. F., & Wagner, H., Jr. (1992). Positron emission tomography evaluation of dopamine D-2 receptors in adults with Tourette syndrome. In T. N. Chase, A. J. Friedhoff & D. J. Cohen (Eds.), *Advances in neurology: Vol. 58. Tourette syndrome: Genetics, neurobiology and treatment* (pp. 233–239). New York: Raven Press.

Smith, S. J. M., & Lees, A. J. (1989). Abnormalities of the blink reflex in Gilles de la Tourette syndrome. *Journal of Neurology, Neurosurgery and Psychiatry, 52,* 895–898.

Solanto, M. V. (1984). Neuropharmacological basis of stimulant drug action in attention deficit disorder with hyperactivity: A review and synthesis. *Psychology Bulletin, 95,* 387–409.

Spanier, G. B. (1976). Measuring dyadic adjustment: New scales for assessing the quality of marriage and similar dyads. *Journal of Marriage and the Family, 38,* 15–28.

Sparrow, S. S., Balla, D., & Cicchetti, D. V. (1984). *The Vineland adaptive behavior scales interview edition.* Circle Pines, MN: American Guidance Service.

Sparrow, S. S., Carter, A. S., Racusin, G., & Morris, R. (1995). Comprehensive psychological assessment through the lifespan: A developmental approach. In D. Cicchetti & D. J. Cohen (Eds.), *Developmental psychopathology: Theory and methods* (Vol. 1, pp. 81–105). New York: Wiley.

Spencer, T. J., Biederman, J., Harding, M., O'Donnell, D., Wilens, T., Faraone, S., Coffey, B., & Geller, D. (in press). Disentangeling the overlap of Tourette's disorder and ADHD. *Journal of Child Psychology and Psychiatry and Allied Disciplines.*

Spencer, T. J., Biederman, J., Harding, M., Wilens, T., & Faraone, S. (1995). The relationship between tic disorders and Tourette's syndrome revisited. *Journal of the American Academy of Child & Adolescent Psychiatry, 34,* 1133–1139.

Spencer, T. J., Biederman, J., Kerman, K., Steingard, R., & Wilens, T. (1993). Desipramine treatment of children with attention-deficit hyperactivity disorder and tic disorder or Tourette's syndrome. *Journal of the American Academy of Child & Adolescent Psychiatry, 32,* 354–360.

Spencer, T. J., Biederman, J., Steingard, R., & Wilens, T. (1993). Bupropion exacerbates tics in children with attention-deficit hyperactivity disorder and Tourette's syndrome. *Journal of the American Academy of Child & Adolescent Psychiatry, 32,* 211–214.

Spencer, T. J., Biederman, J., Wilens, T., Steingard, R., & Geist, D. (1993). Nortriptyline treatment of children with attention-deficit hyperactivity disorder and tic disorder or Tourette's syndrome. *Journal of the American Academy of Child & Adolescent Psychiatry, 32,* 205–210.

Spielman, R. S., McGinnis, R. E., & Ewens, W. J. (1993). Transmission test for linkage disequilibrium: The insulin gene region and insulin-dependent diabetes mellitus (IDDM). *American Journal of Human Genetics, 52,* 506–516.

Spitzer, R. L., Williams, J. B., Gibbon, M., & First, M. B. (1992). The structured clinical interview for *DSM-III-R* (SCID): 1. History, rationale, and description. *Archives of General Psychiatry, 49,* 624–629.

Sprague, R. L., & Sleator, E. K. (1977). Methylphenidate in hyperkinetic children: Differences in dose effects on learning and social behavior. *Science, 198,* 1274–1276.

Sprich-Buckminster, S., Biederman, J., Milberger, S., Faraone, S. V., & Lehman, B. K. (1993). Are perinatal complications relevant to the manifestation of ADD? Issues of comorbidity and familiality. *Journal of the American Academy of Child & Adolescent Psychiatry, 32,* 1032–1037.

Stahl, S. M., & Berger, P. A. (1981). Physostigmine in Tourette syndrome: Evidence for cholinergic underactivity. *American Journal of Psychiatry, 138,* 240–242.

Stahl, S. M., & Berger, P. A. (1982). Cholinergic and dopaminergic mechanisms in Tourette syndrome. In A. J. Friedhoff & T. N. Chase (Eds.), *Advances in neurology: Vol. 35. Gilles de la Tourette syndrome* (pp. 141–150). New York: Raven Press.

Stamenkovic, M., Aschauer, H., & Kasper, S. (1994). Risperidone for Tourette's syndrome. *Lancet, 344,* 1577–1578.

Stanger, C., Achenbach, T. M., & Verhulst, F. C. (1994). Accelerating longitudinal research on child psychopathology: A practical example. *Psychological Assessment, 6,* 102–107.

Stefl, M. E. (1984). *The Ohio Tourette study: An investigation of the special service needs of the Tourette syndrome patients.* Cincinnati: University of Cincinnati.

Steingard, R. J., Goldberg, M., Lee, D., & DeMaso, D. R. (1994). Adjunctive clonazepam treatment of tic symptoms in children with comorbid tic disorders and ADHD. *Journal of the American Academy of Child & Adolescent Psychiatry, 33,* 394–399.

Steketee, G. S. (1993). *Treatment of obsessive-compulsive disorder.* New York: Guilford Press.

Steketee, G. S., Chambless, D. L., Tran, G. Q., Worden, H., & Gillis, M. M. (1996). Behavioral avoidance test for obsessive compulsive disorder. *Behavior Research and Therapy, 34,* 73–83.

Stephens, R., Pelham, W. E., & Skinner, R. (1984). The state-dependent and main effects of pemoline and methylphenidate on paired-associates learning and spelling in hyperactive children. *Journal of Consulting and Clinical Psychology, 52,* 104–113.

Stern, R. A., Singer, E. A., Duke, L. M., Singer, N., Morey, C. E., Daughtrey, E. W., & Kaplan, E. (1994). The Boston qualitative scoring system for the Rey-Osterreith Complex Figure: Description and interrater reliability. *Clinical Neuropsychologist, 8,* 309–332.

Stoetter, B., Braun, A. R., Randolph, C., Gernert, J., Carson, R. E., Herscovitch, P., & Chase, T. N. (1992). Functional neuroanatomy of Tourette syndrome. Limbic-motor interactions studied with FDG PET. *Advances in Neurology, 58,* 213–226.

Stokes, A., Bawden, H. N., Camfield, P. R., Backman, J. E., & Dooley, M. B. (1991). Peer problems in Tourette's disorder. *Pediatrics, 87,* 936–942.

Stone, L., & Jankovic, J. (1991). The co-existence of tics and dystonia. *Archives of Neurology, 48,* 862–865.

Sullivan, R. M., Parker, B. A., & Szechtman, H. (1993). Role of the corpus callosum in expression of behavioral asymmetries induced by a unilateral dopamine lesion of the substantia nigra in the rat. *Brain Research, 609,* 347–350.

Surwillo, W. W., Shafii, M., & Barrett, C. L. (1978). Gilles de la Tourette syndrome: A 20-month study of the effects of stressful life events and haloperidol on symptom frequency. *Journal of Nervous and Mental Disease, 166,* 812–816.

Susser, E. S., & Lin, S. P. (1992). Schizophrenia after prenatal exposure to the Dutch hunger winter of 1944–1945. *Archives of General Psychiatry, 49,* 983–988.

Sutherland, R. J., Kolb, B., Schoel, W. M., Whishaw, I. Q., & Davies, D. (1982). Neuropsychological assessment of children and adults with Tourette syndrome: A comparison with learning disabilities and schizophrenia. In A. J. Friedhoff & T. N. Chase (Eds.), *Advances in neurology: Vol. 35. Gilles de la Tourette syndrome* (pp. 311–321). New York: Raven Press.

Swanson, J. M. (1992). *School-based assessments and interventions for ADD students.* Irvine, CA: K.C. Publishing.

Swedo, S. E. (1994). Sydenham's chorea: A model for childhood autoimmune neuropsychiatric disorders. *Journal of the American Medical Association, 272,* 1788–1791.

Swedo, S. E., Kilpatrick, K., Schapiro, M. B., Mannheim, G. B., & Leonard, H. L. (1991). Antineuronal antibodies in Sydenham's chorea and obsessive compulsive disorder. *Pediatric Research, 29,* 369a.

Swedo, S. E., Leonard, H. L., Garvey, M., Mittleman, B., Allen, A. J., Perlmutter, S., Lougee, L., Dow, S., Zamkoff, J., & Dubbert, B. K. (1998). Pediatric autoimmune neuropsychiatric disorders associated with streptococcal infections: Clinical description of the first 50 cases. *American Journal of Psychiatry, 155,* 264–271.

Swedo, S. E., Leonard, H. L., & Kiessling, L. S. (1994). Speculations on antineuronal antibody-mediated neuropsychiatric disorders of childhood. *Pediatrics, 93,* 323–326.

Swedo, S. E., Leonard, H. L., Kruesi, M. J., Rettew, D. C., Listwak, S. J., Berrettini, W., Stipetic, M., Hamburger, S., Gold, P. W., Potter, W. Z., & Rapoport, J. L. (1992). Cerebrospinal fluid neurochemistry in children and adolescents with obsessive-compulsive disorder. *Archives of General Psychiatry, 49,* 29–36.

Swedo, S. E., Leonard, H. L., Schapiro, M. B., Casey, B. J., Mannheim, G. B., Lenane, M. C., & Rettew, D. C. (1993). Sydenham's chorea: Physical and psychological symptoms of St. Vitus Dance. *Pediatrics, 91,* 706–713.

Swedo, S. E., Pietrini, P., Leonard, H. L., Schapiro, M. B., Rettew, D. C., Goldberger, E. L., Rapoport, S. I., Rapoport, J. L., & Grady, C. L. (1992). Cerebral glucose metabolism in childhood-onset obsessive-compulsive disorder. Revisualization during pharmacotherapy. *Archives of General Psychiatry, 49,* 690–694.

Swedo, S. E., & Rapoport, J. L. (1989). Phenomenology and differential diagnosis of obsessive compulsive disorder in children and adolescents. In J. L. Rapoport (Ed.), *Obsessive compulsive disorder in children and adolescents* (pp. 13–32). Washington, DC: American Psychiatric Press.

Swedo, S. E., & Rapoport, J. L. (1990). Neurochemical and neuroendocrine considerations of obsessive-compulsive disorders in childhood. In S. Deutsch (Ed.), *Application of basic neuroscience to child psychiatry* (pp. 275–284). New York: Plenum Press.

Swedo, S. E., Rapoport, J. L., Cheslow, D. L., Leonard, H. L., Ayoub, E. M., Hosier, D. M., & Wald, E. R. (1989). High prevalence of obsessive-compulsive symptoms in patients with Sydenham's chorea. *American Journal of Psychiatry, 146,* 246–249.

Swedo, S. E., Rapoport, J. L., Leonard, H. L., Lenane, M. C., & Cheslow, D. (1989). Obsessive compulsive disorder in children and adolescents: Clinical phenomenology of 70 consecutive cases. *Archives of General Psychiatry, 46,* 335–341.

Swedo, S. E., Schapiro, M. B., Grady, C. L., Cheslow, D. L., Leonard, H. L., Kumar, A., Friedland, R., Rapoport, S. I., & Rapoport, J. L. (1989). Cerebral glucose metabolism in childhood-onset obsessive-compulsive disorder. *Archives of General Psychiatry, 46,* 518–523.

Sweeney, D., Pickar, D., Redmond, D. E., Jr., & Maas, J. (1978). Noradrenergic and dopaminergic mechanisms in Gilles de la Tourette syndrome [letter]. *Lancet, 1,* 872.

Sweet, R. D., Bruun, R., Shapiro, E., & Shapiro, A. K. (1974). Presynaptic catecholamine antagonists as treatment for Tourette syndrome: Effects of alpha-methyl-para-tyrosine and tetrabenazine. *Archives of General Psychiatry, 31,* 857–861.

Szasz, T. (1995). *Cruel compassion, psychiatric control of society's unwanted.* Canada: Wiley.

Szatmari, P. (1992). The epidemiology of attention deficit hyperactivity disorders. *Child & Adolescent Psychiatry Clinics of North America, 1,* 361–372.

Szatmari, P., Offord, D. R., & Boyle, M. H. (1989). Ontario child health study: Prevalence of attention deficit disorder with hyperactivity. *Journal of Child Psychology & Psychiatry, 30,* 219–230.

Szatmari, P., Saigal, S., Rosenbaum, P., & Campbell, D. (1993). Psychopathology and adaptive functioning among extremely low birthweight children at eight years of age. *Development and Psychopathology, 5,* 345–357.

Szymanski, S., Singer, H., Giuliano, J., Dogan, S., Yokoi, F., Chin, B., Dannals, R., Ravert, H., & Wong, D. F. (1997). *Intrasynaptic dopamine release in Tourette's syndrome.* Abstract.

Takahashi, L. K., Turner, J. G., & Kalin, N. H. (1992). Prenatal stress alters brain catecholaminergic activity and potentiates stress-induced behavior in adult rats. *Brain Research, 574,* 131–137.

Takano, K., & Ishiguro, T. (1993). A study of clinical pictures and monoamine metabolism of Gilles de la Tourette syndrome. *Seishin Shinkeigaku Zasshi— Psychiatria et Neurologia Japonica, 95,* 1–29.

Takei, N., Sham, P., O'Callaghan, E., Murray, G. K., Glover, G., & Murray, R. M. (1994). Prenatal exposure to influenza and the development of schizophrenia: Is the effect confined to females? *American Journal of Psychiatry, 151,* 117–119.

Talairach, J., Bancaud, J., Geier, S., Bordas-Ferrer, M., Bonis, A., Szikla, G., & Rusu, M. (1973). The cingulate gyrus and human behavior. *Electroencephalography and Clinical Neurophysiology, 34,* 45–52.

Tanner, C. M., Goetz, C. G., & Klawans, H. L. (1982). Cholinergic mechanisms in Tourette syndrome. *Neurology, 32,* 1315–1317.

Tannock, R., Ickowicz, A., & Schachar, R. (1991). Effects of comorbid anxiety disorder on stimulant response in children with attention deficit hyperactivity disorder [abstract]. *Proceedings of American Academy of Child and Adolescent Psychiatry, 7,* 56–57.

Tasker, R. R., & Dostrovsky, J. O. (1993). What goes on in the motor thalamus? *Stereotactic & Functional Neurosurgery, 60,* 121–126.

Taylor, E. M. (1959). *The appraisal of children with cerebral deficits*. Cambridge, MA: Harvard University Press.

Taylor, E. M. (1994). Syndromes of attention deficit and overactivity. In M. Rutter, Taylor, & L. Hersov (Eds.), *Child and adolescent psychiatry: Modern approaches* (pp. 285–307). Oxford, England: Blackwell Scientific.

Taylor, S. C. (1980). The effect of chronic childhood illnesses upon well siblings. *Maternal-Child Nursing Journal, 9,* 109–116.

Terry, R., & Coie, J. D. (1991). A comparison of methods for defining sociometric status among children. *Developmental Psychology, 27,* 867–880.

Terwilliger, J. D., & Ott, J. (1992). A haplotype-based "haplotype relative risk" approach to detecting allelic associations. *Human Heredity, 42,* 337–346.

Tew, B., & Laurence, K. M. (1973). Mothers, brothers and sisters of patients with spinal bifida. *Developmental Medicine and Childhood Neurology, 15,* 69–76.

Thelen, E., & Smith, L. B. (1994). *A dynamic systems approach to the development of cognition and action*. Cambridge, MA: MIT Press.

Thomas, E. J., Abrams, K. S., & Johnson, J. B. (1971). Self-monitoring and reciprocal inhibition in the modification of multiple tics of Gilles de la Tourette's syndrome. *Journal of Behavior Therapy and Experimental Psychiatry, 2,* 159–171.

Thomas, J., & Ericksen-Mendosa, H. (1996). *New independent sector study finds giving and volunteering rising. Giving and volunteering press release, independent sector* (http://www.indepsec.org:80/gvrel.html). Washington, DC.

Thomsen, P. H. (1994a). Obsessive-compulsive disorder in children and adolescents. A review of the literature. *European Journal of Child & Adolescent Psychiatry, 3,* 138–158.

Thomsen, P. H. (1994b). Obsessive-compulsive disorder in children and adolescents. A 6–22 year follow-up study. Clinical descriptions of obsessive-compulsive phenomenology and continuity. *European Journal of Child & Adolescent Psychiatry, 3,* 82–96.

Thomsen, P. H. (1994c). Obsessive-compulsive disorder in children and adolescents. A study of phenomenology and family functioning in 20 consecutive Danish cases. *European Journal of Child & Adolescent Psychiatry, 3,* 29–36.

Thomsen, P. H. (1995). Obsessive-compulsive disorder in children and adolescents: A study of parental psychopathology and precipitating events in 20 consecutive Danish cases. *Psychopathology, 28,* 161–167.

Tiffen, J. (1968). *The Purdue pegboard test*. Chicago: Science Research Associates.

Tiger, L., & Fox, R. (1989). *The imperial animal* (pp. vii). New York: Henry Holt.

Tollefson, G. D. (1985). Alprazolam in the treatment of obsessive symptoms. *Journal of Clinical Psychopharmacology, 5,* 39–42.

Tollefson, G. D., Rampey, A. H., Jr., Potvin, J. H., Jenike, M. A., Rush, A. J., Dominguez, R. A., Koran, L. M., Shear, M. K., Goodman, W., & Genduso, L. A. (1994). A multicenter investigation of fixed-dose fluoxetine in the treatment of obsessive-compulsive disorder. *Archives of General Psychiatry, 51,* 559–567.

Tolosa, E. S. (1981). Clinical features of Meige's disease (idiopathic orofacial dystonia). *Archives of Neurology, 38,* 147–151.

Tophoff, M. (1973). Massed practice, relaxation and assertion training in the treatment of Gilles de la Tourette's syndrome. *Journal of Behavior Therapy and Experimental Psychiatry, 4,* 71–73.

Torgerson, S. (1983). Genetic factors in anxiety disorder. *Archives of General Psychiatry, 40,* 1085–1089.

Torup, E. (1962). A follow-up study of children with tics. *Acta Paediatrica Scandinavica, 51,* 261–268.

Tourette Syndrome Association. (1994). *Questions and answers about Tourette syndrome.*

Tourette Syndrome Association. (1996a). Web page, "Who and What We Are" http://TSA.MGH.Harvard.EDU

Tourette Syndrome Association. (1996b). *Annual report: The path to the future* (p. 5). Author.

Tourette Syndrome Association. (1996c, Winter). New brain image study reveals a vital clue to tic severity. *Newsletter, Vol. 24*(No. 3) p. 1.

Tourette Syndrome Association. (1997, Spring). From taunts to tolerance of TS, one student's research transforms student attitudes. *TSA Newsletter, Vol. 24*(No. 4), p. 11.

Tourette Syndrome Association. *An educator's guide to Tourette syndrome* [booklet]. Bayside, NY: Bronheim, S.

Tourette Syndrome Classification Study Group. (1993). Definitions and classification of tic disorders. *Archives of Neurology, 50,* 1013–1016.

Towbin, K. E. (1995). Evaluation, establishing the treatment alliance, and informed consent in child and adolescent psychopharmacotherapy. *Child & Adolescent Psychiatric Clinics of North America, 4,* 1–15.

Towbin, K. E., Leckman, J. F., & Cohen, D. J. (1987). Drug treatment of obsessive compulsive disorder: A review in the light of diagnostic and metric limitations. *Psychiatric Developments, 1,* 25–50.

Towbin, K. E., Riddle, M. A., Cohen, D. J., & Leckman, J. F. (1988). The clinical care of individuals with Tourette's syndrome. In D. J. Cohen, R. D. Bruun & J. F. Leckman (Eds.), *Tourette's syndrome and tic disorders: Clinical understanding and treatment* (pp. 329–352). New York: Wiley.

Tucker, D. M., Leckman, J. F., Scahill, L., Epstein-Wilf, E., LaCamera, R., Cardonna, L., Cohen, P., Heidmann, S., Goldstein, J., Judge, J., Snyder, E., Bult, A., Peterson, B. S., King, R., & Lombroso, P. (1996). A putative poststreptococcal case of obsessive compulsive disorder with chronic tic disorder, not otherwise specified. *American Journal of Child & Adolescent Psychiatry, 35,* 1684–1691.

Turjanski, N., Sawle, G. V., Playford, E. D., Weeks, R., Lammerstma, A. A., Lees, A. J., & Brooks, D. J. (1994). PET studies of the presynaptic and postsynaptic dopaminergic system in Tourette's syndrome. *Journal of Neurology, Neurosurgery and Psychiatry, 57,* 688–692.

Turpin, G. (1983). The behavioural management of tic disorders: A critical review. *Advances in Behavior Research and Therapy, 5,* 203–245.

Ullmann, R. K., Sleator, E. K., & Sprague. R. L. (1985a). A change of mind: Conners' abbreviated rating scales reconsidered. *Journal of Abnormal Child Psychology, 13,* 553–565.

Ullmann, R. K., Sleator, E. K., & Sprague. R. L. (1985b). Introduction to the use of ACTeRS. *Psychopharmacology Bulletin, 2,* 915–919.

Valleni-Basile, L. A., Garrison, C. Z., Jackson, K. L., Waller, J. L., McKeown, R. E., Addy, C. L., & Cuffe, S. P. (1994). Frequency of obsessive-compulsive disorder in a community sample of young adolescents. *Journal of the American Academy of Child & Adolescent Psychiatry, 33,* 782–791.

Valleni-Basile, L. A., Garrison, C. Z., Waller, J. L., Addy, C. L., McKeown, R. E., Jackson, K. L., & Cuffe, S. P. (1996). Incidence of obsessive-compulsive disorder in a community sample of young adolescents. *Journal of the American Academy of Child & Adolescent Psychiatry, 35,* 898–906.

van der Linden, C., Bruggeman, R., & Van Woerkom, T. (1994). Serotonin-dopamine antagonist and Gilles de la Tourette's syndrome: An open pilot dose-titration study with risperidone. *Movement Disorders, 9,* 687–688.

van de Wetering, B. J. M. (1993). *The Gilles de la Tourette syndrome: A psychiatric-genetic study.* Unpublished doctoral thesis, Erasmus University, Rotterdam, The Netherlands.

van Dyck, C. H., Seibyl, J. P., Malison, R. T., Laruelle, M., Wallace, E., Zoghbi, S. S., Zea-Ponce, Y., Baldwin, R. M., Charney, D. S., & Hoffer, P. B. (1995). Age-related decline in striatal dopamine transporter binding with iodine-123-beta-CIT SPECT. *Journal of Nuclear Medicine, 36,* 1175–1181.

Vannucci, R. C. (1989). Acute perinatal brain injury: Hypoxia-ischemia. In W. H. Cohen, D. B. Acker & E. A. Riedman (Eds.), *Management of labor* (2nd ed., pp. 183–243). Rockville, MD: Aspen Press.

van Tol, H. H. M., Caren, M. W., Guan, H.-C., Ohara, K., Bunzow, J. R., Civelli, O., Kennedy, J., Seeman, P., Niznik, H. B., & Jovanovic, V. (1992). Multiple dopamine D4 receptor variants in the human population. *Nature, 358,* 149–152.

van Woert, M., Rosenbaum, D., & Enna, S. J. (1982). Overview of pharmacological approaches to therapy for Tourette syndrome. In A. J. Friedhoff & T. N. Chase (Eds.), *Advances in neurology: Vol. 35. Gilles de la Tourette syndrome* (pp. 369–375). New York: Raven Press.

Varni, J. W., Boyd, E. F., & Cataldo, M. F. (1978). Self-monitoring, external reinforcement, and time-out procedures in the control of high rate tic behaviors in a hyperactive child. *Journal of Behavior Therapy and Experimental Psychiatry, 9,* 353–358.

Veal, D. M., Sahakian, B. J., Owen, A. M., & Marks, I. M. (1996). Specific cognitive deficits in tests sensitive to frontal lobe dysfunction in obsessive-compulsive disorder. *Psychological Medicine, 26,* 1261–1269.

Verhulst, F. C., Akkerhuis, G. W., & Althaus, M. (1985). Mental health in Dutch children (I). A cross cultural comparison. *Acta Psychiatrica Scandinavica Supplement, 323,* 1–108.

Villa, G., Gainotti, G., & De Bonis, C. (1986). Constructive disabilities in focal brain-damaged patients. Influence of the hemispheric side, locus of lesion and coexistent mental deterioration. *Neuropsychologia, 24,* 497–510.

Vitiello, B., & Jensen, P. S. (1997). Medication development and testing in children and adolescents: Current problems, future directions. *Archives of General Psychiatry, 54,* 871–876.

Vitulano, L., King, R. A., & Schahill, L. (1992). Behavioral treatment of children with trichotillomania. *Journal of the American Academy of Child and Adolescent Psychiatry, 31,* 139–146.

Vogt, B. A., Finch, D. M., & Olson, C. R. (1992). Functional heterogeneity in cingulate cortex: The anterior executive and posterior executive regions. *Cerebral Cortex, 2,* 435–443.

Von Economo, C. (1931). *Encephalitis lethargica* (K. O. Newman, Trans.). Oxford, England: Oxford University Press.

Waber, D. P., & Holmes, J. M. (1985). Assessing children's copy productions of the Rey-Osterrieth Complex Figure. *Journal of Clinical and Experimental Neuropsychology, 7,* 264–280.

Wachtel, P. L. (1977). *Psychoanalysis and behavior therapy: Toward an integration.* New York: Basic Books.

Waddington, C. H. (1977). *Tools for thought.* New York: Basic Books.

Wagaman, J. R., Miltenberger, R. G., & Williams, D. E. (1995). Treatment of a vocal tic by differential reinforcement. *Journal of Behavior Therapy and Experimental Psychiatry, 26,* 35–39.

Waizer, J., Hoffman, S. P., Polizos, P., & Engelhardt, D. M. (1974). Outpatient treatment of hyperactive school children with imipramine. *American Journal of Psychiatry, 131,* 587–591.

Walkup, J. T., LaBuda, M. C., Singer, H. S., Brown, J., Riddle, M. A., & Hurko, O. (1996). Family study and segregation analysis of Tourette syndrome: Evidence for a mixed model of inheritance. *American Journal of Human Genetics, 59,* 684–693.

Walkup, J. T., Leckman, J. F., Price, R. A., Hardin, M., Ort, S. I., & Cohen, D. J. (1988). The relationship between obsessive-compulsive disorder and Tourette's syndrome: A twin study. *Psychopharmacology Bulletin, 24,* 375–379.

Walkup, J. T., & Riddle, M. A. (1997). Tic Disorders. In A. Tasman, J. Kay, & J. A. Lieberman (Eds.), *Psychiatry* (Vol. 1, pp. 702–719). Philadelphia: Saunders.

Walkup, J. T., Rosenberg, L. A., Brown, J., & Singer, H. S. (1992). The validity of instruments measuring tic severity in Tourette's syndrome. *Journal of the American Academy of Child & Adolescent Psychiatry, 30,* 472–477.

Walkup, J. T., Scahill, L., & Riddle, M. A. (1995). Disruptive behavior, hyperactivity, and learning disabilities in children with Tourette's syndrome. *Advances in Neurology, 65,* 259–272.

Walter, A. L., & Carter, A. S. (1997). Gilles de la Tourette's syndrome in childhood: A guide for school professionals. *School Psychology Review, 26,* 28–46.

Ward, A. J. (1990). A comparison and analysis of the presence of family problems during pregnancy of mothers of "autistic" children and mothers of normal children. *Child Psychiatry and Human Development, 20,* 279–288.

Ward, I. L. (1984). The prenatal stress syndrome: Current status. *Psychoneuroendocrinology, 9,* 3–11.

Ward, I. L., & Weisz, J. (1984). Differential effects of maternal stress on circulating levels of corticosterone, progesterone, and testosterone in male and female rat fetuses and their mothers. *Endocrinology, 114,* 1635–1644.

Ward, M. F., Wender, P. H., & Reimherr, F. W. (1993). The Wender Utah Rating Scale: An aid in the retrospective diagnosis of childhood attention deficit hyperactivity disorder. *American Journal of Psychiatry, 150,* 885–890.

Warrington, E. K., & James, M. (1967). Disorders of visual perception in patients with localized cerebral lesions. *Neuropsychologia, 5,* 253–266.

Warrington, E. K., James, M., & Kinsbourne, M. (1966). Drawing disability in relation to laterality of cerebral lesion. *Brain, 89,* 53–82.

Weeks, R. A., Turjanski, N., & Brouks, D. J. (1996). Tourette's syndrome: A disorder of cingulate and orbitofrontal function? *Quarterly Journal of Medicine, 89*, 401–408.

Weiss, G., Hechtman, L., Milroy, T., & Perlman, T. (1985). Psychiatric status of hyperactives as adults: A controlled prospective follow-up of 63 hyperactive children. *Journal of the American Academy of Child & Adolescent Psychiatry, 24*, 211–220.

Weiss, G., Hechtman, L., Perlman, T., Hopkins, J., & Werner, A. (1979). Hyperactives as young adults: A controlled prospective ten year follow-up of 75 children. *Archives of General Psychiatry, 36*, 675–681.

Weiss, G., Kruger, E., Danielson, U., & Elman, H. (1975). Effect of long-term treatment of hyperactive children with methylphenidate. *Canadian Medical Association Journal, 112*, 159–165.

Weiss, M., Baerg, E., Wisebord, S., & Temple, J. (1995). The influence of gonadal hormones on periodicity of obsessive-compulsive disorder. *Canadian Journal of Psychiatry, 40*, 205–207.

Weissman, M. M., & Klerman, G. L. (1978). Epidemiology of mental disorders: Emerging trends in the United States. *Archives of General Psychiatry, 35*, 705–712.

Weissman, M. M., Merikangas, K. R., John, K., Wickramaratne, P., Prusoff, B., & Kidd, K. K. (1986). Family-genetic studies of psychiatric disorders: Developing technologies. *Archives of General Psychiatry, 43*, 1104–1116.

Weissman, M. M., Sholomskas, D., & John, K. (1981). The assessment of social adjustment: An update. *Archives of General Psychiatry, 38*, 1250–1258.

Weissman, S. H., & Bashook, P. G. (1986). A view of the prospective child psychiatrist. *American Journal of Psychiatry, 143*, 722–727.

Weizman, A., Mandel, A., Barber, Y., Weitz, R., Cohen, A., Mester, R., & Rehavi, M. (1992). Decreased platelet imipramine binding in Tourette syndrome children with obsessive-compulsive disorder. *Biological Psychiatry, 3*, 705–711.

Welner, Z., Reich, W., Herjanic, B., Jung, K. G., & Amado, H. (1987). Reliability, validity, and parent-child agreement studies of the diagnostic interview for children and adolescents (DICA). *Journal of the American Academy of Child & Adolescent Psychiatry, 26*, 649–653.

Werry, J. S. (1994). Pharmacotherapy of disruptive behavior disorders. *Child and Adolescent Psychiatric Clinics of North America, 3*, 321–330.

Werry, J. S., & Aman, M. (1975). Methylphenidate and haloperidol in children: Effects on attention, memory, and activity. *Archives of General Psychiatry, 32*, 790–795.

Werry, J. S., Aman, M. G., & Diamond, E. (1980). Imipramine and methylphenidate in hyperactive children. *Journal of Child Psychology and Psychiatry, 21*, 27–35.

Werry, J. S., Weiss, G., Douglas, V., & Martin, J. (1966). Studies on the hyperactive child: 3. The effects of chlorpromazine upon behavior and learning ability. *Journal of the American Academy of Child & Adolescent Psychiatry, 5*, 292–312.

Wetzel, H., Hillert, A., Grunder, G., & Benkert, O. (1994). Roxindole, a dopamine autoreceptor agonist, in the treatment of positive and negative schizophrenic symptoms [abstract]. *American Journal of Psychiatry, 151*.

Wever, C. (1994). *Combined medication and behavioral treatment of OCD in adolescents.* Proceedings of the second annual Australian conference on OCD, Sydney, Australia.

Whalen, C. K., Heneker, B., & Granger, D. A. (1990). Social judgment processes in hyperactive boys: Effects of methylphredidate and comparison with normal peers. *Journal of Abnormal Child Psychology, 18,* 297–316.

Wheadon, D. E., Bushnell, W. D., & Steiner, M. (1993, December). *A fixed-dose comparison of 20, 40, or 60 mg paroxetine to placebo in the treatment of obsessive-compulsive disorder.* Paper presented at the 32nd annual meeting of the American College of Neuropsychopharmacology (ACNP).

Whitaker, A. H., Rossem, R. V., Feldman, J. F., Schonfeld, I. S., Pinto-Martin, J. A., Tore, C., Schaffer, D., & Paneth, N. (1997). Psychiatric outcomes in low birthweight children at age 6 years: Relation to neonatal cranial ultrasound abnormalities. *Archives of General Psychiatry, 54,* 847–856.

Wilens, T. E., & Biederman, J. (1992). The stimulants. *Psychiatric Clinics of North America, 15,* 191–222.

Wilens, T. E., Biederman, J., Geist, D. E., Steingard, R., & Spencer, T. (1993). Nortriptyline in the treatment of ADHD: A chart review of 58 cases. *Journal of the American Academy of Child & Adolescent Psychiatry, 32,* 343–349.

Wilens, T. E., Biederman, J. S., Spencer, T. J., & Frances, R. J. (1994). Comorbidity of attention-deficit hyperactivity and psychoactive substance use disorders. *Hospital and Community Psychiatry, 45,* 421–423, 435.

Williams, J. B., Gibbon, M., First, M. B., Spitzer, R. L., Davies, M., Borus, J., Howes, M. J., Kane, J., Pope, H. G., & Rounsaville, B. (1992). The Structured Clinical Interview for *DSM-III-R* (SCID): 2. Multisite test-retest reliability. *Archives of General Psychiatry, 49,* 630–636.

Wilson, C. (1986). Postsynaptic potentials evoked in spiny neostriatal neurons by stimulation of ipsilateral and contralateral neocortex. *Brain Research, 367,* 201–213.

Wilson, F. A., Scalaide, S. P. O., & Goldman-Rakic, P. (1993). Dissociation of object and spatial processing domains in primate prefrontal cortex. *Science, 260,* 1955–1957.

Wilson, R. S., Garron, D. C., Tanner, C. M., & Klawans, H. L. (1982). Behavior disturbance in children with Tourette syndrome. In A. J. Friedhoff & T. N. Chase (Eds.), *Advances in neurology: Vol. 35. Gilles de la Tourette syndrome* (pp. 329–333). New York: Raven Press.

Witelson, S. F. (1993). Clinical neurology as data for basic neuroscience: Tourette's syndrome and the human motor system. *Neurology, 43,* 859–861.

Witzum, E., Bar-On, R., Dolberg, O. T., & Kotler, M. (1996). Traumatic war experiences affect outcome in a case of Tourette's syndrome. *Psychotherapy and Psychosomatics, 65,* 106–108.

Wolf, S. S., Jones, D. W., Knable, M. B., Gorey, J. G., Lee, K. S., Hyde, T. M., Coppola, R., & Weinberger, D. R. (1996). Tourette syndrome: Prediction of phenotypic variation in monozygotic twins by caudate nucleus D2 receptor binding. *Science, 273,* 1225–1227.

Wolff, E. C. (1988). Psychotherapeutic interventions with Tourette's syndrome. In D. J. Cohen, R. D. Bruun, & J. F. Leckman (Eds.), *Tourette's syndrome and tic disorders: Clinical understanding and treatment* (pp. 208–222). New York: Wiley.

Woods, D. W., & Miltenberger, R. G. (1996). A review of habit reversal with child-hood habit disorders. *Education and Treatment of Children, 19,* 197–214.

Woods, D. W., Miltenberger, R. G., & Lumley, V. A. (1996). Sequential application of major habit-reversal components to treat motor tics in children. *Journal of Applied Behavior Analysis, 29,* 483–493.

World Health Organization. (1992). *International classification of diseases* (10th ed.). Geneva, Switzerland: Author.

Wright, K. M., & Miltenberger, R. G. (1987). Awareness training in the treatment of head and facial tics. *Journal of Behavior Therapy and Experimental Psychiatry, 18,* 269–274.

Yazgan, M. Y., Peterson, B. S., Wexler, B. E., & Leckman, J. F. (1995). Behavioral laterality in individuals with Gilles de la Tourette's syndrome and basal ganglia alterations: A preliminary report. *Biological Psychiatry, 38,* 386–390.

Yeates, K. O., & Bornstein, R. A. (1994). Attention deficit disorder and neuropsychological functioning in children with Tourette's syndrome. *Neuropsychology, 8,* 65–74.

Yeates, K. O., & Bornstein, R. A. (1996). Psychosocial correlates of learning disability subtypes in children with Tourette's syndrome. *Child Neuropsychology, 2,* 193–203.

Yepes, L. E., Balka, E. B., Winsberg, B. G., & Bialer, I. (1977). Amitriptyline and methylphenidate treatment of behaviorally disordered children. *Journal of Child Psychology and Psychiatry, 18,* 39–52.

Young, A. B., & Penney, J. B. (1984). Neurochemical anatomy of movement disorders. *Neurologic Clinics, 2,* 417–433.

Young, J. G., Cohen, D. J., Hattox, S. E., Kavanagh, M. E., Anderson, G. M., Shaywitz, B. A., & Maas, J. W. (1981). Plasma free MHPG and neuroendocrine responses to challenge doses of clonidine in Tourette's syndrome: Preliminary report. *Life Sciences, 29,* 1467–1475.

Young, R. (1990). *Mind, brain, and adaptation in the nineteenth century.* Oxford, England: Oxford University Press.

Youngblade, L. M., Park, K. A., & Belsky, J. (1993). Measurement of young children's close friendship: A comparison of two independent assessment systems and their associations with attachment security. *International Journal of Behavioral Development, 16,* 563–587.

Zabriskie, J. B. (1986). Rheumatic fever: A model for the pathological consequences of microbial-host mimicry. *Clinical and Experimental Rheumatology, 4,* 65–73.

Zahner, G. E. P., Clubb, M., Leckman, J. F., & Pauls, D. L. (1988). The epidemiology of Tourette syndrome. In D. J. Cohen, R. Bruun, & J. F. Leckman (Eds.), *Tourette syndrome and tic disorders: Clinical understanding and treatment* (pp. 79–90). New York: Wiley.

Zametkin, A. J., Liebnauer, L. L., Fitzgerald, G. A., King, A. C., Minkunas, D. V., Herscovitch, P., Yamada, E. M., & Cohen, R. M. (1993). Brain metabolism in teenagers with attention deficit hyperactivity disorder. *Archives of General Psychiatry, 50,* 333–340.

Zametkin, A. J., Nordahl, T. E., Gross, M., King, A. C., Semple, W. E., Rumsey, J., Hamburger, S., & Cohen, R. M. (1990). Cerebral glucose metabolism in adults with hyperactivity of childhood onset. *New England Journal of Medicine, 323,* 1361–1366.

Zametkin, A. J., & Rapoport, J. L. (1987a). Neurobiology of attention deficit disorder: Where have we come in 50 years? *Journal of the American Academy of Child and Adolescent Psychiatry, 26,* 676–686.

Zametkin, A. J., & Rapoport, J. L. (1987b). Noradrenergic hypothesis of attention deficit disorder with hyperactivity: A critical review. In H. Y. Meltzer (Ed.), *Psychopharmacology: The third generation of progress* (pp. 837–842). New York: Raven Press.

Zametkin, A. J., Rapoport, J. L., Murphy, D. L., Linnoila, M., & Ismond, D. (1985). Treatment of hyperactive children with monoamine oxidase inhibitors: 1. Clinical efficacy. *Archives of General Psychiatry, 42,* 962–966.

Zausmer, D. M. (1954). The treatment of tics in childhood. A review and followup study. *Archives of Disease in Childhood, 29,* 537–542.

Zeitlin, H. (1986). The natural history of psychiatric disorder in children: A study of individuals known to have attended both child and adult psychiatric departments of the same hospital. *Maudsley Monograph, No. 29.* Oxford, England: Oxford University Press.

Zielinski, C. M., Taylor, M. A., & Juzwin, K. R. (1991). Neuropsychological deficits in obsessive-compulsive disorder. *Neuropsychiatry, Neuropsychology and Behavioral Neurology, 4,* 110–126.

Zohar, A. H., Kaplan, D., Pauls, D. L., Dycian, A., Weizman, A., King, R., Kron, S., Cohen, D. J., Ratzoni, G., & Apter A. (in press). *A test of the stress diathesis model: Adolescents with obsessive-compulsive disorder serving in the military.* Manuscript submitted for publication.

Zohar, A. H., Pauls, D. L., Ratzoni, G., Apter, A., Dycian, A., Binder, M., King, R., Leckman, J. F., Kron, S., & Cohen, D. J. (1997). Obsessive-compulsive disorder with and without tics in an epidemiological sample of Israeli adolescents: Are they distinct subtypes? *American Journal of Psychiatry, 154,* 274–276.

Zohar, A. H., Ratzoni, G., Binder, M., Pauls, D. L., Apter, A., Kron, S., Dycian, A., King, R., & Cohen, D. J. (1993). An epidemiological study of obsessive-compulsive disorder and anxiety disorders in Israeli adolescents. *Psychiatric Genetics, 3,* 184.

Zohar, A. H., Ratzoni, G., Pauls, D. L., Apter, A., Bleich, A., Kron, S., Rappaport, M., Weizman, A., & Cohen, D. J. (1992). An epidemiological study of obsessive-compulsive disorder and related disorders in Israeli adolescents. *Journal of the American Academy of Child & Adolescent Psychiatry, 31,* 1057–1061.

Zohar, J., & Insel, T. R. (1987). Obsessive-compulsive disorder: Psychobiological approaches to diagnosis, treatment and pathophysiology. *Biological Psychiatry, 2,* 667–687.

Zubieta, J. K., & Alessi, N. E. (1993). Is there a role for serotonin in the disruptive behavior disorders? A literature review. *Journal of Child and Adolescent Psychopharmacology, 3,* 11–35.

Author Index

Subject Index

Acetylcholine, 277–278
ACTeRs. *See* ADD-H Comprehensive Teacher
    Rating Scale (ACTeRs)
ACTH, 61
Adaptation/adaptive functioning, 13–16, 18–19,
    108–110, 167, 168, 299–300
  in assessment, 299–300
  level of (risk factor), 167, 168
  selective (Darwinian perspectives), 140–152, 408
ADD-H Comprehensive Teacher Rating Scale
    (ACTeRs), 319
ADHD, tic-related, 63–71
  adaptive traits, 150
  adult, 319–320
  comorbidity, 162, 182–186
  diagnosis, 64–67
  diagnosis, differential, 120, 121, 127–129, 130,
    132, 135, 136, 138
  DSM-IV criteria for (Table 4.2), 66–67
  frequency of, in Tourette's syndrome (Table 4.1),
    65
  genetic factors/vulnerability, 95, 163–165, 199,
    202, 214
  historical perspectives, 64
  IQ tests, with/without Tourette's syndrome, 91
  natural history of, in Tourette's syndrome, 69–71
  pathogenesis, 160, 162
  and peer acceptance/adjustment, 105, 110, 111,
    114
  phenomenology of, in Tourette's syndrome, 68–69
  prevalence (Table 10.5), 187
  research perspectives, 78
  scores on CBCL, 60
  teachers, recommendations for, 365–366
  and Tourette's syndrome, controversy, 63
  treatment, cognitive behavioral, contingency
    management, 347
  treatment, pharmacological (*see*
    Pharmacological/somatic treatment for
    attention-deficit/hyperactivity disorder)
ADHD, tic-related: assessment, 296–298, 327–328
  impairment, 298
  onset and course, 297
  Yale approach, 285–309
ADHD, tic-related:
  neuropsychological/neurophysiological factors,
    80–83, 95–96, 97, 98–99, 141–143, 245–246,
    247–248, 250, 253, 261–281
  basal ganglia, 245–246

cingulate cortex, 253
  dopamine function in, 267
  executive function, 98–99
  neurochemical and neuropeptide systems,
    261–281
  norepinephrine/noradrenergic system, 271
  orbitofrontal cortex (OFC), 250
  premotor and supplementary motor cortices,
    247–248
  serotonin function, 274–275
  stability, 141–143
  thalamus, 247
  visual-motor integration skill (Table 5.1), 83
ADHD Rating Scale, 319
Adult ADHD, 319–320
Advocacy organizations. *See* Voluntary/advocacy
    organizations
Affective disorders, 226, 329. *See also*
    Anxiety/anxiety disorders; Depression/anxiety
Age of onset criterion (controversy), 36
  graph, 39
  and peer acceptance/adaptive functioning,
    111–112
Agoraphobia, 202, 299
AIDS, 12, 128
Akathisia, 123, 124
Akinesia, 123
Alcohol abuse, 201, 300
Alpha adrenergic receptor agonists, 373–374, 395
Alzheimer's disorder, 262
Americans with Disabilities Act (ADA), 407
Amino acid neurotransmitters, 275–277
Amitriptyline (Elavil®), 393, 394
Amygdala. *See* Neuroanatomical circuitry: limbic
    system
Anafranil. *See* Clomipramine (Anafranil®)
Anatomy:
  density of premonitory urges (Figure 2.2), 28
  neural (*see* Neuroanatomical circuitry)
Animal models, 175, 210
Anorexia nervosa, 128
Antiandrogens, 379–380
Antidepressants (for ADHD), 392–395
Antimicrobial and immunological interventions (for
    tic disorders), 380–381
Antisocial personality disorder, 201
Anxiety/anxiety disorders, 164, 165, 167, 200, 226,
    294, 299, 300, 329. *See also* Depression/anxiety
Asperger's syndrome, 130, 299

WMP7 LEC